Clinical Decision Making in Fluency Disorders

Third Edition

Walter H. Manning, Ph.D.
The University of Memphis
Memphis, Tennessee

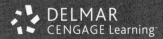

DELMAR
CENGAGE Learning

Australia • Brazil • Japan • Korea • Mexico • Singapore • Spain • United Kingdom • United States

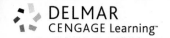

DELMAR
CENGAGE Learning

Clinical Decision Making in Fluency Disorders, Third Edition
Walter H. Manning

Vice President, Career and Professional Editorial:
Dave Garza

Director of Learning Solutions:
Matthew Kane

Senior Acquisitions Editor:
Sherry Dickinson

Managing Editor:
Marah Bellegarde

Product Manager: Laura J. Wood

Editorial Assistant:
Anthony Souza

Vice President, Career and Professional Marketing:
Jennifer McAvey

Executive Marketing Manager:
Wendy E. Mapstone

Senior Marketing Manager:
Kristin McNary

Marketing Coordinator:
Scott A. Chrysler

Production Director:
Carolyn Miller

Production Manager:
Andrew Crouth

Senior Art Director:
David Arsenault

For product information and technology assistance, contact us at **Cengage Learning Customer & Sales Support, 1-800-354-9706**

For permission to use material from this text or product, submit all requests online at **www.cengage com/permissions.**
Further permissions questions can be e-mailed to **permissionrequest@cengage.com**

Library of Congress Control Number: 2009925121

ISBN-13: 978-1-4354-9996-6

ISBN-10: 1-4354-9996-4

Delmar
5 Maxwell Drive
Clifton Park, NY 12065-2919
USA

Cengage Learning is a leading provider of customized learning solutions with office locations around the globe, including Singapore, the United Kingdom, Australia, Mexico, Brazil, and Japan. Locate your local office at:
international.cengage.com/region

Cengage Learning products are represented in Canada by Nelson Education, Ltd.

To learn more about Delmar, visit **www.cengage.com/delmar**

Purchase any of our products at your local college store or at our preferred online store **www.ichapters.com**

Printed in Canada
1 2 3 4 5 6 7 12 11 10 09

Brief Contents

Contents

CHAPTER 4   **Beginning the Assessment Process with Adolescents and Adults**   **145**

The Assessment Process with Young Speakers:
CHAPTER 5   Preschool and School-age Children   239

CHAPTER 9   Facilitating Fluency for Preschool and School-Age Children   423

CHAPTER 10 Assessment and Management for Atypical Fluency Disorders   491

Preface

The writing of the book proved one of its central points: that we write to find out what we know and what we want to say. I thought of how often as a writer I had made clear to myself some subject I had previously known nothing about by just putting one sentence after another—by reasoning my way in sequential steps to its meaning. I thought of how often the act of writing even the simplest document—a letter, for instance—had clarified my half-formed ideas. Writing and thinking and learning were the same process. (p. ix)

William Zinsser (1988). Learning to Write.

A primary goal of this book is to convey to the reader the enthusiasm and creativity associated with assisting people who stutter. I also want to provide the reader with the principles and clinical insight that enable those who stutter to improve their ability to communicate and enhance the quality of their life. Although increasing fluency is, of course, a high priority during treatment, the therapeutic journey is far more expansive. Throughout the book we will also emphasize the primary goals of enhanced communication and the creation of an autonomous and agentic lifestyle.

The readers I have in mind as I write are graduate students who are beginning their first in-depth experience in fluency disorders. I also want to communicate with professional clinicians who want to learn more about this specialty area. The information and ideas discussed in these pages may also be useful for individuals who stutter (and the parents or spouses of people who stutter), for another purpose of this book is to make stuttering less of a mystery and to provide a sense of direction for the process of therapeutic as well as self-directed change.

Stuttering and related fluency disorders are frequently described as a low-incidence problem, although this perception is questionable for young, preschool speakers (Yairi & Ambrose, 2005), as well as for groups of individuals with related communication problems (Bloodstein & Bernstein Ratner, 2008). Nonetheless, working with individuals who stutter is one of the primary responsibilities listed in clinical job descriptions. Based on our professional guidelines and scope of practice, stuttering is a problem that the public expects speech-language pathologists to be able to competently treat (Bernstein Ratner &

Tetnowski, 2006). Unfortunately, stuttering is also one of the least understood communication problems and one that clinicians tend to be uncomfortable with treating.

During the formulation and development of the profession of speech pathology, particularly during the decades from the late 1920s through the 1960s, the area of fluency disorders was a major area of interest in our professional journals and texts. A review of the early issues of the *Journal of Speech Disorders* (published from 1936 through 1946) or the initial volumes of the *Journal of Speech and Hearing Disorders* (published through 1990) confirms that a large proportion of the articles addressed the nature and treatment of stuttering. As the scope of practice continues to expand in the field of communication disorders, fluency and fluency disorders have become but one of many areas that students are expected to learn about during their academic and clinical programs. Graduate students in speech-language pathology are expected to become generalists across the wide range of human communication and related problems. As early as 1994, Henri suggested that "our clinical areas have simply become too substantial" (Henri, 1994). Because clinicians are asked to become knowledgeable about so many different communication disorders and related areas, there is concern that the qualifications of professionals for serving any one disorder are being compromised. One response to this concern, driven in part by consumer demand for better services, is the development of specialty recognition groups by the American Speech-Language-Hearing Association that provide enhanced professional qualifications and continuing education opportunities.

The depth of the field is also changing. Reading the volumes of literature associated with but one specialty area of the field can be intimidating, even for someone who has been a clinician and researcher for many years. It is difficult to negotiate the amount of (sometimes conflicting) information that has become available about the many aspects of stuttering. On the other hand, reading through the thoughtful and often elegant comments of those who have spent a lifetime trying to understand and explain the nature of stuttering onset and development can be an enjoyable experience. One of the most difficult choices in preparing a text is not what to include but, given the space limitations, what to omit. The citations in this text are intended not only to provide support for the ideas that are offered but also to furnish readers additional, more detailed, sources of information about a topic. There is also the wish to pay homage to the people who have preceded us and to credit co-workers in the field for their creative and insightful clinical and research ideas. It is enjoyable to acknowledge the colleagues you feel privileged to be working together with—as Charles Van Riper so often said—in the vineyard of stuttering.

I would like to comment on the writing style of this book. I have used the active voice throughout with the intention of engaging the reader. The "editorial we" has been used for the main body of the text and the first person for boxes titled *Clinical Decision Making* and *Clinical Insight*. Clinical Decision Making boxes are designed to address some of the options a clinician is likely to consider during the assessment and treatment processes. Clinical Insight boxes reflect a particular philosophical view about aspects of therapeutic change for individuals who stutter. On other occasions a third type of (untitled) box is used to provide information that in other ways supplements the text.

As I write I am often thinking of the busy graduate student who (I hope) is under pressure to read hundreds of pages each week in books and journals. Despite the many demands on their time, I would like these students to be instinctively drawn to some of these pages. I hope the words and ideas provide a connection to the individual reader and that, for a textbook at least, the reading is pleasurable.

Related to the style of the writing are choices about some of the terminology used throughout the book. For example, feminine and masculine pronouns are used alternately throughout the chapters to refer to the speech-language pathologist. Although gender pronouns are also alternated throughout the chapters for the person who is stuttering, this is a more complicated issue. It has been suggested that the term *stutterer* is insensitive, too all-encompassing, and serves as a label to negatively stereotype and limit how we define the problem as well as the person. Nonetheless, it is a term that the general public has used and will likely continue to use. Fortunately, there is evidence that the term stutterer has less influence than once assumed in creating a stigmatizing effect (Dietrich, Jensen, & Williams, 2001; St. Louis, 1999). Indeed, many people who stutter have no difficulty referring to themselves as stutterers even when they become highly fluent. Some speakers even show pride in using the term, particularly as they achieve successful management of their stuttering or become actively involved with a self-help group.

The approach I have chosen for this book is to use a variety of terms, including speaker, individual, client, participant, or person who stutters. I also use the term stutterer when it facilitates the clarity of the writing. As we indicate on many occasions throughout the text, this issue has more to do with speakers' interpretations of themselves and the situation rather than the listener's (mis) understanding about stuttering. The view that the person we are assisting is vastly more than someone who stutterers is at the heart of any comprehensive and humanistic approach to the problem.

Some features have been expanded and added to assist both instructors and clinicians. We have refined and expanded the *Clinical Decision Making* and *Clinical Insight* boxes. We have revised the study questions at the end of each chapter to correspond with the new organization of the book and the fresh information included in each of the chapters. A new chapter has been included that addresses the diagnosis and treatment of individuals with atypical fluency problems. Finally, an **online companion** has been (and will continue to be) developed that provides the reader with a variety of materials, including video comments by the author, PowerPoint slides that coincide with the chapters, and video and audio examples of various fluency problems and therapeutic sessions. You may access the online companion via Delmar Cengage Learning's website at http://www. delmarlearning.com/companions, under the Speech Pathology discipline.

This, the third edition of this text, contains 12 chapters. In the following paragraphs the major issues presented in each chapter are described. In addition, each chapter contains a Conclusion that also highlights the basic issues, along with Topics for Discussion and Recommended Readings.

Chapter 1   The Clinician and the Therapeutic Process

As with the first two editions of this book, the first chapter describes the personal characteristics and clinical skills of the effective clinician and their potential impact on the therapeutic process. As others have suggested, I continue to believe that the quality of the clinician is a major factor in a successful therapy experience. Since the publication of the second edition, extensive empirical support has become available that underpins this idea. A new section describes important steps in the development of expertise and the application of principles and rules for making clinical decisions. The final section of this chapter has been updated with recent research concerning the potential value of humor as an important cognitive-affective variable in the process of therapeutic change.

Chapter 2   The Nature of Fluent and Nonfluent Speech: The Onset of Stuttering

In order to fully appreciate the nature of stuttered speech, Chapter 2 begins by describing the salient features of fluent speech as produced by young adult speakers. Definitions and commonly used terms for describing stuttering are provided and factors that influence the onset and development of stuttering are presented. Many of the epidemiological characteristics of early childhood stuttering as reported by Ehud Yairi and Nichole Ambrose (2005) are discussed. This chapter sets the stage for several subsequent chapters describing theories of etiology and assessment procedures intended to distinguish typically fluent from stuttered speech in both younger and older speakers.

Chapter 3   A Historical Perspective of Etiologies

This chapter describes the evolution of the many attempts to explain the onset and development of stuttering. The various related and sometimes contrasting theoretical views provide a historical perspective that places more recent theoretical models into context. The discussion of each theoretical perspective is followed by descriptions of the empirical investigations that provide—to varying degrees—supporting evidence for each point of view. Recent evidence indicating the presence of anatomical and physiological abnormalities under-lying the onset of stuttering is presented, including the findings from recent neuroimaging and genetic investigations.

Chapter 4   Beginning the Assessment Process with Adolescents and Adults

As in previous editions, the assessment and treatment of older speakers is pre-sented prior to discussing younger speakers. We chose this sequence in order to present the features of stuttering as they are manifested in a fully developed form prior to discussing the characteristic features of younger speakers in Chapter 5. Fundamental considerations that are likely to influence the desire for treatment (e.g., the natural variability of stuttering, determining the speaker's desire for change) and basic principles and techniques for determining the extent of the problem are described. While emphasizing self-assessment by the speaker, the diagnostic process is described as a multifactoral approach that includes not only the more obvious overt features of the problem but also important cognitive and affective features of the stuttering experience. The chapter concludes with a dis-cussion of formal assessment measures designed for adolescents and adults.

Chapter 5   The Assessment Process with Young Speakers: Preschool and School-age Children

The evaluation of younger speakers focuses on two major decisions to be made with this population—distinguishing the possibility of stuttering from more common fluency breaks and, given that stuttering is the case, determining the likelihood that stuttering will either subside or persist. The role of the parents and the child's cognitive and behavioral responses to stuttering in making these decisions are emphasized, and the factors that appear to best distinguish chro-nicity are described. A new section describes the possible adverse effects that stuttering can have on a child's educational experience. The importance of the initial (diagnostic) meeting is emphasized, and take home messages for the par-ents are described. The chapter concludes with a discussion of formal assess-ment measures designed for preschool and young school-age children.

Chapter 6   Facilitating the Therapeutic Process

Drawing ideas from a variety of fields, this chapter presents the essential char-acteristics of human behavioral change and provides a context for many of the treatment suggestions found in subsequent chapters. Three primary goals of therapy for individuals who stutter are introduced. Major sections include the cyclical nature of the change process, discussions of stages and processes of change, expected levels of fluency, potential obstacles to change, and the impor-tance of the therapeutic alliance for informing the clinician about the timing and direction of therapy. Key variables that impact the choice of a treatment protocol are suggested. The chapter concludes by addressing issues related to recent calls for evidence-based practice and the applicability of the medical and common factors models for informing the clinician about the process of therapeutic change.

Chapter 7   Counseling and People who Stutter

Regardless of the therapeutic protocol selected for those who stutter, counseling in some form is often an integral part of therapeutic change. This chapter on counseling includes information from the most recent editions of books by authors Gerard Egan and David Luterman for conceptualizing counseling and promoting the process of cognitive change. A description of less useful views of counseling is contrasted with more functional perspectives and includes commentary on the importance of such issues such as empathy, silence, probing, and humor. The importance of the therapeutic alliance is elaborated, along with the metalinguistics of change as reflected in the therapeutic discourse of the client and the clinician. The chapter concludes with a discussion of postmodern counseling approaches, including personal construct theory and a constructivist-narrative approach to counseling.

Chapter 8   Successful Management of Stuttering for Adolescents and Adults

Elaborating on the three primary goals of treatment introduced in Chapter 6, we describe four basic principles of therapeutic change for individuals who stutter. A variety of treatment strategies and techniques for altering the behavioral features of stuttering for adolescents and adults are presented. Also addressed are techniques for assisting the speaker in the process of cognitive restructuring that is so essential for long-term change. A new section describes the rationale and possibilities of a constructivist-narrative approach for assisting those who stutter, including guidelines for reconstructing the speaker's current narrative. The chapter concludes with suggestions for working with adolescent speakers and conducting group therapy sessions for adolescents and adults.

Chapter 9   Facilitating Fluency for Preschool and School-Age Children

Having described interventions for older speakers, we now turn to the variety of treatment options for younger speakers by discussing the rationale and associated techniques for assisting preschool and school-age children. The evolution of procedures for working directly with the child rather than focusing on the child's environment alone is described. A new section describing the Lidcombe program for preschool children is included. Suggestions for assisting the child in responding to and altering stuttering, as well as for enhancing fluent speech, are presented. Counseling techniques appropriate for children are discussed, with particular attention devoted to procedures for helping a child respond to teasing and bullying. The impact of coexisting problems that may impact fluency or, at the very least, make treatment somewhat more complex, are discussed. The chapter concludes with a discussion of transfer and termination, the possibility of relapse, and the importance of informing the child's classroom teacher(s) about the nature of stuttering and the teacher's role in facilitating change.

Chapter 10   Assessment and Management for Atypical Fluency Disorders

This chapter is devoted to both the assessment and treatment of less typical fluency problems. Cluttering, the most common of these problems, is described at the outset. The characteristics of this somewhat neglected (until recent years) fluency problem are described in detail along with a variety of assessment measures and treatment options. Next, fluency disruptions as a result of neurological and psychological factors are described, along with criteria for distinguishing these two forms of acquired stuttering. The chapter concludes with a description of the rarely described but intriguing occurrence of malingering, along with criteria for distinguishing forms of malingering from genuine stuttering.

Chapter 11   Indicators of Successful Change During Treatment

As with earlier chapters concerning assessment and treatment, this description of successful change during the formal treatment process accounts for the multidimensional nature of successful therapy. Successful change is most certainly informed by the speaker along with judgments by the clinicians, often with the assistance of the same devices used to obtain pretreatment assessments. Variables that influence progress are described along with many helpful indicators of successful change (e.g., the speaker's ability to self-monitor, acquire speech naturalness, increase approach behavior, and develop an agentic life style). The chapter concludes with a consideration of factors that inform the appropriateness of terminating treatment.

Chapter 12   Indicators of Successful Change Following Treatment

The characteristics of continued success following the conclusion of treatment are discussed in the final chapter. By appreciating the importance of the speaker's ability to transfer and maintain newly acquired abilities as well as actively confronting the possibility of regression and relapse, the clinician (and the speaker) has the opportunity to predict and enable long-term success. The chapter also includes a commentary of the critical roles that support and advocacy groups play in the maintenance and enhancement of therapeutic change.

Acknowledgements

There are several people who played an important role in the creation of this, the third edition of this book. The constant support, understanding, and encouragement of my wife Cheryl were essential during the many months of ups and downs that typically accompany such a project. I also want to express my sincere appreciation to Anthony DiLollo, Kyungjae Lee, Laura Plexico, and Robert Quesal, who provided thoughtful and insightful suggestions for the initial drafts of this text. In addition, I deeply appreciate several colleagues who have so freely provided their ideas and information, including Nichole Ambrose, Gene Brutten, Jeanna and Glen Riley, Martine Vanryckeghem, and Patricia Zebrowski. Finally, I want to expresses my admiration to the people whose journeys I have been able to share during many therapy sessions over the years. It is with courage and persistence that these individuals who stutter are able to expand their ability to communicate and improve the quality of their lives.

Reviewers

We would like to thank the following instructors and clinicians for taking the time to provide their valuable feedback during the development process:

Anthony DiLollo, Ph.D., CCC-SLP
Assistant Professor
Wichita State University
Wichita, KS

Regina Grantham, M.Ed., CCC-SLP
Associate Professor and Chair, Speech Pathology and Audiology Department
State University of New York College at Cortland
Cortland, NY

Judith B. King, Ph.D., CCC-SLP
Associate Professor
Northern Arizona University
Flagstaff, AZ

Robert W. Quesal, Ph.D., CCC-SLP
Professor of Communication Sciences and Disorders
Western Illinois University
Macomb, IL

Stacy Wagovich, Ph.D., CCC-SLP
Associate Professor, Communication Sciences & Disorders
University of Missouri
Columbia, MO

About the Author

Walt is a professor and associate dean in the School of Audiology and Speech-Language Pathology at The University of Memphis. He teaches courses in fluency disorders and research methods. He has published more than 80 articles in a variety of professional journals and has presented on many occasions to regional, national, and international audiences. He was a member of the Steering Committee of ASHA's Special Interest Division 4 (Fluency & Fluency Disorders) from 1996–2000 and served as vice chair for the Division 4 Specialty Board from 2000–2003. He is an editorial consultant for several professional journals and ad hoc associate editor for the *American Journal of Speech-Language Pathology.* Since 1997 he has been an associate editor for *The Journal of Fluency Disorders.* He is a Board Recognized Specialist in Fluency Disorders, a fellow of ASHA and has received the honors of the Tennessee Association of Audiologists and Speech-Language Pathologists.

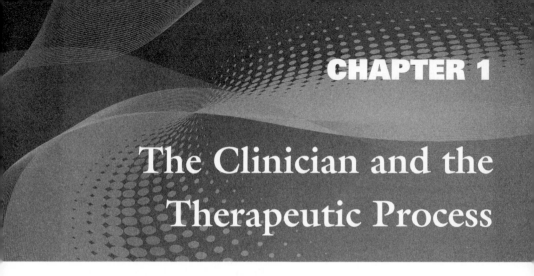

CHAPTER 1

The Clinician and the Therapeutic Process

Perhaps the hardest of all the things a clinician must learn is how to live well. You cannot heal a person's wound if you are a dirty bandage. Unless you are a healthy, strong person, your impact will be minimal, no matter what methods you use. There have been times when I resented my clients' expectations of what I should be, but I have noticed that over the years I have become a much better man than I hoped (or desired) to be. I have found that therapy is a two-edged chisel; it shapes the therapist as well as the client. (p. 140)

Charles Van Riper (1979).
A Career in Speech Pathology.
Englewood Cliffs, NJ: Prentice-Hall.

Chapter Objectives

The purpose of this chapter is twofold. Because the quality of the clinician is a central factor in determining the success of any therapeutic approach, we will begin by examining the characteristics of individuals who are viewed as being especially effective in working with children and adults who stutter. We will discuss the personality attributes, attitudes, and skills that have been suggested as desirable for the clinician who effectively guides a client through the process of therapeutic change. The nature of developing expertise as studied in a variety of human endeavors will be applied to this process and intertwined with the concepts of rule- and principle-based decision making. We will conclude the chapter by describing an attribute of the clinician and the therapeutic relationship that encapsulates many of the essential properties of successful therapeutic change—humor. We will describe how the dynamic nature of behavioral and cognitive change is often echoed in a spontaneously humorous response to the achievement of a conceptual sift and a distancing from and mastery of the problem.

The Effective Clinician

Beginning a book on fluency disorders by discussing the characteristics of the effective clinician is unusual. Typically, the first chapter describes the nature of stuttering, or provides the reader with historical or theoretical views of the problem—topics that are, in fact, presented in the early chapters of this book. But because a primary goal of this book is to emphasize the ability of the clinician to make wise clinical decisions during assessment and treatment, it seems an ideal place to begin. In earlier editions of this book we proposed that as much as, or perhaps even more than, any other component, the clinician is central to the success of the treatment process. Clinical research has since provided support for this idea. Not all clinicians—even those who are clinically certified, specialty recognized, or have years of experience—are equally effective in assisting children and adults with fluency disorders.

Having indicated in the Preface that another primary goal of this book is to convey the enthusiasm and excitement of working with people who stutter, we will now step back a bit and place the learning process into a larger perspective. Following these intense years of formal education, you will soon be on your own. Your role will no longer be that of a graduate student who is continually prodded by your instructors to demonstrate your knowledge and ability. You will be a professional who is likely to be considered the resident expert on the topic of communication disorders in general and stuttering in particular. This change in roles may be difficult because during the years of graduate school, many student clinicians have relatively little exposure to the field of fluency disorders. Most students have the opportunity to take, at most, one course in stuttering and obtain clinical experience with only a few individuals. Student clinicians have the opportunity to observe the progress of clients for only a few weeks or months. When clients achieve success, it is often difficult for the student clinician to know how much of a role he or she played in promoting change. Furthermore, even if the student is fortunate enough to take a course on stuttering that is an especially good one and the clinical experience is instructive, it is only the beginning of learning about the experience of stuttering.

You may occasionally find yourself a little worn out as you successfully negotiate the rigors of a good graduate program. However, in order to become an experienced and wise professional, your learning must continue after graduation. The clinical decisions you will be making one or two decades following graduation will have little to do with some of the information you are currently learning. As described in the Preface, ongoing research and reinterpretation of old data, as well as basic and applied research, continually lead to new constructs and ways of making informed clinical decisions. When people of my generation were students, many things we were taught—including the role of parents in the onset and development of stuttering, the linear development of stuttering through primary and secondary stages, the likelihood of spontaneous recovery in young children, the possibility of relapse following treatment, and the role of genetics in the etiology and epidemiology of stuttering—have since been shown to be partially or completely inaccurate. The evolution of information occurs in all scientific fields, and the shelf-lives of text books are not nearly as long as authors would like them to be. Of course, your instructors are not intentionally providing information that is incorrect. It's just that the profession is still climbing the hills necessary to allow us a more accurate view of the phenomena we are investigating and the people we are attempting to assist.

Carl Sagan's (1996) caution that "One of the great commandments of science is to "mistrust arguments from authority" (p. 28) is probably good advice for many aspects of life. It is good advice for consumers of all information, including the information discussed in this text. As you expand your knowledge through years of clinical experience with many different people and your participation in continuing educational activities, you will begin to create your own principles of change and style of doing things. You will choose new ideas and approaches that will spring from basic and applied research yet to be conceived. Moreover, as you continue to be a student of your field, you will achieve insight, wisdom, and enthusiasm for your work.

The Importance of the Clinician

Experienced clinicians, and—perhaps more importantly—clients who have experienced treatment for stuttering that was more or less successful, have suggested certain clinician characteristics that are more desirable than others. If this is your first exposure to the field of fluency disorders, this initial chapter may help you to determine whether or not helping people with such communication problems is likely to be satisfying, both for you and for your clients.

There is no exclusive set of attributes that defines the ideal clinician. Even if this were the case, no clinician could be expected to possess all or even most of the desirable characteristics described in this chapter. Each client comes to us with different needs and requires, at various points during the treatment process, different attributes of and different roles to be played by the clinician. Furthermore, the professional and personal attributes of the clinician will interact with the characteristics of the client, resulting in a unique and dynamic combination during each therapeutic alliance. After many years of observing both student and professional clinicians, as well as asking clients about their perceptions of their clinicians, it is clear that some clinicians are considerably better than others at supporting and motivating their clients throughout the treatment process. The attitudes and abilities that these clinicians possess distinguish them from the clinicians who are less effective. It is the effective clinicians who are able to select appropriate therapeutic strategies and use or design related techniques. Perhaps more than any other qualities, the best clinicians are uncommonly effective in understanding, encouraging, supporting, and guiding their clients along the path of treatment.

In contrast to the numerous investigations of children and adults who stutter, relatively few questions have been asked about the attributes of the individuals who provide the treatment. Those authors who have considered this side of the therapeutic process, specifically in the area of fluency disorders (Cooper & Cooper, 1985c; Conture, 2005; Emerick, 1974; Guitar, 2006; Hood, 1974; Shaprio, 1999; Van Riper, 1975), provide convincing arguments to support the concept that the clinician is the critical part of the process. For example, regardless of the treatment strategy and the associated techniques, Cooper and Cooper maintain that the person who is administering the treatment is the most important variable in creating the process of change. In Chapter 6 we will discuss empirical evidence indicating that this is also the case in related fields such as counseling and psychotherapy.

The importance of the clinician is perhaps more apparent when a counseling-based treatment is used. Murphy and Fitzsimons (1960) contend that during counseling, the "most important single variable affecting the success in the treatment of stutterers is—the clinician" (p. 27). Even if treatment takes the form of an archetypal program of behavioral modification, Cooper and Cooper (1985b) argue that "it does matter who is doing the conditioning" (p. 21). Regardless of the treatment strategy, authors have consistently found that the clinician plays a critical role in orchestrating a successful treatment program (Emerick, 1974; Hood, 1974; Reeves Shapiro, 1999; Van Riper, 1975; Yaruss, Quesal & Murphy, 2002). For that matter, the clinician often is a major factor in determining whether the client makes the choice to initiate treatment or decides to continue in treatment long enough for meaningful change to take place. Just as in parenting, teaching, and coaching, when treating fluency disorders, it makes a real difference who is serving as a guide and mentor.

Clinician Attitudes About Stuttering and People Who Stutter

Our attitude about those who come to us for help and our understanding of their communication problems have a fundamental influence on how we approach them as people during both assessment and treatment. What the clinician has been told and what he or she has been able to observe about stuttering and people who stutter will determine whether he or she will even have the desire to work with such clients.

One unique characteristic of the field of fluency disorders is that a substantial number of people who stutter (or have stuttered) have gone on to become professional clinicians, often specializing in stuttering. Assuming that clinicians with a history of stuttering have also acquired the necessary academic and clinical knowledge, their life experiences may provide some understanding about a client. The experience of having traveled within the culture of stuttering and survived the many tribulations along the way tends to promote the insight and empathy necessary for guiding others through the process of therapeutic change. It is generally easier to understand and relate to another's experience if we have shared the same or a similar experience (e.g., undergoing surgery, losing and searching for a job, experiencing a divorce). There are many examples of this understanding in the helping professions. For example, ex-addicts often are extremely good therapists in alcohol and drug-addiction programs. They understand from experience the nature of the problem and the many tricks that people use to deny the problem or avoid change.

This does not mean, however, that people who stutter or who have stuttered in the past will be more effective as clinicians or will necessarily have a greater understanding of the stuttering experience. With good preparation and experience, nonstuttering clinicians can have equal understanding and do not have to acquiesce when individuals who stutter offer the challenge "How can you understand? You don't stutter!" (see Manning, 2004b). It may well be that one of these days a client will challenge you in such a way and ask such a question. Will they be correct and how will you respond?

Clinical **Insight**

Speaking as a person with a history of stuttering, I believe that there are many experienced clinicians who, although they have never stuttered, unmistakably understand the experience of those who do. These individuals demonstrate their understanding in the diagnostic procedures they create, the way they measure the success of their interventions, and the research questions they ask. They further their understanding by attending local and national meetings of stuttering support groups and by listening attentively in attempting to understand their clients' stories. Although we can never know all the details of another's experience, we can learn enough so that we can provide accurate and timely help that enables our clients to more effectively cope with their situation.

Investigations of Clinical Preparation

Obviously, at the outset of training, it is perfectly natural for a novice clinician to be uncertain and anxious about how to assist someone with a communication problem. Until the clinician has witnessed success and has taken an active part in facilitating change for many people, it can be difficult to believe that he or she can truly be of any assistance to a person who is struggling to fluently produce even the simplest of utterances. If a clinician has received a quality education and yet continues to be apprehensive about working with people who stutter, such uncertainty is one indication that he or she is not yet qualified to do so. People who stutter will not get the best possible treatment unless they can find a clinician who is not merely competent but also enthusiastic about the process of change.

It is important to appreciate that there are many professional clinicians who feel unqualified and uncomfortable when working with children and adults who stutter. For decades, research has consistently supported this observation (Ainsworth, 1974; ASHA Omnibus study, 2001; Brisk, Healey, & Hux, 1997; Cooper, 1975b, 1985; Cooper & Cooper, 1996; Kelly, Martin, Baker, Rivera, Bishop, Kriziske, Settlery, & Stealy, 1997; Mallard, Gardner, & Downey, 1988; Matkin, Rigel, & Snope, 1983; Reeves, 2006; St. Louis & Durrenberger, 1992; Thompson, 1984; Van Riper, 1992a; Wingate, 1971; Yaruss & Quesal, 2002). The research leaves little doubt that some professional clinicians actively avoid assisting individuals who stutter. As in any specialty in any field, those clinicians who do not find it enjoyable and rewarding to work with people who stutter should not do so, for their lack of enjoyment will show.

The disturbing results of several investigations indicate that some professional clinicians have opinions about the level of their academic and clinical preparation and their ability to assist people who stutter that are not encouraging. The findings of these investigations are consistent and have included large numbers of both student and professional clinicians from many areas throughout the country. The following provides a brief historical pattern and the highlights of these investigations.

- Of 597 certified professional clinicians only 48% of those surveyed felt competent in treating persons who stuttered (Matkin, Ringle, and Snope, 1983).
- 40% of the respondents from ASHA-accredited programs did not believe that their students were being adequately prepared to serve clients with fluency disorders (Curlee, 1985).
- 57% of undergraduate students and 91% of graduate students had the *opportunity* to take a course where fluency disorders was the major topic (St. Louis and Lass, 1981; Lass et al., 1989).
- 97% of 278 school-based clinicians across 20 states reported that they had taken at least one undergraduate or graduate course where fluency disorders

was the major topic. In addition, 90% of those surveyed indicated that they had the opportunity to treat clients who stuttered during their training. The authors also found that 57%, 77%, and 71% of their participants felt confident about evaluating preschool, elementary, and junior/senior high school students, respectively (Brisk, Healey, & Hux, 1997).

- 50% of clinicians working in the public schools had *taken* a course in stuttering; only 6% reported that the coursework emphasized treatment (Mallard, Gardner, & Downey, 1988).

- 12.6% of 1,872 professional clinicians agreed that most speech clinicians are adept in treating stuttering (75.5% disagreed) (Cooper & Cooper, 1992).

- 2.1% of the clinicians agreed that they felt more comfortable in working with individuals who stutter than working with articulatory defective individuals (93.2% disagreed) (Cooper and Cooper, 1992).

- Directors of university programs reported that clinical clock hours for master's degree students in the area of fluency disorders were considerably less (average 20.2 hours, *sd* 18.7 hours) than for language disorders (average 104.2, *sd* 52.8 hours) or articulation-phonology disorders (average 77.4 hours, *sd* 66.3 hours) (Sommers and Caruso, 1995).

- A slight majority of clinicians agreed that they were confident about treating elementary or middle school children (64% and 54%, respectively) who stuttered (Brisk, Healey, and Hux, 1997).

- 54% of bachelor's and 65% of master's students had taken a course that was "entirely or partially" devoted to stuttering. A total of 19% of these students reported that they had never had a course in stuttering. Approximately half of those surveyed indicated that they felt inadequate when attempting to assist people who stutter (Kelly, et al., 1997).

The number of studies on this topic over the years indicates a continuing concern about both the level of academic and clinical preparation and the resulting clinician expertise in the area of fluency disorders. Furthermore, the data over the years suggests an ongoing pattern of preparation that most would agree is less than acceptable. In the following paragraphs we will provide somewhat more detail about the most recent studies on this issue.

Yaruss (1999) surveyed 239 master's-level programs accredited by the American Speech-Language-Hearing Association. A total of 134 questionnaires were returned, for an overall response rate of 56%. Although not all programs completed all questions, the results indicated the following:

- Of 134 programs responding, 101 programs (75%) offered at least one full required course devoted specifically to fluency disorders.

- Of 134 programs responding, 39 programs (29%) offered at least one full elective course devoted specifically to fluency disorders.

- Of 129 programs responding, 23 programs (17.8%) indicated that it was possible to graduate without taking any class specifically devoted to fluency disorders. Of these programs, 19 (97%) reported that fluency disorders are covered as part of some other class.

- Of 128 programs responding, 72 (56%) indicated that diagnostic experience in fluency disorders is not required during clinical practicum.

- Of 128 programs responding, 65 (51%) indicated that treatment experience in fluency disorders is not required.

- Of 128 programs responding, 76 (59%) indicated that it is possible for a student to graduate without any clinical experience in fluency disorders.

The survey also indicated no significant relationships between program size and students' academic or clinical training in fluency disorders. Yaruss concludes that a significant percentage of students graduating from master's-level programs do not have even the most basic academic or clinical background necessary for working with individuals who stutter. Finally, there is some indication that these results may represent a more positive view than is actually the case. That is, although 40% of all accredited programs have a faculty member with enough interest in fluency disorders to join ASHA's Special Interest Division for Fluency and Fluency Disorders (Division 4), 61% of the programs responding to the survey had a faculty member belonging to this Special Interest Division. This suggests that the responses to the survey were more likely to have been completed by programs that had required courses on fluency disorders, greater clinical populations and clinical practicum requirements, and a greater degree of expertise among the faculty.

Yaruss and Quesal (2002) surveyed 159 ASHA-accredited graduate programs and noted that nearly one quarter of the programs (22.6%) permitted students to graduate without a course in fluency disorders. Of the 152 programs who responded to inquires about clinic requirements for individuals who stutter, somewhat less than two-thirds permitted students to graduate without any diagnostic (63.3%) or treatment (64%) experiences. They summarized the results of their survey by reporting "a trend toward fewer required classes taught by less experienced faculty, fewer clinical hours guided by less experienced supervisors, and a great likelihood that students will graduate without academic or clinical education in fluency disorders" (p. 58).

A panel discussion at the Fifth World Congress on Fluency Disorders in Dublin, Ireland, in the summer of 2006 (Kroll, et al., 2006) provided evidence that this less-than-satisfactory situation exists not only in the United States but also in Canada and the United Kingdom. Even in these locations, where one might expect professional preparation of clinicians working with individuals who stutter to be among the best, programs are often able to provide only limited clinical and classroom time. It is clear that many clinicians who are interested in developing expertise in fluency and fluency disorders have to take it upon themselves to seek additional preparation in this area of specialization following graduation.

Compounding the problem of providing quality preparation for clinicians in the area of fluency disorders is the increasing shortage of doctoral-level faculty in speech-language pathology. According to the most recent data available (Oller, 2002) reported that there were 50 unfilled tenure-line positions in 1998 and nearly twice as many in 1999 and 2000. Although there were no specific data for faculty in fluency disorders, the fact that students are not required to take courses or clinical work in stuttering, combined with the ever-expanding scope of practice in our field, makes it increasingly less likely that instructors will be hired in the area of fluency disorders. In fact, many of the best academic programs no longer have doctoral-level faculty teaching and specializing in fluency disorders. This does not mean that individuals with a master's degree do not offer outstanding courses in fluency disorders, for many do. But, it is the doctoral faculty who take a primary role in initiating basic and applied research, directing student research, and mentoring new faculty in fluency disorders.

Finally, a recent survey of 225 school speech-language pathologists by Tellis, Bressler, and Emerick (2008) indicated the lack of adequate preparation provided by undergraduate and graduate programs in the area of fluency disorders. Clinicians working in five northeastern states completed a 49-item Likert-type scale. Of the total, 87.8% had a master's degree and 64.7% had their certificate of clinical competence. The clinicians averaged 16.37 years of experience and, on average, had treated 12 children who stuttered throughout their careers. Some of the results were encouraging in that most indicated a basic understanding of stuttering and the value of parent participation in therapy. However, only 46.9% had taken a one-semester course in fluency disorders and slightly over half (53.5%) of the clinicians were comfortable working with children who stutter. Moreover, the majority of clinicians lacked basic knowledge and skills necessary for assessment and treatment. Many were unaware of current trends in the area of fluency disorders, including how to use new attitude scales to assess stuttering, interventions for bullying, how to contact support groups, and the incidence of stuttering. Few clinicians had attended continuing education courses in fluency disorders, although many of them indicated they would like to attend workshops that addressed assessment (83%) or treatment (92.5%) of stuttering. The authors concluded that improved academic preparation and continuing education for clinicians assisting children who stutter is urgently needed.

How Clinicians Interpret the Disorder

If stuttering is presented as a mysterious disorder—an enigma—clinicians will naturally be wary about treating these clients. Stuttering may indeed be an enigma, for the problem is complex and many of the features lie under the surface. When responding to the suggestion that stuttering is like a riddle, Van Riper stated that "[it] is more than a riddle. It is at least a complicated, multi-dimensional jigsaw puzzle, with many pieces still missing" (1982; p. 1). Sheehan frequently argued the case that stuttering is like an iceberg, with only small portions of the problem visible to those who were unwilling to look below the surface (Sheehan, 1970). Sheehan (1980) also offered the pointed comment that "defining stuttering as [only] a fluency problem borders on professional irresponsibility. It ignores the person. It ignores his feelings about himself" (p. 392).

On the other hand, Ham (1993) argues that stuttering is not significantly more complex than many other human behavioral problems. Much of stuttering behavior is rule governed with cause-and-effect relationships that are understood. Many of the factors that precipitate and maintain stuttering are well known, and many children and adults achieve extraordinary success in modifying both their speech and their handicap as a result of treatment. As students have the opportunity to observe clinicians who understand stuttering and begin to experience success assisting people who stutter, they are likely to become enthusiastic about the assessment and treatment of the problem. Experienced clinicians know what success looks and sounds like, and these changes can be shown to the new clinician. As with most things in life, there is no substitute for experience. Only continual practice of your craft will enable you to learn by your successes as well as your failures. Fortunately, for those who are curious and excited by learning, the process is never complete.

One of the substantial problems faced by students taking part in any clinical experience is that they are not likely to see a long view of progress. This is due, in part, to not being able to follow clients throughout the continuum of change during and following structured therapeutic change. For many practical reasons it is rare, even for a professional clinician, to follow a client for more than a few months or years, particularly in the years following dismissal from treatment. Most students lack the chance to observe and work with a client for a substantial portion of their structured treatment, the time during which the client pays a professional for services, let alone informal treatment, the much longer period when the client gradually develops the "response-ability" required for self-treatment. The window available to student clinicians in graduate programs is a small one. In most instances, student clinicians are just beginning to understand the client and the nature of their stuttering as the semester comes to a close. When the overall picture of behavioral, affective, and cognitive change is unavailable, it is understandable that the treatment process will appear enigmatic. Then again, if student clinicians know what to look for and can be shown indicators of progress during treatment (both for behavioral as well as cognitive-affective change), then helping these speakers will be more likely to be viewed as a positive rather than an aversive experience. A central principle is indicated in the comments of Daly (1988), who noted that the better clinicians tend to be those who hold a belief that their clients have the capacity for success as a result of treatment. Such conviction by the clinician is essential, according to Van Riper (1973), who stated the belief that "out of the therapist's faith can come the stutterer's hope" (p. 230).

Clinician Personality Attributes

The therapeutic relationship has been studied extensively in the fields of counseling and clinical psychology. The results of these investigations began finding their way into the literature in speech-language pathology during the 1960s. Although the therapeutic relationship of the client and the clinician is clearly important in all aspects of clinical intervention, it is especially critical in the area of fluency disorders because of the strong interactive therapeutic component. Research in the fields of counseling and psychology has provided consistent evidence that therapeutic exchanges are more likely to facilitate optimum change or gain if the clinician is able to communicate messages of empathy, positive regard, genuineness, and concreteness (Berenson & Carkhuff, 1967; Carkhuff & Berenson, 1967; Truax & Carkhuff, 1966). Crowe (1997a) cites The American Psychological Association (1947) as recommending the following personal attributes for counselors and psychotherapists: resourcefulness, versatility, curiosity, respect for the integrity of others, awareness of one's own personality traits, humor, tolerance, ability to relate warmly to others, industry, responsibility, integrity, stability, and ethics. As we will discuss in Chapter 7, and as Crowe and others describe in his 1997 text *Applications of Counseling in Speech-Language Pathology and Audiology*, counseling principles are at the core of the assessment and treatment process of all communication disorders.

Van Riper (1975) provided the first comprehensive description of the desirable attributes of clinicians who help children and adults who stutter. He described personality characteristics of *empathy*, an authentic sensitivity for the client; *warmth*, a respect or positive regard for the client; *genuineness*, openness and the ability to disclose oneself as a real person; and *charisma*, an ability to arouse hope, appearing confident yet humble, frank yet tactful. As Van Riper (1973) stated: "Like fishermen, good therapists are optimists. Most of them have come to have profound respect for the latent potential for self-healing that exists in all troubled souls" (p. 230).

A slightly different view of clinician characteristics was proposed by Zinker (1977), who considers therapy as a creative process of changing awareness and behavior. Although Zinker was not discussing therapy for stuttering or describing speech-language pathologists, he views therapy as a creative process and feels that a common malady among therapists is that they fail to see themselves as artists involved in a creative process. As the clinician becomes involved in the dynamic and shared process of change, the opportunity for creativity becomes

Clinical Insight

On a few occasions throughout the book we will include comments from Daniel Goleman's (2006) book *Social Intelligence*. Goleman provides a wealth of supporting data from studies in neuroscience when discussing the concept of *primal empathy*, the ability of individuals to unconsciously employ a "low road" to rapidly scan and interpret another individual for such issues as safety and trust. Neural circuitry connecting such areas as the sensory cortices, thalamus, and amygdala, as well as multiple systems of mirror neurons, allow some individuals to "bridge brains" (p. 43). The "high road," which involves the prefrontal cortex (the brain's executive center) is not involved. Goleman describes how mirror neurons fire in such a way that observing someone else being hurt also feels like being hurt to the observer. People develop an emotional contagion and synchrony as they resonate with another. As the synchrony occurs, individuals' moods begin to match, the timing of verbal and nonverbal communication becomes more coordinated, and participants become more comfortable with silences. The process must be spontaneous and unconscious rather than preplanned and intentional. Fortunately, the process is described as "eminently trainable" (p. 99).

more apparent. As we will discuss in succeeding chapters, the experienced clinician can be seen as a guide who has a map of the territory. The clinician has a sense of direction about where the client may benefit from traveling and a notion of when it might be appropriate to initiate an exploratory trip off the main path. As Zinker suggests, the challenge for the clinician is to "establish an adequate cognitive map which includes the client's experience of himself and then to point to action steps to make the solution possible for the client" (p. 11).

In order to guide a person through successful therapy, Zinker proposes that the clinician possess several characteristics that nurture the creative process. For example, creativity is facilitated by a childlike wonderment and excitement; patience for change without forcing; a love of play; a sense of humor; a positive attitude about risk taking; a willingness to experiment with different approaches and techniques; the ability to distinguish the boundaries between him- or herself and a client; a willingness to push, confront, persuade, and energize another person in order to accomplish the work that needs to be done; and a lifestyle that promotes a rich background with a range of life experiences.

Zinker proposes that blocks to creativity lead to the clinician becoming stuck in a particular theoretical or professional stance or holding to the view that science and art do not mix: a science-versus-art dichotomy. Other blocks to creativity include a fear of failure (playing it safe and not taking risks), a reluctance to play (fear of experimenting with ideas and techniques and of looking silly), over-certainty concerning a particular school of thought (a rigidity concerning the nature of the problem-solving approach), giving up too soon when an approach or a technique does not appear to be "working," a reluctance to push hard enough to help others, or an inability to accept contrasting ways of interpreting things and events (believing that there is only one way or one best way to define success during therapy). It is also worth considering that clinicians should probably not be modeling these blocks to creativity to clients, who may already be experiencing them. Many of these views are nearly identical to those of David Luterman, an experienced counselor and author in the field of communication disorders (see Chapter 7). Luterman (2001) suggests that professional growth is severely limited by the clinician's fear of making mistakes and an unwillingness to assume risks during the therapeutic or counseling process.

Cooper and Cooper (1985b) also provide a description of several desirable attributes of the effective clinician. Many of the attributes described by these authors coincide with their view of fluency treatment as an interpersonal (communication) experience. The effective clinician brings to this interpersonal experience certain desirable attitudes and personality attributes. The Coopers suggest that, especially during the early stages of treatment, the client–clinician relationship should be a major focus. They state that the clinician should be *genuine* and able to openly express both negative and positive feelings to the client. However, as the clinician is expressing these feelings it is important that he or she also indicate a belief in the worth and potential of the client. As treatment becomes challenging and the client is asked to make behavioral, attitudinal, and cognitive changes, the clinician should be continually *honest* in reinforcing the client's feelings of self-worth. Such honesty, the Coopers prudently note, is much easier to manifest when the clinician enjoys working with the client, something which may not always be the case. They warn that the clinician also needs to resist the urge to tell clients how they should feel. As Luterman (2001) cautions, there is a great temptation to try to get the client to feel as we do; something to be avoided if we are to be helpful. The clinician may, however, indicate that although he or she understands a client's feelings (empathy), he or she does not share them (sympathy), or at least does not necessarily agree that they are warranted by the situation. Experienced clinicians are able to indicate the difference between disapproval of feelings expressed by the client and the client's worth as a person.

Cooper and Cooper (1985b) state that the clinician should be "devoid of dogma" and have the ability to adapt the therapeutic approach to the client's uniqueness and needs. This is a fine way of saying that good clinicians are client directed rather than treatment directed. The clinician must be able to recognize subtle client responses that provide cues for direction and indicate progress. Experienced clinicians are not slowed down by a client's negative response to the suggestions and challenges of the therapeutic process. They are, in short, able to be a constant ally and to persevere along with the client when the process of change slows or becomes difficult. Experienced clinicians inform the client by providing information about the latter's status and progress and direction of treatment. Cooper and Cooper submit that clients, at any point in treatment and regardless of age or mental abilities, should be able to describe just where they are in treatment in both behavioral and attitudinal terms. Finally, effective clinicians are able to attend to the technical details of record keeping and report writing.

Undoubtedly, the characteristics we have discussed would be desirable for any clinician working with a person for any reason. They would be valuable characteristics to have in a friend or colleague. Moreover, just as it is possible to be successful as a friend or colleague without all of these attributes, it is possible to be a successful clinician without possessing enormous amounts of each. It is likely, however, that individuals who possess such characteristics not only make the treatment process more effective, they also make it more enjoyable.

Most people come to the professional field of speech-language pathology with many of these personality attributes, attitudes, and abilities. It is not clear whether some or all of these basic characteristics can be created or enhanced as a function of academic and clinical experience. What is clear, however, is that given these personality characteristics, clinicians can achieve proficiency in several intervention skills that increase their effectiveness in treating clients.

Clinician Intervention Skills

Given the aforementioned attitudes and personality attributes, we will now discuss several intervention skills that can be acquired and developed by the student. There is, of course, considerable overlap across each of these abilities.

Becoming Less Inhibited

Becoming desensitized to stuttering is an important first step in understanding the behavior and the person we are treating. Only after the clinician is able to become uninhibited about stuttering in general, and about him- or herself in particular, will treatment proceed (Van Riper, 1982).

To be effective, the clinician must gradually become progressively less inhibited about many aspects of stuttering. First of all, clinicians often need to overcome their concern about doing something "wrong" in therapy that will hurt the speaker and somehow make things worse. This common perspective is most likely related to the notion that there is something psychologically amiss or fragile about the person who stutters and that such individuals are unstable or especially susceptible to emotional trauma. In part, this attitude may be a result of the diagnosogenic view of stuttering etiology advocated during the

Clinical **Insight**

At the outset of my career I had the opportunity to correspond with the charismatic and prolific Dr. Charles Van Riper, clearly a master clinician. I didn't have the opportunity to know him well, but on one occasion we met in his office at Western Michigan University. I remember his primary comment about clinicians. Paraphrasing (for reasons those who knew him well will understand), he said that many clinicians were far too inhibited to be effective with people who stutter. They are afraid of eliciting or creating stuttering. They are afraid of joining in the process of touching and exploring the stuttering. They view stuttering as something to be suppressed and avoided. Likewise, I am always intrigued when I ask students in my class to follow my lead and voluntarily produce some mild to moderate stuttering in front of their peers. The activity indicates the degree to which stuttering is stigmatized and the extent that we must go to decrease our natural inhibitions about approaching and exploring the behavior and the experience of stuttering.

period from the early 1950s through the late 1960s, which held that stuttering was created by inappropriate listener reactions to the fluency breaks of young children (see Chapter 3). Alternately, such a cautious approach may be related to the idea that any increase in the frequency of stuttering is necessarily bad. As we will discuss in later chapters, for a number of reasons, an increase in the frequency of stuttering may be an important indicator of progress, particularly early in treatment. In addition, stuttering is highly variable, and changes in the frequency of the overt behaviors can be attributable to many, sometimes unknown, factors, only one of which is the clinician.

In extreme instances, of course, it may be possible to make the stuttering, or even the person who is stuttering, in some sense worse. If, for example, the clinician is truly an unqualified, uncaring, and insensitive person, the client and, conceivably, the stuttering could become worse. However, a qualified clinician who is inhibited about making a decision during treatment for fear of somehow injuring a client most likely possesses a naive view of the person who is doing the stuttering. Most people who stutter are not fragile. On the contrary, many people who stutter are stable and resilient, particularly those individuals who have the courage to ask for help and initiate treatment. Clinicians with training and experience should not exercise any more caution about doing something "wrong" when assisting a child or adult who stutters than they would with a client with any other communication problem.

The therapeutic relationship or alliance between clinician and client is an important aspect of the process of change during treatment. There is no question, especially with adolescents and adults who stutter, that there is a strong counseling or psychotherapeutic component at the center of the process. As suggested by the quote by Van Riper at the outset of this chapter, there are aspects of this process of change and growth that impact the clinician as well as the client. It is rare that only one person grows during good, interactive treatment. Indeed, such growth is often experienced most clearly during the mixture of personalities and perceptions that take place in group treatment activities. Students have often commented after completing their clinical experiences in fluency disorders that they miss the exciting and challenging experiences provided by group interaction.

Nevertheless, because the process of change and growth is a dynamic one, it is not necessarily something that all clinicians are initially comfortable about entering. One alluring aspect of the behavior modification programs that became popular during the late 1950s, 1960s, and 1970s was the belief that the role of the clinician could be limited to the identification and modification of overt stuttering behaviors. The behaviors that were audible and visible on the surface were the major focus of treatment. Certainly clinicians were making decisions. Frequency counts were made, contingencies were agreed upon or at least implied, and rewards and punishments were dispensed by the clinician based on the client's performance. The often manualized treatment process was clear, goals were explicit, and fluency was charted and altered. The approach was relatively easy to teach to students as well as to clients. Some clients did well, as some clients will do in nearly all reasonable treatment approaches (see Chapter 6). Some even stayed well. However, the point is not whether behavior modification approaches are effective, for they can be. A particular treatment strategy can only be evaluated based on the needs and response of the client. The point is that when using any treatment, including current behavioral modification programs (which tend to encompass more broad-based and multifactorial philosophies and approaches than in the past), the clinician needs to be uninhibited. The clinician needs to be uninhibited about stuttering and the people who are doing the stuttering if he or she expects the client, parents, teacher, or spouse to also approach, understand, and change the problem.

One of the unique aspects about the series of treatment sessions produced by the Stuttering Foundation is that the clinician, Charles Van Riper, demonstrates an uninhibited and interactive therapeutic style with his young adult client, named Jeff (Video # 1080, Therapy in Action). Dr. Van Riper models attributes of empathy, genuineness, warmth, charisma, and particularly frankness throughout the treatment sessions with Jeff. This video series may present some problems that prevent contemporary observers from appreciating Dr. Van Riper's personal attributes. The tapes were made in the 1970s, and because of differences in dress, Van Riper's forthright and sometimes assertive interpersonal style, and current interpretations of "political correctness," it is usually necessary for new clinicians to view the tapes several times in order to fully appreciate the nature of the therapeutic interaction. After viewing the tapes a few times it becomes possible to detect the genuine, humanistic, and supportive nature of Dr. Van Riper's therapeutic interaction. It becomes clear that Van Riper is obviously unafraid of stuttering. As documented by the analysis of verbal patterns of the therapy sessions by Blood et al. (2001), Van Riper simultaneously challenges and supports Jeff and modifies his approach based on Jeff's response. He imparts to Jeff a distinct sense of direction as he helps him to move forward in treatment. There are moments of spontaneous humor on the part of both participants that indicate their synchrony. The tapes also provide a good illustration of how a productive therapeutic relationship is like many successful relationships; they are not always idyllic or characterized by "good rapport."

Another beneficial aspect of this video series is that the student has the opportunity to see an enlarged window of change as the client progresses through treatment. Although the observer is not assisting in the process of change it is encouraging to see that dramatic success is possible during a relatively brief period of therapy. There is some indication that students can increase their level of self-efficacy about clinical performance with fluency clients as a function of academic training (Rudolf, Manning, & Sewell, 1983). There is, however, no substitute for a successful hands-on clinical experience.

Avoiding Dogmatic Decisions

Being able to see beyond the dogma of one particular treatment strategy is a sign of clinical wisdom. Making use of the oft-quoted adage, Egan (1990) cautions that we should "beware the person of one book" (p. 26). The message of a single book or single author can too easily become a calling. It is true that the discovery of *the* method can be empowering and give a sense of direction to the clinician and, therefore, to the client. However, as Egan points out, such devotion to a single treatment path can also lead to a closing down of new ideas and new growth. It is also a path that is likely to lead to boredom. Egan recommends that, for a professional, the foundation for choosing a strategy or technique should not be the treatment protocol, but the nature and needs of the client. As we will suggest throughout this book, clinical decisions should be driven primarily by the needs and goals of the client and the therapeutic context rather than dogma. A technician, particularly an inexperienced one, is likely to make decisions according to the guidelines of the treatment manual. Although this approach is nearly always less thoughtful and creative, it can be much easier and even comforting. It is likely to require less responsibility and fewer decisions on the part of the clinician. As we will see later in this chapter, professionals are more likely to make decisions based on an analysis of the contextual cues of the therapeutic situation. It may be instructive to consider that the most proficient and creative professional chefs rarely follow a cookbook.

Clinical Decision-Making

Several years ago, at a professional meeting of speech-language pathologists, I was a member of a panel that was asked, along with the audience, to view a series of videotapes of children and adults with fluency disorders. The panel's task was to react to these hypothetical clients and speculate about the various strategies and techniques that might be appropriate for them. As we took our turns offering suggestions about each speaker it became apparent that one member of the panel was giving the identical response each time. Regardless of the client's characteristics such as age and severity and nature of the stuttering, this clinician would take her turn at the microphone and say something such as "I believe strongly in the ___ method and feel that this approach would be ideal for this client. I have seen this method work for many clients and would prefer to use this approach with this person." Beyond the highly questionable efficacy of this particular method, the audience witnessed a clear example of a "one book" approach to treatment. The clinician was familiar with a particular approach and this is the approach she believed in. It was apparent that nothing else mattered, including her clients.

Opening Your Treatment Focus

One of the characteristics of learning a new activity is the amount of attention required to focus on the techniques. When first learning a sport such as soccer, for example, it is necessary to learn such techniques as passing, receiving, and shooting the ball. Later, with more experience, one moves beyond the techniques. The accomplished player has a broader, less technical view of the game. With experience, the view includes the strategies of the event and, particularly, an analysis of the other team's strengths and weaknesses. The player's focus begins to open up, allowing a focus on the movements and anticipated actions of the players on the opposing team. Although the techniques remain essential to the accomplishment of the overall strategy, the most important aspect of the process is not so much what to do or how to do it, but when to do it and why. Similar to inexperienced players or coaches, new clinicians tend to focus on accomplishing the techniques of the moment rather than the overall long-term strategies and goals. Even more to the point, new clinicians are more likely to focus on the techniques rather than the person they are trying to help. In part because they know relatively few techniques at the beginning of their career, new clinicians are apt to think to themselves, "What can I do in the therapy session today?" rather than "What does my client need from me now, and how does that fit with our long-term goals of treatment?"

We are not suggesting that specific treatment techniques are unimportant, for we will discuss many of them in succeeding chapters. They are, of course, every bit as essential to treating clients as knowing how to pass and control the ball is to playing soccer. You cannot play the game well if you are not good at the techniques. Techniques are unquestionably important, and the professional clinician must know many of them and know them well. However, they are not the most important aspect of the process. The ability to look beyond the techniques—even beyond the treatment program and see the client is something that distinguishes the experienced clinician from the novice, the technician from the professional.

Just as the new instructor is less likely to vary from prepared notes or stray more than a few steps away from the podium, the less experienced player is more likely to have a rigid, preplanned attack. A preplanned strategy may work for a while, particularly with an easy opponent. However, the plan may not work indefinitely, especially with a challenging opponent. The accomplished participant is flexible; he or she can see what is occurring on the field in a broader sense. The accomplished athlete (or coach) is more likely to be aware of and willing to change strategy based on the circumstances and the level of competition. Decisions and actions are primarily dictated by strengths and weakness of the other players or team. They most certainly are not dictated by a textbook or by dogma.

For decades, Van Riper stated that "the client, not the clinician, is the guide," and certainly not the text or the treatment techniques. There are many paths up the mountain and the path is likely to be different for each person, in part because everyone is beginning the journey from a different place. This seems rather complicated—and sometimes it is. However, before we throw up our hands at the challenges presented to us by each new client, it is important to realize that many individuals who stutter have some similar cognitive and behavioral responses to stuttering. Moreover, there are basic principles of change (see Chapter 8) that contribute to success.

Calibrating to the Client

At the outset of the first several treatment sessions, it is not unusual for clinicians to find that they are presented with a wide range of information by clients. Not only are we introduced to expected surface behaviors that we have seen before in other speakers who stutter but we may also observe some new behaviors that are unique to this particular speaker. Some of these behaviors may be obvious and explicit. Other behaviors may occur rarely or not at all during the initial sessions. Some of the behaviors learned long ago have become part of this person's response to stuttering and will become apparent only during more stressful speaking situations; they are seen only rarely, if at all, during treatment sessions. We will see these coping behaviors only when we accompany the person into daily speaking situations beyond the usual treatment setting. We may also note these behaviors if we call clients unexpectedly or meet them by chance in a social situation. In any case, there are apt to be many surface behaviors that are unique to each speaker, and it will take even the experienced clinician some time to become attuned to them.

In order to fully appreciate the nature of the client's stuttered speech it may be useful to also consider the quality of the person's speech when they are not stuttering. What is it about the subtle surface behaviors of this speaker that indicates to us that they are fluent? Is the client producing truly fluent speech that, as Starkweather (1987) indicates, is characterized by an easy, smooth, relatively effortless flow of information? Or, is their nonstuttered speech characterized by something less than a smooth, effortless quality? Is the client achieving easy, flowing fluency or is the person just "not stuttering"? It may be that the speaker is hesitating, possibly avoiding or exchanging words, sometimes making it difficult for the listener to understand the information the speaker is trying to communicate. It can be useful in calibrating yourself to the client to differentiate at least three levels of fluency: stuttered speech, unstable speech, and truly easy and flowing fluent speech.

One procedure that aids in the calibration process, especially during the first several meetings, is to mimic or imitate the client's speech (Van Riper, 1973). In this way the clinician is able to get a feel (literally) for how the client may, for example, slightly slow his or her speech before a feared sound or word. The clinician can begin to determine whether the speaker scans ahead and "pretastes" words while considering whether to try moving through them. Using audio- or video recordings at the outset of treatment can assist clinicians in tuning in to their new client. The clinician can become calibrated to the client's speech patterns by pantomiming the tapes at the office, at home, or while driving in the car. Although on the surface, the client may appear to be fluent, with time the clinician will be able to detect instances when the client is speaking carefully and making a concerted effort not to stutter. The speech will be unstable, and the clinician will get the sensation that the client is "talking on thin ice"; the client is not stuttering in a technical sense yet seems as though he may fall through the surface of fluency at any moment.

As we become calibrated to the new client, we will begin to notice how the client's speech looks, as well as how it sounds. We can begin to tune in not only to the surface structure, but perhaps even more importantly, to the deep structure of the person. What are the cues signaling that this speaker may be experiencing some loss of control, some helplessness, as he or she approaches, and moves through, moments where he or she expects to stutter? Although the speaker may not have overtly stuttered on a word, he or she was not completely in control of his or her speech. It is as though the stuttering was just under the surface. Until we become calibrated to that person, we are not likely to detect such occurrences. Detecting this loss of control, a key feature of the stuttering experience, is discussed in greater detail in Chapter 4.

Observing Silence

In observing both the surface and deep structures of the client's speech, experienced clinicians are apt to minimize their own talk and maximize observation. This is more likely to occur as the therapeutic alliance matures. One helpful way to tune in to someone is to stop talking. Rather than fill in the silent pauses or providing answers to questions, clinicians use the silence as a time for reflecting on what the client has said. Communication does not cease during silence. Body language, eye contact, and facial expressions tell much about the status of what has been said—and left unsaid. Silence on the part of the clinician may even be thought of as providing the client with a degree of independence. Van Riper (1975) suggested that when the clinician finds him- or herself uttering more than four or five sentences in a row, "warning lights should go off." This is especially true, he suggested, if the sentences contain many I's and we's. Silence on the part of the clinician (or instructor) can force action and response on the part of the client (or students). During the silences by the clinician not only do clients have the opportunity to achieve greater independence, they also have the chance to take responsibility for the pace and direction of treatment.

Clinical Insight

Perhaps more than any other, one of my experiences during a therapy session has remained with me over the years. As a recent college graduate, I had been in therapy for a few months. Although he was not a person who stuttered, the clinician I was working with that day was the first who conveyed to me a real understanding of my plight. The therapy session turned out to be a particularly demanding one. I was being challenged to be introspective and honest about my experience with stuttering and my pattern of avoidance behavior. There were many long and (for me at least) frustrating silences. It was a difficult but productive session. As we neared the end of our time together that day, he quoted a line that went something like "I knew we were friends when we could share the silence." As it turned out, a few years later he was to become my professional mentor and close personal friend.

Modeling Risk Taking

On occasion, we as clinicians must be prepared to take the lead and demonstrate our willingness to take risks. Sheehan (1970) made the insightful comment that "the Achilles heel of most normal speaking therapists who try to work with stutterers is simply that they are not willing to do what they ask their stutterers to do" (p. 283). If we convey anxiety about stuttering and the tasks that await our client on the road to change, how can we expect him or her to follow our recommendations and to move forward? We do not have to do so often, but occasionally we will be called upon to demonstrate our willingness to take risks and to lead the way into speaking situations. Each situation is an opportunity for us to demonstrate that it is possible to be reasonably calm in the midst of stuttering and to openly and easily stutter. Alternatively, depending on how difficult a speaking experience may be for the clinician, it is a chance for him or her to demonstrate that, despite some obvious anxiety, he or she is committed to the client. For example, the clinician may voluntarily stutter to a stranger on the street as the client observes. The clinician can openly stutter on the question, "Pardon me, do you have the ta . . . ta . . . ta . . ." until the listener gives you the time of day. It is one thing to tell the client that you are committed to helping him, but showing him is far better.

It is easy to discuss the variety of therapeutic tasks that can be accomplished. It is another thing to take action, particularly action beyond the relatively secure walls of the clinic environment. As difficult as it can be because of logistical and time issues, the ability of the clinician to accompany clients into some of their daily speaking situations can be critical for functional change. As Peck (1978) suggested, the cornerstone of any clinical relationship is the commitment on the part of the clinician, who must be willing to join in the struggle rather than sitting back and playing a professional role. There will be times during successful treatment when the clinician will be asked to take the field and join in the struggle; not to talk about commitment, but to demonstrate it (see Manning, 1991a; 2004b). If the clinician is able to show that he or she is a stable and understanding ally, the client will be much more likely to go beyond his or her previously established boundaries.

The clinician may also model risk-taking behavior in activities that do not necessarily require speaking. Just as the client is asked to venture outside his or her previously established speech boundaries, the clinician can model behavior that includes presentations to colleagues or other groups. The clinician can take on challenges related to conditioning (e.g., begin a program of walking, running, or swimming), instruction (e.g., enroll in a class to acquire a new skill such as karate or yoga), or professional activities (e.g., coordinate a professional or social event, write an article, pamphlet, or book). By taking risks, the clinician can model new limits for the client and more fully appreciate the risks you are asking the client to take.

Clinical Decision-Making

Several years ago when I was a doctoral student conducting therapy with a young man in his twenties, we left the safety of the clinic in order to obtain some realistic examples of his stuttering behavior as well as typical listener reactions. As we walked across the campus of a large midwestern university, his task was to stop people and inquire about the location of various buildings. Although it was early in the treatment process and he was stuttering severely at this point, he was, nevertheless, willing to take part in the activity. Following a particularly difficult speaking situation, where he found himself completely stuck and unable to say anything, his listener, not knowing what else to do, apologized and walked away. I could see that the young man was devastated and was unable to continue. Perhaps I had asked too much of him. Perhaps I should have done what I was asking him to do. So I took my turn. I asked him what I should say and how I should stutter to the next person we would meet. His task was to verify that I stuttered in the preplanned way and to discover specific listener responses. After we had successfully done this with several strangers, he was more than willing to take the lead in gathering the information we had set out to find.

Challenging the Client

Assuming that we are able to provide the security of a committed therapeutic alliance and a strategy for change with the client, we then must begin assisting the person to move forward. However, change is often difficult even when the motivation exists. Changing the surface characteristics and, especially, the deep structure of stuttering can be difficult, particularly with adolescent and adult speakers. If it were easy, anyone could do it and there would be far fewer people handicapped by the problem of stuttering. However, it is difficult to alter the equilibrium that has been established in one's psyche and in the roles that the stutterer and his listeners have developed over many years. Change involves work; it is time-consuming, and it can be expensive. At the very least, it is an inconvenience.

Because of the difficulties involved, change is not apt to occur without some applied force. The current ways of speaking and thinking about speaking must be moved off-center. There will be times during treatment when the clinician will have to push hard and indicate that specific, concrete tasks be accomplished. Moreover, on more than a few of those occasions, even the most motivated of our clients will not comply. They may be unable to comply because they do not understand the task, because we ask them to move too quickly, because the task seems too difficult, or simply because they do not have the energy to do what needs to be done. Still, on occasion pushing the client—just as in parenting, teaching, or coaching—beyond his previous comfortable levels of performance also shows respect for his potential.

If clinicians, including myself, are to be faulted for any one thing, we are most likely guilty of not pushing our adult clients hard enough. Most adult clients come to us knowing that the task is difficult. They often want us to push them harder, but we are fearful of eliciting a negative reaction. There is some evidence that greater progress in fluency treatment is made when the client is pushed to the point of eliciting negative feelings toward the clinician (Cooper & Cooper, 1965; Manning & Cooper, 1969). As Cooper and his associates have suggested, the dynamic process of change is not likely to yield a consistently positive client–clinician relationship. Just as change is a function of a teacher–student, parent–child, or coach–player relationship, there may be times when progress is especially difficult and the mentor must do what is necessary. Thus there will be times during treatment when the effective clinician will say and demand things that the client does not want to hear or do. Moreover, there will

Clinical Insight

Most of the readers of this book are graduate or undergraduate students who are at the outset of their journey to understanding the nature of stuttering and how to help people who do it. But all of us, no matter how many years we have been at this, must continue to be students of our field. Whether or not continued learning is mandated by our professional association, it is essential that we constantly acquire new information and perspectives about our areas of expertise. The accuracy of the information in any field that is moving forward is characterized by a remarkably brief half-life. Every few years I survey the faculty of our program and ask them to tell me things about their area(s) of specialization that they were taught during their many years of schooling that were later shown to be wrong. They always respond with an extensive and fascinating list of things that they, in turn, taught their students until they discovered new and more accurate information.

It is a sometimes daunting responsibility to become astute consumers of the information in your field. The recent emphasis on evidence-based practice offers some help in this process but it is far from being the answer. Throughout your career you will face the continual goal of sifting the wheat from chaff as you hear presentations and read manuscripts. It is a lifelong adventure to work toward expertise in your areas of interest. Success in any field of endeavor often requires a philosophy that balances enthusiastic curiosity with careful skepticism. It is both demanding and heroic. As we suggested at the outset of this chapter, the clinician is a critical variable in the success of any therapeutic intervention. How is it that some individuals are able to develop exceptional performance?

be periods when, based on our clinical experience and our long-range view of the treatment process, we will have to stand firm in our clinical decisions. It may not be our basic nature and it may feel uncomfortable, but temporarily being the "bad guy" can sometimes be good, especially when it promotes the long-term success for our clients.

Developing Expertise: Implications for Clinicians

The literature describing the ability of individuals to achieve expert performance encompasses a wide variety of human activity, including athletics, dance, chess, and a variety of other domains across the arts and sciences. In general, the research indicates that a minimum of 10 years of intensive preparation is necessary to attain the highest level of performance (Simon & Chase, 1973; Ericsson & Smith, 1991). Berliner (1994), in a summary of the literature on expertise, found agreement with the opinion that 10,000 to 20,000 hours of practice are required in order to perform an activity appropriately and effortlessly, hallmarks of exemplary performance. Although natural aptitude certainly plays a part in the ability to achieve expert performance, empirical evidence indicates that training and preparation are prerequisites for superior performance (Ericsson & Smith, 1991). Berliner (1994) provides a useful explanation of expert performance in his description of a five-stage model proposed by Dreyfus and Dreyfus (1986). (see also Manning, 2006.)

Novices, who are new to an activity, spend much of their time labeling their activities. They tend to act deliberately and pay close attention to context-free rules concerning how things are to be done (e.g., when driving, obeying signs with regard to the speed limit or when to pass other cars). Novices tend to be relatively inflexible and are likely to closely follow such context-free rules and protocols. These attributes are characteristic of students and first-year professionals.

Advanced Beginners are similar to the novice in that they are likely to follow rules. Although they may learn the rules, they are unsure what to do or not to do when new or unusual circumstances occur (e.g., being uncertain about how fast to drive or when to shift gears when driving on ice or snow). Eventually, advanced beginners begin to understand when to ignore or to break the rules when that would be the better thing to do. However, because they are often unsure of the appropriate indicators and patterns to guide them in their decision making, they are likely to respond to new situations by following rules. Because of their relative lack of experience, the advanced beginner will tend to react to new situations by classifying and describing events rather than responding creatively or problem solving. Another interesting sign of the advanced beginner is the tendency to set up barriers to help keep authority in his or her own hands. These attributes are characteristic of second- and third-year professionals.

People who have become *competent* (and not everyone achieves this level) have more than the usual motivation required for gaining additional experience. An important change takes place as competent performers begin making their own choices and developing their own priorities and strategies. Because they are making their own decisions, they tend to have a greater appreciation of the resulting success or failure of their choices and take more responsibility for the outcome of their actions. With continued experience, they further refine and focus their understanding concerning the important indicators and patterns that enable them to make the best decisions. An important hallmark of the competent individual is the ability to develop a better sense of timing and know not only *what* to do but *when* to do it. These attributes are characteristic of professionals with three to four years of experience.

Proficient performers begin to develop what seems to be an intuitive sense of situation. They are able to make micro-adjustments (as when making small balancing adjustments while riding a bike) that less proficient individuals are unlikely to notice. Importantly, they begin taking a *holistic* approach to their performance. This holistic view allows the proficient performer to recognize expansive, reoccurring patterns that others are unlikely to see. As a result they are able to anticipate events with greater precision. These attributes are characteristic of professionals with more than five years of experience.

In order to become an *expert,* it is usually necessary to focus on one or a very few specific domains with great dedication and persistence. This has some implications for our field in general, for one might ask, given the ever-expanding scope of practice for speech-language pathologists, whether or not it is possible for one to become truly competent in more than one or perhaps a few specialty areas. As we discussed above, it takes many thousands of practice hours (10–20 thousand hours for chess players; 10–15 thousand hours of teaching; reading more than 100,000 X-rays) to approach this level of expertise in a given area. Following years of such focused learning, experts appear to develop an intuitive grasp of the situation and seemingly perform effortlessly, "becoming one" with an activity (the car they are driving, the instrument they are playing, the tools or techniques they are using). Experts often appear to be nonanalytic and nondeliberative, as vividly demonstrated by the pianist or the accomplished martial artist; the individual parts of the activity are not easily described as deductive or analytical behavior and performers are able to respond in a rapid and fluid manner. Berliner (1994) cites the vivid example of Wayne Gretsky, the hockey player, who when asked to explain his extraordinary success on the ice, responded by saying, "I don't know; I just go to where the puck is going to be" (p. 9).

A final comment about the nature of expert performance as it applies to a field closely related to the clinical situation. Berliner (1991) was particularly interested in understanding expert performance as it applied to exceptionally adept teachers. He found that expert instructors were flexible in their approach, apt to consider alternative responses to a situation, unlikely to follow a manual, opportunistic about ways to connect with their students (rather than following a pre-planned approach), and often followed the lead of the student. These experts had become integrated individuals who focused less on themselves and more on the student. Additionally, they were unusually sensitive to the affective concerns of their students. We will refer to many of these same characteristics on several occasions throughout this book as we describe the nature of the therapeutic process for individuals who stutter.

Decision Making with Rules and Principles

The reader has undoubtedly noted a trend for the lessening importance of using rules as a guide with increasing levels of expertise. As people improve their ability in the direction of expert performance there is the tendency to make decisions based on principles rather than rules. This is especially the case when the situation is dynamic rather than static. In an analysis of the characteristics of expert psychotherapeutic counselors, Levitt, Neimeyer, & Williams (2004) noted that rule-based approaches have evolved in many areas, including business, education, law, and athletics. That is, *rules* are created and serve as specific guidelines for evaluating an experience—how well something was done and whether or not something was accomplished. Rules are apt to be formalized, unequivocally applied and usually quantitative in nature. *Principles*, on the other hand, are less specific. Decisions based on principles emphasize expert discretion, intuition, and personal knowledge and are often contextual and qualitative.

Levitt et al. (2004) cite John Braithwaite (2002), a professor of law in Australia, who discusses the rules–principles continuum. Braithwaite suggests that the application of rules without regard to the context of the situation or action works best when the type of activity is stable and relatively simple. In such cases, rules tend to help us to understand and respond to the circumstances with greater certainty than principles. Conversely, Braithwaite makes a convincing case that when the type of situation being considered is dynamic and complex, principles tend to help us respond with greater certainty than rules. Braithwaite suggests that using rules to regulate dynamic activities results in lower consistency and validity and cites several examples in a wide variety of situations, including the management of nursing homes, banks, and nuclear energy facilities. For example, he describes how the strict application of rules for regulating nursing homes in Australia and the United States resulted in vastly reduced quality of care. In a variety of examples he illustrates how the sharp edges of rules can be used as "an interpretive strategy to defeat the purpose of a rule"(p. 71). Although the intent of the rules is to insure best practice, the strict interpretation of the rules far too often results in limiting options for the workers. Braithwaite describes how in case after case the situation improved for the residents of the nursing homes when intelligent people found ways to honor the principles that justified the rules rather than strictly following the rules themselves. Braithwaite recommends the implementation of nonbinding rules backed by binding principles for obtaining greater consistency and effectiveness for making decisions about relatively complex phenomena. Braithwaite's primary interests have to do with the consistent application of the law. He suggests that in order to accomplish consistency it is necessary to understand that, in many instances, the cultures and processes involved are best understood not as a rulebook but a storybook. Many of the comments throughout this book will reflect a greater emphasis on *principles* over *rules* when seeking avenues of therapeutic change.

To illustrate Braithwaite's point we offer a common example of the contrast between the application of rules and principles for simple (less dynamic) and complex (more dynamic) situations. When driving a car during relatively stable and usual circumstances (a clear day with good road conditions) rules provide reasonable guidelines for making decisions (what speed to drive, when to turn or pass). However, when driving in dynamic and unusual situations (a stormy day with snowy or icy road conditions), the normal rules may not serve us well and principles may provide better guidelines for making decisions. In such conditions the normal guidelines for passing, turning, and what speed to maintain are likely to be adjusted in order to achieve the binding principle of our safety.[1]

The characteristics of experts described by the above authors are remarkably similar across many fields (Ericsson & Smith, 1991). Furthermore, and particularly important for our discussions in subsequent chapters concerning therapeutic intervention, we will see that many of the attributes of experts are predicted by the Common Factors Model of treatment, a model we will discuss in Chapter 6. As we will see, the research that led to this model indicates that the expertise of the clinician is a key ingredient in successful therapy; far more influential, in fact, than particular therapeutic protocols and associated specific techniques. Coinciding with our comments earlier in this chapter, Berliner's analysis indicates that although expert instructors imparted information and techniques, they did so by responding in non-dogmatic and creative ways to the unique characteristics of the person and the situation, rather than forcing their own teaching agenda. They made use of their extensive experience and insight by allowing themselves the flexibility to experiment with procedures rather than following a pre-planned approach. They considered alternative responses.

---

[1]For example, a U.S. Department of Transportation report (no. FHWA/RD-85/096) indicates that the safest speed to drive is approximately 10 miles per hour faster or slower than the average speed of the surrounding traffic, rather than the posted speed limit. That is, if the principle is safety, the wisest decision may require breaking the rule.

Their focus was on the client, rather than on themselves or the techniques. They were also particularly attuned to the affective concerns of the other person.

Mahoney (2000) provides similar thoughts concerning the development of expertise and the decision-making process based on rules and principles. In describing the professional training of psychotherapists, Mahoney indicates that new trainees are impatient for simple answers to complex questions. He suggests that an important theme in their development is the cultivation of "patience and a respectful tolerance of ambiguity and complexity" (p. 731). Explaining that many important clinical and life decisions must be made with incomplete information and limited control, Mahoney and his colleagues have found that as clinicians accumulate more experience they report an increased tolerance for ambiguity. It is interesting to note that clinicians experienced in fluency disorders have much the same opinion. For example, both Conture (2001) and Zebrowski (2006) comment on the importance of developing a tolerance for ambiguity combined with a devotion to a lifetime of self-education.

Specialty Recognition in Fluency Disorders

One of the ways for clinicians in the area of fluency disorders to achieve expertise is to engage in the process of specialty recognition. The Specialty Board on Fluency Disorders and the website at *stutteringspecialists.org* provide the guidelines for obtaining recognition as well as valuable information for consumers and helpful links to related sites. Clinicians indicate a variety of benefits as a result of becoming a specialist, including improved visibility in the professional community and increases in referrals, requests for assistance from other clinicians, and the number of fluency clients in their caseloads (Donaher, 2006). In addition, the annual meeting of the Division of ASHA's Special Interest Division 4 (Fluency and Fluency Disorders) and the Division's peer-reviewed quarterly publication *Perspectives on Fluency and Fluency Disorders* offer a variety of information and opportunities for learning.

We now move to the final section of this chapter to discuss a variable that, perhaps to the surprise of some, has been associated with successful therapy and exceptional clinicians. In this section we are suggesting that the recognition of humor provides an overarching indicator of many successful clinicians as well as a sensitive metric of successful therapeutic change for many individuals undergoing therapy for stuttering.

Humor and the Clinician

As indicated throughout the earlier sections of this chapter, many experienced professionals suggest that humor is a valuable characteristic of clinicians and a natural part of a dynamic therapeutic process. The primary focus of our discussion about humor in the following paragraphs concerns a range of clinician attributes that have frequently been associated with a successful therapy outcome. However, our discussion also relates to how our clients interpret themselves and their circumstances and how humor both impacts and reflects therapeutic change. It is clear that a sense of humor is helpful, sometimes even essential, for coping with life on a daily basis. For example, Brissette, Scheier, and Carver (2002) found humor, acceptance, and positive reframing to be three functional coping responses. This can be true for the clinician who is working to help people with serious communication problems as well as the speaker who, at least at the outset of treatment, is often overwhelmed with his or her problem.

A Historical Perspective

In order to advocate for the importance of humor in the process of change, we will place the discussion of this uniquely human characteristic into an historical perspective. Kuhlman (1984) reported that during the first two decades of behavior therapy (1950–1970) there was not a single reference to humor in the literature. Beginning in the early 1970s, there was a substantial and progressive increase in the therapeutic use of humor, particularly in the professional fields of clinical psychology, counseling, and allied health. In 1977, McGhee & Goldstein reported that humor began to be recognized as a legitimate part of the human healing process—a way to maintain both physical and psychological health. A review of even a portion of the literature on humor, especially in the area of "therapeutic humor," clearly indicates that there are some valuable concepts for the speech-language pathologist. The fact that, in the early stages of research on the topic, humor was positively correlated with such personality characteristics as enthusiasm, playfulness, hopefulness, excitement, and vigorousness and negatively correlated with fear, depression, anger, indifference, and aloofness (McGhee & Goldstein, 1977) should have alerted clinicians to the possible importance of humor during the therapeutic process. Subsequent research by Thorson and Powell (1993b) confirmed many of these relationships and added a few more. Using a Multidimensional Sense of Humor Scale (MSHS) developed by the authors (1993a), Thorson and Powell found that MSHS scores positively correlated with exhibition, dominance, warmth, gregariousness, assertiveness, excitement seeking, creativity, intrinsic religiosity, arousability, positive emotions, extraversion, and cheerfulness. Humor scores correlated negatively with neuroticism, pessimism, avoidance, negative self-esteem, deference, order, endurance, aggression, depression, death anxiety, seriousness, perception of daily hassles, and bad mood.

In the field of fluency disorders there was a corresponding lack of interest in the therapeutic value of humor. In 1973, Van Riper commented briefly about the significance of humor for the person who stutters, describing it in terms of an antiexpectancy device used to lessen the severity of stuttering. He referred to Bryngelson (1935), as well as Luper and Mulder (1964), who recommended that people who stutter learn to joke about their stuttering in order to help others feel more at ease and to help themselves develop more optimistic attitudes about their problem. There are also several examples of humor occurring throughout the videotapes of Van Riper's therapy sessions with Jeff mentioned earlier. In 1995, based on a review of the literature on therapeutic humor, Manning & Beachy proposed that humor should be taken seriously as a variable in the therapeutic process for individuals who stutter. Guitar (1997) suggested using humor during the transfer stage of treatment with children as a way of showing them how to become open about their stuttering.

Kuhlman (1984) suggested that trying to define and understand humor is like trying to do so for the concept of "learning." Attempts to understand the essence of humor and its therapeutic potential have evolved through at least three stages of research. The initial stage of research on humor has been defined by Goldstein (1976) as the pre-theoretical stage. This stage began during the early part of the 20th century and continued until about 1940. Published manuscripts during this period consisted largely of correlational and observational studies of laughter and smiling; when and how people responded to humor-producing stimuli. There were relatively few attempts to develop or test a particular theory. Goldstein termed the next stage of humor research the psychoanalytic phase. Beginning in the 1940s and continuing until the 1970s, this phase was concerned almost exclusively with Freudian theory of wit and humor. Sigmund Freud viewed humor as a potential reducer of stress and placed it alongside the neurotic and psychotic disorders as a basic mechanism of adaptation to human suffering. The essential difference was that humor was thought of as a nonpathological adaptation. In addition, Freud (1928, 1961) asserted that perceived humorousness is related to the degree with which one is able to empathize and assume the role of the person who is the focus of humor.

Alport (1937, 1961), Maslow (1968), Rogers (1951, 1961), and Combs and Snygg (1959) all identified humor as an essential attribute of a healthy and fully functioning person. Burton (1972) stated the issue clearly: "One thing every therapist must have is a feeling for the comic. This balances his feeling for the tragic. I am suspicious of any therapist who never laughs" (p. 93). Zinker (1977), in describing the creative nature of Gestalt therapy, argues that a love of play is a fundamental aspect of the creative life and essential for change. In a similar vein, Rosenheim (1974) commented on the therapeutic potential of humor by saying that the unique value and potency of humor in psychotherapy derives mainly from its intrinsic attributes of intimacy, directness, and humaneness. Humor helps to draw the patient and therapist into a closer alliance than is often possible through a more formal, purely rational modality. Laughing with a patient "puts to the test and strengthens the accurate perception of both internal and interpersonal realities" (p. 591).

As indicated earlier in this chapter, Zinker (1977) viewed a sense of humor as an important characteristic of an effective clinician. Humor enables us to "turn the world upside down, to make the familiar strange" (p. 45). He indicates that humor has allowed him to view the action of the treatment session with a broader view or from a different angle than would have otherwise been possible. It also enabled him to laugh at his own self-importance. Humor can open a gate for taking a behavior or event and turning it just enough to see the humorous colors. Sometimes it can help loosen what is stuck.

The third and current stage of research on humor began during the 1970s and stressed the cognitive foundations of humor: what it is that causes a person to interpret a particular event as humorous. The change from a Freudian view of humor to a cognitive approach corresponded to the loss of interest in the psychoanalytic view of human behavior and a corresponding increase in Jean Piaget's cognitive-structural view of humor development and behavior.

The research on humor in general, and especially as applied to various forms of treatment for human physical and behavioral problems, increased dramatically during the mid-1970s. The increasing interest in the potential of therapeutic humor may have occurred, at least in part, because of an increased interest in the humanistic tradition and a renewed appreciation of the cognitive aspects of behavioral intervention in psychology, counseling, and related fields. The publishing of Norman Cousins's book, *Anatomy of an Illness*, in 1979 (describing his recovery from the life-threatening disease of ankylosing spondylitis) provided a major impetus for the appreciation of the therapeutic potential of humor by the general public as well as researchers in many areas of human development. Formal and informal networks of professionals interested in the potential of humor in human growth and adjustment were formed (Robinson, 1991). Subsequent years have seen the formation of many groups with associated newsletters and meetings, all with an interest in promoting the benefits of humor in various aspects of personal and professional life. Although it is evident that empirical support continues to be necessary, the benefits are often striking and the therapeutic potential is obvious.

Also in the 1970s, the field of psychotherapy saw an increased call for clinicians who were empathic, spontaneous, flexible, and creative (Kuhlman, 1984). It was reasoned that selecting such a person was the best way to increase the likelihood of creating an effective professional through the academic and clinical training processes. Most of us would choose as a colleague someone who possessed these characteristics—and most clients would be likely to choose such a clinician. As we will see, the characteristics proposed by Kuhlman are closely related to the ability to recognize and appreciate humor with yourself and with others. Morreall (1982) noted that a person with a sense of humor is more likely to interact well with others than a person lacking humor. Individuals with a sense of humor tend to be more imaginative and flexible and correspondingly less likely to become obsessed with a particular issue or approach to a problem. In addition, a person with a sense of humor is more likely to be open to suggestions from others and more approachable (Morreall, 1982). Subsequent research has resulted in support for these concepts and we will provide a few examples in an effort to encourage similar studies in the field of communication disorders.

Graham (1995) gave the Situational Humor Response Questionnaire (SHRQ) (Martin & Lefcourt, 1984) to 160 college students (80 males and 80 females). Participants were paired with unfamiliar partners according to gender (both same and opposite) and according to sense of humor scores. The participants were asked to interact with each other for 30 minutes. The college students with a high sense of humor on the SHRQ were rated on a second scale as significantly more *socially desirable* by conversational partners more than those with low sense of humor scores. Graham also found that those with a high sense of humor were more likely to reduce anxiety and uncertainty in their partners more than those with a low sense of humor. She also found no effects for gender of the conversational partners. In light of these results Graham argued that an individual's sense of humor is likely to facilitate the development of an interpersonal relationship.

In a series of studies, Hampes found significant correlations of humor with a variety of characteristics suggested by Kuhlman in 1984. Hampes (1992) also used the Situational Humor Response Questionnaire to examine the relationship between *intimacy* and humor with 32 male and 71 female undergraduates, ranging in age from 18 to 52 years. Hampes (1992) found that intimacy scores were higher for those with higher humor scores than those with lower humor scores ($F = 15.97$, $p < .001$). No significant differences were found between male and female participants.

Hampes (1994) employed a more comprehensive humor assessment scale, the Multidimensional Sense of Humor Scale (MSHS) (Thorson & Powell, 1993a) in a systematic replication of his 1992 investigation. In this case, 20 male and 40 female undergraduate students were given the MSHS. A significant difference was found between humor scores for those in the high intimacy and low intimacy groups ($t(58) = 2.28$, $p < .05$). Again, no significant difference was found between the scores of the male and female participants.

Hampes (1999) also used the MSHS to investigate the relationship between humor and *trust* with 89 college students ranging in age from 16 to 54 years. Hampes found significant positive correlations between measurements of humor and trust. In 2001, Hampes used the MSHS to examine the relationship between humor and *empathy*. In this case, the participants were 124 undergraduate volunteers (71 females, 53 males) ranging in age from 17 to 48 years. Hampes found significant positive correlations ($p < .05$) between the empathy and the MSHS scores. The author suggested that an individual's ability to show empathetic concern is enhanced by the individual's ability to use humor to reduce stress.

Humke and Schaefer (1996) used the MSHS in their investigation of the relationship between sense of humor and *creativity*. They administered the MSHS and the Franck Drawing Completion Test (Anastasi & Schaefer, 1971), a measure of the nonverbal aspect of creativity, to 51 female and 35 male mental health professionals. The authors found support of their experimental hypothesis in the form of a significant positive correlation ($r = 0.77$, $p = .01$) between humor and creativity. That is, individuals who scored high on the MSHS also tended to score high on the Franck Drawing Completion Test creativity scale. The authors speculated that humor and creativity are positively related because they both involve risk taking and the production of unexpected and unusual responses.

Acknowledging Humor During Therapeutic Change

To some clinicians, treatment is "serious business", an unlikely place to find humor. One can imagine some people reacting to the suggestion of acknowledging humor during the treatment of a handicapping problem by saying, "Be serious! Change is difficult, even painful, so how can you possibly imply that there is something humorous about such an overwhelming problem?" Not surprisingly, clients also may have this initial question about the appropriateness of humor during treatment. However, there are clinicians who argue that a humorous view of the circumstances presented to us by life could be considered an appropriate issue for the process of treatment (Schimel, 1978).

It is important to consider the way we think about humor in a therapeutic sense. The phrase "using humor" suggests that humor is a device that the

Clinical Insight

On many occasions we have asked the members of a group therapy session to see if they can recall instances when their stuttering has resulted in a humorous experience. The newer members of the group typically respond with some strange looks, and it's not unusual for a participant to question the veracity of such a request. The more experienced group members, however, are more than happy to tell what often have become their favorite stories, stories that are unique and truly humorous. These are individuals who have clearly achieved some distance from the original experience and have achieved a conceptual shift concerning their previously embarrassing circumstances. They have also achieved a good deal of mastery over their speech.

clinician brings to the treatment session in the same way that one might bring a questionnaire or treatment technique. To think in terms of using humor may give the impression that a clinician will arrive at the treatment session with a well-rehearsed series of jokes (Kuhlman, 1984) or perhaps wearing a red clown nose. Rather than thinking of using humor in this sense, Kuhlman (1984) proposed that humor is more appropriately viewed as an integral part of the interactional aspects of treatment. Rather than a device or tool, humor is best conceived as one aspect of the client–clinician relationship and to the sense of timing therein. He suggested that *spontaneity* is the essence of all effective humor, and certainly this can be true of the therapeutic alliance. Accordingly, until the clinician is calibrated to the client and until some level of intimacy has been established in the therapeutic relationship, humor is less likely to serve a beneficial purpose. This perspective is also taken by Simmons-Mackie and Schultz (2003) based on their analysis of both verbal and nonverbal therapeutic interactions with adults who have aphasia. These authors found that humor effectively enhanced the interpersonal interaction between clinician and client. Like Kuhlman (1984), these authors made the important distinction that spontaneous humor, rather than preplanned humor, is most effective in promoting and managing therapy interactions.

Humor and laughter frequently take place during successful treatment, including treatment for fluency disorders. There is, during effective treatment, the enthusiasm and excitement of exploration. The resulting change in insight often leads to an expression of humor, and conversely, humor can lead to insight. E. B. White (1954/1960) wrote that "humor at its best is a kind of heightened truth—a super truth." Therapeutic protocols seek to expand the client's awareness of and insight about the problem that brought him to treatment. Alport (1961) demonstrated the close relationship between insight and humor, finding a positive correlation of .88 between the two. He further noted that insight and humor were related to an individual's capacity for self-objectification and the ability to construe oneself as both subject and object (Kuhlman, 1984). That is, humor reflects a person's ability to step away and distance himself from his situation in order to gain a degree of insight. The distance provides for a degree of objectivity that allows us to see ourselves from a new angle or with a "God's eye" view. As a result of three basic characteristics (conceptual shift, distancing, and mastery) humor can be an effective facilitator of therapeutic change.

The Conceptual Shift

Two similar views of humor provide a good beginning for appreciating the possibilities for intervention with individuals who stutter. Morreall (1982) suggested that laughter is the natural expression of the feeling of amusement in response to a sudden conceptual shift. He suggested that the essence of humor is found in the enjoyment of incongruity. Associated with an appreciation of incongruity is a conceptual shift (not necessarily an emotional one) in the way we consider an event. For maximum effectiveness, the conceptual shift must be immediate and the change relatively large. When the shift is predictable or anticipated the degree of humor decreases accordingly.

Davis and Farina (1970) advance a similar explanation for a humorous event. They include as basic features of humor contradiction or incongruity, as well as the sudden integration of contradictory ideas or concepts. Furthermore, this new insight often results in an objective—in contrast to an emotional—experience of the concepts. As Davis and Farina (1970) explain, "We may say that on the cognitive side, laughter results from the sudden insightful integration of contradictory or incongruous ideas, attitudes, or sentiments which are experienced objectively" (p. 307).

Such conceptual shifts are not likely to take place early in the therapeutic relationship. The initial treatment sessions often are spent gathering information such as acquiring baseline performance, obtaining demographic data, developing procedural guidelines, and becoming calibrated to the client. During these initial stages, the clinician is becoming attuned to the client and his or her story. Once the therapeutic relationship matures and the client begins to understand that the clinician is capable of providing a secure and supportive environment, humor is more likely to become a feature of the dialogue. As the sessions continue, an interactional environment will begin to be established in which spontaneity and expressions of concepts beyond the preliminary aspects of the relationship begin to occur. As more intimacy is established in the relationship, the limits of appropriate humor can expand, as well as the number and severity of the taboos that may be violated in safety (Kuhlman, 1984). Accordingly, humor leads to a relaxed atmosphere that encourages communication, particularly on sensitive matters (McGhee & Goldstein, 1977). Although humor is but one dynamic in the process of promoting clients' conceptual shifts about themselves and their situation, it can play an important role in the process.

As humor facilitates insights about an old problem, the client may respond with pleasure or laughter. A kind of catharsis may take place, and for the first time, a new way of looking at the problem may result. Kuhlman (1984) suggests that the client's laughter, if spontaneous and genuine, can be taken as a sign of validation of a change in insight. On occasion, a client's initial reaction to a new view of the problem or the situation may be one of anger. He or she may not like the view that the new insight provides, especially if the old, habitual view is comforting. Consequently, the appropriateness of a humorous interpretation of an event must be judged within the context of the therapeutic relationship at a particular moment. To be appropriate as well as effective, the timing of the humorous response must be both accurate and spontaneous.

It has often been suggested that an integral part of a comprehensive behavioral treatment strategy involves the client's development of a new belief system—a paradigm shift—about him- or herself and the problem (e.g., Botterill & Cook, 1987; Cooper, 1993; Covey, 1989; Dilollo, Neimeyer & Manning, 2002; Fransella, 1972, Fransella & Dalton, 1990; Hayhow & Levy, 1989; Kuhlman, 1984; Peck, 1978; Plexico, Manning & Dilollo, 2005; Van Riper, 1973). Changing perspective may be difficult, and the client may tend to ward off the clinician's alternative views of the problem. As Kuhlman (1984) suggested, although people seek treatment in order to feel better, they are often less than enthusiastic about the behavioral and cognitive changes necessary to achieve the goals of treatment. It is common for the client to cling to established perspectives and belief patterns because they are familiar, comfortable, and self-protective. The client is often too close to the situation, especially a threatening or emotionally laden one, to see it any other way. He or she may have viewed the situation for so long from a particular perspective that no other view seems possible. As Kuhlman (1984) stated, before clients are able to adopt a new belief system, they must acknowledge and dismiss the old one as being in error in some way. Although humor does not have to be a part of the process, it can be an effective and pleasurable way to facilitate and share the changes that are occurring.

Distancing with Humor

In order to facilitate the development of a new cognitive perspective and begin to form a new belief system about both oneself and the problem, it is often helpful to step away from the situation somewhat (Kuhlman, 1984). It is not necessary to step back a great distance, only far enough to see its paradoxical aspects. Until the person is able to move back somewhat, especially from a threatening experience or a problem that creates anxiety, the paradoxical aspects of the situation will not be readily apparent. However, as the client, with the clinician's assistance, is able to achieve greater distance, it will be possible to gradually gain objectivity by viewing the problem with the "third eye" of humor. Rather than endlessly reliving earlier experiences with the old view, new interpretations will become possible. Humor promotes the possibility that the client will begin to play with the possibilities and have fun considering a variety of new interpretations of the experience.

Morreall (1982) also discussed the role of distancing in humor. He suggested that humor has a liberating effect. Often something is funny because it violates what is supposed to be sacrosanct; it goes against the rational or accepted order of things. Morreall made the observation that humor enables us to achieve some distance and perspective. This occurs not only in situations where we are failing, but also in situations where we are succeeding, for humor can prevent us from overrating our achievements. The more developed a person's sense of humor,

Clinical **Insight**

One afternoon during our group therapy session, Marcy was reporting to the others that she had finally, after many failures, willed herself to order something at a drive-through restaurant. Since we were at the early stages of treatment, the goal of this activity was simply to do the task regardless of any stuttering that might occur. In vivid detail, Marcy described her fear as she approached the enclosed microphone-speaker and her attempt to place her order. The typical semi-intelligible voice asked for her order, and she promptly responded by saying, "I would like an order of fries, a coke, and a ham- ham- hambur- hambur- hamburger." The group responded with applause at her courage for taking such a risk and carrying out an action that she had rigorously avoided for many years. She thanked us all but added that the only real problem she had was when she pulled around to receive her lunch. The cashier handed her an order of fries, a coke, and five hamburgers. The laughter of Marcy along with the other members of the group suggested that she had achieved some distance from an event that had always been thought of as an absolutely dreadful experience.

the wider the range of situations in which the clinician can achieve the distance required to promote laughter. For the clinician, and certainly for the client, it is important to appreciate that to the extent that we can achieve this distance from the practical aspects of a situation, we will be free from being dominated by it. Moreover, to the degree that a person can appreciate the humor in his or her own personal situation, that person will be liberated from the dominance of emotions and more likely to develop a more objective view.

Mastery and Humor

Lefcourt and Martin (1989) found that the expression of humor is also related to a feeling of mastery of a task or situation. Their interpretation of this relationship relates to the view of humor as a reducer of stress. As Kuhlman (1984) pointed out, the relationship between mastery and humor is readily observed in children as they face problem-solving situations. Laughter is often a by-product of children's shifts from one cognitive stage to another as they master a new problem. Problem solving, especially when the experience is a new one, is exhilarating (Levine, 1977). The client's subsequent behavior change suggests that some reorganization of internal reality (insight) has been achieved, which allowed the problem to be solved.

This perspective of humor and mastery also coincides with the view of humor suggested by Freud (1928). That is, the humor process includes a cognitive reorientation in the face of stress (Martin & Lefcourt, 1983; Nezu, Nezu, & Blissett, 1988). The ability to appreciate as well as use humor has been shown to be related to a person's internal locus of control, which provides an indication of how much the individual perceives events as a consequence of his or her own behavior (Craig, Franklin, & Andrews, 1984). Subjects who hold an internal locus of control were found to smile and laugh more in the face of stress (Lefcourt, Sordoni, & Sordoni, 1974). Martin and Lefcourt (1984) found that people with better internal locus of control scores demonstrate greater ability to take multiple perspectives when problem solving as well as to resist the effects of persuasion. People whose locus of control is more internally based are more able to consider alternative constructions for their experiences. Though having multiple perspectives regarding an issue does not necessarily lead to humor, the experience of humor is believed to require a person's ability to view a situation or event from multiple perspectives (Lefcourt & Martin, 1989).

Lefcourt and Martin (1989) suggested that in order to have a greater ability to entertain alternative interpretations for experiences, one must perceive oneself as an actor, a determiner of one's fate, and an active maker of choices. Only by making choices among available options can one be free. In the absence of choice, one is more likely to feel controlled and constrained. Thus, in the exercise of choice and the ability to consider alternative interpretations, there is a connection between a sense of mastery and the potential for humor (Lefcourt & Martin, 1989).

Everyone has experienced relief following the successful completion of a particularly daunting activity. Sometimes with adults (and even more so with children) accomplishment and the associated relief is often accompanied by laughter. Laughter is also frequently present in the retelling of the experience. As people who stutter achieve the ability to vary and change their behavior they are likely to report humorous reactions and experiences that would not have been regarded as humorous only a short time earlier. This relief is also the case for nonstuttering clinicians who are asked to take the role of a person who is stuttering in order to understand the fear and avoidance that is part of the experience.

Conclusion

In this chapter we have addressed a critical component of the treatment process for people who stutter: the clinician. We have considered the impact of the clinician's attitudes and skills on the treatment process and described the characteristics of the experienced and effective clinician. Although it is apparent that the current state of academic and clinical preparation for clinicians is less than acceptable, it is possible for dedicated professionals to develop high levels of expertise in assisting those who stutter. We found that experts in many areas tend to be guided by principles rather than sharp-edged rules. Experts are less likely to follow a preplanned strategy or a manually driven approach. Rather, they were more likely to follow the lead of the individual they want to assist. They are flexible and opportunistic in considering alternative responses, and they are sensitive to that person's affective and cognitive response. Table 1-1 provides a summary of several continuums that help to distinguish the technician from the professional.

Corresponding to these clinician characteristics, we also introduced the variable of humor, as both a clinician characteristic as well as an indication of cognitive change as people achieve mastery, distance, and a conceptual shift concerning their situation. The clinician's ability to recognize and respond to humor may be an overarching indicator of a clinician's ability to lead the way in viewing the client's current circumstances from different angles. The results of many investigations provide convincing evidence of the relationship of humor to many personality characteristics (e.g., creativity, risk taking, intimacy, empathy) that positively influence the therapeutic alliance and the ability of the clinician to impact a successful therapeutic outcome.

It is good to have a guide when beginning a new adventure. The experienced guide is able to provide help that is both timely and insightful. It takes energy and optimism on the part of the clinician, as that guide, for the work is sometimes demanding. Each client provides a challenge that may test us repeatedly, and it is necessary and appropriate that we ask ourselves if we are up to the task. Burnout is a frequent problem in the helping professions. However, if we view our journey with each client as an adventure and as an opportunity for a continual process of learning and growth, we renew ourselves with continuing opportunities for personal enrichment. Much of our growth comes from the people we are trying so hard to assist. The best clinicians recognize that clients have much to teach us and that we often benefit nearly as much from the treatment process as they do. Although we have traveled along paths of therapeutic change before, the territory and timing of the steps will be new for our companion, to whom we must attend closely with both determination and esteem.

Table 1-1 Continuums that distinguish clinical decision making by a less experienced technician and by a more experienced, professional clinician.

Technician	Professional
Narrow focus on problem	Open focus on person
Guided by rules	Guided by principles
Preplanned procedures	Flexible procedures
Dogmatic treatment	Treatment alternatives
Technique directed	Client directed
Intolerant of ambiguity	Tolerant of ambiguity

Topics for Discussion

1. What are the justifications for beginning this book with a chapter about the clinician?

2. What are some of the reasons why far too many clinicians are resistant to providing treatment for people who stutter?

3. Aside from a graduate course, where can one obtain information and insight about the nature and treatment of stuttering?

4. Which of the personality characteristics of clinicians described in this chapter do you feel that you possess? Which characteristics would you like to enhance and why?

5. Which of the clinician intervention skills described do you feel are the most challenging?

6. Given each of the talents and skills you have achieved, where would you place yourself on the novice–expert continuum described in this chapter?

7. Using a variety of everyday or clinical circumstances, consider whether rules or principles may provide better problem-solving strategies.

8. Describe the difference between "using" humor and being open to spontaneously responding to humorous interpretations of events.

9. What, in your opinion, are the most convincing arguments that the ability to construct a humorous interpretation of an event is an indication of cognitive change?

10. Provide at least two examples of past experiences or situations that were embarrassing or frightening at the time but have since become humorous. Explain this change in perspective in terms of distance, mastery, and paradigm shift.

Recommended Readings

Cousins, N. (1979). *Anatomy of an illness.* New York: Norton.

Mahoney, M. J. (2000). Training future psychotherapists. In C. R. Snyder & R. E. Ingham (Eds.), *Handbook of Psychological Change,* (pp. 272–735). New York: John Wiley & Sons, Inc.

Manning, W. (2004). "How can you understand? You don't stutter!" *Contemporary issues in Communication Science and Disorders, 31,* 58–68.

Van Riper, C. (1979). *A career in speech pathology.* Englewood Cliffs, NJ: Prentice Hall Inc. (see chapters titled, "The Clinician's Skill," pp. 103–114; "The Rewards of Therapy," pp. 115–138.)

CHAPTER 2

The Nature of Fluent and Nonfluent Speech: The Onset of Stuttering

When I asked my mother what she thought caused me to stutter, she told me about my Aunt Helen and about everything the psychologists and therapists she and my father consulted had told them, and then added, "You know, when you were very little, still a toddler, and were living on 178th Street in the Bronx, you were playing on the floor in the living room, and this mouse ran right past you. I had the superintendent come and plug up the hole, and it never happened again, but I always wondered." (p. 32)

Marty Jezer (1997).
Stuttering: A Life Bound Up in Words.
New York, NY: Basic Books.

Chapter Objectives

In this chapter we will describe ways of considering the many characteristics of fluent and nonfluent speech in adults and children. A brief historical perspective of the terms used to describe both fluent and stuttered speech will be provided and a variety of attempts to define stuttering will be described. With this information in mind, we will then consider recent information concerning the onset of developmental stuttering and the essential characteristics that distinguish stuttering from typically fluent speech. The speaker's sense of an anxiety-producing loss of control and helplessness is described as a core feature of the stuttering experience, which compels many of the coping responses in the form of avoidance and escape behaviors. Beyond the more overt, behavioral features on the surface we will also begin to see that stuttering has many layers and is manifested in a variety of ways according to the individual's response to his or her difficulties in producing naturally spontaneous and fluent speech. Finally, we will describe conditions that appear to be more (or less) influential in contributing to the onset of stuttering.

The Characteristics of Normal Fluency

Just about everyone has some basic understanding of what stuttering looks and sounds like. Even if you haven't been acquainted with a family member, classmate, or friend who has stuttered you have observed the ways that stuttering has been portrayed in the movies or on television (a good topic for a group therapy discussion). But, of course, most people never consider the nature of fluent speech, for they speak habitually and effortlessly, taking their fluency for granted.

Although our understanding is increasing, we know relatively little about the fluency characteristics of normally fluent children and their responses to fluency-disrupting stimuli. We know even less about changes in fluency throughout the life cycle, particularly for older speakers who stutter (Katz, Lincoln, & McCabe, 2008; Manning, Dailey, & Wallace, 1984; Manning & Shirkey, 1981). Furthermore, comparatively few data have been accumulated about fluency characteristics as a function of variables such as gender, race, culture, and socioeconomic level. Given the rapidly changing demographics of the United States, there are many important questions that could be asked concerning these variables in order to provide the best assistance to those who stutter (Cole, 1986, 1989; Cooper & Cooper, 1991b; Satcher, 1986; Waldrop & Exter, 1990).

In order to fully appreciate the characteristics of speech that is interpreted by the speaker or the listener as less than fluent, it is necessary to appreciate the dimensions of fluent speech. Even the most accomplished speaker performing under ideal conditions can experience disruptions in the flow of their sounds and words. Language and speech production is a complex task and it takes many years of experience to do it well, especially under conditions of communicative or emotional stress. As authors have pointed out, it is probably fortunate that humans have the opportunity to practice speech as much or more than nearly any other activity (Van Riper, 1982; Starkweather, 1987).

Starkweather (1987) provides a comprehensive assessment of the research on the dimensions of fluent speech in both children and adults. The term fluency, derived from the Latin for "flowing," describes what the listener perceives when listening to someone who is truly adept at producing speech. The speech flows easily and smoothly in terms of both sound and information. There are no disruptions in the sequence of sounds and words and the listener can attend to the message rather than considering how the message is being produced. As pointed out in Chapter 1, the seemingly effortless nature of an accomplished performance can be observed in athletic feats that require complicated sequential movements, such as gymnastics, ice skating, swimming, and martial arts. The impression when observing such athletic displays is one of smoothness and ease. The individual segments of the performance are blended together, with no obvious transition from one movement to the next. There is a consistency to the behavior, and little or no tension is evident. It often appears as though the performer is relaxed and unencumbered by the force of gravity and that relatively little effort being expended. These examples have much in common with the production of flowing speech; the notion of fluent speech as a continual and effortless flow of both movement and information. This is an important concept that will be emphasized in later chapters when assessment and indicators of successful intervention are discussed.

Fluency in Adult Speakers

Starkweather (1987) suggests that fluency can be thought of having both language and speech components. Citing the work of Filmore (1979), Starkweather (1987) suggests the four components of *linguistic fluency*: syntactic, semantic, phonologic, and pragmatic fluency. Speakers who are syntactically fluent are able to construct highly complex sentences using a variety of complex forms. Speakers who are semantically fluent possess and are readily able to access large vocabularies. Speakers who are phonologically fluent are able to pronounce long and complicated sequences of sounds and syllables, including nonsense and foreign words. Those with pragmatic fluency are adept at making timely and appropriate verbal responses in a variety of social and cultural contexts.

Starkweather (1987) defines *speech fluency* in terms of continuity, rate, duration, coarticulation, and effort. Continuity relates to the degree to which syllables and words are logically sequenced, as well as the presence or absence of pauses. If the semantic units follow one another in a continual and logical flow of information, the speech is interpreted as fluent. However, despite a continual flow of sound and the absence of pauses, the speech is not thought of as fluent if unnecessary or illogical sounds or words are present, as in the following paragraph offered by Starkweather:

> What I mean, what I mean is, that, uh, when you, you, go to the, uh, store because, uh, you, you want some, need some, uh, food or supplies or something, and, and, uh, the storekee—the man, clerk, who, who waits, well not waits, but serves, you know, gets some—something for you is, well, if he, if he, well if he is sort of, well, stern, or you know angry or something, then, well, then, I find it, well, I find it difficult to talk. (p. 19)

Another aspect of continuity has to do with a disruption in the flow of sound in the form of pauses. Clark (1971) differentiates pauses as conventional and idiosyncratic. Conventional pauses are used by speakers to signal a linguistically important event. Idiosyncratic pauses, on the other hand, reflect hesitation or uncertainty on the part of the speaker. These pauses indicate a decision-making process concerning upcoming word choice, style, or syntax.

Pauses also have been considered as unfilled or filled. Unfilled pauses are characterized by a silence lasting longer than approximately 250 milliseconds (ms) (Goldman-Eisler, 1958). This duration is suggested as a convenient threshold for normal silent intervals during fluent speech, since normal word junctures rarely exceed this duration (e.g., the juncture necessary to distinguish "night rate" from "nitrate"). Filled pauses are characterized by essentially meaningless sounds such as "ah," "er," "uh," and "um." With filled pauses, the flow of sound continues, but, again, the flow of information does not.

Rate of speech also signals the perception of fluency. Most people talk about as fast as they can, as indicated by Tiffany (1980), who noted that the maximum and ordinary rates of speech tend to be similar. Young adult speakers of English average approximately five syllables per second (Pickett, 1980; Stetson, 1951; Walker & Black, 1950). The rate of speech varies considerably according to such factors as formality of the speaking situation, time pressure, and interference from background noise or competing messages. There appears to be a reasonably wide range of acceptable rates in the judgment of fluency. It is well known that if communication failure is likely, such as when speaking in a noisy environment, speakers are likely to slow down (Longhurst & Siegel, 1973). Likewise, if a speaker is producing a lengthy utterance, the rate of speech is likely to be more rapid (Malecot, Johnston, & Kizziar, 1972). It is not surprising, then, that listeners provide speakers with a great deal of latitude in their judgments of nonfluency based on rate alone. That is, simply because the speaker is producing speech at a slow rate, everything else being equal, the speaker is not likely to be evaluated as being nonfluent. Conversely, simply because a speaker is producing speech at a rapid rate, he or she is not likely to be evaluated as being especially fluent. Although the rate of speech production is obviously one aspect of fluency, it does not appear to be a primary dimension. The flow of speech and information is based not only on rate, but on a combination of many factors, particularly the ease of production.

The final dimension of fluency—and perhaps the most important, particularly as it relates to stuttering—is effort. Starkweather (1987) distinguishes two types of effort: effort associated with linguistic planning and that associated with muscle movement. Clinically, it may be that the listener's perception of effort is the most sensitive indicator of fluent speech. As Starkweather suggests, "Fluent speech is effortless in two distinct ways: It requires little thought, and it requires little muscular exertion" (p. 37). Fluent speech is characterized by little attention being paid to the process of production; speaking is "automatic." The focus is on what is being said—the message being communicated from one person to another. To the degree that the focus of the speaker is on how speech is being produced, there is the corresponding chance that attention will be taken away from the message. Starkweather (1987) also suggests that the perception of effort is closely related to the force of contact between opposing articulators. Fluent speech is characterized by little sensation of opposition of the articulators or constriction of airflow. The air, the movements, and the sounds are produced with evident ease and smoothness. On the other hand, people who stutter are typically at the opposite end of this continuum of effort. Greater effort is associated with all the following: greater contact between articulators; greater impedance between the flow of air and the structures of the vocal tract, beginning with the vocal folds; and greater subglottic air pressure. With the speaker producing speech in this fashion, it is likely that speech will be judged by both the speaker and the listener as nonfluent, and the focus will be on how the speech is being produced.

Ingham and Cordes (1997) viewed effort in much the same manner as Starkweather by describing both the cognitive effort necessary for concentrating on the message and the muscular effort or exertion necessary for producing speech. Although recognizing that the perception of listeners plays a role in determining the extent of fluency, they also stressed the key role of the speaker in determining the quality of fluency. A series of quantitative and qualitative investigations provide support for these views, indicating that normally fluent speech:

- Sounds natural to listeners (Finn, 1997).
- Contains normal disfluencies (interjections, revisions, whole-word repetitions) (Finn, 1997).
- Is associated by listeners with faster speech rates within the normal range (Finn, 1977).
- Is perceived by speakers to be associated with less cognitive effort (Finn & Ingham, 1994).
- Is associated by speakers with faster rather than slower (and less natural) speech (Finn, 1997).
- Is associated with little cognitive effort by speakers (Finn & Ingham, 1994).
- Is associated by speakers with feeling good (or neutral) about speaking (Finn, Howard, & Kubala, 2005).
- Is associated with speakers who are focused on communicating a message rather than paying attention to the process of speaking (Finn, Howard, & Kubala, 2005).

Defining Stuttering and Related Terms

Prior to offering generally accepted definitions of stuttering, we will introduce some of the related terms and concepts (see Table 2-1). For example, the term *stammering* can be found in some early literature in this country, where it tended to be used interchangeably with stuttering. While currently the term *stuttering* is used in the United States, stammering is often used in Europe to mean the same thing. The major self-help group in Great Britain, for example, is called the British Stammering Association.

The term *disfluent* is often used in the literature to indicate the fluency breaks of normal speakers, while the term *dysfluent* is used to describe the abnormal fluency breaks of people who stutter. According to a variety of medical dictionaries, the prefix *dis* means reversal, separation, or duplication. The prefix *dys*, on the other hand, means difficult, impaired, painful, bad, or disordered. Because of the potential confusion of the words and because of a degree of overlap in the fluency breaks found in stuttered and normally fluent speech, the majority of authors use the term disfluent.

In order to provide a context for the findings by Yairi and his colleagues at the University of Illinois Stuttering Research Program presented later in this chapter, we will briefly describe two terms that, while frequently used in the past, are much less common now. Originally suggested by Bluemel (1932), *primary stuttering* was thought of as a transient phenomenon characterized by a child's easy repetitions of syllables and words. The child is typically unaware of these events and displays no special effort or tension during speaking. These initial motoric behaviors taking place in the speech production mechanism have been referred to as core (Van Riper, 1982), alpha (Conture, Rothenberg, & Molitor, 1986), or pure (Bluemel (1932) fluency disruptions. It was not until the speaker became aware of and responded to these core behaviors that "real" or "secondary stuttering" began. For many years it was generally agreed that secondary behaviors were learned responses resulting from the child's attempt to cope with the initial breaks in speech flow. A key assumption of this view

Table 2-1   Equivalent terms commonly used for describing stuttering and associated behavior.

Stuttering	Stammering	
Fluency	Normal speech	
Disfluency	Dysfluency	
Primary behaviors	Core behaviors	Alpha behaviors
Secondary behaviors	Accessory behaviors	Coping behaviors

was that the initial "pure" or primary stuttering was essentially normal and the secondary stuttering that followed was distinctly abnormal, or "real" stuttering. As we will see in the following chapter, this was a widely held view and a major factor in guiding diagnostic and intervention decisions for many years.

Definitions of Stuttering

The variety of definitions of stuttering that have been offered over the years indicates the many ways of viewing this problem. Sometimes the definitions reflect the author's view of etiology rather than actually defining the problem. Johnson's 1946 definition, for example, reflected his view of etiology when he argued that stuttering was what the person who stutters does to avoid stuttering (Johnson, 1946). As we will illustrate in Chapter 8, although there is much to be said for taking this view of how older children, adolescents, and adults who stutter cope with their situation, it does not provide an accurate understanding of stuttering onset for the youngest speakers.

During the 1940s and 1950s Johnson and his associates came to define stuttering as an anticipatory, apprehensive, hypertonic avoidance reaction. This view held that stuttering was a learned response to environmental events and was something that the person (a) does, rather than something that happens to him or her; (b) expects to or anticipates will occur; (c) is fearful or apprehensive about doing; (d) is tense (hypertonic) about; and (e) tries to keep from happening again (avoidance). This was a somewhat restrictive definition, as stuttering can occur in the absence of some or even many of these attributes.

Another definition of stuttering was provided by the World Health Organization (WHO) in 1977. This definition points out, in contrast to the perception of many nonprofessionals, that the person who is stuttering knows what he or she wants to say. Although we all experience word finding problems on occasion, telling a person who stutters to "stop and think what it is you want to say" indicates a lack of understanding about the nature of the problem. The person who stutters generally knows exactly what he or she wants to say but is unable, however, to move through a sound or make the transition from one sound to another. The WHO states that stuttering includes "disorders in the rhythm of speech in which the individual knows precisely what he wishes to say, but at the time is unable to say it because of an involuntary, repetitive prolongation or cessation of a sound" (p. 202). There are aspects of this definition that will reoccur throughout this text. For example, the word "disorders" implies that the symptoms of stuttering can take many forms and have more than one etiology (hence the title of this text). Furthermore, many of the behaviors seen in stuttering are involuntary.

Views of stuttering as classical or operant conditioned behavior are reflected in Brutten & Shoemaker's 1967 definition that "stuttering is that form of fluency failure that results from conditioned negative emotion" (p. 61). Conversely, for those who view stuttering as a type of primary neurosis, a symptom of a basic emotional or psychological conflict, there is the tendency to define stuttering by citing the presumed source of the conflict (cause) rather than by describing the stuttering behavior (symptom). Coriat (1943), for example, described stuttering as a psychoneurosis characterized by the persistence of early, pregenital oral nursing, oral sadistic, and anal sadistic elements. Taking a similar approach, Glauber (1958) described stuttering as "a symptom in a psychopathological condition classified as a pregenital conversion neurosis" (p. 78). Perhaps the most memorable explanation of this type was offered by Fenichel in 1945, who stated, "Stuttering is a pregenital conversion neurosis in that the early problems of dealing with retention and expulsion of feces have been displaced upwards into the sphincters of the mouth" (as cited in Van Riper, 1982, p. 264).

One of the most frequently cited operational definitions is that of Wingate (1964). For many years this definition has been used to describe subjects in clinical studies, since it provides a comprehensive list of both behaviors and attitudes that the clinician can expect to see across a variety of clients.

> The term "stuttering" means: 1. (a) Disruption in the fluency of verbal expression, which is (b) characterized by involuntary, audible, or silent repetitions or prolongations in the utterance of short speech elements, namely: sounds, syllables, and words of one syllable. These disruptions (c) usually occur frequently or are marked in character and (d) are not readily controllable. 2. Sometimes the disruptions are (e) accompanied by accessory activities involving the speech apparatus, related or unrelated body structures, or stereotyped speech utterances. These activities give the appearance of being speech-related struggle. 3. Also, there not infrequently are (f) indications or reports of the presence of an emotional state, ranging from a general condition of "excitement" or "tension" to more specific emotions of a negative nature such as fear, embarrassment, irritation, or the like. The immediate source of stuttering is some incoordination expressed in the peripheral speech mechanism; the ultimate cause is presently unknown and may be complex or compound. (p. 488)

In 1980, the handicapping nature of an impairment was addressed within the classification scheme proposed by the World Health Organization (WHO, 1980). The International Classification of Impairments, Disabilities, and Handicaps (ICIDH), developed by the WHO, described separate but related levels of a disease or disorder: impairment, disability, and handicap. More recently, the WHO provided a revised framework for describing the consequences of disorders, which resulted in the *International Classification of Functioning, Disability, and Health* (ICF; WHO, 2001). Yaruss and Quesal (2004) interpret this revision and its implications for the experience of stuttering. The new ICF

Clinical **Insight**

What does the most recent ICF revision mean to clinicians? It means that clinicians and researchers have a much broader interpretation of the stuttering experience. It means a greater appreciation for the fact that individuals who stutter are likely to respond in unique ways according to the internal and external factors that influence their experience. It means that a basic goal of assessment is to understand and monitor the wide variety of external and internal factors that uniquely impact the disability and handicap of each individual. It means that the goals of treatment involve helping people to not only change the obvious, relatively overt behaviors of stuttering but to also improve the quality of their lives, with increased involvement at all levels of interaction relative to their environments. It means that, as clinicians, if we are not already doing so, we pay attention to the many cognitive and affective features of the stuttering experience and that we include this information in our interpretation of treatment efficacy.

framework acknowledges that all disabilities involve more than the observable behaviors. An important difference in this revision to the 1980 edition is that no distinction is made between the concept of the "disability" (the difficulty performing tasks) and the "handicap" (disadvantages experienced in the ability to achieve life goals). Furthermore, the revision construes both environmental and personal factors as central to the disorder. That is, beyond the observable features of the problem of stuttering (e.g., repetitions, prolongations, blocking of airflow and voicing); environmental influences (e.g., support from others, attitudes of society, communication services, support organizations, educational services); and the individual's response to his or her ability to participate across many aspects of life (e.g., social, education, work, employment, civic involvement) are included.

Distinguishing Stuttering from Normal Fluency Breaks

The fact that all speakers experience disruptions in their fluency brings up the question of whether it is possible to distinguish between the breaks of normally fluent speakers and those who stutter. Whether or not the fluency breaks of stuttered and nonstuttered speech are categorically different or can be thought of as being on the same continuum has long been a historical point of contention in the field. Even the semantics of what to call the fluency breaks of normal and stuttering speakers has created difficulty. At the center of the controversy is whether the fluency breaks of nonstuttering speakers are qualitatively different than those of stuttering speakers. It is also important to understand that most of the research has been conducted with older speakers with, until recently at least, little information about the features of stuttering in children at the point of, or shortly following, onset. We will first provide an overview of what have been considered to be the distinguishing characteristics of both fluent and stuttered speech in adolescent and adult speakers. We will then consider the nature of these characteristics in young, preschool-age children, who provide an understanding of the situation near to the onset of stuttering.

Distinguishing adults who stutter from those who do not is not as easy as it might appear. Some people who stutter do not do so in any easily observable way; at least, they do not do so by producing the repetitions, prolongations, or blocking behavior of traditional stuttering. They may speak very carefully, avoiding sounds, words, people, or, in some instances, cease speaking altogether, choosing to be electively mute (as described by James Earl Jones in his 1993 book *Voices and Silences*) or pretending to be deaf. As we will see in succeeding chapters, if the focus of our decision making during assessment and intervention is on the person who is doing the stuttering, it is clear that we must go beneath the surface and consider not only the more obvious behavior characteristics of the person's speech but also the affective and cognitive features of how the person is coping with their problem.

Some authors have suggested that it is best to consider the fluency breaks of all speakers as falling along the same continuum (Bloodstein, 1992; Starkweather, 1992). After all, it has been suggested that people who stutter are making use of essentially the same speech-production system as normal speakers. Even given some difficulties at one or more levels of the system, one might expect that there would be considerable overlap in the nature of the speech produced by stutters and nonstutterers alike. Others have suggested that the fluency breaks of those who stutter and those who are normally fluent are categorically different (Hamre, 1992; Yairi, 2004; Yairi & Ambrose, 2005). Although there is considerable overlap in the surface features of adult stuttered and nonstuttered speech (e.g., the frequency and type of breaks), the core feature of helplessness and lack of control discussed earlier is generally absent from the experience of fluency disruptions of normally fluent speakers. As we shall see in a moment, the differences between stuttered and nonstuttered speech appear to be even more distinguishable in young children.

Van Riper (1982) suggests criteria for differentiating normal from abnormal fluency breaks (see Table 2-2). These often-cited guidelines distinguish stuttering and normal disfluency on the basis of speech characteristics and reaction of the speaker to forms of stress and awareness of the problem. It is apparent that more than the overt speech attributes must be considered when differentiating between a typically fluent speaker and someone who is stuttering.

Table 2-2   Guidelines for Differentiating Normal from Abnormal Disfluency.

Normal Behavior	Stuttering	Disfluency
Syllable Repetitions:		
a. Frequency per word	More than two	Less than two
b. Frequency for 100 words	More than two	Less than two
c. Tempo	Faster than normal	Normal Tempo
d. Regularity	Irregular	Regular
e. Schwa vowel	Often present	Absent or rare
f. Airflow	Often interrupted	Rarely interrupted
g. Vocal tension	Often apparent	Absent
Prolongations:		
h. Duration	Longer than one second	Less than one second
i. Frequency	More than 1 per 100 words	Less than 1 per 100 words
j. Regularity	Uneven or interrupted	Smooth
k. Tension	Important when present	Absent
l. When voiced	May show rise in pitch	No pitch rise
m. When unvoiced	Interrupted airflow	Airflow present
n. Termination	Sudden	Gradual
Gaps (silent pauses):		
o. Within the word boundary	May be present	Absent
p. Prior to speech attempt	Unusually long	Not marked
q. After the disfluency	May be present	Absent
Phonation:		
r. Inflections	Restricted; monotone	Normal
s. Phonatory arrest	May be present	Absent
t. Vocal fry	May be present	Usually absent
Articulatory Postures:		
u. Appropriateness	May be inappropriate	Appropriate
Reaction to Stress:		
v. Type	More broken words	Normal disfluencies
Evidence of awareness:		
w. Phonemic consistency	May be present	Absent
x. Frustration	May be present	Absent
y. Postponements	May be present	Absent
z. Eye contact	May waver	Normal

From a historical perspective and for our subsequent comments about assessment, it is important to understand that many of the categories used by Van Riper were influenced by the work of others who developed one of the first systems for categorizing fluency breaks, and one that was used for many years (Johnson, 1961; Johnson & Associates, 1959; Williams, Silverman, & Kools, 1968). This scheme placed some of the surface behaviors of stuttering into the seven categories of part-word repetition[1], single and multisyllabic word repetition, phrase repetition, interjections, revision-incomplete phrase, disrhythmic phonation (sound prolongations within words, unusual stress or broken words), and tense pause (barely audible heavy breathing and other tense sounds between words).

Yaruss (1997a) provides a summary of terms that have more recently been used to categorize the fluency breaks of individuals who do stutter and those who do not (Table 2-3). The fluency breaks of speakers who stutter tend to be characterized by *within*-word motoric breakdowns in producing syllable and word-size units. The breaks of normally fluent speakers tend to reflect difficulty in formulating the content of the message. These breaks tend to occur *between* larger word and phrase units of language production. The other basic characteristic is the extent of both the duration and tension of the break, with both being noticeably greater during stuttered speech. Throughout this text we will adopt terminology used by Yairi and his colleagues of *stuttering-like disfluencies* (SLD) and *other disfluencies* (OD).

As the above attempts to differentiate the nature of stuttered and normally disfluent speech indicate, there appears to be some influence of motoric and formulative factors in the inability of humans to generate completely fluent speech. Van Riper (1982) and Perkins (1983) suggest, for example, that a fluency break is more likely to be considered normal or nonstuttered if it is the result of "linguistic uncertainty." That is, the speaker is hesitating because he has not yet formulated how to express himself. Stuttering is more likely to be occurring when formulation is not the major issue and if there is a physical constriction or closure of the vocal tract. Drawing from comments of these authors as well as the writings of Starkweather (1987); Bloodstein (1974); Yairi and Clifton (1972); and Gordon, Hutchinson, and Allen (1976), Manning and Shirkey (1981) suggest the use of two categories for describing the continuum of fluency breaks among speakers. Formulative fluency breaks are characterized by (a) breaks (usually in the form of repetitions) between whole words, phrases,

---

[1]For the large majority of fluent as well as nonfluent speakers, part-word repetition occurs at the outset of the word. Repetitions that occur in medial- or final-word positions are not characteristic of developmental stuttering. They have been reported for individuals with disorders of executive function such as traumatic brain injury (LeBrun & Leleux, 1985), developmental delay (Stansfield, 1995), and Asperger's syndrome (Scott & Sisskin, 2007).

Table 2-3 Ways of categorizing disfluencies. Fluency breaks characteristic of individuals who do stutter are listed in the first column. Fluency breaks characteristic of individuals who do not stutter are listed in the second column.

Within-Word Disfluencies	Between-Word Disfluencies
Monosyllabic whole-word repetition	Phrase repetition
Sound/syllable repetition	Polysyllabic whole-word repetition
Audible prolongation	Interjection
Inaudible prolongation	Revision

Stuttering-Like Disfluencies (SLD)	Other Disfluencies
Part-word repetition	Interjection
Monosyllabic word repetition	Phrase repetition
Disrhythmic phonation	Revision/Incomplete phrase

Stutter-Type Disfluencies	Normal-Type Disfluencies
Part-word repetition	Whole-word repetition
Prolongation	Phrase repetition
Broken word	Revision
Tense pause	Incomplete phrase
	Interjection

Less Typical Disfluencies	More Typical Disfluencies
Monosyllabic word repetition (three or more repetitions)	Hesitation
Part-word syllable repetition (three or more repetitions)	Interjection
	Revision
Sound repetition	Phrase repetition
Prolongation	Monosyllabic word repetition (two or fewer repetitions: no tension)
Block	Part-word syllable repetition (two or fewer repetitions: no tension)

From Yaruss, 1997a (page 19); ASHA.

and larger syntactic units and (b) interjections between whole-word or larger syntactic units. The fluency breaks are characterized by little or no effort or tension. These breaks are typical of normally fluent speakers and are found, somewhat less often, in the speech of adults who stutter. Formulative fluency breaks are the result of linguistic planning or uncertainty and may provide the speaker time to organize the remainder of the sentence. Motoric fluency breaks are characterized by (a) breaks between sounds or syllables (part-word breaks), (b) obvious effort or tension (often focused in but not limited to the vocal tract), (c) pauses with a possible cessation of airflow and voicing, and (d) an excessive prolongation of sounds or syllables. These breaks are more typical of speakers who stutter but may occur in normally fluent speakers during conditions of communicative or emotional stress.

The fluency breaks of young adults who stutter are made up almost entirely of motoric fluency breaks. In fact, there appears to be a notable absence of formulative (or normal) fluency breaks, a characteristic that may be used to distinguish adults who stutter from normally fluent speakers (Manning & Shirkey, 1981). Although there is little research on how the quality of a speaker's fluency changes during and following treatment, it may be that progress in treatment is sometimes signaled by an increase in the frequency of formulative fluency breaks to levels typical of normal speakers. That is, as the person who stutters begins to consider the variety of ways of expressing a thought rather than dealing with the short-term problems inherent in avoiding or struggling through a motoric fluency break, formulative breaks may increase in frequency to normal or near-normal levels. The relatively few studies conducted with older normal speakers provide preliminary evidence suggesting that formulative fluency breaks tend to increase somewhat during late adulthood, and that motoric fluency breaks continue to be infrequent (Gordon, Hutchinson, & Allen, 1976; Manning & Monte, 1981; Yairi & Clifton, 1972).

The Speaker's Loss of Control

It is unfortunate that many definitions of stuttering include the perceptual effect of the stuttering on a listener but fail to consider the reaction of the speaker that occurs before, during, and following the most obvious aspect of the stuttering moment. Van Riper acknowledged this when, in 1982, he stated that "stuttering occurs when the forward flow of speech is interrupted by a motorically disrupted sound, syllable, or word, *or by the speaker's reactions thereto* [italics added]" (p. 15).

As much or more than anything else, it is the speaker's response to the breaks in fluency that differentiates people who stutter from those who experience normal and usual disruptions of fluency. Several authors agree that the involuntary nature of the problem and the associated loss of control and helplessness felt by the speaker are a crucial feature that is at the core of the experience of being a person who stutters (Bloodstein, 1987; Cooper, 1968; Manning, 1977; Manning & Shrum, 1973; Perkins, 1983; Van Riper, 1937). Van Riper stated that "the stutterer feels he has no control over his stuttering performance" (p. 151). Bloodstein felt that for the person who stutters, the fundamental difference between real and fake stuttering is the awareness of tension and being out of control associated with real stuttering. Perkins (1983) also argues that the involuntary nature of stuttering is at the core of any definition of the stuttering experience. It is this loss of control that makes stuttering categorically different from more typical fluency breaks (Perkins, 1990). He points out the shortcomings of definitions that depend exclusively on listener perception. Although the listener may be able to identify the acoustic features of the fluency break, he or she may not distinguish the cognitive and affective experience of the event.

> The essence of stuttering, in my view, is not what is perceived by listeners as stuttering in the acoustical signal, but rather what occurs in the production of stuttered speech. . . . Stuttering is the involuntary disruption of a continuing attempt to produce a spoken utterance. . . . From the stutterer's vantage point, however, the judgment is categorical: Either involuntary blockage has or has not occurred to some degree. If it has not occurred, then what sounds like stuttering to the observer would not feel like stuttering to the speaker. The reason that this distinction is categorical is because the proposed definition posits that loss of control of the ability to voluntarily continue a disrupted utterance is the essence of stuttering. If the disruption is not involuntary to some degree, then it is not a stuttered disfluency. Moreover, the stutterer would not react to it with apprehension, struggle, or avoidance if it were stuttered. (p. 376)

When discussing the handicapping effects of stuttering, Silverman (1996) suggests that how speakers react—what they tell themselves about their stuttering experience (or even the possibility of stuttering)—helps to define themselves and their speech. Silverman maintains that the number of choices and activities that stuttering prevents the person from doing defines the degree of handicap. Citing several personal accounts (Attanasio, 1987; Carlisle, 1985; Johnson, 1930; Murray & Edwards, 1980; Shields, 1989; Sugarman, 1980; Van Riper, 1984), Silverman points out that the actual handicap that can result from being a person who stutters can be considerably different (often greater) than the surface features of the stuttering would indicate. It is not uncommon for the handicapping effects associated with stuttering to result from the speaker's reaction to his situation and his attempts to alter or adapt to the problem, often in less than effectual ways.

While the idea of losing control of one's speech can be difficult for the observing clinician or researcher to identify and quantify (Martin & Haroldson, 1986; Moore & Perkins, 1990), Manning and Shrum (1973) argue that such a loss of control can be extremely identifiable and specific. The client is able to know whether he or she or the stuttering is "in charge" of his or her speech. Many people who stutter are able to consistently indicate whether or not they have achieved control of their speech. The experience is somewhat analogous to tipping back and forth between losing and regaining one's balance. Once calibrated to a speaker, the experienced clinician can become adept in identifying such control or the lack of it.

In summary, although the surface features of stuttering are often obvious and quantifiable, it would appear that some of the most telling features lie under the surface and reside in the more subtle cognitive and affective layers of the syndrome. Sometimes these subtle features of psychosocial discomfort are reflected in a variety of nonverbal features, such as body movement (Conture, 1990). But as Starkweather (1999) points out, efficacious therapies should deal with all levels of the disorder for, in many cases, the less observable features are often more important (particularly for the speaker) than the more obvious ones.

In order to provide the reader with the perspective that informs many comments throughout this book, the following indicates the current view of the present author in defining the nature of stuttering. Although the experience of speaking is complicated by communicative stress, as it is for most speakers, the person who stutters is able to linguistically formulate what he or she wants to say. Stuttering appears to be the result of a combination of cortical and subcortical neurological and physiological characteristics that result in a speech production system that is susceptible to fluency breaks. For many individuals, these characteristics appear to be genetically influenced. The resulting interaction of these characteristics typically becomes apparent as young speakers begin to produce sequences of two or more words. These intrinsic characteristics interact with environmental influences during early language and speech development, providing the opportunity for stuttering development. Breaks in fluency typically result in the fragmentation of words or syllables and are often accompanied by physical tension that further limits the efficient and coordinated functioning of the systems involved in fluent speech production. Many of the overt behaviors that are characteristic of stuttering are learned, usually natural but often maladaptive coping behaviors that the speaker uses to avoid, postpone, or escape from the stuttering experience. In many instances, the breaks in fluency are accompanied by a profound sense of helplessness and loss of control. Listeners are often able to observe the occurrence of stuttering in the speech of an individual, a surface event that provides a point estimate of stuttering. However, the speaker's cognitive and emotional experience of stuttering often begins well before and continues well after the overt disruption of his or her fluency. The experience of stuttering is likely to restrict many options for verbal communication and negatively influence many facets of an individual's quality of life.

Soon after the onset of stuttering, the speaker will begin devising ways of coping with the situation. The speaker develops subtle and sophisticated ways of avoiding and escaping from communication situations associated with fear and the penalty brought about by the stuttering experience. Speakers begin to interpret themselves and their ability to communicate in specific ways, and, to varying degrees, they learn to play the role of a person who stutters (Sheehan, 1970). On the surface of the problem are an assortment of avoidance and escape behaviors that become accessories to the experience of the fluency breakdown. Avoidance behaviors are related to the anticipation of stuttering. Anticipating a difficult speaking situation, the speaker chooses to avoid or completely postpone the situation by using starter sounds or words ("Ah, let me see") or timing and distraction devices (finger or head movement, audible or inaudible movements of the articulators). The point is that these behaviors gather around the initial fluency break, making it ever more complex, distracting, and handicapping. Escape behaviors, on the other hand, are attempts to get away from the stuttering moment that is currently occurring and include a multitude of possible responses, including eye blinks, head nods, interjections, and a wide variety of often tense struggle activities. As the speaker is able to move away from the moment of helplessness or through the sentence, the behavior that facilitated the ability to escape is rewarded. A powerful link is formed between these responses that allow the speaker to avoid or escape from stuttering; one that, not surprisingly, can be difficult to weaken.

The Fluency Breaks of Children

Because of the variety of studies, theoretical models, and research methods used, there has been considerable controversy over the differences, or lack thereof, in the fluency breaks of young stuttering and nonstuttering children. Much of the controversy stems from the fact that the very early stages of stuttering have been difficult to investigate. Out of necessity, investigations were retrospective in nature and relied on parent accounts about the timing and features of stuttering onset. In some instances, months or years had passed from the onset of disfluency and the first opportunity to interview the child's parents and observe the child. As Yairi and Ambrose (2005) suggest, until recently there were relatively few qualified clinicians with the necessary interest or capability for observing and recording early stuttering and high quality recording equipment for recording, storing, and analyzing speech samples. These problems have undoubtedly contributed to the conflicting results and interpretation of data giving rise to the suggestion both that the fluency breaks of young children who stutter are indistinguishable from those of normal speakers (Glasner & Rosenthal, 1957; Johnson & Associates, 1959; Johnson & Luetenegger, 1955) and that they are different in many important ways from normal speakers (Bloodstein, 1974; McDearmon, 1968; Van Riper, 1982 Yairi & Ambrose, 2005). As we will see in the next chapter, this issue has several important implications for the theoretical principles that guide our clinical decisions. We will also see in the following paragraphs that more recent empirical information indicates that the fluency characteristics of young stuttering children and their normally fluent peers have many important differences.

Because much of what follows (both in this chapter as well as Chapter 5) is based on the work of Ehud Yairi and his colleagues (in particular Nicoline Ambrose; see Yairi and Ambrose, 2005), we will take a moment to briefly summarize their work at the University of Illinois.

Beginning in 1980, these researchers and their colleagues have conducted a series of longitudinal investigations concerning the onset and development of stuttering in children. Inclusion criteria for the children required that they were 6 years of age or younger and that their parents believed that their child stuttered, with parent ratings of disfluencies at least a 2 on an 8-point scale (0 = *normal*, 7 = *very severe*). In addition, it was required that both Yairi and Ambrose agreed that the child was stuttering, rating them greater than 1 (borderline) on a similar scale. Furthermore, the children had to exhibit a minimum of three stuttering-like disfluencies (SLDs) per 100 syllables of spontaneous speech and have no history of neurological disorders. Three SLDs is widely considered to be a threshold between stuttering and typically fluent children (Ambrose & Yairi, 2005). The authors also obtained corresponding ratings on these criteria in selecting a normally fluent control group of 59 children.

The authors were especially interested in finding children who had begun stuttering less than one year prior to their first evaluation. As a result of their efforts, a total of 163 children were identified. Of this total, 146 (101 male, 45 female) were seen within 12 months of stuttering onset (a mean age of 5 months post onset). This group of children was termed the Early Experimental Group and comprised the major group of children studied. A second group of children (Later Experimental Group) included children who were first seen somewhat more than one year following onset. This group was composed of 17 children (10 male, 7 female). The control group of 59 normally fluent children was composed of 40 males and 19 females.

Yairi and Ambrose and their colleagues obtained 40-minute audio and video recordings of 1000–2000 syllables. They were able to achieve good inter- and intra-judge agreement (average of 86%) for both frequency counts for type and location of the stuttering-like disfluencies. They also administered a comprehensive battery of speech, language, hearing, motor, psychological, and other tests. Follow-up recordings were achieved for the children either locally or by speech-language pathologists located in areas where some of the children and their families had moved. Fortunately, over the course of the investigation they were unable to obtain follow-up information for only 5% of the original participants, an unusually low participant mortality rate for a longitudinal study.

Characteristics at the Onset of Stuttering

Readers should note that much of the information presented in the following section represents the highlights from the 2005 Yairi and Ambrose text *Early Childhood Stuttering: For Clinicians by Clinicians,* and readers are urged to consult this rich source of information concerning the dimensions of stuttering onset. In the following three sections, the epidemiological attributes (i.e., the factors contributing to the incidence and prevalence of a problem, the possibility of the problem remitting or becoming chronic, and changes in symptomatology and subtypes) of stuttering onset in young, preschool children will be described in terms of the major factors that help to distinguish children who are experiencing the onset of stuttering from their normally fluent peers.

Age and Gender

Stuttering rarely begins after the early childhood years. For this reason, stuttering has often been called a disorder of childhood (Bloodstein, 1995; Conture, 1990; Van Riper; 1982). In those cases where the onset of stuttering takes place in adulthood, it is referred to as *acquired stuttering* and is described in Chapter 10. It is important to understand that, as Yairi and Ambrose have pointed out (Yairi & Ambrose, 1992b; 2005), in the vast majority of cases stuttering begins after a period of normally fluent speech. That is, following a brief period of fluent speech the child experiences the *loss* of the ability to achieve fluency. This experience is distinctly different from the inability to originally develop a skill that is characteristic of other more common language, phonological, or articulatory problems—a difference that the authors suggest may impact the child's awareness of and response to his or her situation. In addition, the loss of fluency often occurs rather suddenly, also in contrast to the gradual realization by the child and the parents that an expected skill has failed to occur.

The 163 children studied by Yairi and Ambrose (2005) demonstrated a range of onset, with children becoming disfluent as early as 16 months and as late as 69 months of age. The authors' analysis indicated that mean (and median) age of onset was 33 months, about 9 months earlier than the mean age of onset calculated from 11 previously published studies (Yairi, 1997a). Both the 101 male and the 45 female participants in the Early Experimental group showed nearly identical mean age of onset at 34.02 and 34.24 months, respectively.

Although there were more males than females included in the total sample of 163 children, the pattern of onset for both genders was similar. Yairi and Ambrose (2005) found that the onset of stuttering for 85% of the boys and girls occurred by 42 months, with 95% occurring by age 4; only 5% of the children began stuttering beyond age 4. The majority of the onsets were concentrated between 24 and 42 months during the third year of life.

Rate and Uniformity of Onset

The nature of the fluency characteristics at onset is closely related to the rate of onset. Dating back to the 19th century, the long-held view was that stuttering developed gradually and followed a uniform pattern of development (e.g., Froeschels, 1943; Bluemel, 1932), the gradual and linear development of stuttering associated with the earlier description of primary and secondary stuttering described earlier in this chapter. This understanding of stuttering onset and development was a common feature of recent textbooks including, to some extent, the earlier editions of the one you are reading. As it turns out, the detailed analysis provided by the longitudinal studies by Yairi and colleagues indicates that the onset of developmental stuttering is not necessarily gradual or uniform. A few investigators had noted that children sometimes experienced sudden onset and presented with what had been previously considered to be advanced (secondary) behaviors (Van Riper, 1971; Yairi, 1983; Yairi & Ambrose, 1992b). In some instances, children began stuttering within a single day, demonstrating at the outset disfluencies that were unusual and obviously different to the more common fluency breaks of other young, normally fluent speakers.

The children studied by Yairi and Ambrose (2005) showed a wide variety in the rate of onset, ranging from sudden (1 day to 2–3 days), intermediate (1–2 weeks), and gradual (3–5 weeks and 6 or more weeks). Parental report indicated that nearly 30% (29.6%) experienced onset over the course of one day. When including those reported to have begun stuttering in 2–3 days, those experiencing sudden onset reached just over 40% (40.7%). Intermediate onset was reported at 32.1% and gradual onset at 27.1%. As with the age of onset, there was no significant difference for boys or girls across the three categories of sudden, intermediate, and gradual onset. Based on their interviews with the parents who participated in their investigation, Yairi and Ambrose obtained vivid examples of parents' ability to provide discrete and detailed descriptions of their child's first instances of stuttering. In several instances, the parent's recall was aided by the fact that onset had taken place only a few months or days prior to the interview.

Stuttering-Like Disfluencies

Another important issue at onset is whether or not some disfluencies are particularly unique to young children who stutter. If this were the case, these specific form types would aid clinicians in differentiating those children who are stuttering from those who are experiencing the more common disfluencies characteristic of normally fluent preschool children. We will provide a brief historical perspective describing the importance of this issue and then summarize some of the investigations that have identified the fluency breaks that are particularly unique to children who are beginning to stutter.

One of the theories that dominated the research and clinical practice in the field through the middle of the 20th century was the diagnosogenic (or semantogenic) theory on stuttering onset (Johnson and Associates, 1959) described in detail in Chapter 3. A primary tenet of this view was that children who stutter begin speaking normally (including normal speech disfluencies) and then slowly progress through a transitional phase to a continuum of increasing abnormal forms of disfluency. Based on an analysis of the early disfluencies of children who had begun to stutter, Johnson and his associates felt that the initial disfluencies were essentially normal fluency breaks (e.g., easy repetitions) that had been misdiagnosed as stuttering by significant others in the child's environment (typically the parents). However, a reanalysis of Johnson's data by McDearmon (1968) indicated that many of the disfluencies present at the outset of stuttering were far from normal. Subsequent research by Yairi (1983), who interviewed the parents of 22 young children six months after they had begun to stutter, found that the children were producing a variety of unusual or abnormal fluency breaks, including blocks, facial contortions, repetitions that included three to five iterations, and sound prolongations. Only 35% of the parents described their child's stuttering as easy repetitions.

As Yairi and Ambrose (2005) point out, Johnson and his associates regarded three to four repetitions per stuttering event as brief and essentially normal fluency breaks. In fact, that many repetitions are considerably greater than the 1.1 iterations found by Ambrose and Yairi (1995) for normally fluent children. Ambrose and Yairi (1995) analyzed 1,000 syllables of 29 children recently diagnosed (mean of 2.14 months post-onset) as children who stuttered (average age, 34.76 months) and 29 control subjects (average age, 35.57 months). The young stuttering children demonstrated a significantly greater number of units per repetition ($p < .002$). The frequency per 100 syllables of disfluencies containing two or more repetition units for the experimental subjects was 3.70 (SD = 3.77), and for the control subjects it was 0.21 (SD = .20).

In one of the earliest studies to result from the University of Illinois Research Program, Yairi and Lewis (1984) analyzed the fluency breaks of 2- and 3-year-old children within two months after stuttering onset. Ten children with stuttering (CWS) (five boys and five girls) were matched with a group of children who did not stutter, or children with no stuttering (CWNS). There was considerable overlap in the types of fluency breaks of the two groups, especially for interjections and revision-incomplete phrases. The most frequent fluency breaks for children who were normally fluent were, in order, (1) interjection, (2) part-word repetition, and (3) revision-incomplete phrase. The most frequent fluency breaks for the stuttering children were, in order, (1) part-word repetitions, (2) disrhythmic phonation, and (3) single-syllable repetitions. In addition, the CWS produced more than three times the number of fluency breaks of the normally speaking children (21.5 and 6.2 breaks per 100 syllables, respectively). The CWS had significantly more fluency breaks ($p < .05$) for part-word repetitions and disrhythmic phonations. Finally, Yairi and Lewis found that while the normally speaking children rarely repeated a part-word repetition more than once (range of 1–2), the stuttering children typically repeated a portion of the word two or more times (range of 1–11).

A comparison of the speech of 23 children from the Early Experimental Group who were seen within 1 month of onset was made with normative data obtained by Ambrose and Yairi (1999). Yairi and Ambrose (2005) indicate that sound and syllable repetitions occurred more than nine times per 100 syllables and disrhythmic phonations (prolongations and stoppages of airflow) occurred more than three times for 100 syllables. Taken together, these totaled 12.63% Stuttering-like disfluencies (SLDs), far more than the number of SLDs for normally fluent 2- and 3-year-olds (Ambrose and Yairi, 1999). The mean number of times a segment was repeated during each repetition was just under 1.75 for the CWS, which was more than 5 standard deviations above the mean number (1.10) of normally fluent children. Yairi and Ambrose (2005) conclude by stating their conviction that "a large number of long disfluencies (e.g., repetitions containing two or more iterations) plays a major role in parents' decisions that their child has begun stuttering" (p. 68).

Another important distinction of the disfluencies for the young stuttering children was noted by Throneberg and Yairi (1994). When comparing the disfluencies of 20 preschool children who stuttered and a control group of 20 nonstuttering children, these authors found that the CWS produced shorter silent intervals between repeated units and thus a more rapid rate of iterations than the CWNS. These results supported the findings of Yairi and Hall (1993), who found that children in the early stages of stuttering tend to repeat at a faster rate than children who do not stutter.

The rapid rate of iterations produced during stuttering results in both complex and interesting findings concerning the duration of stuttering-like disfluencies for young speakers. There are many investigations indicating that disfluencies that are longer than 1 second are more likely to be perceived as stuttering. As a result, the duration of stuttering events have been used both to differentiate stuttering from nonstuttering (Van Riper, 1972) and in determining the severity of stuttering (Riley, 1994). The majority of the investigations concerning the duration of stuttering involved a variety of participant ages and measurement techniques. The Throneburg and Yairi (1994) study cited earlier indicated that when disfluencies were limited to repetitions of syllables and monosyllabic words, the CWS produced significantly *shorter* disfluencies than the controls. Analyzing the speech of 30 children (27–59 months of age, 3 months post-onset of stuttering, no history of clinical intervention), Yairi and Ambrose (2005) found that children with more severe stuttering (based on the frequency of SLDs) produced shorter duration of three-unit repetitions (because they repeat faster) than children with mild or moderate stuttering.

As we have seen in this section, the form types that distinguish children who are experiencing the onset of stuttering appear to be disfluencies that are both quantitatively and qualitatively different from the disfluencies of their normal speaking peers. As indicated earlier, these types have been referred to (particularly by Yairi and his colleagues) as Stuttering-like disfluencies or SLDs. Stuttering-like disfluencies are composed of three basic types of disfluencies: part-word repetitions, single-syllable word repetitions, and disrhythmic phonations, which include sound prolongations or blocks of airflow and voicing. Other disfluencies include interjection, revision, and phrase repetition. Table 2-4 provides the mean frequency and standard deviation of (SD) of stuttering-like and other disfluencies per 100 syllables for the experimental and control groups of children studied by Yairi and Ambrose (2005).

Clustering of Disfluencies

Several researchers have noted the tendency for children who stutter to produce a sequence of disfluencies in close proximity to one another (Colburn, 1985; Hubbard & Yairi, 1988; LaSalle & Conture, 1995; Silverman, 1973). This tendency for the spatial grouping of disfluencies, or clustering, has been defined by Yairi and Ambrose (2005) as "two or more consecutive disfluencies that occur within the same word, on adjacent words, or on a word and an adjacent between-word interval" (pp. 125–126). Hubbard & Yairi (1988) found that 15 children (age 2–4 years) who stuttered produced 57% of their disfluencies in clusters. In contrast, a control group of 15 normally fluent children produced 66% of their disfluencies in isolation. In addition, the CWS produced more than six times as many clusters as the CWNS. LaSalle and Conture (1995) found similar results when comparing 300-word conversational speech samples

Table 2-4   Mean Frequency and Standard Deviation *(SD)* of Disfluencies Per 100 syllables for Experimental and Control Groups.

Disfluency Type	Experimental Group Frequency (SD)	Control Group Frequency (SD)
Stuttering-Like Disfluencies		
Part-word repetitions	5.64 (4.28)	0.55 (0.43)
Single-syllable word repetitions	3.24 (2.01)	0.79 (0.74)
Disrhythmic phonations	2.42 (2.62)	0.08 (0.12)
Total	11.30 (6.64)	1.41 (0.96)
Other Disfluencies	5.79 (2.75)	4.48 (2.41)

From *Early Childhood Stuttering* (p. 114), by E. Yairi and N. G. Ambrose, 2005, Austin, TX: PRO-ED. Copyright 2005 by PRO-ED, Inc. Reprinted with permission.

of 30 young (average age of 4 years, 3 months) children who stuttered with a control group of normally fluent children. The children who stuttered produced clusters containing two disfluencies an average of 32% of the time, while the normally fluent children never produced such clusters. They also found that the occurrence of clusters containing within-word disfluencies was positively correlated with greater severity of stuttering.

Awareness and Reaction of the Child to Disfluency

The extent to which a young speaker who is beginning to stutter is aware of his or her disfluencies is an intriguing question and one that has proven difficult to answer. Yairi and Ambrose (2005) have also studied this issue and point out that because fluency is highly variable and the child's awareness of his or her disfluencies is momentary, it depends not only on how children are asked to indicate their awareness but when. Of course, parents are able to provide indirect indications of their child's difficulty in achieving fluency. Some children respond to their difficulty in more subtle ways such as withdrawing from speaking or showing signs of facial tension. Other children react more obviously by crying in frustration or saying things such as "I can't talk." The extent and nature of a particular child's response to the onset of stuttering is undoubtedly related to his or her level of maturity and temperament.

Yairi and Ambrose (2005) found that early awareness can and does occur but is highly variable. In their classic 1994 "puppet study" they asked 2–6-year-old children who stuttered and a control group of 20 nonstuttering children (matched by age and gender) to observe a series of videotaped statements by two puppets. Children were asked to identify with a fluent or disfluent puppet ("Point to the puppet that talks the way you do") (Ambrose & Yairi, 1994; p. 233–234). Approximately 15% of the children who stuttered indicated some degree of awareness. More recent data (Yairi & Ambrose, 2005) using this same videotaped procedure indicate that almost 10% of 64 children who were within 12 months of stuttering onset showed indications of awareness of their stuttering.

As would be expected, as children mature they become increasingly aware of their fluent and disfluent speech. Also using video-puppet procedure, Ezrati-Vinacour, Platzky, and Yairi (2001) found that normally fluent children show consistent awareness of speech fluency by about age 5. Interestingly, Yairi and Ambrose (2005) note that only after children have been stuttering for 3 years is there positive correlation between clinician ratings of stuttering severity and awareness by the child. And in a related issue, the percentage of children who are aware of their stuttering increases with age, especially between the ages of 4 and 5. It is also worth noting that a variety of measures designed to indicate anxiety in children failed to show any link between the awareness of disfluencies and the presence of anxiety (Yairi & Ambrose, 2005).

Given that some children are aware of their stuttering, do they necessarily assign a negative valuation to their situation? Using the Communication Attitude Test (CAT; Brutten & Dunham, 1989), many authors have demonstrated that by age 6 children are not only aware of their disfluent speech but have developed a negative attitude about speaking (Vanryckeghem and Brutten, 1997). With the goal of determining whether such negative attitudes about communicating might exist in younger children who were beginning to stutter, Vanryckeghem, Brutten and Hernandez (2005) used a modified version of a self-report measure designed for preschool children (The KiddyCAT; Vanryckeghem & Brutten, 2002) to obtain self-report responses from 45 children who stuttered (3 years, 0 months to 6 years, 5 months, mean 4 years 4 months) and 63 fluent children. These authors found that preschoolers and kindergartners who stutter are significantly ($p < 0.0001$; effect size of 1.44) more likely to assign a negative attitude about speaking than their nonstuttering peers. There were no significant effects across age and gender. The results support the studies described earlier (Ambrose & Yairi, 1994, Yairi & Ambrose, 2005, Ezrati-Vinacour et al., 2001) indicating that children ages 3 and 4 who are at the outset of stuttering are not only aware of their disfluencies but they are also experiencing a negative attitude about speaking in comparison to normally fluent children. These results are in contrast to traditional views that very young speakers are unaware and unconcerned about communicating. As it turns out, some children who have recently begun to stutter are aware of their situation and are beginning to react negatively. In subsequent chapters we will describe the clinical and theoretical implications of these results.

Conditions Contributing to Onset

This section will consider two sets of conditions that have been related to the onset of stuttering. These are issues that clinicians are frequently questioned about by clients and parents. The wide diversity of conditions at onset argue against a unitary or simple explanation for the etiology of the stuttering problem (see also Chapter 3). The many conditions that have been associated with stuttering onset may complicate the task of diagnostic decision making for the clinician. Furthermore, many of these conditions interact with one another (e.g., age and gender), and it is difficult to categorically suggest that some factors are more influential than others. Given that caveat, we will first describe a set of conditions that appear to have a greater influence on onset. The second set of conditions, while sometimes mentioned in the literature, has comparatively less influence. Although these factors may be prominent aspects of the child's life, they are more likely to simply temporally coincide with the initial observation that the child is beginning to stutter. It is also important to understand that many investigations of young stuttering children are descriptive in nature and do not allow an assumption of cause-and-effect relationships between the speaker or environmental characteristics and the onset of stuttering behavior. While there may indeed be some relationship between these factors, the fact that they covary in some manner may only signify that one or more other factors are causing this relationship. Many of these factors, particularly the more influential ones, will be discussed in considerably more detail in the following chapters.

More Influential Factors

These factors appear to have a somewhat greater influence on the likelihood of stuttering, although, in many instances, their precise impact remains unclear. In some cases it may be best to think of some of these conditions as predisposing factors that can place a child at greater risk for both precipitating and maintaining stuttering (Silverman, 1992).

Age

Andrews (1984) suggests that the risk of developing stuttering drops by 50% after age 4, 75% after age 6, and is virtually nil by age 12. A different assessment was noted by Yairi and Ambrose (2005), who studied a younger sample of children and found that 60% of the children began to stutter prior to age 3 and more than 85% by age 3 1/2 years of age. They noted that stuttering onset was unlikely after age 4 and especially unlikely after age 6. Nevertheless, Bloodstein and Bernstein Ratner (2008) indicate that a number of studies have reported stuttering onset occurring during early adolescence. Plexico, Manning, and DiLollo (2005) found that it is not usual for adolescents and adults to report that the first time they remember realizing that they stuttered was just prior to or during their early teenage years. In some instances, it may be that while the actual onset took place during the preschool years, the stuttering was present in a mild and less than handicapping fashion. It was not until the speaker experienced the social penalties and associated social and educational disadvantages associated with stuttering that it became a problem. As indicated earlier in the chapter, the onset of acquired stuttering during the middle or late adult years is relatively rare and is likely to occur in cases of neurological or psychological origin (see Chapter 10). In an epidemiological study of stuttering across the entire life span, Craig and colleagues (2002) found the lowest prevalence (0.37%) for the group of individuals who were 51 years of age and older.

Gender

Kent (1983) discussed the fact that the higher occurrence of stuttering in adult males is one of the few consistencies about the disorder. Stuttering in school-age and adult males has been estimated in ratios that range from 3:1 to as high as 6:1. However, at the time of onset, stuttering has been found to occur with approximately equal frequency for males and females, with ratios ranging on the order of 1:1 or 2:1 (Yairi, 1983; Kloth, Janssen, Kraaimaat, & Brutten, 1995). This disparity across gender and age can be accounted for by the fact that females are more likely than males to experience a natural recovery from stuttering. As mentioned earlier, patterns of onset age are similar for males and females, with 95% of onsets occurring by age 4 (Yairi & Ambrose, 2005). It is also important to appreciate that speaker gender and age interact in a number of ways. In addition, there are gender-related genetic influences that may result in males being more susceptible to stuttering and females having a higher threshold, with more factors required for stuttering onset (Kidd, 1984). Based on the results of several studies, Yairi and Ambrose (1999a) suggest that gender and genetics interact in such a way that young females who stutter are much less likely to persist in stuttering than young males.

Genetic Factors

As described in the previous chapter, there is a long history of documentation that stuttering occurs with much greater than usual frequency in some families. Bloodstein and Bernstein Ratner's (2008) review indicates that the percentage of people who have relatives on the maternal or paternal side who stuttered ranges from 30 to 69%. Studies concerning the genetics of stuttering have focused on the occurrence of stuttering in families, particularly in instances where there is a high density of stuttering in the first- and second-degree relatives. Research during the past few decades has indicated a genetic component in selected groups of people who stutter (Cox, Seider, & Kidd, 1984; Falsenfeld, 1997; Johnson & Associates, 1959; Kidd, 1977; Kidd, 1884; Kidd, Heimbuch, Records, Oehlert, & Webster, 1980; Pauls, 1990; Poulos & Webster, 1991; Sheehan & Costley, 1977; Yairi, 1983). As suggested earlier, genetics and gender appear to interact in predictable patterns during stuttering development. As Ambrose (2004) points out, if stuttering onset were completely determined by genetics, when one identical twin stuttered the other would also. It is apparent therefore that environmental factors are also influential. At this point it is reasonably clear that the onset as well as the persistence (and recovery from) stuttering have strong genetic components and that environmental factors also play an important role (see also Chapter 3).

Twinning

Because of genetic influences, there is a clear relationship between twinning and stuttering. Approximately one-third of all twin pairs are monozygotic (MZ) and are genetically identical. The remaining twin pairs are dizygotic (DZ), or fraternal, and share about half of their polymorphic genes. A child is more likely to stutter if he or she is a member of a twin pair in which the other twin also stutters (Howie, 1981). This is especially true if the twins are monozygotic. It is less likely that both members of a fraternal twin pair will stutter (Howie, 1981). These findings seem to be explained by a genetic predisposition to stuttering (Howie, 1981; West & Ansberry, 1968) but family and environmental factors also have an influence.

Cognitive Abilities

The general cognitive abilities of children who stutter are similar to and perhaps somewhat better than those of their nonstuttering peers (Yairi & Ambrose, 2005). On the other hand, it is well documented that individuals who possess less than normal cognitive abilities tend to have more fluency problems (Andrews & Harris, 1964; Otto & Yairi, 1976). Van Riper (1982) summarized the results of seven independent studies indicating prevalence figures ranging from a low of 7% (Schaeffer & Shearer, 1968) to a high of 60% for clients with Down's syndrome (Preus, 1973). Averaging across all seven studies Van Riper found a prevalence figure of 24% (SD = 18.1). Of course, with this population there is also a much higher occurrence of many speech and language problems, including cluttering (see Chapter 10). In addition, it can be difficult to distinguish motor speech and language problems (particularly word finding) from fluency breaks, and developmental delays can mask the identification of fluency disorders.

Motor Abilities

Because the production of fluent speech requires skilled motor ability, any delay or lack of coordination among the various levels of the speech production system is likely to adversely affect the development of normal fluency. The majority of the research concerning motor function of individuals who stutter has focused on adults. The research with children has indicated only subtle differences in laryngeal function, speaking rate, and articulatory movement.

Riley and Riley (2000) found that from a sample of 50 children who stuttered, 68% showed evidence of speech motor difficulties (50% severe and 18% moderate) for accuracy of voicing, coarticulatory movements between syllables, and diadochokinetic rate for syllable production (versus 2% severe and 8% moderate for normally fluent children). Hall & Yairi (1992) found some evidence of instability of laryngeal control (fundamental frequency, jitter, and shimmer values) in the fluent syllabic utterances of 10 male preschool CWS as compared to 10 fluent males. Zebrowski, Conture, and Cudahy (1985) found indications of a lack of appropriate interaction between laryngeal and supralaryngeal behaviors during fluent speech in young children who stutter, which was subsequently confirmed by Borden, Kim, and Spiegler (1987).

Hall, Amir, and Yairi (1999) acoustically analyzed the articulatory rate (number of fluently produced syllables and phones) uttered per second and found that preschool children close to the onset of stuttering produced significantly slower rates than their fluent peers. Subramanian, Yairi, and Amir (2003) found that articulatory movements were significantly smaller (as indicated by the frequency shifts of second formant transitions) for children who had recently begun to stutter. These findings coincide with the notion that stuttering is a reflection of problems in performing the temporal and spatial requirements necessary for fluent speech (Kent, 1984). Similar results have been found for children who stutter by Zebrowski, Moon, and Robin (1997) in a kinematic investigation of children's ability to perform tracking of acoustic signals by jaw movement.

The evidence that adults who stutter have somewhat greater difficulty in fine motor integration of speech production is even more convincing (Riley & Riley, 1984, 2000; Starkweather, 1987; Van Riper, 1982). As with children, adults who stutter also demonstrate more obvious coarticulatory instability during the production of fluent utterances, as indicated by analysis of their second formant (F2) fluctuations compared to normally fluent adult controls (Robb & Blomgren, 1997; Robb, Blomgren, & Chen, 1998) as well as adults who have undergone successful stuttering treatment (Robb, Blomgren, & Chen, 1998). Finally, Archibald and De Nil (1999) studied the oral kinesthetic ability of four adults with very mild and four adults with moderate-to-severe stuttering (as determined by the Stuttering Severity Instrument, Riley, 1980). Participants were instructed to make the smallest possible jaw movements from a defined starting position in response to a series of short tones. The participants performed the task with and without visual feedback. When only proprioceptive information was available to the subjects with moderate/severe stuttering, they took significantly longer than either the subjects with mild stuttering or the non-stuttering controls. The findings provide additional support for the notion that some adults who stutter to a moderate or severe degree may have an oral kinesthetic deficit.

Speech and Language Development

There is an obvious interplay of all the above factors in the development of speech and language skills. Traditionally, there has been general agreement that children who stutter typically achieve lower scores than their peers on measures of receptive vocabulary, the age of speech and language onset, mean length of utterance, and expressive and receptive syntax (Andrews & Harris, 1964; Berry, 1938; Guitar, 1998; Kline & Starkweather, 1979; Murray & Reed, 1977; Peters & Guitar, 1991; and Wall, 1980). More recent investigations suggest that the relationship of stuttering and expressive language and phonological abilities is far from simple. Watkins, Yairi, and Ambrose (1999) studied 62 preschool children who recovered from stuttering and 22 who persisted in stuttering. Spontaneous language samples of 250–300 utterances were used to examine the children's expressive language skills (lexical, morphological, and syntactic measures). Both groups of children (those who recovered from and those who persisted in stuttering) displayed expressive language abilities near or above developmental expectations. For both groups of children, those who were the youngest when entering the investigation (2 to 3 years old) had expressive language scores well above normative values.

Yairi and Ambrose (2005) summarize their findings on the language abilities of children shortly after the onset of stuttering by stating that many such children have average or above-average expressive language skills. They also conclude that many of these children who have begun to stutter appear to have language skills that exceed their capabilities for producing fluent speech. As described in greater detail in Chapter 5, these expressive language skills tend to reduce to more age-appropriate levels as a consequence of natural recovery as well as successful therapy. Yairi and Ambrose further indicate that the likelihood of the recovery from or persistence of stuttering appears to have little to do with a child's language ability. Conversely, linguistic variables such as grammatical complexity and loci of stuttering events (especially as related to language planning units) do appear to be important factors for understanding the occurrence of disfluencies for all speakers, regardless of whether they stutter or not.

The co-occurrence of delayed phonological development and stuttering in children has been noted by many authors over several years. A review of the literature on the co-occurrence of phonological (and articulation disorders when including investigations conducted prior to the 1970s) and stuttering by Yairi and Ambrose (2005) indicates that this co-occurrence is approximately 30%–35% for children seen in clinical settings and less than 30% for the general population (Throneberg, Yairi, & Paden, 1994). Yairi and Ambrose (2005) point out that there are some issues to be considered when interpreting the phonology–stuttering connection; for example, the fact that boys are more likely to stutter than girls (generally 2:1 at the outset) and, especially for young children, boys are also more likely to exhibit phonological deficits. Even studies of relatively young CWS are likely to miss children who stuttered for a few months and then recovered. In spite of a number of well-constructed investigations, there is no strong evidence that there is any relationship between the production of phonologically difficult words and the occurrence of stuttering (see Yairi & Ambrose, 2005, pp. 197–234 for a review).

Yairi & Ambrose (2005) summarize their findings about the connection between phonological development and the onset and development (including recovery from) stuttering for preschool children by stating:

- Soon after onset, children who stutter tend to be behind normally fluent children in phonological development.

- Children who will eventually persist in stuttering are apt to be slower in phonological development than those who will eventually recover.

- In spite of this delay, phonological skills alone are insufficient to predict the further course of stuttering.

- The difference in level of phonological acquisition seen near stuttering onset between children whose stuttering will be persistent and those for whom it will be transient will probably have disappeared within two years.

- The phonological delay that is associated with stuttering will be overcome much sooner than earlier research would have predicted.

- The phonological development of children who stutter is similar in order of progression and strategies used to those of normally fluent children.

Yairi and Ambrose (2005) also point out that the stuttering–phonology connection is not necessarily linear in that there is no clear relationship between stuttering severity and the level of phonological skills.

Response to Emotional Events

There have been a number of interesting reports associating the rapid onset of stuttering (within one or two days) and unusual and possibly traumatic emotional events (see Mower, 1998). Although this is not generally viewed as a common occurrence, there is some justification for considering this form of onset as a subtype of stuttering. Yairi and Ambrose (2005) found that over 40% of the parents in their Early Experimental Group indicated that their child experienced events that emotionally upset the child shortly before onset. In addition, more than 50% of the parents indicated that their children appeared to be undergoing some stress as a consequence of their rapidly developing language skills. Nevertheless, Yairi and Ambrose (2005) found no significant differences between the persistent, recovered, and control groups on anxiety scales designed for children—although the children in the persistent group had the higher mean scores (greater anxiety).

Guitar (2006) provides a particularly interesting interpretation of the research on the temperamental characteristics of children and the possible interaction with the regulation of emotion in the two cerebral hemispheres as it may relate to children who stutter. Guitar cites research by Davidson (1984) and

Kinsbourne (1989) indicating hemispheric specialization for emotions; the left hemisphere is involved with regulating emotions associated with approaching, exploring, and taking action and the right hemisphere is specialized for emotions that accompany avoidance, withdrawal, and arrest of action. Furthermore, Calkins and Fox (1994) and Davidson (1995) found that sensitive children are right hemisphere-dominant for emotion. Combined with the information presented in Chapter 3 indicating an overactive right hemisphere for at least some individuals who stutter (albeit adults), this suggests that at least some individuals who stutter may be more temperamentally reactive. Kagan, Reznick, and Snidman (1987) found that more sensitive children react to novel or threatening stimuli by generating higher levels of physical tension, especially in laryngeal muscles. Of course, not all children who are sensitive or reactive turn out to be children who stutter. But if a child also possesses familial characteristics leading to an unstable speech production system this combination of factors may result in the onset of stuttering. Guitar, as well as Yairi and Ambrose (2005), considers the possibility that the presence of higher levels of anxiety may be associated with children who persist in their stuttering.

There are, of course, many forms of both emotional and communicative stress for families and children. However, there is no indication that children who stutter have a greater number of emotional conflicts than their normally speaking counterparts (Adams, 1993; Andrews & Harris, 1964; Bloch & Goodstein, 1971; Bloodstein, 1987; Johnson & Associates, 1959; Van Riper, 1982). Various forms of communicative stress, such as time pressure and verbal competition, undoubtedly enhance the possibility of breakdowns in the motor sequencing of speech. This may be particularly true if the temperamental nature of some children who stutter results in their being more susceptible to these forms of stress (Anderson, Pellowski, Conture, & Kelly, 2003). It can be difficult to connect a stressful event with the onset of stuttering, for as both Van Riper (1982) and Silverman (1996) point out, in many cases the initial signs of stuttering often precede the suspected event. Rather than being a cause of the stuttering, an event that happens to occur at approximately the same time as the stuttering was first observed may serve as a marker of that time period. Parents may report the onset of stuttering associated with an event without knowing that their child had been stuttering for some time in school and other locations outside the home. Examples of events that have been mentioned in the literature as being associated with stuttering onset include parental divorce, moving, separation from the mother, birth of a sibling, attending daycare centers, and imitating stuttering (Glasner & Rosenthal, 1957; Mower, 1998; Yairi & Ambrose, 1993). Mower's (1998) case study of sudden onset and subsequent remission in a young boy (age 30 months) provides a detailed example that seems to be best explained by factors of insecurity and sensitivity to such environmental changes.

Clinical **Decision-Making**

We recently had the opportunity to observe a young girl (age 30 months) who also responded to a series of environmental changes. This situation was unique for two reasons. This young female was one of two identical twin girls, and the differential response of the children to environmental factors in spite of similar genetics seems to illustrate the interaction of genetics and environment. In addition, the mother was an experienced counselor and was able to provide detailed information prior to and following our initial contact with the family.

The initial contact with the family occurred via e-mail and telephone on November 6 with the mother. The parents had a 5-year-old son and the identical twin girls, aged 2.5 years. Both girls had acquired speech early, had a large vocabulary, and were extremely verbal and outgoing, interacting with others easily. The family had recently moved to Memphis from Seattle. The mother explained that, along with all the events associated with the move, their lives had been moving at a faster pace than usual for the last few months, but with no apparent stress on the children.

During the initial phone call, I asked the mother about when her daughter had begun to stutter, to which she replied, "Three Thursdays ago at noon." She explained that she and her husband had been looking for day-care centers for their children. Following the return from a visit to one site, one of the girls (whom we will call Ellen) experienced an immediate onset of stuttering. The mother was with her children during the visit and nothing out of the ordinary had occurred. When her husband arrived home from work at 8:00 he immediately noticed Ellen's stuttering (her sister maintained her highly verbal and fluent speech). Ellen's stuttering gradually increased, and over a three-week period, the mother estimated that it increased in severity by 30%; a retrospective rating by the mother using a 1–10 scale rated the initial stuttering at a 6–7, with severity increasing to a rating of 8. The parents described the stuttering as consisting of elongated first letters and repetition (5–6 repetitions) of single-syllable words (I-I-I) and parts of words. No blocking was reported, but some facial grimacing was noted. The parents noted that Ellen also began to decrease her speech output, abandon words she struggled with, and refuse to answer questions unless she was asked numerous times. During the following two weeks the parents went on a trip while the grandparents stayed with the children, and Ellen's stuttering continued to worsen during this time. There was no known history of stuttering in the family. I encouraged the mother (and, by extension, the father) to slow their speech somewhat by increasing pause time, to acknowledge the disfluencies during obvious struggle or frustration by Ellen, to maintain eye contact during the stuttering, and to not ask the child to produce the words fluently. I also suggested some choral reading together, along with encouragement for the child to say words that she was beginning to avoid or abandon.

(continues)

The parents supplied us with a videotape that they recorded a few days later and which we reviewed on November 12. We noted 22% words stuttered, examples of pitch rise, glottal fry, word and part-word repetitions, a few phrase repetitions, blocking, and facial tension/grimacing. Some repetitions were as long as 17 iterations, and the longest disfluencies were 10 seconds in duration. There were some examples of abandonment of words following initial blocking as Ellen attempted to say some words. When observing the tape, we noted that the mother was frequently interrupting the child, using demand speech with many "why" questions. Although the style of communication may have only been typical of this taping, the mother was using complex language. The mother would ask questions and the child would comply in response and there was relatively little conversational speech.

On November 14, the parents brought both girls in for a formal evaluation. The children interacted easily with the parents and the three examiners. The parents reported that the day prior to the evaluation Ellen experienced an increase in fluency. This was confirmed by a neighbor who often kept the children. The improvement occurred over a 24-hour period and continued for a week. During this time the parent rated Ellen's stuttering at a 2–3 on a 10-point scale (except for one day when the parents gave her a rating of 6). The parents reported, however, that Ellen continued to "hold her mouth awkwardly and elongate the first letter of words." The parents also reported that they had been diligent about slowing their speech by increasing pause time, asking fewer questions, and using choral speech when reading together.

Observation and video recording during the evaluation indicated a severity of 3–4 with some posturing and whole-word repetitions and 1–2 second prolongations. The mother noted, however, that Ellen continued to be unusually quiet and was not as outgoing as in the past. Along with the suggestions from the previous week, we asked the parents to use less demand speech, including "why" questions if this was typical, and to follow the child's lead during conversational speech. The parents agreed to follow our recommendations, obtain video samples of both girls, and to keep weekly/daily severity ratings on a 1–10 scale.

On November 25, the mother reported to us that Ellen had regained complete fluency within two days following the formal evaluation and had experienced no other episodes. Both girls were now equally verbal and outgoing with no examples of stuttering behavior. On December 21, the mother again reported "absolutely no stutter" other than "very minor elongations of initial sounds, at most, two times a day." The mother reported that she was thrilled with Ellen's progress.

During the first week of April the following year, the mother reported via e-mail that Ellen spontaneously began stuttering again. The stuttering was "fairly significant," and she rated it at 6–7 on the 10-point scale. The stuttering lasted all day and was exactly like before. The stuttering continued like this for approximately two and one-half weeks and then stopped "fairly abruptly" (within two days). During the month of May, Ellen produced very little to no stuttering. As of this writing (30 months later), Ellen continues to have the same highly fluent speech as she did prior to the initial call two years ago.

Less Influential Factors

Physical Development and Illness

Children who stutter have the same general physical makeup as normally fluent children. There is no evidence that children who stutter are distinctive in
terms of general developmental milestones such as ages of teething and wean-
ing, or in developing the ability to dress and feed themselves, acquire bowel
and bladder control, sit, creep, stand, and walk (Andrews & Harris, 1964;
Cox, Seider, & Kidd, 1984). Yairi and Ambrose (2005) did note that 14%
of the parents in their Early Experimental Group reported that their children
experienced illness or excessive fatigue just prior to stuttering.

On occasion, parents will indicate that stuttering began following an illness.
As Silverman (1996) points out, if the illness affects the central nervous system, a
cause-and-effect relationship between the illness and the onset of stuttering may
be possible. However, children who stutter do not appear to have more illnesses
than those that do not (Andrews & Harris, 1964; Johnson & Associates, 1959).
Illness may, however, influence the nature and severity of stuttering in those
who already stutter. It is difficult for children to maintain the energy to monitor
speech production and use fluency-enhancing techniques when they are sick and
resistance and energy are low (Luchsinger & Arnold, 1965; Van Riper, 1978).

Culture, Nationality, and Socioeconomic Status

Some descriptive research has found a higher occurrence of stuttering in African-
American than Caucasian populations (Gillespie & Cooper, 1973; Dyker &
Pindzola, 1995). However, Proctor, Duff, Patterson, and Yairi (2001) surveyed
3,404 preschoolers, including 2,223 African-Americans, 943 European-
Americans, and 239 others. Using individual speech screenings and teacher
reports, they found prevalence figures of 2.46% overall with no group
differences for African-American and European-American or other minorities.
A comprehensive review describing the relative occurrence of stuttering
according to both culture and race is provided by Van Riper (1982).

The relatively few data that are available concerning the possible effect of
a child's socioeconomic status suggest that stuttering is present at the same
frequency of occurrence in all socioeconomic groups. Undoubtedly, factors of
socioeconomic level and race interact with—and cloud—this issue. A lack of
diagnostic and treatment services is likely to result in an underestimate of the
occurrence of stuttering for certain populations in lower socioeconomic categories. It may also be that those in upper socioeconomic categories are more
informed about and economically capable of obtaining assistance. Bloodstein
(1987) suggests that the occurrence of stuttering may be related to the imposi-
tion of high standards for the achievement of status and prestige, along with the

intolerance of deviancy; values that may vary depending on the socioeconomic status of families. At this point, there appears to be no convincing evidence of socioeconomic influence.

The occurrence of stuttering in technologically developed countries is typically reported at approximately 0.7–1.0% of the population. The occurrence is somewhat higher in several cultures throughout the world, possibly due to a combination of limited gene pools and differing cultural responses to disfluency (Bullen, 1945; Lemert, 1953, 1962; Morgenstern, 1956; Snidecor, 1947).

Bilingualism

A review of the literature by Van Borsel, Maes, and Foulon (2001) includes the estimate that 50% of the world's population is (at the very least) bilingual. Given that prevalence figures for currently stuttering people and lifetime incidence figures (currently stuttering or in the past) are consistently reported across cultures and countries to be 1% and 5%, respectively, it does not appear that learning to speak two or more languages is likely to dramatically increase the possibility of stuttering. However, early research did suggest that this was the case. Travis, Johnson, and Shover (1937) analyzed reading and conversational speech samples of 4,827 public school children (2,405 boys, 2,422 girls; average age of 8.5 years) in East Chicago, IN. The researchers found a higher occurrence of stuttering in both bilingual (2.8 %) and trilingual (2.4 %) speakers compared to monolingual (English speaking) children (1.8 %). Likewise, Stern (1948) (cited in Bloodstein and Bernstein Ratner, 2008) surveyed 1,861 children and also found a higher occurrence of stuttering in bilingual children (2.16 %) than monolinguals (1.66 %).

More recent investigations have failed to support these earlier findings. For example, Au-Yeung, Howell, Davis, Charles, & Sackin (2000) used a self-report procedure on the Internet and found that of 656 respondents (82.6 % bilinguals; 17.4% monolinguals). The results indicated exceptionally similar incidence figures among monolingual (21.74%) and bilingual (21.65%) respondents. However, Van Borsel et al. (2001) point out several methodological problems with the Au-Yeung study, including the lack of a definition of stuttering, which may have led to the inclusion of many other types of typical formulative or common disfluencies, as well as the possibility that many respondents were individuals with other fluency problems who were attracted to a website having to do with stuttering/ stammering. Although several authors have recommended additional study, given the equivocal results and the methodological problems of the relatively few published investigations on this issue, Bloodstein and Bernstein Ratner (2008) concluded that there was no solid indication that being a bilingual speaker is a risk factor for stuttering.

Based on their review of the literature, Van Borsel et al. (2001) did conclude that stuttering is probably more prevalent in bilingual than in monolingual speakers, although there are many possible factors that could contribute to such differences (e.g., the child being exposed to mixed linguistic input or being placed in a new cultural or living situation). Van Borsel et al. offer some preliminary diagnostic and therapeutic guidelines. Indicators of bilingual stuttering include disfluencies occurring in both languages, the presence of secondary behavior and/or negative feelings and attitudes about communication, and a family history of stuttering. In instances where bilingual children are found to be stuttering in one or more languages, it is advisable for the clinician to acquire the assistance of a native speaker of the language that the clinician has not mastered in order to distinguish stuttering from more typical or formulative disfluencies. There have been a few case study presentations indicating that treatment may be more effective if it is initiated in the speaker's predominant or most proficiently mastered language (Shenker, Conte, Gingras, Courcey & Polomeno, 1998; Scott Trautman & Keller, 2000). Finally, Van Borsel et al. conclude that there is inconclusive evidence that a successful therapy outcome is more or less likely for bilingual speakers who stutter than for monolingual speakers.

Imitation

Although it is not unusual for clinicians to be asked if their child could be stuttering as a result of hearing a playmate who also stutters, there is little evidence to support this possibility. In his review of clinical cases, Van Riper (1982) indicated that although there were several instances where imitation appeared to be involved in the onset of stuttering, only one case appeared to be finally attributed to this cause. However, Otsuki (1958, as cited by Silverman, 1992) reported that in Japan, imitation was viewed as a major causal factor in 70% of his cases. The strongest arguments against imitation are the unique characteristics of each individual's pattern of stuttering and that the early forms of stuttering are frequently dissimilar from the more advanced forms.

Conclusion

The many attempts to provide a definition of stuttering can provide a confusing picture to students and professionals alike. For individuals seeking information so that they may help themselves or their children in dealing with the problem, the search is even more daunting and often frustrating. The different interpretations of what stuttering is (and is not) indicates the complexity of the problem. The stereotypes assigned to people who stutter, as with most stereotypes, may convey some elements of truth, but are generally inaccurate and naïve concerning the true nature of the problem. Newer descriptions by such organizations as the World Health Organization provide more comprehensive and accurate explanations of stuttering by incorporating the cognitive and affective features of the problem.

The features of stuttering that are on the surface are the primary characteristics that most listeners use to differentiate speakers who are stuttering from those that are not. The stuttering-like disfluencies (SLDs) of young speakers at the outset of stuttering are, for the most part, distinguishable from the more usual fluency breaks of their typically fluent peers. Beyond these more obvious characteristics, however, are many important cognitive and emotional reactions to the experience of stuttering that begin to occur even for young speakers. Young children who are just beginning to stutter are not only aware of the difficulties they are having in generating a fluent sequence of sounds and words but they are also likely to assign a negative emotional valuation to the experience. For many years, a common sequence of development was thought to prevail for children who had begun to stutter with young speakers gradually moving from effortless fluency breaks to progressively greater awareness, effort, and struggle. More recent longitudinal investigations, particularly from the University of Illinois Stuttering Research Program, indicate that many children begin stuttering abruptly (within one or two days) and with obvious awareness and struggle.

Many factors have been associated with both onset and development that appear to have little influence on the development of stuttering. Other factors, particularly those of speaker gender, age, familial genetic factors, and phonological ability, appear to play a stronger role in influencing the nature of how the problem develops. As we will see in the following chapters, as stuttering continues to evolve, the speaker's manner of coping with the problem can have an extensive and sometimes negative impact on the individual's self-interpretation and response to nearly all aspects of life. Having begun to describe some of the basic concepts and terminology, we now begin to consider models of etiology in more detail.

Topics for Discussion

1. Describe some common stereotypes that listeners often have about people who stutter. Based on your experience, how well do these views describe people that you know who stutter?

2. Write a description of the "the look" you receive from several listeners as you portray a speaker with moderate-to-severe stuttering behavior.

3. What are the various dimensions of speech fluency suggested by Starkweather? What are your thoughts about your ability across each of the dimensions?

4. What are the primary categories that help to distinguish stuttering from more usual fluency breaks in young children?

5. While counting from 1 to 10, produce examples of clustering behavior.

6. What nonverbal behaviors may be useful for distinguishing between children who are stuttering and those with more usual fluency breaks?

7. What conditions or events, although they have not been shown to be particularly influential in the etiology of stuttering, may be associated with stuttering onset by parents?

8. Select a definition of stuttering and describe why you think it would be the best one to use when explaining stuttering to the parents of a stuttering child.

9. Develop two brief definitions of stuttering based on (a) your understanding prior to reading this chapter and (b) your understanding having considered the explanations provided in this chapter.

Recommended Readings

Guitar, B. (2006). Developmental, environmental, and learning factors, Chapter 3 (pp. 71–103). In Guitar, B. (2006). *Stuttering: An integrated approach to its nature and treatment* (3rd ed.). Baltimore, MD: Williams & Wilkins

Yairi, E. (2004). The formative years of stuttering: A changing portrait. *Contemporary Issues in Communication Science and Disorders, 31*, 92–104.

Yairi, E., & Ambrose, N. G. (2005). The Onset of Stuttering, Chapter 5 in *Early Childhood Stuttering: For Clinicians by Clinicians*, Austin, TX: Pro-Ed.

CHAPTER 3

A Historical Perspective of Etiologies

Scientists often strive for special status by claiming a unique form of "objectivity" inherent in a supposedly universal procedure called *the* scientific method. . . . This image may be beguiling, but the claim is chimerical, and ultimately haughty and divisive. For the myth of pure perception raises scientists to a pinnacle above all other struggling intellectuals, who must remain mired in constraints of culture and psyche. (p. 148)

Stephen Jay Gould (1995)

Slavish adherence to a theoretical protocol and maniacal promotion of a single theoretical approach are utterly in opposition to science. (p. 217)

Bruce Wampold (2001)

. . . no model or theory will get it right all the time, and in practice, often a single theory (approach) explains only a small amount of the variance in targeted behaviors. (p. 66)

Jill Cockburn (2004)

Chapter Objectives

This chapter is intended to provide a historical context for the evolution of the many theoretical perspectives of stuttering as well as the most recent empirical advances that inform current theories. Because the variety of explanations for stuttering onset and development can be confusing to even the most seasoned of clinicians, another goal for this chapter is to describe what appear to be kernels of reality in the many different theoretical views. As it is for those who conduct research, it is also important for the clinician to have a theoretical perspective when assisting those with the problem of stuttering.

The reader will note that many of the concepts found in past theories occur again—often taking a somewhat different form—in current theories as technological advances allow increasingly more refined and sophisticated views of the human ability to produce language and speech. Each of the theoretical perspectives described will be followed by examples of empirical investigations that provide evidence more (or less) in support of each view. Another objective of this chapter is to describe the recent advances in neuroimaging and genetic research as applied to stuttering. A final overarching theme of this chapter is to suggest, as many have, that stuttering onset and development is best understood from a multifactorial perspective.

The Importance of a Historical Perspective

One of the first and most frequently asked questions of the clinician by clients, parents, and other professionals is, "What causes stuttering?" The clinician's response to this question will be the first opportunity to demonstrate his or her competence and understanding concerning the problem. The clinician's response will set the stage for the client's interpretation of him- or herself and his or her speech. Informing the speaker (and his or her spouse or parents) that stuttering is a symptom of a psychological conflict resulting from a pregenital conversion neurosis is likely to have a considerably different effect than explaining that stuttering is likely the result of a combination of genetic and physiological influences. The clinician's understanding about the possible etiologies of the problem will also have an influence on the clinician's treatment decisions. If the clinician believes that fluency failure is a result of excessive communication demands that exceed the speaker's capacity for speech and language production, some treatment recommendations will be judged more appropriate than others. The clinician's explanations concerning etiology will also influence the parents' response to their child, including how they deal with any guilt or shame they associate with their child's speech and how they respond when their child speaks fluently or stutters.

Perhaps no other disorder of human communication has been described in so many different ways. Stuttering has been called, among other things, a mystery, an enigma, a puzzle, and a riddle (Bluemel, 1957). Stuttering can look and feel very different depending on one's experience, perspective, and particularly whether one is a person who stutters—reminiscent of the often-cited analogy by Wendell Johnson (1958) about a group of blind men describing an elephant. Each arrived at a very different conclusion because they were examining a different aspect and so were unable to see the entire structure of the animal.

Similarly, because a large portion of the stuttering experience lies beneath the surface and is not readily apparent to most observers, stuttering also has been aptly equated to an iceberg with only the tip showing (Sheehan, 1970). These characterizations argue that stuttering is a complex disorder composed of many levels or factors. However, they also suggest reasons for the different perspectives and disagreements the problem holds for even the most experienced researchers and clinicians in the field. While there appears to be increasing accord concerning appropriate methods for intervention, the etiologies of the various forms of developmental stuttering and related fluency problems that humans manifest continue to be an appealing mystery as well as an attractive challenge for dedicated researchers.

The uncertainties concerning the etiology of stuttering are such that it could be argued that one sign of the competent clinician is that he or she does not casually provide an answer to the question of etiology. Glib and persuasive answers about such a complex problem may be one sign of a less than knowledgeable (or ethical) professional. Throughout history, there has been no shortage of people who were comfortable proposing simplistic solutions concerning the etiology of stuttering. Today, someone exploring the Internet does not have to travel far before coming face-to-face with such claims. These are typically accompanied by testimonials of former clients who now profess to be as fluent as someone anchoring the national news. Silverman (1996) makes the barbed—but accurate—comment that should any so-called authority propose to understand the cause, let alone a cure for all those who stutter, all but the most naïve clinicians should be highly suspicious of anything else the person may say. Some of the best experts in the field have reflected on the ambiguity of this multidimensional human problem that can so dramatically detract from one's ability to communicate with others. For example, on two occasions Conture commented about this issue.

> I don't know what causes stuttering. I also don't know the best way to treat it. I don't even know if there is one way. I'm not sure if anyone else does either. Of one thing I am sure, however: The history of stuttering reflects a multidimensional problem that has repeatedly and successfully defied unidimensional solutions. (1990, p. 1)

More recently Conture makes an even stronger statement by saying that:

> . . .stuttering is a multidimensional problem that has defined a variety of unidimensional explanations. . . . It would certainly be nice to say, for example, that we will tell our readers what causes stuttering. Yes, that would be comforting, reassuring, and a minimally ambiguous thing to say. However, to suggest that we know, in any absolute or certain fashion, what causes stuttering would be intellectually, ethically, and professionally dishonest. (2001, p. 2)

Even though clinicians and researchers may not yet have a complete answer about the etiology of the problem, it is important for the clinician to have an opinion. The clinician should have, at the very least, a reasonable response to the questions of causation and development. In a few select cases we are able to identify, with reasonable certainty, a likely cause. For example, there are instances of sudden onset, such as acquired stuttering, where it is possible to identify specific environmental or neurologic events that appear to have precipitated the problem (see Chapter 10). But even then we do not fully understand the precise cause-and-effect relationships between these events and the onset of the speaker's fluency problems. The possible reasons for the onset of developmental stuttering are even less certain, for there appear to be combinations of several factors that come together within a requisite time interval during the early phases of speech and language acquisition that contribute to the etiology of stuttering. Furthermore, the combination of factors that precipitate stuttering may vary for different people and subgroups of people who stutter. The problem, especially for adolescents and adults, is plainly not a simple one. If there were a single or obvious reason why people stutter, the answer would probably have been found long ago. Many intelligent and dedicated people have spent lifetimes (see, for example, Van Riper, 1979, 1990) searching for a cause.

Fortunately, in most cases, it is not necessary for the clinician to know the precise cause of the problem in order to provide the speaker with substantial help. Fish (1995) suggested that efforts to determine the causes of many current human problems may be unnecessary, misguided, or even counterproductive. And as Guitar (2006, p. 4) indicates, although one could spend a lifetime and not know all there is to know about stuttering, it is not necessary to understand everything in order to be of assistance to people who stutter. Moreover, although explanations about etiology vary, there are probably seeds of truth in many of them.

Although stuttering is a complex phenomenon, it nevertheless holds a fascination for most people. Students of the field only have to mention to one or more people that they are taking a course on the topic in order to elicit a flood of queries about stuttering. The initial questions will usually center on etiology, the psychological components of the problem, and the possibilities of treatment. Individuals who stutter appear with some regularity as characters in movies and books. No doubt much of the interest about stuttering centers on the mystery of the etiology and the unique, sometimes humorous, situations that stuttering can create. It is also worth noting that, as with many characterizations of the human condition, the understanding of many individuals is based on the way people who stutter are portrayed in books, television, and movies.

Stereotypes of People Who Stutter

A wide variety of groups, including speech-language clinicians, teachers, and naïve listeners, have consistently assigned negative stereotypical responses to persons who stutter (Cooper & Cooper, 1996; Crowe & Walton, 1981; Doopdy, Kalinowski, & Armson, 1993; Horsley & Fitzgibbon, 1987; Lass et al., 1992; Lass et al., 1994; Lass, Ruscello, Panbacker, Schmitt, & Everly-Myers, 1989; Ruscello, Lass, Schmitt, & Panbacker, 1994; St. Louis & Lass, 1981; Turnbaugh, Guitar, & Hoffman, 1979; Woods & Williams, 1976; Yeakle & Cooper, 1986). Several reasons have been suggested for the formation of these negative stereotypes. One possibility is that the normally fluent individuals have limited personal experience with individuals who stutter. Their views of a person who stutters may be influenced by the way that these individuals are portrayed in books, movies, and the news media. For example, Benecken (1995) argues that books, movies, and newspapers often depict individuals who stutter as possessing neurotic or even psychopathologic characteristics. It may also be that the greater mental effort required by listeners to both recall and comprehend information from stuttered speech may elicit a negative behavioral response from listeners (Panico & Healey, 2008).

Another possibility for the often negative reaction to stuttering was proposed by White and Collins (1984) and subsequently by both Doopdy, Kalinowski, Armson, and Stuart (1993) and Guntupalli, Kalinowski, Nanjundeswaran, Saltuklaroglu, and Everhart (2006). These authors suggested that normally fluent speakers interpret stuttering in terms of the negative internal states (e.g., self-consciousness, anxiety, and stress) associated with their own speech disfluencies. That is, fluent speakers infer from their own experiences of disrupted fluency that people who stutter (PWS) are chronically anxious or nervous.

This view is supported by Mackinnon, Hall, and MacIntyre (2007), who used an anchoring and adjustment model (Tversky & Kahenman, 1974; Epley et al. 2004) to explain how listeners tend to make such inferences about people who stutter. Mackinnon et al. (2007) had 183 male and female participants use a 25-item semantic differential scale (Woods & Williams, 1976) to rate two hypothetical adult male speakers. One speaker was described as an "uncontrollable trait stutterer" and one a normally fluent speaker who "temporarily stutters." The results coincided with the anchoring-adjustment model, which suggests that when people must make a rapid judgment about another person they begin by anchoring their understanding from an egocentric perspective. The researchers found, as did White and Collins (1984), that the observers interpreted stuttering by relating the behavior to their own disfluent experiences and associating the experience with emotions of being nervous, fearful, tense, and anxious. The results also indicated an adjustment process as the participants altered their understanding until a plausible (but typically insufficient) explanation was achieved. That is, there was small but significant adjustment resulting in a less negative and less emotionally extreme rating assigned to the temporally disfluent speaker. The listeners, however, because of a lack of understanding about the nature of stuttering, failed to make a full adjustment in the case of the PWS, interpreting their experience as similar to the reactions of the typical, fluent speaker (too negative). Mackinnon et al. suggested that providing listeners with a more accurate explanation of stuttering and the people who do it may help to further the adjustment process in order to understand that the speaker who stutters is basically no different than the typical fluent speaker.

What clinicians believe about the etiology of stuttering has a profound influence on the various stereotypes held by the general public (Silverman, 1992; Van Riper, 1982). A review of the research on the personality charac-teristics of individuals who stutter by Bloodstein and Bernstein-Ratner (2008) noted that the typical person who stutters is not neurotic or maladjusted in the usual meaning of these terms. Little evidence has been forthcoming indicating that those who stutter possess a particular set of character traits. In fact, there is great overlap between groups of people who stutter and those who do not in terms of adjustment and emotional health. To be sure, the experience of coping with stuttering is apt to impact the ability of most people to participate in daily activities, and for some this pattern of avoidance can be extreme. However, the natural manner of humans to conceptualize any group of people by stereotyping them limits understanding as well as the ability to provide assistance.

Clinical **Insight**

If you, the reader, have doubts concerning the attitudes and reactions of listen-ers to someone who stutters, challenge yourself to do the following. Assume the role of a person with moderate-to-severe stuttering and enter into a variety of daily speaking situations. If possible, elicit the support of a partner. With your partner to help you record your responses as well as those of your listeners, make a series of telephone calls and enter into face-to-face speaking situations. Note both the verbal and nonverbal responses of your listeners. See if you are able to elicit "the look" from listeners that people who stutter are all too famil-iar with. Rate your level of anxiety in each situation and determine if you are able to achieve some desensitization as you experience at least 10 speaking situations during a single outing. With increased desensitization you will begin to appreciate the dynamics of the situation for a person who stutters. You will also find that some listeners will react to you as though you are, at the very least, unintelligent. Listeners may respond minimally, for stuttering tends to act as a behavioral depressant (McDonald & Frick, 1954). Listeners may respond by

(continues)

being overly helpful, speaking slowly, and using excessively simple vocabulary and syntax. Some listeners may attempt to avoid you completely or respond minimally and quickly exit the conversation. Others will demonstrate both understanding and empathy.

As you consider your reactions to this experience, you will realize that you avoid certain people and speaking situations and approach others that, for one reason or another, provide less of a threat. You will, quite naturally, begin making decisions based on the prevention and avoidance of embarrassment as you present yourself as a person who stutters. You will begin to appreciate the challenges that you are asking your clients to face each day as you encourage them to change their response to their stuttering. You will realize that successful therapeutic change is about more than becoming fluent. It is also about developing the courage that is necessary to change ways of conceptualizing oneself and the experience of communicating with others.

The Variety of the People We See

Sometimes our theories result in our considering people who stutter in an abstract and stereotypical fashion. At times, our research has tended to promote a homogeneous view of the stuttering experience. Although there are likely to be some cognitive, emotional, and behavioral characteristics that commonly occur across our clients, most people who stutter are vastly more different than they are the same. Some have one or more obvious or perhaps subclinical problems that can make successful treatment more difficult. Others have many talents and abilities and are very likely to find success with many forms of intervention, or even perhaps on their own. It is important to enjoy this diversity and to appreciate the context of our clients' histories and their stories so that we can help to create a match between what they need and what we are able to provide. The following Clinical Insight box offers two examples that indicate the range of people we encounter.

Clinical **Insight**

John, was a 16-year-old who obviously stuttered. He avoided many communication situations, and the possibility of stuttering was a dominant theme in his life. John was intelligent, mature, and had a high level of self-esteem. His family was supportive and well-educated. Both John and his parents consistently attended our sessions and were responsive to my suggestions. John was willing to practice the things we discussed in his daily school and social environments.

(continues)

After seven months of weekly and bi-weekly sessions (a total of 15 sessions), he was doing well and was ready to be on his own. He continues to do well, he is fluent, and even more importantly, the possibility of stuttering is not a major theme in his life.

Sarah, on the other hand, was a young woman who demonstrated no obvious stuttering but was concerned about her high anxiety in many communication situations. She had excelled in college and was now considering graduate school. While in college she had roles in school plays and took part in debates. During our initial meeting she spoke continually for nearly three hours with relatively few instances of overt stuttering. Aside from several short pauses, during which she appeared to be formulating her thoughts, there were several instances of brief but tense prolongations. It was clear that she was adeptly avoiding certain sounds and words and, by speaking carefully, she managed to hide her stuttering. Her detailed descriptions of her communication style indicated clear patterns of avoidance and a person whose life was governed by the possibility of stuttering.

She eventually asked for my opinion about the nature of her problem, which her physician (an internist) had identified as a "social anxiety disorder." I informed her that her descriptions, as well as her speech behavior, indicated that she was a person who stuttered. I thought she might be pleased to hear my opinion. However, she refused to accept that option, in part, I believe, because of her family history as well as her cultural background. Because of her extremely negative reaction to my diagnosis, as well as out of curiosity, I asked her how she would respond to a forced choice question: "Would you rather have stuttering or cancer?" Without a moment's hesitation she chose cancer. She explained that cancer was more socially acceptable and possibly curable. I presented a choice between stuttering and AIDS and she immediately selected AIDS. It was only when I presented the options of stuttering and leprosy (which I explained in somewhat graphic terms) that she—after some consideration—chose stuttering. She indicated that she was going to seek other opinions, and that was the last I saw of her.

Theories of Etiology—A Historical Perspective

A recent summary of the many theoretical perspectives concerning the onset of stuttering by Bloodstein and Bernstein Ratner (2008) points out the many unique aspects of developmental stuttering that differentiate stuttering from other communication problems. These aspects include a relatively sudden onset between the ages of 2 and 4 (often following a period of fluent speech) and the recovery of as many as 80% of children who stutter, especially females. In addition, the reason(s) for the onset of stuttering may not be the same as the explanations for the development and evolution of stuttering as speakers cope with their disrupted fluency. That is, the behaviors and attitudes that, as clinicians, we seek to understand and treat may have little to do with the reasons for the inception of the problem. In addition, Bloodstein and Bernstein Ratner point out that while some theories focus on the onset or etiology of stuttering, others attempt to explain the nature of the stuttering event. Furthermore, many more recent theories are really earlier theories with a new conceptual framework. As these authors suggest, even in the absence of an acceptable accounting of why humans begin to stutter, a complete understanding of a speaker's experience of stuttering may allow the implementation of effective treatment procedures.

Some readers may not value the historical context provided by earlier theoretical perspectives of stuttering etiology. Silverman provides a fine justification for such reflection when he says:

> Our present views on both the etiology and management of stuttering are built upon the experience of the past. Clinicians who are unaware of how stuttering has been treated in the past are more likely to use intervention strategies that have been shown again and again to be of little or no long-term value than are those who have this knowledge. These strategies may produce a rapid reduction in stuttering severity, but the vast majority of clients on whom they are used are likely to relapse within five years following termination of therapy. (Silverman, 1996, p. 10) In commenting on theoretical perspectives of stuttering and evidenced-based practice, Ambrose states:

> The current thrust toward evidenced-based practice demands that clinicians take a position and provide an objective rationale for their treatment regimes.... Not only is the nature-nurture debate pointless and artificial, the division between researchers and clinicians is equally fruitless. (2004; pp. 88–89)

Another factor that tends to influence the nature of theories is the notion of what is currently popular. Wingate (1968) suggests that the questions that are asked in a field are influenced by the *zeitgeist* (the spirit of the times). What is published is driven, to some degree, by what is fashionable as much as it is by the decisions of reviewers and editors. Those issues that are considered important enough to be supported by available funds are influenced by the zeitgeist. Questions are researched and the results of investigations generate further considerations along a line of inquiry. The zeitgeist gradually changes and the pendulum swings back and forth, often returning to views that were thought to have outlived their usefulness. Sometimes the published articles—particularly review articles—summarize research that has pursued a particular direction for a time. These review articles, in turn, have their own influence on the zeitgeist. However, review articles may simply reflect and document changes in the zeitgeist that have already occurred. For example, views of stuttering as a neurophysiological problem that were popular during the first third of the 20th century have again achieved favor as a result of new understanding concerning normal speech and language acquisition, as well as technological advances. New research methods such as qualitative research and technologies such as neuroimaging and genetic engineering, provide new ways of asking old questions that advance our understanding of the stuttering experience and anatomical and physiological characteristics that may explain the onset and development of stuttering.

There is some measure of support as well as conflicting evidence for nearly all attempts to explain the onset of stuttering. The many attempts to formulate models that explain stuttering suggest that we are investigating a multidimensional problem. Understanding the impediments that humans encounter when attempting to produce speech fluently is complicated by the fact that fluency problems take many forms and are often highly variable. There are no absolute criteria for differentiating stuttered speech from fluent speech. Conture (1990) compares stuttering to the common cold. Despite years of trying, no one has come up with a simple cause or solution to the problem, although there is a variety of explanations and remedies. For some people, sometimes, a remedy will work. In other instances, possibly because of the interaction of the remedy and the person—or the timing of this interaction—the remedy is less effective. Each theoretical viewpoint and resulting treatment recommendations come with their own cadre of supporters. There is one major difference, however, between the common cold and stuttering. The likelihood of successfully treating a relatively brief cold is considerably better than altering an often well-established network of behaviors and attitudes that are united by the helplessness and fear found in stuttering. Excellent, comprehensive descriptions of the long and fascinating history of proposed stuttering causation are provided by Bloodstein and Bernstein Ratner (2008), Van Riper (1982), and Silverman (2004).

Perhaps the oldest view is that stuttering is a form of punishment for wrongdoing or sin on the part of the child or the parent. Undoubtedly this view continues to be held today in some cultures and socioeconomic groups throughout the world. Stuttering has been around for a long time throughout human history. There is, in fact, discussion about the possibility that Moses was a person who stuttered (Attanasio, 1997; Bobrick, 1995; Fibiger, 1994; Goldberg, 1989; Silverman, 2004).

The earliest recorded indication of stuttering is provided by the Egyptians, who used a sequence of hieroglyphics to represent the term *nitnit* or *njtjt,* which meant "to talk hesitantly" (Faulkner, 1962). The verb "to stutter" appeared in a

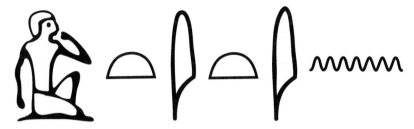

Figure 3-1   Reading from right to left are the Egyptian hieroglyphic symbols from the Middle Kingdom indicating "impediment," followed by the determinative designating human speech. From L. H. Corcoran and A. Webb, Institute of Egyptian Art and Archaeology, The University of Memphis. Reprinted with permission.

papyrus copy of a narrative dating from the Middle Kingdom of Egypt titled "The Tale of the Shipwrecked Sailor" (DeBuck, 1970, p. 100). Reading Figure 3-1 from right to left, the symbols represent the concept of "impediment" or "to impede," and the final portion, the determinative, indicates human speech. This reference to stuttering is the earliest known evidence of a human communication disorder.

The references to stuttering in this narrative tale of a high official returning to the royal court after a failed expedition include the sentences: "You must speak to the king with presence of mind. You must answer without stuttering! A man's mouth can save him. His speech makes one forgive him" (p. 212). In addition, as a sailor in the story makes his way about the island on which he is shipwrecked, he encounters a large snake who repeats phrases: "Who brought you, who brought you, fellow, who brought you? Don't be afraid, don't be afraid" (Lichtheim, 1973).

Many anatomical structures of the body, particularly those associated with speech production, have been implicated as a cause of stuttering. Examples include—but are not limited to—dryness of the tongue or problems in the hyoid bone, the hard palate, the uvula, the root of the tongue, the larynx, various aspects of the hearing mechanism including the higher auditory pathway, assorted bones of the head, the endocrine and autonomic nervous systems, and the central nervous system. The tongue, as primary articulator and often involved during moments of stuttering, has often been implicated. According to Silverman (2004), the belief that stuttering results from an abnormality in the tongue's structure, function, or both, appears to have been the most widely held view between the time of Aristotle and the Renaissance, approximately 1500 C.E.

Since many anatomical structures used in speech were thought to be the source of the problem, it was not uncommon to recommend various forms of surgery for those who stuttered. Believing a spasm of the glottis to be responsible for stuttering, Johann Dieffenbach, a German surgeon, performed more than 250 operations on the tongues of people who stuttered in France and Germany in 1841. Performed without anesthesia, the operation involved making a horizontal incision at the base of the tongue and excising a triangular wedge. As self-proclaimed experts in stuttering are fond of doing, Dieffenbach claimed that his technique was highly successful—except, of course, for those who died as a result of infection. As his claims failed to be confirmed by others, the technique was abandoned by the end of the same year (Hunt, 1861). (Interestingly, the common houseplant Dieffenbachia, known for its bitter-tasting leaves, is named after this infamous surgeon.)

Other "cures" for offending parts of the anatomy included severing the hypoglossal nerve, piercing the tongue with hot needles or blistering it with fluids, encouraging smoking as a sedative for the vocal folds, and both tonsil- and adenoidectomies. According to Blanton and Blanton (1936), such procedures continued in the United States through the first few decades of the 20th century. There is also a long history of placing objects in the mouth or next to a variety of locations in the vocal tract (both externally and internally) in order to elicit fluency. The first reported example of such an approach may be that of Demosthenes, who was told to place pebbles under his tongue and practice speaking loudly to the sea. During the past several centuries there have been a multitude of devices (see Silverman, 2004; Van Riper, 1982) that facilitated fluency by both distracting the speaker from his or her habitual method of speech production and creating altered forms of phonation, articulation, timing, and proprioception. With few exceptions, however, these devices provide, at best, only temporary fluency.

At the most basic level, models of stuttering can be separated into (1) psychological theories suggesting that stuttering behaviors are a symptom indicative of an underlying psychological or emotional neurotic conflict; (2) learning theories proposing that at or near the onset of stuttering the speaker learns that speaking is difficult and subsequently learns to anticipate stuttering and struggles when attempting to produce fluent speech; (3) physiological theories proposing that the speaker's ability to produce fluent speech breaks down, particularly in response to various forms of stress; and (4) multifactorial views that consider combinations of factors that result in the onset and development of stuttering (see Table 3-1). There is considerable overlap between many of the theoretical perspectives, with some providing better explanations of the onset of stuttering and others providing explanations of the subsequent development of the problem. Some explanations are not fully developed and do not provide relationships among variables and make predic-

Table 3-1   Types of theories explaining the onset and development of stuttering described in the following sections

Physiological	Cerebral Asymmetry
	Temporal Processing
	Linguistic Processing
	Cybernetic Dysfunction
	Genetic Factors
	Modified Vocalization
Psychological	Psychosexual
	Repressed Need
Learning	Diagnosogenic
	Anticipatory Struggle
	Classical and Operant Conditioning
Multifactorial	Multifactorial-Dynamic Model
	Demands and Capacities Model

tions and therefore are difficult to test. We will discuss the basic ideas of each view in the next section followed, in turn, by examples of investigations that speak to the veracity of each viewpoint.

Stuttering as a Symptom of Repressed Internal Conflict

Van Riper, after many decades of treating thousands of children and adults who stuttered, wrote an engaging article in what was then called the *Western Michigan University Journal of Speech Therapy*. Written in 1974, the article was titled "A Handful of Nuts" (see also Van Riper, 1979). From the many hundreds of clients he had seen up to that point in his career, Van Riper found only a very few who had severe emotional problems. These people, while they most certainly stuttered, also had emotional problems that were considerably more handicapping. His description of these clients makes for some interesting reading. However, as we shall see, there are relatively few people who stutter that have such deep-seated emotional problems.

Through the first several decades of this century, many people who treated stuttering in this country were physicians, and some of these individuals held a psychoanalytic view of the problem. This perspective was that stuttering is a psychopathology and that the overt stuttering behaviors are symptomatic of a deep-seated psychological disorder. Bannister describes this point of view in the following manner:

> . . . psychoanalytic theories seem to suggest that man is basically a battle-field. He is in a dark cellar in which a well-bred spinster lady and a sex-crazed monkey are forever engaged in mortal combat, the struggle being refereed by a rather nervous bank clerk. (1966; p. 21)

With the development of university speech and hearing centers and the creation of the National Association of Teachers of Speech in 1925 (the precursor of the American Speech-Language-Hearing Association) (Paden, 1970), fewer physicians provided treatment. The new clinicians, who were trained in the behavioral sciences, were less likely to hold a psychoanalytic view of stuttering.

The neurotic or psychoanalytic explanation of stuttering also has been termed the repressed-need hypothesis (Bloodstein & Bernstein Ratner, 2008; Silverman, 2004). That is, stuttering is seen as a neurosis, and individuals who stutter do so as a result of a repressed, neurotic, unconscious conflict. Stuttering behavior is seen as a symptom that is symbolic of this conflict. The origin of the conflict is a central question, and there has been no shortage of suggestions about the possible source. Some theorized that the source was psychosexual, a fixation of psychological development at an oral or anal stage of infant sexual development (Glauber, 1982). It was proposed, for example, that one who stuttered had not experienced oral erotic gratification as an infant, possibly due to a disturbance in the mother–child relationship. Others proposed a neo-Freudian view that the source of conflict was the result of inadequate interpersonal relationships (Barbara, 1965, 1982; Wyatt, 1969). Other unconscious and repressed needs that have been suggested take the form of stuttering to gain attention, sympathy, or to avoid responsibilities.

Many of these opinions sound strange and even preposterous to most current speech-language pathologists. The chapter by Travis, "The Unspeakable Feelings of People with Special Reference to Stuttering," that appears in the two editions of his *Handbook of Speech Pathology* (1957, 1971) provide lucid examples of this viewpoint. This chapter may represent the high-water mark of this psychoanalytical perspective. It is unlikely that a client or parent will have access to the opinions about stuttering etiology expressed in these chapters. However, the experienced clinician should be aware of these views and be able to respond to this manner of conceptualizing stuttering.

Silverman (2004) indicates that an American physician Edward Scripture (1931) was one of the first to combine psychotherapy and speech treatment that focused on changing specific speech habits. This combined approach is similar to that of more recent clinicians who are psychoanalytically based (Barbara, 1982; Freund, 1966; Glauber, 1982). According to Silverman, there has been relatively little success reported by those using a psychoanalytic approach for treating stuttering. Brill (1923) indicated that after 11 years of treating a total of 69 individuals who stuttered through psychoanalysis, he was able to claim only 5 persons cured, 1 of whom was reported to have subsequently relapsed. There is a suggestion that even Freud himself (Freund, 1966) did not believe that psychoanalytic techniques were particularly helpful in treating stuttering.

Evidence from Empirical Investigations

The psychological status of children who begin to stutter, and particularly the psychological characteristics of their parents, has received considerable attention in the literature. In order to determine the possibility that the parents of children who stutter are emotionally or psychologically different from parents of nonstuttering children, Adams (1993) reviewed 35 articles that contrasted the attitudes, traits, emotions, psychological adjustment, and child-rearing practices and behaviors of parents of children who stutter. Adams found some limited support for the notion that the parents of young children who stuttered may possess some attributes that could have a negative effect on young children who stutter. For example, Zenner, Ritterman, Bowden, and Gronhovd (1978) found that parents of young stuttering children may exhibit higher than usual levels of both trait and state anxiety. Gildston (1967) noted that parents were perceived by some of the children who stuttered as being slightly less accepting. Quarrington, Seligman, and Kosower (1969) found that parents of young children who stutter set lower goals for their children than those of normally speaking children. However, Adams found that the vast majority of investigations indicated no differences between the experimental and control parents. In fact, some investigations identified characteristics in the parents of young children who stuttered that are generally viewed as psychologically healthy—for example, parents of stuttering children were found to be less possessive and less likely to exert hostile control (Yairi & Williams, 1971).

Adams (1993) summarized his findings by addressing three questions concerning the home environment of children who stutter:

1. Do children who stutter grow up in a home environment that can validly be described as blatantly pathologic or unhealthy emotionally? Adams's answer was a certain no.

2. Do children who stutter grow up in a home environment that can validly be described as "emotionally unsatisfactory or conducive to maladjustment?" Adams's answer to this question was that he found little support for this idea.

3. Do children who stutter grow up in a home environment that, although not obviously pathologic, is nonetheless unique or different from the home environment of youngsters who develop normal speech? Adams's answer to this final question was also a certain no.

In a review of studies that have investigated the influence of both home environment and parent–child interaction, Yairi (1997) also found that the evidence failed to support the view that parents of children who stutter have abnormal personalities and emotional or adjustment problems. Yairi concludes that "it is clearly time to declare that the belief that parents' personalities or attitudes are causally related to stuttering is null and void for purposes of counseling and treatment" (p. 44). More recently, based on many years of longitudinal data, Yairi and Ambrose (2005) conclude that parents of stuttering children do not perceive their children appreciably differently than the parents of fluent children.

A series of editions of Bloodstein's *A Handbook on Stuttering*, including the most recent sixth edition by Bloodstein and Bernstein Ratner (2008), indicate that scientific support for a psychogenic perspective of stuttering onset in children is lacking. Finally, Yairi and Ambrose (2005) suggest that as part of the information provided to parents about their child who is stuttering, clinicians may considering the following:

> The best research has failed to show that people who stutter, as a group, are more neurotic or have more other psychological disorders than those who do not stutter. We do not think that your child began stuttering because of any serious emotional difficulties. (Yairi & Ambrose, 2005, p. 387)

Stuttering as a Learned Anticipatory Struggle

This view of stuttering onset has been termed the anticipatory-struggle model (Bloodstein & Bernstein Ratner, 2008; Silverman, 2004). The essence of this model is that stuttering is a learned behavior. Bannister (1966) provides this succinct, if basic, view: "Learning theory seems to suggest that man is basically a ping-pong ball with a memory." This view, at least in an informal sense, also has a long history. Amman (1700/1965) was one of the first to state that stuttering was, in fact, a bad habit. In a precursor to the learning theories of the 20th century, in the 1800s, Erasmus Darwin (grandfather of Charles Darwin) attributed stuttering to emotionally conditioned interruptions of motoric speech. Arnott (1928) believed that stuttering resulted from a learned "spasm of the glottis." According to Van Riper (1982), this was the most popular view of stuttering onset and development in both the United States and Great Britain from the middle to the end of the 19th century. For example, during this time Alexander Melville Bell (grandfather of Alexander Graham Bell) wrote a number of books suggesting that stuttering was learned. One important implication of this view was to place the problem within the arena of the educator rather than a medical professional (Bell, 1853). Dunlap (1932) also considered much of stuttering to be learned and recommended weakening the behavior by having the speaker purposely or voluntarily stutter. However, these views of stuttering as a learned behavior were the exception during the early part of the 20th century.

After several decades in which the zeitgeist favored physical and psychoanalytical views of stuttering etiology, during the middle third of the 20th century (beginning approximately in 1930) there began a gradual change toward viewing stuttering as learned behavior. Many people were entering the field at this time with backgrounds in psychology, and the majority had received their training at the University of Iowa. Many of these scholars had a profound influence on the general field of communication disorders. This concentration of researchers, clinicians, and authors led to what has been termed the "Iowa Development" (Bloodstein, 1995). A second generation of clinicians included such individuals as Hugo Gregory, Joseph Sheehan, David Williams, and Dean Williams.

The Diagnosogenic Theory

A most influential result of the Iowa development was the diagnosogenic theory of stuttering onset as proposed by Wendell Johnson. At the time, this theory provided one of the most comprehensive theories of both stuttering onset and development. Having been influenced by the writings of Alfred Korzybski in his book *Science and Sanity* (1941) and his work in general semantics, Johnson developed a "semantic theory" of stuttering. General semantics is the study of the ways in which people use words to explain their lives and solve problems. Johnson's theory also became known as the semantogenic or interactional theory (Perkins, 1990), and it had both a profound and lengthy impact in the area of fluency disorders. A key aspect of a general semantic approach to events and behavior is our interpretation of the events and our choice of labels for these occurrences. The theory held that stuttering evolves from normal fluency breaks to which the parents (or other significant people in the child's environment) overreact and mislabel as "stuttering." Two sentences contained in Johnson's "An Open Letter to the Mother of a Stuttering Child" state the essence of this view:

> The diagnosis of stuttering—that is, the decision made by someone that a child is beginning to stutter—is one of the causes of the stuttering problem, and apparently one of the most potent causes. Having labeled the child's hesitations and repetitions as "stuttering," the listener—somewhat more often the mother than the father—reacts to them as if they were all that the label implies. (Johnson, 1962, p. 2)

The theory assumed that many children, including those who eventually stutter, experience a period of effortless fluency breaks. Furthermore, when children are penalized (typically by their parents) for producing these normal disfluencies, the result is both greater anticipation and increased struggle behavior. Stuttering, therefore, is created by the listener as normal breaks in fluency are shaped into stuttering. Eventually, the speaker "learns" to stutter in his unique manner and the problem becomes self-reinforcing, eventually affecting many aspects of life.

Evidence from Empirical Investigations

As with other explanations of stuttering onset and development, there are several studies that provide support and several that do not. That is, normally speaking preschool children do tend to repeat and hesitate (Johnson & Associates, 1959; Yairi, 1981, 1982). A central question, however, is whether these early fluency breaks are normal or are the stuttering-like disfluencies (SLDs) described in the previous chapter. Although Johnson and Associates (1959) tried to make the case that the initial fluency breaks are essentially normal, the vast majority of subsequent researchers and authors (Ambrose & Yairi, 1999; Bloodstein, 1958; McDearmon, 1968; Thorneberg & Yairi, 1994; Van Riper, 1982; Wingate, 1988; Yairi, 1997; Yairi & Lewis, 1984; Yairi & Ambrose, 1999; Yairi, Ambrose, & Niermann, 1993) indicate that at the onset of stuttering, the original fluency breaks are far from normal, both in terms of quantity and quality. In addition, an extensive review of the literature concerning the role of parents of young children who stutter by Nippold and Rudzinski (1995) found little evidence that parents of children who stutter differ in the ways they respond to their children.

One of the more compelling attempts to determine if stuttering could be created by labeling normal fluency breaks as "stuttering" was an unpublished master's thesis by a student, Mary Tudor, at the University of Iowa in 1939. The investigation, titled "An Experimental Study of the Effects of Evaluative Labeling on Speech Fluency," was conducted under the direction of Wendell Johnson. It is important to emphasize that the investigation was conducted some three years prior to the initial development of the diagnosogenic theory and was not, therefore, an attempt to provide support for the theory. The goal of the study was simply to see if labeling someone as a stutterer would temporarily alter a young speaker's fluency. Although available at the University of Iowa library to anyone, it was generally unknown until described by Silverman as "The Monster Study" in 1988 (see Silverman, 1988b). In response to the reaction created by the publication in 2001 of a newspaper article describing the study and the alleged long-term effects on some of the children who participated, a thorough re-analysis of the design and analysis of the data was conducted by Ambrose and Yairi in 2002.

Contributing to the emotional impact of the newspaper account, the investigation involved children living at the Soldiers and Sailors Orphans' Home in Davenport, Iowa, a population that was frequently studied by researchers from several fields. For the Tudor study, five judges trained in speech pathology used a 5-point scale to rate 3-minute samples of each child's speech. From a total of 256 children, 12 fluent children were randomly selected. In addition, 10 children identified as stuttering were chosen. The children were divided into four groups. Group IA included five children who were determined to stutter. All five children were males, with an average age of 12.4 years. They were informed that they did not stutter and during a period of "treatment" sessions attempts were made by judges to remove the label of "stutterer" from these children. Group IB included five children who were determined to stutter. Two were males, one was female, and two were of unknown gender. The mean age of these children was 12 years. During the treatment sessions the children were informed that they stuttered and were labeled as "stuttering." Group IIA included six children who had been determined to be fluent speakers. Four were females and two were males, with a mean age of 10.7 years. During treatment these children were informed that they stuttered and were labeled as stuttering. Group IIB included six fluent speakers. Two were males, one female, and two of unknown gender. The mean age for these children was 10.7. During treatment these children were informed that they had good speech.

The four females and two males in Group IIA are of particular interest for, having been identified as possessing normal fluency, they were informed that they stuttered and efforts were made to assign the label of stuttering to these children. The study lasted for three months. During this time, the children in the Group IIA were told that they were demonstrating classic signs of stuttering and this label was reinforced by selected members of the staff. The initial instructions to the children were particularly graphic.

> The staff has come to the conclusion that you have a great deal of trouble with your speech. The type of interruptions which you have are very undesirable. These interruptions indicate stuttering. You have many of the symptoms of a child who is beginning to stutter. You must try to stop yourself immediately. Use your will power. Make up your mind that you are going to speak without a single interruption. It's absolutely necessary that you do this. Do anything to keep from stuttering. Try very hard to speak fluently and evenly. If you have an interruption, stop and begin over. Take a deep breath whenever you feel you are going to stutter. Don't ever speak unless you can do it right. You see how (the name of a child in the institution who stuttered rather severely) stutters, don't you? Well, he undoubtedly started this very same way you are starting. Watch your speech every minute and try to do something to improve it. Whatever you do, speak fluently and avoid any interruptions whatsoever in your speech. (pp. 10–11)

The teachers and staff were informed that the children in Group IIA showed definite symptoms of stuttering and were consulted a minimum of once each month in order to reinforce this label. Staff members were told that "the types of interruptions these children were having very frequently turn into stuttering. . . . Watch their speech all the time very carefully and stop them when they have interruptions; stop them and have them say it over. Don't allow them to speak unless they can say it right" (Tudor, 1939, pp. 12–13). However, Tudor reported that it was doubtful that these instructions to teachers and staff were carried out, due to their generally "low esteem" for the children (Ambrose & Yairi, 2002).

Dictaphone recordings were made of all children during reading and mono-logue samples both at the outset and conclusion of the study. The five judges rated the speech of all children using a 5-point, perceptual-fluency rating scale, and disfluencies were tabulated and placed into categories of syllable repetition, word repetition, phrase repetition, interjection, and pauses. Apparently no count was made of silent or audible prolongations.

Tudor provided a subjective analysis of the subjects from Group IIA by stating that by the end of the investigation, all six children showed varying degrees of speech disruptions and concern about their speech. According to Tudor:

> They were reluctant to speak and spoke only when they were urged to. . . . [T]heir rate of speaking was decreased. They spoke more slowly and with greater exactness. They had a tendency to weigh each word before they said it. . . . [T]he length of response was shortened. . . . [T]hey became more self-conscious. They appeared shy and embarrassed in many situations. . . . They accepted the fact that there was something definitely wrong with their speech. Some hung their heads, others gasped and covered their mouths with their hands. (pp. 147–148)

The re-analysis of the original study by Ambrose and Yairi (2002) indicates a very different understanding of both the nature and results of the study. In their concluding comments, Ambrose and Yairi suggest that the investigation provides a good example of how the quality of an investigation must be considered when interpreting and accepting the results. Although the original study presented only group means, Ambrose and Yairi provide a thorough statistical analysis of both perceptual and disfluency data. In addition, they point out the many fatal flaws in both the design and interpretation of the original data.

Of the many problematic aspects of the Tudor study, participant selection was primary. Several of the children placed in group IIA at the outset of the study—designated as fluent children who were informed that they stuttered—actually showed indications of stuttering prior to the study. The speech of participant #11, for example, contained nearly 7% stuttering-like disfluencies (SLDs) (including 5.3% syllable repetitions), and it is likely that this female, assigned to this normal-speaking group, was stuttering at the outset. In addition, no reliability measures were obtained for either the perceptual or disfluency analyses that were conducted. Furthermore, all forms of disfluencies, including those not currently considered as SLDs (word and phrase repetitions, interjections and pauses), were counted as stuttering.

Statistical analysis of the perceptual data obtained by the five judges indicated no significant differences in the ratings of the children in the four groups at the beginning or the end of the study, and no significant pre–post differences for the children in each of the groups were found. In fact, none of the judges indicated that any of the children in Group IIA (normal speakers labeled as stuttering) were found to stutter at the end of the study. Part-word repetitions, considered as indicative of stuttering, stayed the same or decreased for this group of children. Furthermore, the trends in the perceptual data indicated that the children in Group IIA *improved* their fluency while the children in Group IA (children identified as stuttering and labeled as normal) *decreased* their fluency. Statistical analysis of the *disfluency* data also showed no significant differences pre- and post-treatment for any of the experimental groups. On the other hand, all children showed a pre–post increase in the number of interjections, and four of the six children increased in the frequency of pauses. These results and the notes taken by Tudor concerning the post-treatment response of the children in Group IIA indicate the development of a hesitancy to communicate, low self-esteem, a general inhibition about communicating, and a tendency to speak slowly and carefully. The indications of emotional reactions of the children labeled as stuttering reported by Tudor are impossible to interpret because no baseline information was obtained.

Ambrose and Yairi (2002) point out that the investigation was not published, not because of any attempt to conceal ethical issues, but because it failed to confirm any of the research questions. Furthermore, the issues that today would be seen as inappropriate and deceptive and which would clearly fail to meet the current standards of internal review boards for conducting research are best placed in the context of the research community in the 1930s. The development of recent standards for the protection of human participants began in the years following WWII and, in spite of valiant efforts, did not become mandated until the early 1990s in the United States. Finally, it is clear that the investigators, Tudor and Johnson, did not intend to cause harm. As Ambrose and Yairi explain, the investigators attempted to induce a temporary disruption in fluency rather than a long-term effect, something that many investigators, for a variety of reasons, have done and continue to do. If anything, the study demonstrated that labeling someone as a "stutterer" does not have a long-term influence.

The Continuity Hypothesis

Another explanation of stuttering as learned behavior is the continuity hypothesis as described by Bloodstein (1961, 1993, 1995) and by Shames and Sherrick (1965) in their explanation of normal disfluencies increasing as a result of reinforcement. Like the diagnosogenic theory, this view also proposes that stuttering develops from the normal fluency breaks produced by young children. However, misdiagnosis and negative reactions by one or more significant listeners are not seen as part of the problem. Bloodstein suggests that both the tension and the fragmentation of fluency breaks increase as a result of communicative pressure. The development of stuttering is not a consequence of the child's trying to avoid normal fluency breaks that have been mislabeled, but as tension and fragmentation increase, especially for part-word repetitions, the pattern becomes chronic and the child is more likely to be identified as someone who stutters.

Models of Stuttering as an Operant Behavior

During the late 1950s and early 1960s, there was increasing interest in conceptualizing stuttering in terms of classical (respondent) conditioning or operant (instrumental) conditioning. Both approaches hold that the speaker gradually learns to stutter, but for slightly different reasons. With classical conditioning, the speaker learns to associate speaking with emotional arousal and the involvement of the autonomic nervous system (just as a dog salivates having learned that a ringing bell is associated with the dispensing of food). That is, through a reinforcement schedule, a previously neutral stimulus (a bell) is associated with the food. Just how negative emotion may be associated with speaking is unclear, although some children—not necessarily those who are eventually diagnosed as stuttering—may have physical or personality characteristics that make it more difficult for them to achieve fluency. In addition, some children may have a reactive personality that sensitizes them to stressful environmental events. In any case, the child learns that speaking is often difficult and begins to both anticipate fluency disruptions and struggle during fluency breaks in the manner of classical conditioning. Whether or not the initial fluency breaks are normal has been a major issue. If the initial breaks are normal, then the argument that stuttering is principally a learned behavior is strengthened. If the initial or core breaks in fluency are not normal, learning would take on somewhat less importance suggesting that—at least at the outset—the child's speech production system is unable to function normally. As we discussed in the previous chapter, the investigations of Yairi and his associates indicates that the initial fluency breaks (the SLDs) are distinctly different to the usual disfluencies of young children.

Models of operant conditioning are based on B.S. Skinner's concepts of experimental analysis of behavior (Skinner, 1953). The primary association in operant models is between a behavior and the consequence of the behavior. A reinforcement is seen as positive when the occurrence of the behavior (the operant) increases and negative when the behavior decreases. Operant models of stuttering propose that the fluency breaks of young children are shaped by the response they elicit. These theories propose that listener response to the child's fluency breaks reinforce their occurrence. The moments of disrupted fluency are then gradually shaped into greater abnormality, with associated struggle and secondary characteristics. Operant models do better in accounting for the evolution of stuttering and the great variety of avoidance and escape behaviors that often develop than they do in explaining the onset of the problem. Speaker responses to listener reactions tend to shape somewhat distinctive coping behaviors. The fact that these coping or secondary behaviors are not regularly reinforced makes them particularly resistant to change, since an intermittent schedule of reinforcement tends to strengthen behaviors, making them more difficult to extinguish. Over time, the learned or secondary behaviors such as eye blinks, head movements, tongue protrusion, or gasping for air become part of an integrated and tightly bound pattern of behavior.

Brutten and Shoemaker (1967) attempted to combine classical-conditioning and operant-conditioning models in a two-factor approach. They suggested that the initial fluency breaks occur as a result of classically conditioned negative emotion being associated with the act of speaking (and the participation of the autonomic nervous system). The negative emotion results in a disruption of the cognitive and motor sequencing of speech production. The secondary responses that help the speaker to avoid and escape from stuttering are the result of operant conditioning and soon become part of the problem.

The high-water mark for traditional learning theories was likely a review article by Gerald Siegel published in 1970. One of the foremost researchers in the field of behavioral science, Siegel pointed out that operant-conditioning models fail to adequately explain stuttering behavior in the laboratory, let alone in the real world. Although research has shown that it was clearly possible to manipulate the secondary behaviors of stuttering, clinicians had much less success in explaining the development of the core behavior of the problem: that is, the cause of the fluency breaks in the first place.

Evidence from Empirical Investigations

The early work of researchers provided encouraging results indicating that stuttering was an operant behavior and that stuttering could be unlearned based on positive or negative consequences. For example, Flanagan, Goldiamond, and Azrin (1958, 1959) and Martin and Siegel (1966a, 1966b) found that stuttering could be reduced when immediately followed by punishing loud noises or electric shocks. However, there were also many investigations showing inconsistent results that did not follow the outcomes predicted by the operant model (e.g., Williams & Martin, 1974; Martin, St. Louis, Haroldson, & Hasbrouck, 1975). No acceptable explanation has been offered for why stuttering behavior increases or decreases as a result of contingent responses. This is most likely due to the complex interaction of the speaker's many possible reactions to the wide variety of factors present in most speaking situations. Several researchers have found that responses contingent on stuttering serve to distract or highlight the occurrence of stuttering, allowing the speaker to change his or her behavior

(Cooper, Cady, & Robbins, 1970; Daly & Kimbarow, 1978; Siegel & Martin, 1966). As we will see in Chapter 9, the response of parents contingent upon the fluency or disfluency of their children has been shown to be effective in promoting fluency in young speakers. There are, however, a variety of other explanations for this effect.

Problems with the Speaker's Anatomical and Physiological Systems

The Possibility of Cerebral Asymmetry

In the 1920s a number of anecdotal reports suggested that individuals who stutter are more likely to be left-handed or ambidextrous than nonstutterers and that the onset of stuttering had occurred in conjunction with attempts to change their handedness in some way (Bloodstein & Bernstein Ratner, 2008). In response to this concept and the early understanding that, for most individuals, speech and language appeared to be associated with left-hemisphere dominance (Geschwind & Galaburda, 1985), Samuel T. Orton proposed a theory of stuttering that would become known as the "Cerebral Dominance" theory (Orton, 1927). The subsequent publication of a text by one of his students, Lee Edward Travis, popularized Orton's theory (Travis, 1931).

Orton and Travis theorized that because the muscles of the speech mechanism receive nerve impulses from both the left and right hemispheres of the brain, it is necessary for one hemisphere to be dominant over the other in order for speech movements to be properly synchronized and proposed that the left hemisphere was the more dominant in this process. They suggested that the nervous system of people who stutter had not matured sufficiently to achieve left hemispheric dominance over speech movements, and that this maturational failure resulted from hereditary influences, disease, injury, or even emotional arousal and fatigue.

Initially, research on the theory focused on investigating the handedness of individuals who stutter, and the results were encouraging. By the 1940s, as investigations yielded inconsistent findings, interest in the cerebral dominance theory subsided because there was little support for the idea that people who stutter as a group differed from nonstuttering speakers on measures of handedness or sidedness. The inconsistent results prompted researchers to develop new ways of studying the innate "sidedness"—rather than simply the handedness—of individuals.

Evidence from Empirical Investigations

The Wada Test

By the 1960s, new interest in the cerebral dominance theory emerged with the development of procedures that could more precisely examine hemispheric dominance for language functions. For example, the Wada test involved injecting sodium amytol into the left and right carotid arteries of a conscious speaker, resulting in a temporary loss of the ability to produce speech. Wada and Rasmussen (1960) found that four patients who stuttered demonstrated transient aphasia regardless of either right or left side injection, suggesting a lack of cortical dominance for speech. Follow-up studies (e.g., Andrews, Quinn, & Sorby, 1972; Branch, Milner, & Rasmussen, 1964) failed to find significant differences between those who stuttered and those who did not with regard to hemispheric dominance for language. Little research has continued using the Wada test, in part because of the discouraging results, and in part because the procedure can have potentially harmful side effects for the patient.

Dichotic Listening Procedures

Dichotic listening tasks involve the simultaneous (competing) presentation of two different signals to opposite ears, with subjects being required to repeat back what was heard in one or both ears (Mueller & Bright, 1994). As the auditory-cortical system is taxed by the simultaneous presentation, auditory processing via the primary (contralateral) pathways indicate accuracy and response time advantages for stimuli presented to right-ear–left-hemisphere or left-ear–right-hemisphere pathways. Studies employing this technique with individuals who are fluent speakers have reported a significant right-ear advantage (REA) in the recognition of linguistic stimuli (e.g., Broadbent & Gregory, 1964; Kimura, 1961; Lowe-Bell, Cullen, Berlin, Thompson, & Willett, 1970) while other studies (e.g., Kimura, 1964) have reported a left-ear advantage (LEA) for the recognition of dichotically presented melodic tones. These findings have suggested hemispheric dominance for certain psychological phenomena such as speech and language, which have been associated with left-hemisphere processing (Kimura, 1961; Studdert-Kennedy & Shankweiler, 1970) for most right-handed individuals. Furthermore, numerous studies have found REAs for both right- and left-handed subjects (e.g., Berlin, Lowe-Bell, Cullen, Thompson, & Loovis, 1973; Kimura, 1961; Studdard-Kennedy & Shankweiler, 1970) although results have not been as consistent as with the Wada test. Nonetheless, it was a logical step to employ various dichotic paradigms with individuals who stutter.

The cerebral dominance theory of stuttering (Orton, 1927; Travis, 1931) suggests that due to the stutterer's lack of a dominant hemisphere for language, his or her performance on a dichotic listening task should demonstrate a reduced or nonexistent REA or perhaps an LEA. Curry and Gregory (1969) were the first to use a dichotic listening approach with speakers who stuttered. They presented both verbal and nonverbal dichotic stimuli to adults who stuttered and a group of nonstutterers and found that on a verbal task 75% of the nonstutterers demonstrated an REA, whereas 55% of the participants who stuttered demonstrated an LEA. They reported that no differences were found between the two groups on the nonverbal tasks. Similar results have been found by other researchers (Brady & Berson, 1975; Moore, 1984; Moore & Haynes, 1980; Sommers, Brady, & Moore, 1975) using meaningful words as stimuli.

Hall and Jerger (1978) also found differences between the performance of individuals who stuttered and fluent speakers on a dichotic listening task (the staggered spondaic word test) given as part of a central auditory processing (CAP) test battery. They stated that their results indicated that participants who stuttered demonstrated a mild CAP dysfunction not associated with hemispheric specialization but found in the area of the brain stem. This finding has received support from other researchers (Dietrich, 1997; Hageman & Greene, 1989; Liebetrau & Daly, 1981; Toscher & Rupp, 1978) who found differences between stutterers and nonstutterers on selected central auditory processing subtests. Toscher and Rupp, for example, found a statistically significant difference between stutterers and nonstutterers on one of three subtests (the Ipsilateral Competing Message Subtest) of the Synthetic Sentence Identification test. They concluded that this was the only subtest that was sufficiently difficult to activate the central integrative functions of the central auditory system.

Conflicting evidence regarding the performance of stutterers relative to nonstutterers on dichotic listening tasks was found by Sussman and MacNeilage (1975). Sussman and MacNeilage used a dichotic listening task and a pursuit auditory tracking task to assess the hemispheric specialization in a group of 28 stutterers and 31 nonstutterers. The pursuit auditory tracking task was similar to that used by Sussman (1971) and Sussman et al. (1974, 1975), where subjects are asked to match a control tone presented to one ear with a target tone presented to the other ear that is controlled by either movements of a speech articulator (tongue or jaw) or by the subject's dominant hand. In their initial studies, Sussman et al. found that fluent speakers demonstrated a significant REA on this task. Sussman and MacNeilage found that those who stuttered demonstrated an REA similar to nonstutterers on the dichotic listening task, but failed to demonstrate a significant REA on the pursuit auditory tracking task. These results led them to conclude that stutterers may differ from nonstutterers in terms of hemispheric specialization for speech production but not for speech perception. However, Berlin et al. (1973) and Berlin and McNeil (1976) proposed an interpretation of Sussman's original work with pursuit auditory tracking that suggested the existence of a left-hemisphere speech analyzer involved in analysis of acoustic events that contain rapid gliding motions of the vocal tract. This interpretation suggests that the stimuli used by Sussman and MacNeilage did not possess the appropriate characteristics to activate this speech analyzer.

Pinsky and McAdam (1980) also found conflicting evidence regarding the cerebral laterality of speakers who stutter. They performed a comprehensive study of five speakers who stuttered and five fluent speakers using four experimental paradigms: dichotic listening, alpha localization, contingent negative variation, and readiness potential. Results indicated a left-hemisphere dominance for language in 9 of the 10 subjects, prompting the authors to state that "no support was found for the Orton-Travis hypothesis of a contribution of bilaterality to dysfluent speech" (p. 418). This conclusion was also supported by the results of studies by Dorman and Porter (1975) and Liebetrau and Daly (1981), both of which failed to find differences in performance on dichotic listening tasks between speakers who stuttered and those who did not. The results of other studies indicate that for individuals who stutter, control of speech production, perception, or both may be shared by both hemispheres (Cerf & Prins, 1974; Curry & Gregory, 1969; Haefner, 1929; Oates, 1929; Ojemann, 1931).

One possible explanation for these discrepancies was presented by Moore (1976, 1984). Moore suggested that differences in the dichotic verbal stimuli (e.g., syllables, digits, words) between the various studies may have influenced the results. He stated that studies that employed meaningful linguistic stimuli rather than syllables in their dichotic listening tasks (e.g., Curry & Gregory, 1969; Sommers, Brady, & Moore, 1975) did indicate that stutterers as a group failed to demonstrate an REA.

Similarly, Molt and Brading (1994) questioned the accuracy of dichotic listening measures of hemispheric specialization that used consonant-vowel (CV) syllables. They compared the performance of a group of stutterers to a group of nonstutterers on a dichotic listening task that used CV-syllables, while also measuring hemispheric activity via recording of event-related potentials (ERP). They found no significant differences between the groups on the dichotic listening measure, but they did note laterality differences between the groups based on the ERP recordings, a finding that they suggested was "especially notable in that the scalp-recorded electroencephalographic activity should reflect actual hemispheric patterns to a greater extent than dichotic ear advantage measures" (p. 149).

Evidence from Electroencephalography (EEG) and Event-Related Potentials (ERPs)

In order to provide support for his theory, Travis and his colleagues conducted a number of investigations using *electroencephalographic* (EEG) studies (see Bloodstein & Bernstein Ratner, 2008, pp. 128–132) to compare the cortical potentials of individuals who stuttered with those of typically fluent speakers (e.g., Travis & Knott, 1936, 1937; Travis & Malamud, 1934). These authors used what became the first of many techniques that represent the characteristics of neurological systems. Electroencephalography indicates neurological activity as reflected in the waxing and waning of electrical signals from tens of thousands of neurons in the cerebral cortex (Guenther, 2008). The alpha wave (8–10 Hz) is one of many EEG waveforms obtained from the cerebral cortex that indicate changes in event-related potentials (ERPs) between separated points on the scalp (Bhatnagar & Andy, 1995). Neural activity following the presentation of a stimulus is indicated by a suppression of the rhythmic activity of the waveforms. For example, the rhythmic activity alpha potentials disappear or are greatly attenuated in the presence of active cognitive processes. *Magnetoencephalography* (MEG) also measures many neurons in the cortex by employing *superconducting quantum interference devices* (SQUIDs) that provide sensitive readings of magnetic fields produced by neuronal activity (Guenther, 2008).

Several investigators have consistently found asymmetry of EEG patterns with greater suppression of alpha waves in the right hemisphere of adults who stutter (Boberg, Yeudall, Schopflocher, & Bo-Lassen, 1983; Moore & Lang, 1977; Moore & Haynes, 1980). Although many studies have indicated increased activity of the right hemisphere for adults, there have been few investigations of younger speakers who stutter. Fitch and Batson (1989) used EEG to investigate alpha-wave suppression with young (ages 10–15) stuttering speakers during auditory-verbal, auditory-nonverbal, visual-verbal, and visual-nonverbal tasks. While the 12 fluent male participants indicated no evidence of hemispheric asymmetry, the 12 young men who stuttered (with Stuttering Severity Instrument (SSI) (Riley, 1972) ratings ranging from moderate to severe) showed small but significant ($p < .001$) right-hemisphere asymmetry. In another investigation of younger speakers who stuttered, Khedr, El-Nasser et al. (2000) found evidence of both slower and more asymmetric EEG rhythms for individuals age 6 to 25.

Evidence of Cerebral Asymmetry from Neuroimaging Techniques

Guenther (2008) points out that the generation of language and speech is one of the most complex of all cognitive and motor tasks and that many cortical and subcortical portions of the brain are active during even the smallest of speech activities. Areas of the cerebral cortex in the temporal, parietal, and frontal lobes are involved in auditory, somatosensory, and motor activities. In addition, many subcortical portions (the cerebellum, basal ganglia, thalamus, and brain stem) of the brain contribute to the neural control of speech. Determining the precise contribution of any one area is confounded by the variability in the location of specific brain functions, the anatomical variability between subjects (brain size, shape, and gyral patterns), and the adaptability of the brain, as well as the data averaging/spatial smoothing procedures often necessary when analyzing images.

Structural and Functional Neuroimaging

Structural neuroimaging studies identify anatomical structures of the brain using *computed tomography* (CT) and *magnetic resonance imaging* (MRI) techniques. CT (originally called *computed axial tomography* or CAT) uses a narrow X-ray beam and computerized reconstruction to create "thin slice" images of cross-sections of the body. Structures that are denser (e. g., bones of the skull) result in lighter images than softer tissues (e.g., the brain, muscles) resulting in absorption maps of the structures (Bhatnagar & Andy, 1995; Guenther, 2008). CT scanning indicates the structural characteristics of cortical and subcortical regions indicating lesions and cerebrovascular disease. MRI creates brain images by using the magnetic properties of hydrogen atomic nuclei. The structure to be imaged is placed into a strong magnetic field and shortwave radio-frequency pulses are directed toward it. Transmission of these pulses temporarily aligns the normal random polarity of the hydrogen atoms. When the pulses cease, the atoms return to their previous alignment, and in doing so discharge electromagnetic signals. These signals are converted by a computer into shades of black, gray, and white. Because of the varying water (and therefore hydrogen) content of brain structures, MRI provides greater resolution of brain tissue than does CT scanning (Bhatnagar & Andy, 1995; Kertesz, 1989).

Functional brain imaging includes radiographic techniques that investigate the physiological and biochemical properties of the brain and include *functional magnetic resonance imaging* (fMRI), *regional cerebral blood flow* (rCBF), *positron emission tomography* (PET), and *single photon emission computed tomography* (SPECT). Functional imaging allows for better spatial resolution for cortical as well as subcortical areas; however, temporal resolution is not as good as with the previously described event-related potentials (ERP).

Based on the brain's uptake of oxygen leading to increased blood flow during activity of a region (the hemodynamic response), positron emission tomography (PET) scanning, like rCBF, uses a radioactive isotope to measure physiological events in the brain (Guenther, 2008). PET uses a positron-emitting isotope "tagged" to a natural body substance (e.g., water or glucose) that will be metabolized by cells in the brain. Brain activity/metabolism occurs in response to stimuli or tasks. As radiation is released, changes in blood flow are associated with particular areas or regions of interest (ROI) of the brain (Bhatnagar & Andy). According to Bhatnagar and Andy (1995) and Kertesz (1989), PET scans allow the study of physiological activity within the brain that directly reflects cognitive functioning. Single-photon-emission computed tomography (SPECT) also makes use of radioactive tracers (Bhatnagar & Andy, 1995) and is functionally similar to PET while not providing as much detail. SPECT has been used to determine dopamine transport and therefore has been used to study motor function in the basal ganglia in individuals who stutter (Guenther, 2008). Recordings provide images of thin cross-sections of the brain from multiple directions and indicate biochemical and physiologic properties. Radioactive iso-topes can only be used with adults and allow for a limited number of scans. In addition, the resulting signal is low-level, requiring averaging of responses over tasks and individuals.

Functional MRI (fMRI) combines the structural imaging techniques described previously with real-time representation of physiological activity in the brain (Bhatnagar & Andy, 1995), but, the scanning process involves the generation of loud noises that can be disturbing to the client. This form of imaging provides better spatial resolution than PET. There is also less risk to participants since the injection of radioactive isotopes is not necessary. Both PET and fMRI make use of subtraction analysis whereby levels of brain activity recorded during the participant's performance of a task are compared to those during a resting state or baseline task (Guenther, 2008). The results from the fMRI can be combined with magnetoencephalography (MEG) to improve the temporal resolution of fMRI. However, the fMRI procedure can easily be influenced by minimal movements of the participant. Summaries of these functional imaging techniques are provided by Bloodstein and Bernstein Ratner (2008), De Nil (2004), Guenther (2008), and Ingham (2004). De Nil explains that the objectives of investigations using these imaging technologies involve (1) detecting differences in brain activity during speech/language perception and production in normally fluent and stuttering speakers, and (2) identifying cortical patterns characteristic of stuttered versus fluent speech.

Indications of Structural Differences

The majority of the structural differences noted in the cortical and subcortical areas relate to aspects of hemispheric asymmetry described earlier. Using MRI scans of 16 adults with persistent developmental stuttering and a matched (age, gender, handedness, and general level of education) group of controls, Foundas et al. (2001) found evidence of atypical anatomy in the stuttering individu-als. Both the right and left planum temporal areas were significantly larger in the adults who stuttered, and the extent of planar asymmetry (typically larger in the left hemisphere of fluent individuals) was reduced. In addition, there were significant gyral variants along the superior bank of the sylvian fossa in the adults who stuttered. These signs of anomalous anatomy in the perisylvian fissure speech and language areas region indicate multiple loci for putting an individual at risk for stuttering. These findings of atypical anatomical structures may also suggest a form of neurological compensation for a long history of stut-tering. In other words, the anatomical differences may be the cause or the effect of stuttering.

Sommer et al. (2002) used a form of MRI termed *diffusion tensor imaging* (DTI) that provides image intensities based on the local microstructure characteristics of water molecule diffusion. DTI allows the determination of axonal projections, providing information about connectivity among different areas of the brain (Guenther, 2008). Investigating adults with persistent developmental stuttering (PDS), they noted atypical levels of gray and white matter in the area of the rolandic operculum (an area close to the portion of the motor strip that controls oral tract function) as well as the arcuate fasciculus, which links Broca's and Wernike's areas of speech production and perceptual processing. Given an observed reduction in white (transmission) matter in the left hemisphere for speakers with PDS, the authors offered the possibility that these differences result in decreased signal transmission and sensorimotor integration for speech production. A similar study using MRI technology by Jancke, Hanggi, and Steinmetz (2004) found increased volume of white matter in the right hemispheric structures (e.g., planum temporal, inferior frontal gyrus, and precentral gyrus and anterior frontal gyrus) of 10 adults who stuttered compared to 10 fluent adults. Fluent participants had greater white matter asymmetry favoring the left auditory cortex while the PWS had greater symmetry for left and right auditory cortices.

Preibisch et al. (2003) conducted fMRI scans with 16 adult male speakers (age 19–51 years) with persistent developmental stuttering and 16 controls. Participants performed both a passive (silent) viewing of a synonym judgment task and a reading aloud task. During the reading tasks 14 of the 16 PDS speakers showed activation in the right frontal operculum (RFO) (BA45), a pattern that was not observed in any of the controls. Levels of activation in the RFO were negatively correlated to stuttering severity, which the authors interpreted as suggesting compensation rather than a primary dysfunction. The authors reasoned that if RFO activation were associated with stuttering in a causal fashion, activation would have increased with the severity of stuttering. Conversely, the negative relationship suggests that overactivation corresponds with successful compensation. RFO activity was also noted when experimental participants read aloud without stuttering. Finally, an overactive response of the RFO also occurred during the passive task, indicating RFO compensation in the absence of motor speech output. The RFO was the only region of the brain that was consistently overactivated in both experimental conditions (reading aloud and passive viewing). The authors point out that the RFO, being the right hemisphere homologue of Broca's area, is a "good candidate to compensate for deficient signal transmission between Broca's area and the left-sided articulatory motor representations" (p. 1361).

Watkins, Smith, Davis, and Howell (2007) used a combination of structural and functional (fMRI) brain-image analysis with 12 speakers (eight male, four female) who stuttered (ages 14–27, with a mean age of 18 years) and 10 age- and gender-matched controls. They also scanned eight participants (five individuals who stuttered and three controls) with diffusion imaging. The participants read sentences out loud under three feedback conditions (normal, delayed by 200 milliseconds, and upward frequency-shifted by one octave). All participants demonstrated similar fMRI responses under each of the feedback conditions. Comparisons of the controls and the speakers who stuttered showed overactivity in the anterior insula and the cerebellum and midbrain bilaterally and underactivity in the ventral premotor area, rolandic opercular and sensorimotor cortex bilaterally, and Herschl's gyrus on the left. The authors interpreted these results as being similar to the meta-analysis of functional imaging results by Brown et al. (2005). Two additional findings included abnormal function of the midbrain in the region of the basal ganglia associated with excessive dopamine and underactivity of the cortical motor and premotor areas (areas responsible for the timing of speech articulation). In addition, the integrity of the white matter underlying the underactive areas in the ventral premotor cortex was reduced in the individuals who stuttered. Disruption of white matter tracts underlying the ventral premotor cortex is likely to interfere with the integration of sensory feedback and execution of articulatory movements necessary for fluent speech production. Although the authors indicate that a history of stuttering for these adult speakers may have influenced the development of white matter tracts, they argue that their results "support the conclusion stuttering is a disorder related primarily to disruption in the cortical and subcortical neural systems supporting the selection, initiation and execution of motor sequences necessary for fluent speech production" (p. 50). The results provide some support for models discussed in the following section (Alm's Dual Premotor Systems Hypothesis and Howell's EXPLAN theory).

With the purpose of following up on evidence of white matter deficiencies and reversed right–left asymmetries in adults who stutter, Chang et al. (2008) studied three groups of children: eight children with persistent stuttering (average age 132 months), seven children who had recovered from stuttering between 2 and 3 years of age (average age of 130 months), and a control group of seven fluent peers (average age of 130 months). All participants were right-handed boys with no other speech or language problems. Using MRI optimized voxel-based morphometry to determine gray matter volume (GMV) and diffusion tensor imaging to measure fractional anisotropy (FA) in white matter tracts, the authors found that in contrast to the fluent children, both the children with persistent stuttering and those who had recovered showed reduced GMV in speech-relevant regions, the left inferior frontal gyrus, and bilateral temporal regions.

As Sommer et al. (2002) had found with adults, Chang et al. noted that white matter integrity was reduced for the left rolandic operculum, an area related to oral-facial motor regions in the left hemisphere. They also found reduced left white matter tracts underlying motor regions for face and larynx in the persistent stuttering group. Although the stuttering groups had reduced gray matter volume in the left superior temporal gyrus (STG) compared to their fluent peers, the children with persistent stuttering had greater gray matter volume than the recovered children in both the left and right STG, a finding consistent with the investigations of Foundas et al. (2001) with adults. However, unlike Foundas et al., they did not find evidence of greater right–left asymmetry. The authors suggested that the increased volume in STG for children with persistent stuttering may be the result of continuing to stutter for 6–9 years following onset. As many others have suggested, the anatomical increases in the right-hemisphere structures of adults may indicate neuroplasticity as a result of long-term persistent stuttering.

The authors concluded that the decreased "gray matter development in the left inferior frontal area (Broca's area) and the STG may be specific regions of differences in children who stutter" (p. 1342). Children at risk for stuttering onset may have deficiencies in left gray matter volume while those who experience persistent stuttering may have reduced white matter integrity in the left hemisphere areas associated with the speech system. Stuttering seems to be related to the lack of development of white matter tracts underlying the oral facial motor regions on the left and corresponding reduced gray matter growth in the inferior frontal region of the left hemisphere (Broca's area).

Indications of Functional Differences

Pool, Devous, Freeman, Watson, and Finitzo (1991) collected single-photon-emission computed tomography (SPECT) to obtain regional cerebral blood flow (rCBF) data (also during a resting state) for the same 20 adult developmental stutterers studied by Finitzo et al. (1991). Their results indicated a reduction in blood flow to the frontal and left temporal lobes of the individuals who stuttered when compared to a control group. The rCBF asymmetries observed in the stutterers were consistent with cortical areas usually identified as being involved in speech motor control. Watson, Pool, Devous, Freeman, and Finitzo (1992) performed SPECT/rCBF scans on 16 adult males with developmental stuttering (a subgroup of the experimental subjects from their previous studies) and compared them to the subjects' performance on a laryngeal reaction time (LRT) task. The authors found extreme asymmetry with reduced blood flow in the left and middle temporal regions, suggesting a subgroup of the stuttering subjects for whom premotor processing is impaired.

Ingham, Fox, and Ingham (1994) reported PET/rCBF data for four adults with developmental stuttering and four normal speakers during resting, solo reading, and choral reading conditions. Their data indicated that the adults who stuttered showed increased blood flow to the supplementary motor area (left greater than right) and the superior lateral premotor cortex (right greater than left) during the solo reading condition, but that "activation" of these regions was significantly reduced during the fluency enhancing choral reading condition.

Wu et al. (1995) also studied PET scans of stuttering and fluent adults in solo and choral reading conditions. Four adults who stuttered were compared to their performance during choral speech (a fluency-enhancing condition) and to normal-speaking controls. The speakers who stuttered showed decreased cerebral activation in several unilateral and bilateral regions, including Broca's and Wernicke's regions in the left hemisphere. These results coincided with Pool et al.'s (1991) observations for stuttering speakers during a resting state. They identified a left caudate region in the basal ganglia indicating hypometabolism that was observed during both stuttering and induced fluency and suggested that this was a "trait characteristic" of a "functional neuroanatomical circuit" that may be basic to stuttering. They also identified hypoactivity in Broca's area, Werneke's area, the superior frontal cortex, and the right cerebellum and hyperactivity in the substantia nigra/ventral tegmental areas and the limbic system, which they described as "state-dependent" characteristics of the circuit, meaning that they occurred only during stuttering and not during induced fluency.

Fox et al. (1996) performed a functional-activation study with 10 adult males with developmental stuttering and 10 adult male nonstutterers, matched for age and handedness. They took three 40 second PET scans for each of three conditions: solo reading, chorus reading, and eyes-closed rest. Their results indicated significant differences between stuttering and nonstuttering subjects in both activations and deactivations for areas of both brain hemispheres. Fox et al. state that the findings suggest that the neural systems of stuttering include a diffuse overactivity of the cerebral and cerebellar motor systems, a right dominance of the cerebral motor system, a lack of normal self-monitoring activations of left anterior superior temporal phonological circuits, and a deactivation of a verbal fluency circuit between left frontal and left temporal cortex.

Not all investigators have found evidence of cerebral asymmetry for speakers who stutter. The Pinsky and McAdam (1980) investigation using dichotic listening procedures mentioned earlier also employed EEG techniques to study the possibility of differences in cerebral laterality. In their comparisons of five adults who did and did not stutter, alpha tracings from all five individuals who stuttered indicated consistent patterns of cerebral laterality indicative of localization of speech function in the left (rather than the right) hemisphere. Ingham et al. (1996) performed a systematic replication of the Pool et al. (1991) study but utilized a more up-to-date imaging (PET) technique. Participants for this study were 10 adult males diagnosed with chronic developmental stuttering and 19 adult males who did not stutter. The groups were rigorously matched for age and "body-dominance." All participants underwent three 40-second PET-acquisition scans and a full-brain MRI scan. MRI data were used to accurately identify regions of interest (ROIs) for each individual subject. Results indicated a lack of evidence for any functional or anatomical lesions in the brains of men who stutter. Ingham et al. state that their findings "do not support theories or previous research findings using other methodologies indicating that developmental stuttering is associated with, or due to, focal functional lesions (e.g., Pool et al., 1991). Nor do the present findings support the postulate that developmental stuttering is associated with an absence of normal asymmetry between the cerebral hemispheres" (p. 1222).

Changes in Asymmetry as a Result of Fluency-Inducing Activities and Treatment

An especially intriguing finding from a number of investigations is that as a result of fluency-inducing activities or treatment speakers who stutter show a change from prominent right-hemisphere asymmetry to the more typical left-hemisphere asymmetry noted in fluent speakers.

Fluency-Inducing Conditions. Ingham, Fox, and Ingham (1994) found that when four adults with developmental stuttering took part in a fluency enhancing choral reading condition, PET/rCBF analysis indicated changes in the direction of more typical activation of the supplementary motor area superior lateral premotor cortex. Wood, Stump, McKeehan, Sheldon, and Proctor (1980) reported SPECT results during resting and reading aloud conditions for one male adult and one female adult who stuttered. Analysis was conducted prior to and following a two-week trial of Haloperidol, a psychoactive drug used in the treatment of some neurogenic motor control and psychiatric disorders. The researchers found severe stuttering and significant differences in cerebral blood flow (right greater than left) between specific regions of the hemispheres for both subjects in the unmedicated reading-aloud condition and less severe stuttering and a reversal of comparative cerebral blood flow (left greater than right) for both subjects in the medicated reading-aloud condition.

DeNil, Kroll, Kapur, and Houle (2000) used PET scanning procedures to investigate 10 right-handed male adults who stuttered and a control group of fluent individuals. Participants were asked to read single words silently or aloud. Between- and within-group differences were obtained by subtracting the functional brain images obtained during the two reading tasks and a baseline nonlinguistic task. During oral reading, both stuttering and nonstuttering speakers showed bilateral cortical and subcortical activation. However, nonstuttering speakers showed greater left-hemisphere activation while stuttering speakers showed greater right-hemisphere activation. During silent reading, speakers who stuttered showed increased activation in the left anterior cingulate cortex (ACC), while typically fluent speakers did not. Stager, Jeffries, and Braun (2003) used the fluency-producing activities of singing or paced speech, finding that both fluent and stuttering speakers showed greater bilateral activation of auditory association areas and motor control areas. The speakers who stuttered showed increased activation in the left hemisphere, suggesting that recruitment of the left hemisphere may be required for the production of fluent speech.

Foundas, Bollich et al. (2004) studied 14 adults with developmental stuttering and a group of normally fluent speakers matched for age, sex, education, and handedness. MRI scans supported previous research indicating typical leftward asymmetry of the planum temporal (PT) portions of the auditory cortex for the fluent speakers and atypical, rightward asymmetry for the majority of the stuttering speakers. The stuttering individuals with atypical PT asymmetry demonstrated greater stuttering severity during baseline measures than those with typical asymmetry. Furthermore, stuttering individuals with atypical PT asymmetry experienced significantly ($p < 0.0005$) increased fluency when speaking with delayed auditory feedback (DAF), while the stutterers with typical PT asymmetry did not experience a change in fluency. The authors suggested that atypical (rightward) PT asymmetry may alter the speaker's auditory feedback and that speaking with DAF may provide the speaker with a way to compensate.

Treatment. Some especially interesting investigations have indicated a reversal of hemispheric processing following treatment resulting in increased fluency. In 1982, McFarland and Moore measured alpha-wave suppression for a group of adults who stuttered and were treated using a biofeedback design. Pretreatment recordings indicated right-hemisphere alpha suppression. However, as fluency increased with the use of the biofeedback treatment, a gradual and consistent suppression of left-hemisphere alpha waves was noted. Boberg, Yeudall, Schopflocher, and Bo-Lassen (1983) used an EEG technique to gather alpha-wave suppression data for verbal tasks with a group of stuttering clients before and after fluency shaping treatment. As expected, the typically fluent speakers demonstrated alpha suppression in the left hemisphere for linguistic tasks (Moore, 1990). Also as expected, prior to treatment the participants who stuttered demonstrated decreased alpha suppression over the right posterior frontal region. However, following a short period of treatment emphasizing fluency enhancement, Boberg et al. found normal EEG results (left posterior frontal alpha suppression).

The use of PET imaging by Kroll et al. (1997) suggested that neural remodeling may occur for adults following successful treatment. The results indicated that, prior to treatment, adults who stuttered showed a preponderance of widely distributed right-hemisphere activation in the primarily and secondary cortical motor regions. Following intensive fluency-shaping treatment the adults showed increased activation in the cortical motor regions of the left hemispheres. The authors interpreted this shift from right- to left-hemisphere activation as an indication of greater volitional control over their articulatory movements.

More recently, De Nil, Kroll, Lafaille, and Houle (2003) obtained PET scans on male speakers (13 who stuttered and 10 who were fluent) during a baseline visual stimulation task, a silent single-word reading task, and an oral single-word reading task. Participants were matched for educational level and handedness. Compared to the nonstuttering participants, baseline scans of the stuttering speakers showed elevated cortical activity, particularly in the right hemisphere for areas associated with speech motor control (the inferior frontal gyrus, precentral gyrus, and cerebellum). This high level of neural activation occurred even when no articulatory movements were taking place (silent reading), a finding coinciding with the suggestion that speakers who stutter recruit a wide range of neural resources even during simple speech-related tasks.

The adults who stuttered received three weeks of the Precision Fluency Shaping Therapy Program (PFSTP) (Webster, 1974) (see Chapter 8) followed by a gradually reducing series of one-year follow-up sessions. Mean disfluency during reading reduced from 6.07% pre-treatment to 0.76% post-treatment (7.07% to 1.61% during monologue). Immediately following treatment, neuroimaging results indicated that the overall level of activation for the participants who stuttered decreased. Activation in the precentral gyrus, right-lateralized during pretreatment, became bilateral post-treatment and left-lateralized after one year. Previously bilateral activation in the inferior frontal gyrus was replaced by a unilateral left activation. At one-year follow-up, brain activation during speech tasks, although not completely normalized, was more similar to that of typically fluent speakers.

Neumann et al. (2005) used fMRI with nine male adults who stuttered prior to and within 12 weeks of receiving a modified version of the Precision Fluency Shaping Program (Webster, 1974). All participants reduced their stuttering to 20% or less of their pretreatment levels. Prior to therapy, fMRI imaging during an overt sentence-reading task indicated higher activation in the right middle frontal cortex. Following therapy, increased activation was most prominent in frontal speech and language regions and the temporal areas of both hemispheres, particularly on the left side. The post-treatment increases in activation were adjacent to the areas identified by Sommer et al. (2002) as displaying decreased amounts of white matter. Neumann and her colleagues suggest that fluency shaping therapy may help to reorganize neuronal connections for speech motor planning and motor execution in the left hemisphere and reduce compensatory activity of the right.

A Summary of Neuroimaging Evidence

The results of many neuroimaging studies indicate consistent differences between fluent and stuttering speakers, with wide-ranging patterns of over-activation in the right hemisphere and under-activation in the left hemisphere for adults who stutter. Atypical activity for individuals who stutter are most likely to occur in regions of the brain responsible for motor planning and execution as well as monitoring of feedback (De Nil, 2004; De Nil, Jokel, & Rochon, 2007). Furthermore, the patterns of atypical activity indicate that fluency failure is more closely associated with physiological problems than affective or cognitive factors (Ingham, 2004).

A meta-analysis by Brown et al. (2005) of several neuroimaging studies indicates activation patterns for fluent speakers in the left, primary motor cortex, premotor cortex, supplementary motor area, operculum, cerebellum, and auditory processing areas. For speakers who stutter the patterns showed over-activation of motor areas (e.g., primary motor cortex, supplementary motor area). As noted by Preibisch et al. (2003) and Van Borsel et al. (2003), the activation of the right frontal operculum was lateralized to the right. The Brown et al. (2005) meta-analysis also indicates a pattern of greatly depressed activation for self-monitoring of speech.

Ingham et al. summarized the structural differences of adults with persistent stuttering by describing three consistent findings:

(1) a loss, reversal, or reduction of asymmetry between cerebral areas;

(2) aberrant features of white matter tract connectivity and tract size; and

(3) abnormal patterns of perisylvian cortical folding, including aberrant sulcal patterns and increased gyrification (Ingham et al., 2007; p. 63).

Ingham et al. also summarized the meta-analysis results across eight neuroimaging studies of cerebral blood flow using PET and fMRI technology:

(1) In comparison to fluent speakers, individuals who stutter show over-activation especially in the right anterior insula (BA 13) as well as the cerebellar vermins and frontal eye fields (BA 8).

(2) Anomalous right-dominant lateralization of the above areas and additional motor and nonmotor areas of activation not seen in the fluent speakers occur in those who stutter.

(3) An absence of auditory activations bilaterally (BA 21/22) was noted in those who stuttered.

(4) A small level of left basal ganglia activation was noted in the fluent speakers (mostly in the putamen) but was not observed in those who stuttered. (Ingham et al., 2007; pp. 59–60).

Finally, Ingham et al. (2007) suggest some thought-provoking therapeutic implications based on the current understanding of the anatomical and functional characteristics of individuals who stutter. These include the possibility of identifying the neurophysiological changes that coincide with individuals who have achieved successful management of their stuttering (including the possibility that some neurophysiological markers of stuttering persist), the possibility of pharmacological intervention to alter and normalize the levels of activation in the regions of interest (ROIs) associated with stuttering, the possibility of altering the connectivity of the ROIs via transcrainal direct-current stimulation (tDCS), the use of behavioral treatments that employ techniques shown to result in changes in brain function as described earlier in this chapter, and the use of biofeedback training employing real-time neurophysiological information in order to assist the speaker in increasing or decreasing activation levels.

As the reader has undoubtedly noted, the vast majority of studies of developmental stuttering have used adults rather than young speakers near the onset of stuttering. As noted earlier, many investigators have suggested that the asymmetric structural and functional differences that have been found may be the result of a compensatory or recruitment mechanism in the right hemisphere (Bakker & Brutten, 1989; Braun et al., 1997; Bloodstein & Bernstein Ratner, 2008; Blomgren et al., 2003; Chang et al., 2008; De Nil, 1997; Foundas et al., 2001; Neumann et al., 2005; Preibisch et al., 2003; Sommer et al., 2002; Van Borsel et al., 2003).

The many advances in both structural and functional imaging in the recent past have resulted in greatly increased understanding of the contributions of cortical and subcortical areas of the brain in the production of speech. The most recent investigations with adults and young children have been particularly useful in helping to explain the possible anatomical and functional differences that may contribute to the onset and development of stuttering. As combinations of technologies and procedures lead to better spatial and temporal resolution, greater understanding of the neural basis for typical as well as impaired speech will undoubtedly be forthcoming. Perhaps most exciting are the possibilities of cross-disciplinary studies and computational neural modeling. For example, Guenther and his colleagues have developed the Directions Into Velocities of Articulators (DIVA) model designed to replicate "the brain's transformation of the desired movement directions in sensory space into velocities of the articulators" (Guenther, 2008, p. 13). Using equations or algorithms to model electrical activity and synaptic weights of neural networks, the program is able to simulate combinations of neural systems that can be used to understand developmental skills of speakers as well the possible causes of communication disorders. Simulations of the model can then be verified using experimental results from several disciplines with the goal of providing an integrated account of behavioral findings.

Evidence from the Human Genome

For many years it has been noted that stuttering tends to run in families suggesting a genetic link for the disorder. This supposition for stuttering onset gained scientific support during recent decades and undoubtedly has implications for the studies of structural and physiological characteristics of individuals who stutter. Investigators of patterns of expression of stuttering in families, particularly in twin pairs, suggest that there are genetic influences that at least predispose a person to develop stuttering. *Concordance* is the occurrence of a trait in both members of a pair of twins. When this is not the case, the twins are said to be *discordant.*

Investigators who have considered the occurrence of stuttering in identical (MZ) with identical genetic makeup and fraternal twins (DZ) sharing only about half of their genes have found stuttering to occur more often for both children in monozygotic pairs than in dizygotic twins (Andrews, Yates-Morris, Howie, & Martin, 1991; Howie, 1981). Although concordance occurred more often in monozygotic than in dizygotic twin pairs, some identical twins were discordant, suggesting the influence of environmental factors. Howie (1981) found, for example, that 6 out of 16 identical twin pairs did not result in concordance for stuttering. In a series of investigations, Kidd and his associates (Kidd, 1977; Kidd, Kidd, & Records, 1978; Kidd, Reich, & Kessler, 1973) found convincing evidence that the occurrence of stuttering follows familial patterns, which the authors suggest can be explained by a combination of both genetic and environmental factors. Adoption studies suggest that stuttering is more closely related to whether or not a child's biological parents stutter than whether the adoptive parents stutter (Felsenfeld, 1997).

From a large population of twins in Australia, Felsenfeld et al. (2000) identified 91 twin pairs in which one or both members stuttered. Diagnostic information obtained via telephone for 457 of these individuals verified self-reporting of stuttering. Monozygotic twins were concordant for stuttering 45% of the time and dizygotic twins were concordant 15% of the time. The authors determined that approximately 70% of the variance-associated liability for stuttering was attributable to additive genetic effects, with the remainder (30%) due to nonshared environmental factors.

Dworznski et al. (2007) investigated the genetic and environmental influences for both persistence and recovery for young male and female twins. Using longitudinal information from a large study of twins in the United Kingdom, the authors used reports of stuttering by parents when the children were 2, 3, 4, and 7 years old to determine persistence and recovery. Incidence, prevalence, and gender ratios for stuttering coincided with those found in previous studies. The majority of children reported to be stuttering at age 2 were no longer reported by their parents to have the problem at age 7 (a 69% recovery rate at age 2 and 79% and 53% rates for recovery at ages 3 and 4, respectively). As expected the monozygotic twins were more concordant for all ages than dizygotic twin pairs. Liability threshold modeling indicated that both the heritability of stuttering as well as early recovery from stuttering was influencing the occurrence of both transient and persistent stuttering with estimates similar to those of Andrews et al., 1991 and Felsenfeld et al. (2000). Dworznski et al. (2007) did find several instances where monozygotic twins were discordant for stuttering, suggesting that environmental factors or differences in how the children respond to such factors may also be influential.

Studying the pattern of occurrence of stuttering in families can also indicate the form of genetic transmission. Non-sex chromosomes are referred to as autosomes. Many genetic diseases are transmitted as single gene autosomal traits, which can be either dominant (e.g. Huntington Disease) or recessive (e.g. cystic fibrosis) in their mode of inheritance. Some disorders such as hereditary deafness can be caused by mutations in many different genes, some inherited as dominant and some inherited as recessive. Common familial disorders, such as stuttering, typically involve many genes, acting individually or in concert, or genes plus environmental factors, in which case they are referred to as complex traits.

Andrews and Harris (1964) traced the family history of 80 stuttering children. They found that males were more likely to stutter than females, that females were more likely to have relatives who stuttered than males, and that those who stuttered were more likely than fluent speakers to have stuttering relatives. Several experimenters found that the risk to first-degree male relatives of an individual who stutters is about fivefold greater than in the general population (Kay, 1964; Ambrose, Yairi, & Cox, 1993; Kidd, 1984). A model based on the results of Ambrose and Cox (1997) indicated that females who stuttered were likely to have a parent who stuttered 19% of the time, while males who stuttered were likely to have a parent who stuttered 67% of the time.

Pedigree analysis makes use of a family tree diagrams across several generations to determine genetic relationships and modes of inheritance. Diagrams are created using symbols to indicate family members (boxes for males, circles for females), and vertical lines extend down to children and subsequent generations. Individuals possessing a trait in question are indicated by shaded symbols. The pedigree is drawn from the point of view of the person who first called the family to the researcher's attention—referred to as the *proband. Segregation analysis* is a statistical method for determining whether an observed trait is compatible with a particular mode of inheritance. In an analysis of the familial distribution of stuttering in the relatives of 69 school-age children who stuttered, Ambrose, Yairi, and Cox (1993) found evidence suggesting a single major gene locus for the familial transmission of stuttering (see also Ambrose, Cox, & Yairi, 1997).

Using data from a previous multigenerational pedigree analysis of 56 adult probands of European origin with persistent developmental stuttering (Viswanath et al., 2002), Viswanath, Lee, and Chakraborty (2004) used complex segregation analysis to determine a model that would provide a best fit for the original data. The authors reasoned that because stuttering appears to be the result of complex genetic traits rather than a simple mode of inheritance, a possible mutation in the major gene is expressed in the phenotype only when certain combinations of environmental and other polygenic factors are present. This combination of factors may obscure the disease penetrance of the mutation and introduce non-Mendelian disease-transmission probabilities. Based on their statistical modeling, they found that the most parsimonious model for explaining the earlier pedigree results (Viswanath et al., 2000) was an autosomal dominant Mendelian transmission where the penetrance of the dominant *allele* (one of the genes from the two parents) is influenced by two covariates: sex and the affection status of the parents. In addition, complex segregation analysis indicated that "When there is no affected parent the disease penetrance for the carrier is 38% for males and 7% for females. With addition of an affected parent, the male and female risk becomes 67% and 19% [respectively]" (p. 408). A power calculation based on linkage simulation resulted in a LOD score of 6.8 for 10 cM density genome scan markers when the model was applied to 47 pedigrees. An LOD score (a logarithm of the odds to the base 10) is a statistical estimate of the probability that two genetic loci are physically near each other on a chromosome and thus likely to be linked (inherited together). A desirable threshold for LOD scores is 3.0 (indicating odds of 1,000 to 1) and is considered to indicate linkage. These findings of a significant major gene combined with multifactorial polygenic effects (a mixed model) agree with those of Ambrose et al. (1993); however, this may only be the case for the phenotype used in this study, persistent developmental stutterers.

The *genome* is an organism's complete set of DNA, from the smallest organism (about 600,000 base pairs) to the largest (humans have about 3 billion base pairs—although so do mice). The human genome is arranged into 23 pairs of chromosomes (including a pair of sex chromosomes), physically discrete molecules of varying sizes. Each chromosome contains many *genes,* each with specific sequences that encode instructions for making *proteins.* A major research goal is to understand how the genes interact with one another and the environment. The human genome is estimated to have 20,000–30,000 genes. For more than 50% of the genes that have been discovered, the functions are unknown.

In 1990, the Human Genome Project was initiated with the goal of mapping the human genome. The project was sponsored by the United States Department of Energy and the National Institutes of Health (NIH) and was conceived as a 15-year project. With the involvement of 18 countries and with unexpected progress, in the spring of 2003, on the 50th anniversary of the fundamental description of the structure of DNA by James Watson and Francis Crick, the human DNA sequence was completed. For further information, see the website for the Human Genome Project Information, particularly the Education link: *http://www.ornl.gov/sci/techresources/Human_Genome/ education/education.shtml*

One of the many research sections of the Human Genome Project is found within the NIH's National Institute on Deafness and other Communication

Disorders (NIDCD). Coordinated by Dr. Dennis Drayna, the goal of the Family Research Project on Stuttering is to identify regions of the human genome using linkage analysis. *Linkage analysis* utilizes DNA samples to determine which variants of known markers are co-inherited with stuttering within a family. These markers are typically single nucleotide polymorphisms (SNPs). *SNPs* are variations that occur when a single nucleotide (A, T, C, or G) in a sequence is altered. For example, a SNP might change the DNA sequence AAGGCTAA to ATGGCTAA. For a variation to be considered a SNP, it must occur in at least 1% of the population. Linkage analysis determines the genes that are in proximity to one another on a chromosome (often expressed as a LOD score as described earlier). Genes found to be close to one another are more likely to be inherited together.

Understanding how inherited (genotypic) traits are manifested in behavioral (phenotypic) responses is a primary goal of the project. In addition, scientists have begun to address the ongoing discussion of the role of the nature-nurture continuum as it applies to the onset and development of stuttering. A number of linkage studies have been completed as of this date and are reported below.

Shugart et al. (2004) performed a genome-wide linkage of 68 families and 226 probands of European ancestry. These investigators obtained maximal statistical support for markers on chromosome 18 (NPL score of 5.143/LOD = 1.50). The authors state that the findings implicated a region of genes on chromosome 18 known to be associated with intercellular communication and involved with speech production in the brain. The authors also suggest that given the lack of linkage on chromosome 18 in studies of other populations, the possibility of locus heterogeneity exists mostly for groups of genetically isolated populations.

Riaz et al. (2005) investigated 46 highly inbred Pakistani families where stuttering was identified across two or more generations. Stuttering was confirmed via video and audio recordings of speech samples, and scores on the SSI were obtained from two clinicians who specialized in stuttering. Participants were required to have a minimum of 4% stuttered words or syllables. The investigators performed a genome-wide linkage analysis on 144 probands. The results indicated significant linkage to chromosome 12q (LOD = 4.61) as well as indication of linkage to chromosome 1q (LOD = 2.93). No evidence of linkage was obtained for chromosome 18 as noted by Shugart et al. (2004), leading the authors to suggest that "stuttering, like numerous Mendelian and non-Mendelian genetic disorders, can be caused by mutations at many different loci" (pp. 649–651).

In summarizing studies employing both pedigree and segregation analysis, Suresh et al. (2006) determined that transient and persistent stuttering are not genetically independent and that, as Ambrose et al. (1997) suggested, individuals with persistent stuttering may require transmission of additional genetic factors. Suresh and colleagues used whole-genome scans and high density SNP maps (e.g., >10,000SNPs vs. microsatellite markers averaging ~10cM) to detect genetic variation related to stuttering in 100 families of European descent. Of 585 individuals,

362 were males (233 adults and 129 minors) and 223 were females (182 adults and 41 minors). Speakers' stuttering was determined to be persistent if they had stuttered for a minimum of 4 years and stuttered into later childhood and adulthood. The results indicated sex-specific evidence for linkage, with females linking to chromosome 21 (LOD = 4.5) and males to chromosome 7 (LOD = 2.99). There was also some evidence suggesting linkage for chromosome 9 (LOD = 2.3 at 60 cM) and modest evidence for persistent stuttering found on chromosomes 15 (LOD = 1.95) and 13 (LOD = 1.72). One interesting finding for the linkage for chromosome 7 to males is that this chromosome has also been implicated in studies of specific language impairment and autism.

Wittke-Thompson et al. (2007) reported findings of a linkage analysis of stuttering in a Hutterite population found in South Dakota. The population is an example of a founder population, a community of people that has evolved from a small initial population and which promotes intermarriage and isolation from outsiders. Such populations are ideal for linkage mapping because these conditions promote the loss of genetic variation. Although the results did not indicate any region with highly significant statistical support, an area of chromosome 13 had the highest linkage. This is the same area associated with specific language impairment, autism, and Tourette's syndrome.

These various results, combined with a subsequent meta-analysis of the Hutterite population and a Caucasian population (Suresh et al., 2006), indicate little support for a single major gene locus contributing to stuttering. Rather, the findings provide support for a polygenic explanation whereby several genes of varying influence increase the susceptibility to stuttering.

The behavioral studies of Yairi and Ambrose (2005) described in Chapter 2, along with the most recent genetic studies, indicate that a strong family history is the single most reliable predictor of persistence or recovery. However, the issue of what is being genetically transmitted is complex and compounded by the variety of technical approaches that are used, subtle and inconsistent findings of genetic influence, interaction with possible gender effects for those who stutter (e.g., Suresh et al., 2006; Viswanath et al., 2004), and the issue of whether or not speakers who experience transient and persistent stuttering represent the same or different genetic conditions (Ambrose et al., 1997, 2004; Seider et al., 1983; Viswanath et al., 2004). Based on the frequency and length of disfluencies, Suresh et al. (2006) found no genetic distinction related to severity of stuttering. Also at issue is whether it is stuttering itself that is inherited or, more likely, a combination of physical, physiological, or cognitive-emotional characteristics that interact with developmental and environmental factors that set the stage for stuttering (Dworznski et al., 2007; Felsenfeld et al., 2000). As of this writing, only marginally statistically significant linkages have been identified, and even these appear to make modest contributions in accounting for the occurrence of stuttering in the populations being studied. These results are similar to many studies of complex diseases, with few examples of replicated findings (Suresh et al., 2006). Although intriguing progress is being made, the status of research to identify genes that influence or at least predispose individuals to stutter indicates that clinical application of genetic research is still in the future.

Several researchers have found that the disproportionate ratio of males who stutter indicates a genetic loading for the likelihood of onset as well as recovery (Yairi & Ambrose, 1999). The skewed male sex bias in the prevalence of stuttering suggests that males are more susceptible to stuttering, females are more resistant to it, or both. It may be that females will stutter only with a higher degree of genetic loading, and will also be more likely to pass it on to their offspring. Similar findings have been noted in the familial history of cluttering (Weiss, 1964) and the co-occurrence of stuttering and other related speech and language problems has often been noted. People who stutter are far from a homogeneous population, and it appears that some, particularly those with a strong familial history of stuttering, may possess a strong neurophysiological loading for the disruption of speech fluency. As noted in subsequent chapters, these findings have strong implications for treatment and post-treatment success as well as the possibility of relapse.

Disruption of Cognitive-Linguistic and Motor-Sequencing Processes

Some investigators have suggested that people who stutter experience somewhat more specific problems in processing the various features of higher-level organization and lower-level implementation of language and speech. Some models incorporate internal or external loops for monitoring speech and language output. In addition, most models relate the variety of difficulties that may impact the ability of humans to fluently express themselves to suspected anomalies in the structure and function of the cortical and subcortical neural system. Or as Bannister (1966) whimsically explains, some models of the many problems that humans experience are those of "a digital computer constructed by someone who had run out of insulating tape" (p. 22).

Kent (1983) proposed that stuttering originates in a central nervous system disturbance that results in a "reduced ability to generate temporal patterns, whether for sensory or motor purposes, but especially the latter" (p. 252). Speakers who stutter appear to lack the ability to smoothly sequence the movements or gestures of speech. There is some indication that people who stutter perform less well than fluent controls on tasks requiring the discrimination of subtle temporal differences in signals (Hall & Jerger, 1978; Kramer, Green, & Guitar, 1987; Toscher & Rupp, 1978). Individuals who stutter may be demonstrating a lack of central nervous function that allows for the control of both incoming and outgoing signals.

Other investigators have considered the abilities of individuals who stutter on nonspeech activities such as auditory and visual tracking, finger tapping, and reaction time. Several researchers have found that subjects who stutter perform less accurately or slower on these activities than those who do not. Related to this general line of thinking is the fact that many more males than females are found to stutter, with ratios from 3:1 to 5:1 often cited (American Psychiatric Association, 1994; Andrews & Harris, 1964; Beech & Fransella, 1968; Bloodstein, 1987; Van Riper, 1982). The findings of Geschwind and Galaburda (1985) suggest the possibility that because of the secretion of testosterone during fetal development, males have more disorders involving less-than-ideal development in the left hemisphere. The result is less obvious hemispheric dominance for speech activities, and thus, a central nervous system that is more vulnerable to fluency disruptions.

The Modified Vocalization Hypothesis

It was popular during the late 1960s and 1970s to attribute an inefficiency or over-adduction of the vocal folds as a core aspect of stuttering etiology. Wingate's (1969) publication titled "Sound and pattern in 'artificial fluency'" and his proposal of a "modified vocalization hypothesis" led to many investigations of vocal fold function during both stuttered and fluent speech. Starkweather (1995), although not specifically implicating the vocal folds, stated that "elevated muscle activity is itself the proximal cause of stuttering behavior" (p. 91).

Evidence from Empirical Investigations

Subsequent findings by several investigators (Caruso, Gracco, & Abbs, 1987; Conture, McCall, & Brewer, 1977; Denny & Smith, 1992; McClean, Goldsmith, & Cerf, 1884; Smith, 1989; Smith, Denny, & Wood, 1991; Smith, Denny, Shaffer, Kelly, & Hirano, 1996) failed to support the notion of a consistent pattern of vocal fold adduction or abduction during stuttering or excessively high intrinsic muscle activity during either fluent and/or nonfluent speech of adults who stutter. In a review of pharmacological approaches for treating stuttering, Bothe, Davidow, Bramlett, Franic, & Ingham (2006) cite additional investigations of laryngeal fold physiology that are not consistent with the modified vocalization hypothesis (Brumfitt & Peake, 1988; Ingham, 1998).

The Dual Premotor Systems Hypothesis

Alm (2004, 2005) expands on the role of the basal ganglia in stuttering by emphasizing their motor functions. Drawing from the work of authors in the early 1900s and the more recent work of Goldberg (1985) and Ludlow et al. (1987), Alm explains that the basal ganglia are subcortical structures in the center of the brain that receive input from many areas of the cerebral cortex and the limbic system. Tracts extend from the basal ganglia to the frontal cortex. The basal ganglia play a key role in the automatization of fast motor sequences and provide timing cues to the supplementary motor area (SMA), which in turn plays a key role in motor control and timing for many activities, including speech.

Important to the model are two associated pathways, the first a direct, medial pathway that includes the basal ganglia and the SMA and the second a lateral, indirect pathway including the lateral premotor cortex and the cerebellum. The medial system is associated with self-initiated actions, and in connection with the limbic system, motivational factors. The lateral system functions in response to sensory input based on feedback control and is associated with voluntary and conscious control. As an example, Alm associates the medial system with the production of spontaneous speech (similar to the emotionally based response of a true smile), while the lateral system is associated with speech that is mediated by external stimuli (similar to the nonemotional or "staged" smile). Normally, the medial and lateral pathways work in synergy to modulate the activity of the frontal cortex. Importantly, the two pathways function with different dopamine receptors, D1 and D2, requiring a high ratio of D1/D2 for motoric functioning. A high number of D2 receptors results in reduced inhibition of the cortex. A peak in dopamine receptors in the basal ganglia occurs at age 2.5 to 3 years, approximately the same time of stuttering onset in young speakers. It has also been suggested that the D1/D2 ratio is lower in boys. A decreased function of the direct (D1/D2 ratio) pathway results in deficient activation of the desired action, such as initiating speech movements. Impairment of the indirect pathway prohibits diffuse inhibition of the cortex, resulting in unintended movements and the impaired release of intended movement.

Stuttering occurs when various factors affecting the medial premotor system are present—impaired input from motor cortex regions to the basal ganglia, a low ratio of D1/D2 dopamine receptors in the striatum, focal lesions of the striatum or other parts of the medial system—as indicated by the findings of structural or functional anomalies that impair input from the left motor cortex (Foundas et al., 2001, 2004; Jancke et al., 2004; Sommer et al., 2002; Watkins et al., 2007). The basal ganglia are dependent on input from left lateral motor regions in order to produce timing cues for initiation of the sequential motor segments. With input to the basal ganglia disturbed or disrupted, the input from the limbic system has a disproportionately greater emotional influence on the basal ganglia, making speech fluency more vulnerable to distressing emotional input. The dual premotor theory proposes that most of the fluency inducing conditions such as singing, unison (choral) reading, and altered feedback create a shift in the dominance of speech motor timing from the impaired medial pathway to the lateral system, bypassing the instability of the medial system.

Evidence from Empirical Investigations

Individuals who stutter have been found to be somewhat slower in starting and stopping a sound when they hear a buzzer (Adams & Hayden, 1976; Freeman & Ushijima, 1975, 1976; Starkweather, Hirschmann, & Tannenbaum, 1976). Individuals who stutter also have been found to be somewhat slower when reacting to respiration (during exhalation) and articulation (lip-closing) movements. The results of a number of studies (see Bloodstein & Bernstein Ratner, 2008, pp. 166–174; Silverman, 2004, pp. 56–57) consistently indicate that people who stutter have slower phonatory reaction times (the time it takes to initiate or terminate phonation in response to a signal). In a related study, Cross and Luper (1983) found that speakers who stutter took longer than control subjects to perform nonspeech movements, such as finger tapping. In addition to the many experimenters that have reported slower responses for speech and nonspeech tasks, there are also reports of decreased accuracy for achieving articulatory targets. There have also been many investigations suggesting that adults who stutter have a neurophysiological deficit that results in an inability to achieve accurate articulatory targets or move their articulators as quickly as their nonstuttering counterparts (e.g., Alfonso, Watson, & Baer, 1987; Caruso, Abbs, & Gracco, 1988; De Nil & Abbs, 1990; Zimmerman, 1980, 1981). This seems especially to be the case for people who stutter more severely.

The Covert Repair Hypothesis

The covert repair hypothesis (CRH) (Kolk & Postma, 1997; Postma, Kolk, & Povel, 1990; Postma & Kolk, 1993) proposes a psycholinguistic perspective involving both production and perception to account for fluency breaks (see also Levelt, 1989). The model proposes that internal or covert monitoring allows speakers to detect errors in phonological encoding prior to the implementation of articulatory commands. As errors are detected, the planning of the phonetic sequence is interrupted and the correct plan is reinitiated. As a result of this error detection and subsequent covert repair of the speech plan, fluency breaks occur. While this internal monitoring and repair occurs for all speakers, Kolk and Postma propose that individuals who stutter possess an abnormally slow rate of phonological encoding, requiring more time to activate a target and resulting in a greater chance of error. Furthermore, individuals who stutter tend to begin speech rapidly, not allowing time for their slowed phonological encoding system to select phonological targets. The process of detection-and-repair, in combination with a system that is not adept in selecting the correct phonological target before it, produces stuttering behavior.

Postma and Kolk suggest that this covert process may be thought of in much the same way as overt self-repairing. That is, the process involves an interruption of speech production and a revising of the necessary movements, followed by a new attempt with a revised plan. This hypothesis nicely explains many of the disfluencies of normal speakers and has been extended to explain the fluency breaks in stuttering speakers, for both loci (the beginning of words and syllables) and type of intrasyllabic disfluencies (part-word repetitions and pauses). It also coincides well with a number of reports of phonological-processing abilities of subjects who stutter (Bosshardt, 1990; Bosshardt & Nandyal, 1988; Postma, Kolk, & Povel, 1990; Wingate, 1988).

Evidence from Empirical Investigations

The covert repair hypothesis (CRH) appears to offer a number of testable ideas and has generated a good deal of research. However, as with other models, the reasoning is somewhat circular (Yaruss, 2000) in that the CRH assumes that individuals who stutter put demands on their phonological encoding mechanism that exceeds their (assumedly diminished) ability to rapidly and precisely select correct phonological units. Nevertheless, some studies and clinical observations have provided partial support for the CRH. Louko, Edwards, and Conture (1990) found that children who stutter also produced a greater number and variety of phonological processes (systematic or rule-governed sound changes). Authors have found that some children show an increase in speech disfluencies when undergoing treatment for articulation and phonological disorders (Hall, 1977; Ratner, 1995). LaSalle and Conture (1995) analyzed the disfluencies produced by preschool children who stuttered, providing preliminary support for the notion that both overt and covert self-repairs may interact with a child's ability to perform phonological encoding in a timely manner. Yaruss and Conture (1996) studied nine boys who stuttered with normal phonology and nine boys who stuttered and exhibited disordered phonology. All the children were approximately five years old. The researchers found that both groups were similar in their speech disfluencies, nonsystematic speech errors, and self-repair behaviors. Both groups of children exhibited similar speaking rates, and there was no association between faster speaking rates and more speech disfluencies. Neither group of children repaired their systematic speech errors during conversation, suggesting that these deviations from adult speech were not considered as errors by these children. Some support for the CRH was noted in that there were co-occurrences of disfluencies and speech errors for nonsystematic "slip-of-the-tongue" errors. That is, utterances containing nonsystematic speech errors were significantly more likely to contain within-word speech disfluencies for both groups of children, a finding similar to LaSalle and Conture (1995). A recent review of the evidence by Brocklehurst (2008) found that while the rate of phonological encoding is similar for stuttering (CWS) and nonstuttering children (CNS) there are differences in the way that CWS organize lexical information that may contribute to some occurrences of stuttering. Brocklehurst concludes that although there is not strong support for the Covert Repair Hypothesis, error repair requiring monitoring and restarting of encoding sequences may play a role for speakers with persistent developmental stuttering.

The Execution and Planning (EXPLAN) Model

In many ways, the EXPLAN model (Howell & Au-Yeung, 2002; Howell, 2004) elaborates the covert repair hypothesis by suggesting independent linguistic and motor processes. However, EXPLAN is presented as an autonomous model in that this sequence of production is not linked to internal or external monitoring. Speech is initiated by an internal cognitive-linguistic system that covertly plans (PLAN) the syntactic, lexical, phonetic features in serial order. The motor process organizes and executes (EX) the output. Fluent speech occurs when the motor system receives and executes the linguistic sequences in order. If the linguistic system experiences difficulty in generating a linguistic (syntactic, lexical, and phonetic) sequence, the motor system is unable to execute fluent speech. As a result—and this is the case for all speakers—breakdowns in fluency occur at the language–speech interface; although one linguistic plan is completed the next plan is not ready for execution. Speakers may respond by stalling and either repeating speech already produced (whole words) or pausing, allowing time for the completion of the linguistic plan. Speakers may also continue with the linguistic sequence that is available and attempt to advance forward. However, without sufficient time speakers are likely to prolong the first part of the word (e.g., "ssssister"), repeat the first syllable (as in "suh-suh-sister"), or insert a pause (as in "s-ister") (Watkins, et al., 2007).

Howell and his colleagues argue that although children who stutter are similar to controls in syntactic ability (Howell et al., 2003; Nippold (1990, 2001), there are several studies suggesting that speakers who stutter have difficulties with motor timing (Caruso, Abbs, & Gracco, 1988; Max, Caruso, & Gracco, 2003; Smith & Kleinow, 2000; van Leishout, Hulstijn, & Peters, 1996), a problem that is exacerbated as linguistic complexity increases. As with several of the models discussed in this section, the results of recent neuroimaging studies provide support in the form of structural and functional differences found in adults and children who stutter (e.g., anomalous white matter tracts in the ventral premotor cortex and functional difficulties in cerebellum).

Evidence from Empirical Investigations

Anderson and her colleagues devised novel procedures to consider the possibility that young children who stutter experience slowness, inefficiencies or dyssynchronies with lexical phonological and syntactic encoding (Anderson & Conture, 2000, 2004; Anderson, Wagovich & Hall, 2006; Anderson, Pellowski, & Conture, 2005). For example Anderson & Conture (2000) found that children who stutter (CWS) may have disparities in their lexical and syntactic abilities suggesting an imbalance among different language formulation processes.

Anderson and Conture (2004) used a computer-based sentence-structure priming task with simple active affirmative declarative (SAAD) sentences along with a speech reaction time measure. The procedure determined the time from the onset of a picture to the onset of a child's verbal response in the absence and presence of semantically unrelated SAAD priming sentences. Children who stutter (N = 32) not only exhibited slower speech reaction times in the absence of the sentence priming task, but also tended to benefit more from the syntactic primes than the 32 children who did not stutter. Although Anderson (2008) found some evidence indicating that the semantic-phonological connections of CWS are not as strong as those of the non-stuttering peers, she suggests that any problems that CWS have with speech-language production may be more likely related to lexical or phonological encoding, morpho syntactic construction or a combination of processes.

Watson, Freeman, Devous, Chapman, Finitzo, and Pool (1994) reported SPECT rCBF data for 16 adult male developmental stutterers and 10 adult male nonstutterers. These groups represented subgroups of both stutterers and controls from the Pool et al. (1991) study. Individuals who stuttered were further separated into groups that performed at normal or below normal levels on linguistic tasks. The SPECT rCBF data were compared to performance on a discourse (linguistic) task. Findings identified three ROIs related to language processing (superior temporal, middle temporal, and inferior frontal). No rCBF differences were found between nonstutterers and stutterers who performed normally on the linguistic task. However, significant rCBF differences were found between the linguistically impaired stutterers and the normal controls in the middle temporal and inferior frontal ROIs. Watson et al. (1994) suggested that these findings indicate a subgroup of stuttering speakers who have involvement of linguistic processing areas of the brain. However, the studies by the Watson et al. research group have been criticized on methodological grounds (e.g., Viswanath, Rosenfield, & Nudelman, 1992; Fox, Lancaster, & Ingham, 1993) regarding the appropriateness of control groups used, analytical techniques chosen, and accuracy of scanning procedures.

In a series of studies using event-related potentials (ERP) to investigate linguistic function, Weber-Fox and her colleagues found evidence of difficulty in lexical or syntactic processing for individuals who stutter. Weber-Fox (2001) found that in contrast to fluent speakers, nine individuals who stuttered showed lower ERP amplitudes, suggesting differences in functional brain organization. Subsequent ERP data from Cuadrado and Weber-Fox (2003) suggested that individuals who stutter have atypical syntactic analysis abilities even when not required to produce spoken language. Weber-Fox, Spencer, Spruill, and Smith (2004) found right-hemisphere asymmetry during judgments of rhyming for word pairs with contrasting phonologic and orthographic characteristics that did or did not rhyme.

Salmelin et al. (2000) using magnetoencephalography (MEG) found that while fluent speakers first processed the articulatory planning of nonstuttered words in Broca's area followed by motor execution in the central sulcus and premotor area, participants who stuttered indicated a partially reversed pattern of activation for these areas.

Cybernetic and Feedback Models

The nature of auditory feedback in those who stutter is another feature that has been the subject of research. Cybernetic theory has to do with the automatic control inherent in many mechanical and biological systems. Many such systems incorporate various forms of feedback that are used to regulate the output of a system—similar, for example, to a thermostat that is part of a closed-loop arrangement that controls the temperature of a building. The goal of such a system, termed a *servosystem,* is to match the intended output to the actual output and reduce any differences that are detected between the two—the error signal—to zero. If for some reason there is a distortion of the information arriving via the feedback loop, the error signal will be incorrect. When this occurs, the system tends to go into oscillation. Fairbanks (1954) and Mysak (1960) described the nature of such systems and interpreted many aspects of speech production in this manner. The basic idea was that for speakers who stutter, the distorted feedback creates the misconception that an error has occurred in the flow of speech. Stuttering occurs when the speaker attempts to correct an error that has, in fact, not occurred.

Evidence from Empirical Investigations

Subsequent studies (Black, 1951; Lee, 1951; Neeley, 1961; Yates, 1963) provided some indication that what was occurring for speakers who stuttered was a distorted auditory feedback signal. They noted that for normal speakers, altering the auditory feedback by delaying the signal tended to produce stuttering-like behavior. For example, it was generally agreed that fluent speakers who stutter speak under conditions of delayed auditory feedback (DAF) in much the same way people do when they stutter. That is, the effect of DAF on normal speakers is to produce repetitions and prolongations of sounds, slowing of speech, pitch increases, and greater vocal intensity. In order to "beat" the effect of the delayed feedback, the speaker must disregard that signal, slow his or her speech, and focus attention to the undistorted tactile and proprioceptive feedback that is available from articulatory movements. When speakers who stutter respond (with or without DAF) in this manner, there tends to be a reduction in the severity of stuttering. Depending on how these fluency breaks are considered, there may also be a reduction in the frequency of stuttering (Hayden, Scott & Addicott, 1977). Because of these effects of DAF, some treatment programs have employed it as a way to establish fluency in some speakers (Ryan & VanKirk, 1974; Shames & Florance, 1980). Once the speaker learns to maintain improved fluency under the distorted feedback, the delay intervals are varied in the direction of instantaneous or normal feedback, and the speaker, although now weaned from the device, continues to use the slow speech along with emphasizing proprioceptive feedback.

Postma and Kolk (1992) investigated the effects of error monitoring in 18 adults who stuttered and a group of control subjects. The speakers were asked to detect self-produced phonemic errors under normal and masked auditory feedback conditions. The results failed to indicate that the experimental (stuttering) speakers performed less well than nonstuttering speakers in either the accuracy or speed of their error detection. They concluded that rather than possessing an error in the feedback loop, speakers who stutter possess a deficit in their ability to self-monitor the accuracy of their speech production. They further speculated that rather than a deficit in any speech-monitoring ability, speakers, and particularly those who stutter, may be experiencing pre-articulatory errors, which they are attempting to covertly repair as described above by the covert repair hypothesis.

Multifactorial Models

As suggested earlier in this chapter, simplistic and unidimensional approaches to understanding stuttering onset and development, while they may be easy to explain and understand, are far from adequate. As authors and researchers have increasingly appreciated the multidimensional nature of stuttering, there has been an increase of such models that describe the many intrinsic and extrinsic factors that influence one's ability to produce fluent speech (Andrews et al., 1983; Andrews & Neilson, 1981; Cooper & Cooper, 1985c; De Nil, 1999; Neilson & Neilson, 1987; Riley & Riley, 1979, 1984; Smith, 1990, 1999; Smith & Kelly, 1997; Wall & Myers, 1984). Multifactoral models by their nature involve many factors, are complex, and are therefore more difficult to understand and to test than simple models. However, they have led to many empirical investigations as well as clinical techniques. It seems reasonable to heed Cockburn's (2004) view that

> No single theory dominates behavioral change and health promotion. Many concepts in different models overlap, and some aspects of behavioral-change models have a stronger evidence base than others. The most useful approach is to combine concepts from more than one theory to address a problem. . . . no model or theory will get it right all the time, and in practice, often a single theory (approach) explains only a small amount of the variance in targeted behaviors. (p. 66)

The Demands and Capacities Model

The demands and capacities model (DCM) is appealing, particularly for clinicians, because it includes many of the factors that seem to influence fluent and nonfluent speech. From a clinical standpoint, it provides a straightforward explanation for parents of children who may be stuttering (see Curlee, 2000 and Gottwald & Starkweather, 1999). Variants of this model were first proposed by Andrews and colleagues (Andrews et al., 1983; Andrews & Neilson, 1981; Neilson & Neilson, 1987; Riley & Riley, 1979, 1984). For example, based on their accumulated diagnostic data, Riley and Riley propose a component model that describes factors that distinguished the ability of children to produce fluent speech. These components include attending, auditory processing, sentence formulation, and oral motor ability. Their assessment and treatment approaches concentrate on enhancing a child's ability to improve performance in one or more of these components rather than altering environmental demands (see Chapter 5). Other authors (Adams, 1990; Gottwald, 1999; Gottwald & Starkweather, 1999; Starkweather, 1987; and Starkweather & Gottwald, 1990) have provided theoretical elaboration.

The demands and capacities model considers both the capacities of the individual and the effects of both internal and environmental "demands" in the development of the stuttering. The model proposes that children who stutter possess genetically-influenced tendencies for fluency breakdown that interact with environmental factors to both originate and maintain the problem. The model also addresses, in a preliminary way, the fact that human genotypes (the fundamental hereditary constitution of an individual) interact with the environment to create what we observe as the phenotype (the outward, visible expression of a specific person). Recent advances in the understanding of the nature–nurture interaction (epigenesis) have yielded explanations of the multiple interactions influencing this process (see Kelly, 2000; Smith, 1999; Smith & Kelly, 1997).

In the demands and capacities model the deterioration of fluency is viewed as reflecting an imbalance between the child's current capacities or abilities for producing fluent speech and the demands placed on the child. Capacities are viewed as inherited tendencies, strengths, weaknesses, and perceptions, which may influence a child's ability to speak fluently. They are dynamic and changing rather than static. Capacities include—but may not be limited to—the general categories of motoric (the ability to initiate and control coarticulatory movements smoothly, rapidly, and with minimal effort), linguistic (the ability to formulate sentences), socioemotional (the ability to produce smooth movements when under communicative or emotional stress), and cognitive (the ability to use metalinguistic skills).

Demands take the form not only of environmental demands (external) but also self-imposed demands (internal). Examples of external demands are fast-speaking rates used by parents and other adults, time pressure to respond quickly, and competition and lack of turn-taking by other speakers. Examples

In his book *Social Intelligence,* Daniel Goleman (2006) describes the nature of epigenetics, or the understanding of how our experiences with our environment influence how genes function. Genes "express" themselves via their signature proteins only through interplay with the environment. This interaction results in the activity of genes being sped up or slowed down or even in genes being turned on or off. Citing the work of Plomin and Crabbe (2000), who describe how genes affect behavior (behavioral genomics), Goleman states that, in fact, "It is biologically impossible for a gene to operate independently from its environment: genes are designed to be regulated by signals from their immediate surround, including hormones from the endocrine system and neurotransmitters in the brain—some of which, in turn, are profoundly influenced by our social interaction." (p. 151)

of internal demands include overstimulation of language centers and demand for language performance, including the need to formulate complex sentences; excitement and anxiety; and cognitive requirements for expressing complicated thoughts. If the internal or external demands exceed the capacities of a particular child, stuttering is more likely to occur. The model is dynamic in that internal or external demands interact with the speaker's skills at a given moment. Although the child is not viewed as possessing a disorder or deficit, the skills that allow fluent speech production change as the child grows both physically and cognitively, just as internal and external demands change over time. As Starkweather and Gottwald (2000) describe, when the positive forces (either environmental or internal) outweigh the negative ones, the person will be fluent; when the negative forces outweigh the positive ones, fluency will break down. Since these internal and environmental variables have been identified in the literature as making it more or less likely that a person will speak fluently, it is reasonable to suggest that a threshold may be present that varies for different speakers.

The demands and capacities model, despite its intuitive appeal, has received criticism from those who suggest that for a variety of reasons it is not possible to test the model (Ingham & Cordes, 1997; Siegel, 2000). That is, the capacities that are suggested as being necessary for producing fluent speech are not directly measurable, and specific requirements for mismatches between demands and capacities are not defined. In addition, no thresholds are indicated for when mismatches may lead to the disruption of fluency. Finally, these authors suggest that the model invites circular reasoning: Stuttering occurs when demands exceed capacities indicating that demands are too great for the child (Ingham & Cordes, 1997).

Siegel (2000) suggests that reconfiguring the model as a "demands and performance model" would lead to empirical testing of the proposed relationships of a child's ability and behavior. However, others have questioned the necessity or value of such a change (Curlee, 2000; Kelly, 2000; Ratner, 2000; Starkwather & Gottwald, 2000; Yaruss, 2000). As Kelly (2000) indicates, performance (the execution of an action or a reaction to stimuli) may be more measurable than capacities (faculties or potential), but the interaction of the two is clear and has been inferred in many areas of scientific study, including the behavioral sciences. The demands and capacities model brings together many of the complexities that have been observed about stuttering and the people who speak in this fashion.

Ratner (1995, 1997; 2000) describes support for the model in the form of a trading relationship between fluency and associated speech and language capacities in children. She notes that a proportion of children's fluency breaks evolve from linguistic pressures that exceed their productive capacities. That is, a fluent child sometimes begins to "stutter" following intervention to enhance expressive language or phonological skills (Hall, 1977; Meyers, Ghatak, & Woodford, 1990). Furthermore, Winslow and Guitar (1994) demonstrated a relationship between conversational turn-taking and fluency for a 5-year-old child during family dinnertime interaction. Fluency increased when conversational demands were lessened with turn-taking, while stuttering increased when turn-taking rules were withdrawn. Yaruss et al. (1995) found that nine nonstuttering children exhibited a strong positive correlation between their articulatory speaking rate and their diadochokinetic (DDK) rate ($r = .81$), indicating that these children speak at rates in line with their abilities. On the other hand, the nine children who stuttered showed a mild negative correlation ($r = -.24$) between speaking rate and DDK, suggesting that children who stutter may attempt to use speaking rates that exceed their ability to rapidly and precisely move their articulators. Yaruss (1997b) found a trade-off between production rate and DDK accuracy. Children exhibiting faster DDK rates also produced more errors than children with slower DDK rates, again suggesting that children who produced more errors were actually exceeding their ability to rapidly and precisely move their articulators in a speech-related task.

Additional study may help to specify the relationships between a child's capacities (such as diadochokinetic ability) for responding to demands of rapid speech. Of course, understanding the relationships between capacities and demands and determining thresholds for fluency disruption may be particularly difficult for socioemotional and cognitive domains. Likewise, specifying and quantifying self-imposed demands will require creative research designs. Defining and testing the model will likely lead to capacity–demand relationships that are unique to particular children at different points in their development.

The Dynamic-Multifactorial Model

In an attempt to create a unified strategy for communicating about the disorder, Smith (1990; 1999) and Smith and Kelly (1997) provide a novel way of describing the multifactorial nature of stuttering within a nonlinear, dynamic framework (see Figure 3-2). They suggest that viewing stuttering by tabulating a linear sequence of disfluency units provides only a record of the surface events. Although tidy and simplistic in nature, the problem with this approach is that stuttering is a complex and dynamic disorder with many processes that underlie the surface behaviors. Using an analogy from the scientific study of volcanoes that fits nicely with stuttering, the authors explain that early volcanologists concentrated on the surface characteristics of volcanoes. That is, they counted and classified volcanoes based on the shape of the landform and type of eruptive materials. After decades of this approach, researchers began to understand that classifying volcanoes by their surface characteristics failed to explain the dynamic nature of the phenomena. A true understanding of volcano activity only began once the volcanologists began to apply the theory of plate tectonics to the problem. This explanation of what was occurring under the surface provided a unified framework for studying the many aspects of volcanic activity. Likewise, Smith and Kelly suggest that a major impediment to developing a global theory of stuttering is the belief in the "reality of the units of stuttering" (1997; p. 29). These surface units of stuttering are akin to the smoke of the volcano and fail to provide insight to the true dynamic nature of the phenomenon.

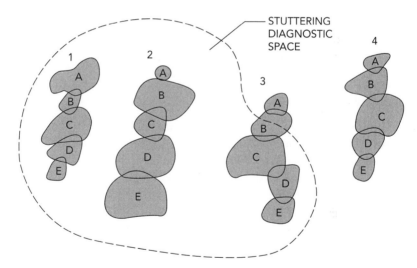

Figure 3-2   The stuttering diagnostic space is indicated by the broken lines. Each collection of the shaded areas represents an individual. Individuals 1 and 2 are both diagnosed as stuttering; however, each of these individuals has a different weight on the factors that underpin the disorder. Individual 3 has many of the contributing factors but moves in and out of the diagnostic space, while individual 4 has many of the contributing factors but is not diagnosed as stuttering. The essence of the model, then, is that stuttering emerges from the complex, nonlinear interaction of many factors. No single factor can be identified as "the cause" of stuttering. From Smith A., & Kelly, E. (1997). Stuttering: A dynamic, multifactorial model. In R.F. Curlee & G.M. Siegel (Eds.) The nature and treatment of stuttering: New directions (2nd ed.) (p. 83). Reprinted with permission of Allyn & Bacon.

Moreover, concentrating on the surface behaviors of stuttering will continue to obscure our understanding of the multifactoral nature of the disorder.

Perhaps the best argument in favor of this view is the fact that the stuttering experience occurs for the speaker even when a listener is unable to perceive the surface behaviors in the form of a traditional moment of stuttering. As we discuss at several points in this book, it is possible for profound stuttering events to take place in the complete absence of any observable stuttering events. As Smith and Kelly point out, even though stuttering "events" may appear to be highly specific on the surface of the speaker's behavior, the dynamic processes influencing the relative level of fluency–disfluency are distant in time and space from the event that is perceived as stuttering. That is, there are many neurological and physiological events that occur long before the placement of some arbitrary timing mark suggesting the onset or termination of the stuttering event. Even though precise identification of those stuttering events on the surface may be possible, at best it provides an artificial boundary for segmenting the dynamic process of speech production. Additionally, there is no one-to-one relationship between traditional classifications of fluency breaks and many of the underlying events. Commenting on the use of traditional fluency form types in analyzing stuttering, Smith states:

> Requiring researchers to use these units, to use "reliable means" of classification, and to interpret their data in relation to these units is analogous to asking the scientist who is recording seismic activity around volcanoes to interpret the data in relation to the pattern of smoke rising from the surface of the volcano. (1999; p. 30)

For those who live with it, the notion that stuttering is a multifactorial problem is clear, and it has frequently been compared to the many layers of an onion. During treatment (or self-directed change) the many layers must be peeled away in order to get at the core characteristics of the problem.

Smith also provides other important insights that impact the way we look at theories of stuttering onset and development. She attempts to integrate the nature and nurture views of onset. Although the genetic and physiological aspects of the CNS are being implicated in the etiology of stuttering, no single gene locus has been identified. Smith points out that the mammalian brain is constantly changing in response to environmental stimuli. Both the structure and the function of the brain are remodeled not only during the early years of development but also, as a result of experience and learning, throughout all stages of life. Nearly all the recent neurological and genetic research suggests the interactive and dynamic nature of the organism with the environment, supporting Smith's premise that understanding the onset and development is not a nature vs. nurture issue. The two perspectives are essentially one and the same, an organic–learning combination.

Smith also employs the concept of "attractor states" from dynamic systems theory to understand the development of both normal nonfluency and stuttering in children. Attractor states are observed when systems self-organize into models of behavior that are preferred, even though they may be very complex or even undesirable. Once the system is in a deep or stable attractor state, it takes more energy to move away from that state. Although during childhood the skills necessary for producing fluent speech are developing and are influenced by both nature and nurture, instability of speech is predictable. Children move between fluent and nonfluent attractors during development. Following years of development, the fluent young adult demonstrates a highly stable attractor for fluent speech and few unstable or disfluent attractors. For those who stutter, however, there is a combination of both fluent and disfluent attractors, resulting in instability and perpetuating a breakdown in speech motor control. Furthermore, adults who stutter may have stable patterns of neuromuscular activity during stuttering (as in a tremor). The ultimate goal of this modeling is to study the factors that influence speech motor performance and "to understand the dynamic interplay of these factors as the developing brain seeks the stable, adaptive models of interaction among neural networks that generate . . . fluent speech" (p. 42).

Finally, as Smith (1999) explains, "Successful behavioral therapy essentially helps the child to establish adaptive, stable patterns of operation and interaction among the widely distributed neural networks involved in language production" (p. 37). Fortunately, the mammalian brain is plastic and continually changing. Although the structure and cortical functioning of the brain are rapidly changing during early development, this remodeling also continues throughout life, resulting in an experience-determined plasticity in the adult brain. This view of therapeutic change is similar to the neurological findings resulting from successful therapy described earlier in this chapter by Boberg et al. (1983), De Nil et al. (2003), Foundas et al. (2001), Kroll et al. (1997), and Neumann et al. (2005).

The Neurophysiological Model

De Nil and his colleagues describe a model that provides a comprehensive and unifying model of stuttering (De Nil, 1999). This model also includes capacities or skills similar to those noted in the demands and capacities model. In addition, De Nil proposes that just as nature and nurture are not separate phenomena, psychological and neurophysiological processes are not independent entities. This model emphasizes the dynamic interplay among three levels of influence on human behavior and on stuttering in particular: processing (central neurophysiological processes), output (motor, cognitive, language, social, and emotional processes), and contextual (environmental influences). Bidirectional dynamic feedback takes place across all levels and continually influences output. That is, environmental stimuli and behavioral consequences are filtered through neurophysiological processes and vary both between individuals and within individuals over time. Long-term modification of behavior necessitates the modification of how information is processed centrally.

Conclusion

We have considered several perspectives of people who stutter and why it is that some speakers have more difficulty than others producing fluent verbal communication. It seems best to view those who have such problems on a continuum with their fluent peers rather than categorizing them into distinctly different stereotypes. On several occasions throughout this book we note that there are many more similarities between fluent and nonfluent speakers than there are differences. Playing the role of a person who stutters in daily speaking situations illustrates this to even the most fluent speaker by bringing forth natural coping responses common to everyone. It is also clear that people who stutter are far from a homogeneous group. This may be one reason why there have been so many explanations for stuttering onset throughout history. It also may help to explain why some speakers are more apt to recover than others, why treatment techniques that work well with one person do not work as well with another, and why relapse is an especially important issue for some people.

The wise clinician should have an understanding for many views concerning etiology that have been proposed in the past as well as the more current models. Certainly the experienced clinician should have an appreciation for the lack of support for certain perspectives and understand, for example, that individuals who stutter are no more neurotic than their typically fluent peers. The ebb and flow of theories reflects an interaction between the current zeitgeist and the published research, and the process moves forward in directions that are sometimes unpredictable. The long history of viewing stuttering as a combination of learned behaviors has helped to explain many of the responses that can be more (and often less) helpful for those who stutter. The once-influential diagnosogenic theory found little support in subsequent empirical literature. Incorporation of classical (respondent) conditioning and operant (instrumental) conditioning models began to inform the decision making of clinicians, particularly in the 1960s and 1970s.

In this chapter we have selected a relatively few investigations from the long list of studies indicating that adults who stutter demonstrate many unique speech and non–speech-related characteristics. Many experimenters have identified subtle motoric and temporal characteristics suggesting variability or instability for those who stutter. Ever more technologically sophisticated investigations continue to identify unique structural and functional differences in cortical and subcortical neural systems of these speakers. Reading through the literature one can easily begin to wonder how adults who stutter can function at all during daily activities. Until recently, nearly all of these investigations have been conducted with adults, and many have suggested that the findings indicate the effects of years or decades of compensating for and adjusting to one's stuttering. More recent studies have begun to use children, with results suggesting that some of the anatomical–physiological and motoric–acoustic characteristics may also be present shortly following the onset of stuttering.

Early conjectures and evidence of anomalies in the central nervous system of those who stutter, especially in the form of cerebral asymmetry, have received continued support in recent research employing advanced technologies. These investigations are increasingly informing our understanding of both structural and functional characteristics that distinguish individuals who stutter from their fluent peers, even during the earlier years of language and speech development. Indications of normalization of brain asymmetry as a result of treatment are particularly intriguing and may eventually prove helpful in assisting the speaker to alter his or her neurological functioning (brain plasticity). New etiological models such as the dual premotor systems hypothesis and EXPLAN may spur new research designs and comprehensive explanations for stuttering onset. Studies using advancing techniques of neuroimaging, neural modeling, and genetic linkage, along with investigations of cognitive and behavioral factors, provide support for the utility of multifactorial models for developing a broad and deep perspective about the nature of stuttering. It may be that the successful outcome of the research in the areas neuroscience and genetics will go a long way toward building a consensus about the etiology of the problem.

Some may be frustrated by the complexity of stuttering and would like to have a clear, unequivocal answer as to how and why stuttering is a universal characteristic of human communication. But, as we suggested in Chapter 1, it is probably best for the clinician to cultivate a tolerance for ambiguity and espouse a broad perspective for the many accounts of stuttering. Having many views for what seems on the surface to be essentially the same problem would seem to detract from our credibility as a profession. However, although we do not know all that we need to know, we have good information about what to do when faced with children or adults who stutter. Assessment and treatment protocols and techniques have been shown to be effective and, as a profession, we have been and will continue to be of great assistance to children and adults who stutter. Even so, the obvious complexity of the problem we call stuttering requires— as Conture (2006) aptly recommends—that the clinician approach the problem with a Swiss army knife rather than a hammer in hand.

Topics for Discussion

1. How will you respond when you are asked by the parents of a young stuttering child the inevitable question, "Why is my child stuttering?"

2. How can you demonstrate your competence as a clinician given the multiple explanations and current status of the research on stuttering etiology?

3. Of the various etiological theories discussed in this chapter, which one is most appealing to you?

4. How would you respond if a friend commented that "Stuttering is mostly a psychological problem, isn't it?"

5. Access the Stuttering Home Page *http://www.mnsu.edu/comdis/kuster/stutter.html* on the Internet and look up examples of how characters who stutter have been portrayed in books, movies, and television.

6. Give several examples of times when you experienced a "loss of control." Describe the emotional and cognitive characteristics of each experience.

7. Which investigations described in this chapter do you feel provide the strongest support for the idea that stuttering has a neurophysiological basis?

8. What are the basic similarities and differences in the three examples of multifactorial models presented in this chapter (capacities and demands, the multifactorial-dynamic model, and the neurophysiological model)?

9. Develop a response about the nature of stereotypes about stuttering to an adolescent who tells you that "Everyone thinks I'm stupid!"

10. Discuss why it is important to have a historical context for understanding the various theoretical perspectives of stuttering etiology. What factors appear to influence current perspectives?

Recommended Readings

Ambrose, N. G., & Yairi, E. (2002). The Tudor study: Data and ethics. *American Journal of Speech-Language Pathology, 11,* 1190-203.

Ingham, R. J., Cykowski, M., Ingham J. C., & Fox, P. T. (2007). In R. J. Ingham (Ed.), *Neuroimaging in Communication Sciences.* pp. 53–85. San Diego: Plural Publishing Inc.

Conture, E. G., (2001). Chapter 6, Conclusions, (pp. 327–378). In *Stuttering: Its nature, diagnosis and treatment.*

Smith A., & Kelly, E. (1997). Stuttering: A dynamic, multifactoral model. In R. F. Curlee & G. M. Siegel (Eds.), *The nature and treatment of stuttering: New directions* (2nd Ed.). (pp. 204–217). Needham Heights, MA: Allyn & Bacon.

Van Riper, C. (1974). A handful of nuts. *Western Michigan Journal of Speech Therapy, 11 (2).*

Van Riper, C. (1990). Final thoughts about stuttering. *Journal of Fluency Disorders, 15,* 317–318.

CHAPTER 4

Beginning the Assessment Process with Adolescents and Adults

"When you stutter you are always in a country where you don't speak the language."

Kevin, an adult who stutters

"Not everything that can be counted counts, and not everything that counts can be counted."

Albert Einstein[1]

Chapter Objectives

The first of two chapters on the assessment of stuttering describes the features of stuttering as manifested in a fully developed form in adolescents and adults. The sequence of describing the assessment and treatment of older speakers prior to presenting the characteristics of younger speakers was chosen because the nature of stuttering is more clearly manifested in older speakers, thus providing a comprehensive view of the many overt features and the speaker's cognitive and affective response to his or her circumstances. Over the course of this and the following chapter, the differences between the assessment of speakers who have traveled the often bumpy road of stuttering for many years and those younger speakers who may or may not be starting (or continuing) on the road of stuttering, will become apparent.

The primary objectives of this chapter are to describe strategies for determining the surface and intrinsic characteristics presented by the speaker

---

[1]Robins, G. www.cs.virginia.edu/~robins/quotes.html

during the initial assessment. The variability and depth of the behavioral, cognitive, and affective layers of the stuttering experience for each speaker requires some time to fully appreciate, and the clinician often finds that this process will continue well into the early treatment sessions. This chapter provides examples of the procedures and tools available to clinicians, which—along with essential input from the speaker—begin the process of mapping the surface features of the problem as well as the discovery of speakers' abilities to cope with their situations in ways that positively or negatively influence the quality of their lives. In determining the severity of the problem, the importance of a multidimensional approach (beyond the basics of stuttering frequency and quality) is emphasized. Another major focus is the value of the clinician's close attention to how speakers interpret and describe themselves and their ability to communicate during the early baseline assessment period so that subsequent therapeutic change may be documented. The following box provides an overview of the most basic aspects of the assessment process for older speakers.

Factors and Procedures to Consider When Assessing Adolescents and Adults

Keep in mind the great variability of stuttering.

Why is the person seeking assistance now?

What is the person's level of motivation?

Remember, stuttering frequency is but one indicator of severity.

The surface features: What does the speaker do *when* stuttering? Consider:

- Frequency
- Tension and duration
- Avoidance
- Substitution
- Postponement

The intrinsic features: What does the speaker do *because* of stuttering? Consider:

- Loss of control
- Cognitive and affective factors
- Restricted lifestyle

The value of the speaker's self-assessment.

Formal measures of surface and intrinsic features.

Fundamental Considerations of Assessment

The Unique Sample of Our Clients

The vast majority of people who stutter do not seek treatment. Rather, they make it through life by coping with the problem in more or less effective ways. For one reason or another, most choose not to seek professional help. They may not be aware that help is available, and for many who are, the time and cost of treatment may be prohibitive. For others, the challenges of treatment are so unappealing that they refuse assistance even if they are able to afford it. For many who stutter, however, it may be the case that although the problem is apparent, it is not sufficiently great to promote action.

Although there are no data to indicate the proportion of individuals who stutter who never seek formal help, there is little doubt that the majority of individuals who stutter never make contact with professional treatment centers. Consequently, these people never serve as participants for the research on which we base our understanding of the problem and form the rationale for most of our clinical decisions. It seems reasonable to suggest that our knowledge about people who stutter is based on a nonrepresentative, perhaps even biased, sample of the total population of people who stutter. The sample we observe is most likely skewed in the direction of people who, for whatever reasons, come to recognize not only that they need help but are also able to seek and obtain assistance.

As with many undesirable human conditions, those who stutter are sometimes able to achieve successful change on their own. Still, some strategies and techniques are likely to be more effective than others, and an experienced guide or coach can show the way or, at the very least, make the journey more efficient and often more pleasant. There are useful strategies and techniques that, while helpful, are nevertheless counterintuitive and not something that most people who stutter would consider—voluntary stuttering being, perhaps, the best example. Without the assistance of a good instructor, the novice is apt to select less effective or even counterproductive options. Without good coaching, swimmers will try to raise their head above the water rather than turn their head and breathe efficiently; soccer players will kick the ball with their toe rather than their instep; kayakers will pull away from a wave or rock rather than leaning into it. Likewise, most people who stutter instinctively make every effort not to stutter. When they do stutter, they tend to expend ever more effort attempting to push through a sound or word and to "control" their stuttering. Without an experienced coach, teacher, or clinician few people will be aware of the best techniques or why, how, and when to use them.

Clinical Insight

At a reception a woman I was speaking to introduced me to her husband. He was a young man in his early thirties who was a successful businessman. He was extremely pleasant and outgoing. He also appeared to be spontaneously fluent. As we discussed my field and my interest in stuttering, he volunteered that he too had stuttered as a child and, on occasion, still had difficulty with certain words. His brother had also stuttered, and his description of the impact his stuttering had on his life as a young child and teenager left no doubt that he truly was a member of the clan of the tangled tongue. Although he had experienced some teasing about his speech, his close friends had been understanding and supportive. During his elementary school years he had been seen for a brief time by a clinician who emphasized speaking slower, something he felt provided little help. Now, as a young adult, he explained that, for the most part, he had "gotten over it." He described that actually, rather than stuttering (repeating sounds and words), he stammered (blocking and "getting stuck" on words).

When I asked what he had done to get over his stuttering, he informed me that he had several specific techniques that he used. He had learned to adeptly change words or topics as he anticipated stuttering on a feared sound or word. He had adopted an assertive approach and "went for it" in many aspects of his life, including all communication situations. It was clear that although stuttering had been a traumatic experience for him when was younger, he wasn't going to let something like that get in his way. He had been an outstanding athlete and had a broad circle of friends. By any standard he was successful. He explained that "everyone has their faults" and that he just happened to stutter.

Not all speakers would be satisfied with this approach to their stuttering. This young man adjusted his approach and, with a history of success in other areas of his life and the support of others, was able to elaborate a confident and assertive approach to communication situations. However, it was apparent that his stuttering continued to impact his life. He chose to describe his fluency breaks as stammering because that term, in this country at least, has less stigma associated with it than the word stuttering. His statement that "everyone has their faults," while an accurate and generally healthy comment, indicated that he viewed stuttering—to some degree at least—as a "fault." His strategy of changing words prevented him from being as spontaneous as he might have otherwise been and required that he scan ahead for feared stimuli that might result in stuttering. Word avoidance and substitutions detract from the precision of the message and for some speakers can be highly exasperating. It is possible that the quality of this man's life would have been enhanced by learning more about and becoming desensitized to stuttering. He may have experienced some relief from his goal of hiding his stuttering by giving himself permission to easily stutter on some occasions.

Clinical **Decision-Making**

On occasion it becomes apparent, either during the initial assessment or early in the treatment process, that individuals who seek our help are addicted to alcohol and/or drugs. Some individuals have become addicted to pain medications. Some individuals who stutter are prescribed medications such as Xanax by their physicians to control their anxiety or "social anxiety disorder." In my own experience, and as a result of reading clinical exchanges on the Internet and discussing this issue with other clinicians who specialize in fluency problems, the general consensus is that such individuals are unlikely to achieve consistent or long-term success in treatment. The motivation, judgment, and general cognitive functioning of these individuals are likely to be inconsistent or impaired. Until the person has successfully completed a program of detoxification and rehabilitation, treatment for his or her fluency problem—particularly in the long term—is not likely to be beneficial.

The Variability of Fluency and Stuttering

Even for typically fluent speakers, fluency is a speech characteristic that varies greatly—perhaps more so than any other—depending on the communicative situation. Most speakers appear to speak with little effort or thought, with words flowing smoothly and effortlessly. But even for accomplished speakers, particularly when communicative or emotional stress is introduced, the smoothness often begins to disappear and breaks in the flow of speech are likely to occur. For those who stutter, the variability is often especially pronounced, because, given their past experiences with fluency failure, these speakers are apt to react sooner and to a greater degree to fluency-disrupting stimuli such as time pressure and difficult speaking situations than fluent speakers. In addition, people who stutter are sometimes able to "turn on their fluency." By avoiding feared sounds and words or—with heightened energy and emotion, momentarily "rising to the occasion"—it is not unusual for speakers who typically stutter to achieve uncharacteristically fluent speech.

The variability of both the frequency and quality of stuttering is one of the hallmarks of developmental stuttering. Although this variability is typical and to be expected, it contributes as much as anything else to the mystery of the problem.[2] It is difficult for many listeners to understand how people can be speaking fluently one moment and then a moment later struggle dramatically as they attempt to say a word they have already said fluently. The "natural"

---

[2]As we will see in Chapter 9, some forms of "atypical" fluency disorders do not show such great variability, a characteristic that helps to identify these problems.

variability of stuttering can make it difficult for a listener to adapt to and become accustomed to a speaker. Such variability also presents a predicament for the person doing the stuttering. That is, the person who stutters cannot always be certain of the amount and degree of difficulty he or she will experience in a given speaking situation. This, of course, makes it difficult for the speaker to compensate for a problem that is so inconsistent and unpredictable. Of the many communication problems that people may experience, perhaps none is more variable than stuttering.

This variability of fluency both within and between speakers can make the assessment of fluency more formidable than it may first appear. As Bloodstein (1987) states, "The great variability of stuttering from time to time under different conditions is liable to result in assessments that are unrepresentative" (p. 386). For most speakers, a single assessment protocol obtained at a particular time will provide only a glimpse of the depth and breadth of the problem. Many aspects of the fluency disorder will go undetected unless the assessment process is conducted in a variety of speaking situations. We are not likely to observe the variety of overt behaviors and covert coping responses during one or even several meetings. The more these situations simulate the speaker's daily communication situations the more apt we are to obtain a true indication of the problem.

Is it Stuttering?

On occasion a person will seek our help and it is not immediately apparent that the problem has anything to do with stuttering. In an attempt to lessen the impact of stuttering on their lives, adult speakers will sometimes shape their speech and overall behavior into a pattern of symptoms that resemble other

Clinical Insight

On several occasions I have had the experience of running into a client while entering places such a restaurant or a movie theater. It is not unusual for the unexpected meeting in a context far from the clinical environment to yield examples of stuttering and associated behaviors that I have not seen before and, perhaps, that the speaker has not produced for many months or years. During such encounters individuals who stutter sometimes reach back into their past repertoire of coping responses. Although the responses may not have been used for some time, it's clear that they are especially well-learned and still present under the right circumstances. It can be informative and useful to include these behaviors as we construct a map of the person's stuttering.

problems such as motor-speech disorders, voice disorders, language disorders, social anxiety, or even emotional disturbances. For example, because of tension in a speaker's voice or the fact that he or she is speaking in a careful, slow, or labored manner, it may appear as though the person has a voice or word-finding problem. In order to protect him- or herself from the social penalties and suffering associated with stuttering, the person may refuse to speak or choose to speak in a way that, although it is obvious that something is amiss, it is not clear that stuttering is the problem.

Some speakers who are particularly adept at avoiding feared sounds and words, specific people, or speaking situations, may rarely if ever be perceived as a person who stutters. The person may, however, be thought of as someone who is introverted, shy, lazy, or at the very least, somewhat peculiar. He or she may be seen as a person who is a bit strange because, due to avoidance and word substitutions, he or she uses usual syntax, speech rates, or intonation patterns that are idiosyncratic or inappropriate. For example, one client described how he answered his office telephone by saying "Hi" rather than saying "Hello" followed by his name and the name of the company. The person may not always respond in expected ways to simple questions, pretending he did not hear a question or does not know an answer when it is obvious that he does. He may avoid saying his own name or introducing friends or relatives when it is expected and appropriate to do so. He may make excuses so that he will not have to participate in projects at work, school, or engage in social activities. In other words, this person will do the same things normal speakers do when they want to avoid aversive stimuli. As speakers develop such ways of adjusting to stuttering, they are sometimes able to mask the stuttering entirely, or at least obscure the true nature of their situation and therefore the actual severity of their problem. In general, we have found that the more successful the speaker is at covering up the stuttering behavior, the more difficult it will be to let go of these coping responses and experiment with alternative choices during treatment, some of which are likely to expose his or her stuttering.

Most adults who come to a clinician for assistance know that the problem is stuttering, and the basic problem is obvious at the outset. Others attend the assessment interview and display little or no obvious stuttering. Even though the stuttering may not be overt or obvious, if the person really is someone who stutters there will be ample indicators. On occasion the speaker's body language will "leak" his or her anxiety as he or she approaches or attempts to use certain words or sounds. The cues provided by the speaker's body language are likely to be subtle and unique to each speaker, and we are more likely to detect these features once we have the opportunity to become calibrated to the person and his or her patterns of communicating. Some individuals may reveal their anxiety by subtle nostril flaring or by a slight alteration in the rate or tempo of their speech. We may ask ourselves such questions as "Is the speaker producing speech that, although not clearly stuttered, is also not entirely fluent? Is the speech being produced carefully with a monotonous, measured nature, with a tense and constricted vocal tract? Are there brief, "sticky" moments that are distinguishable from the other syllables and words? Are there signs of word switching or substitution?" In some cases a person's speech may be "fluent" in a traditional sense, but it is really just "not stuttered." As the clinician tries to imitate the client's speech characteristics, it will become apparent that, although the person is not stuttering in a technical sense, he is "talking on thin ice." As a clinician gradually becomes calibrated to the person, it is possible to sense that he or she is not completely in control of his or her speech. The speaker may not necessarily be trying to hide his or her stuttering but rather that this way of coping with the problem has become habitual.

After the clinician has several sessions with a client, she will begin to understand how the person is apt to express himself during periods of fluent speech. Not only will she begin to anticipate the rate and tempo of the client's speech, but she will begin to predict what sentence structure and vocabulary the speaker is going to use. Moreover, when these usual patterns are not part of the client's speech, we may guess, often correctly, that he has avoided or substituted a word, or that he has scanned ahead, is anticipating difficulty, and is speaking cautiously. The following exchange between a client and a clinician taking place after several treatment sessions is such an example.

Client: "We had a wonderful time. We drove to [the speaker slightly slows his speech and indicates minimal tension in the jaw] my hometown in Indiana for the weekend."

Clinician: "Did you avoid the word of your hometown just now?"

Client: *(smiling)* "Yes. How did you know?"

Clinician: "Because you slowed your speech, it sounded just a little sticky, and because I know that is one of your feared words."

Such exchanges take many forms but occur with regularity for most speakers who stutter. As the clinician gradually becomes attuned to the client's characteristics, these important events become more transparent.

Many authors have described the experience of losing control and associated helplessness as a central feature of the stuttering experience (Bloodstein, 1987; Cooper, 1968, 1987, 1990; Manning, 1977; Manning & Shrum, 1973; Perkins, 1990). In describing this experience, Guitar (2006) cites the work of Mineka (1985), who suggested that anxiety is closely associated with the sense of losing control and leads to fear-based responses. Speakers feel they are out of control and unable to stop the behavior. As Prins (1997) suggests, the essence of the difference between real and voluntary stuttering is the experience of being out of control that accompanies real moments of stuttering.

Clinical **Insight**

My experience as a school-aged child who stuttered illustrates the importance of appreciating the intrinsic aspects of stuttering. I think that all the clinicians who worked with me over the years knew about stuttering. They could identify stuttering moments and categorize the overt aspects of my surface behaviors. They helped me to understand, monitor, and—to some degree—modify these behaviors. However, most of the clinicians failed to indicate to me that they understood anything about what I was experiencing as the person who was struggling with his speech and his life. It seems to me that the fear and helplessness that were so strongly influencing my choices as they related to my speech were not apparent to them. Because the clinicians knew about the surface features of stuttering, that is what we focused on. At least, I suspect that was the reason. Fortunately, later on I encountered clinicians who not only knew about the surface features of the problem but also showed me that they had insight about how this problem influenced my responses to my predicament. Although they themselves did not stutter, they understood something about the deep structure and the intrinsic nature of the problem. They knew that at the center of my daily decision making was the fact that I often felt helpless. I had little or no sense of being able to control my speech. Sometimes I had what felt like "lucky fluency," which, at that time, I regarded as a good thing. But a moment later I would be unable to communicate even my most basic thoughts. Even when I wasn't overtly stuttering, I still experienced the problem as I often altered my choice of words and constricted my options due to even the possibility of stuttering. In many instances, stuttering never reached the surface, but the choices I was making were examples of profound moments of stuttering even though they were not being tabulated by the clinician as a repetition or prolongation.

Surface and Intrinsic Features

Another basic characteristic of stuttering is that most of the features that we see and hear indicate only the surface features of the problem. The typical listener naturally tends to focus on the obvious characteristics such as the frequency, duration, and tension associated with the stuttered moments, as well as the sometimes dramatic accessory features the speaker uses to postpone or escape from stuttering. Although there is usually some consistency in these features across speakers, the diversity and sometimes unique nature of coping responses of individuals who stutter may require some exploration. Despite these issues, it is necessary for the clinician to identify the quantity and quality of the surface features presented by the client, for these behavioral characteristics provide one indication of the severity of the problem and provide evidence of behavioral change during treatment.

However, even with younger speakers—and certainly with adolescents and adults—we must look below the surface of the speaker's behavior in order to obtain a complete appreciation of the problem. As interesting—even fascinating—as the surface features may be, it is good to keep in mind that these behaviors also indicate the nature of the dynamics taking place under the surface. It is beneath the surface of the overt behaviors that we find the intrinsic features, the deep structure of stuttering. Although these are less apparent aspects of the stuttering experience, they are, to varying degrees, normal and expected components. A primary aspect of the assessment process is to begin to identify both the surface and intrinsic features that are unique to each speaker, something we will describe in some detail later in this chapter.

Determining the Speaker's Desire for Change

Virtually all clinical authorities agree that the motivation of the person who stutters is a key feature of a successful treatment outcome (Van Riper, 1973). Motivation can also be regarded as a covert aspect of stuttering, for—as with the sense of loss of control—motivation can be difficult to identify and quantify. The person's commitment to change and growth should be assessed prior to, as well as throughout, the therapeutic process. Depending on past successes and the client's response to new and sometimes difficult challenges, motivation will vary greatly between and within clients.

One thing that does not accurately—or at least not completely—reflect a person's level of motivation are the statements made during assessment and treatment sessions. Many clients make sincere and honest statements of commitment, saying things that lead us to believe they are highly motivated. These are similar to the announcements we make when deciding to do things like diet or train for an event such as a marathon or triathlon. While it may be pleasant to hear these declarations of commitment during the assessment interview, by placing too much importance on such statements, we are likely to be deceived. It is often best to be cautious of statements that indicate that the person is overly committed. It is one thing to plan and discuss an arduous journey and quite another to persistently take each step along the way.

It is both natural and necessary to be motivated at the outset of treatment. As the process gets underway, there are many interesting things to learn about the nature of stuttering and about the speaker's history of dealing with the problem. However, the initiation of treatment can be both exciting and anxiety-producing, as it is whenever we challenge ourselves with a new task such as taking a class, starting a new job, or expanding the envelope of our lives in any sense. There is an element of risk as well as the possibility of partial or complete failure.

It is good to enter the process with some level of self-esteem and energy. Nevertheless, when evaluating a potential client it is useful to consider their degree of "mental toughness" or "psychic energy" (Cooper, 1977). This is not to suggest that we only enroll highly motivated people in treatment, but the client's true level of motivation—whatever that may be—does provide an indication of the progress we can expect once treatment is initiated. As clinicians we can provide a measure of reassurance, security, and support. But, as much as anything, it is the speaker's motivation and determination that determine the rate of change.

It is often helpful to take some time during the initial meeting to provide an overall picture of the treatment process to the speaker and interested others. The speaker may be overly enthusiastic, in part because he or she does not fully understand the nature of the journey. The speaker may believe that it is the clinician's role to "fix" or provide a "cure" for the problem when, in reality, it is the speaker who must do the largest share of the work. As the speaker begins to appreciate the focus and effort it will take to alter his or her response to the problem, the initial high level of motivation may fade somewhat (sometimes referred to as the "honeymoon effect"). Of course, we do not want to compromise the person's level of motivation, for he or she will need to draw upon this reserve. We do, however, want to provide the potential client with a realistic view of the journey.

One practical suggestion for determining a person's level of motivation is to describe examples of the activities that will occur during treatment. Of course, we don't want to discourage potential clients or scare them off by overly emphasizing the rigors associated with therapeutic change. But a cautious explanation or demonstration may be worthwhile for a realistic estimate of the speaker's determination. In addition, there are questions that the clinician can ask in order to tap into a potential client's level of motivation, questions that will force a realistic consideration of his or her current priorities. For example, we can ask the person how much treatment is worth. Aside from the fees associated with the treatment center, how valuable—in real money—is this experience at this time? Would the potential client be willing to pay $5, $25, $50, or $100 per hour? How far would he or she be willing to drive to receive treatment—5, 50, 100 miles each way? Such questions may at first appear to be contrived, possibly even unethical. However, we have found that these thresholds of money or distance can provide a surprisingly precise indication of the eventual level of motivation that clients demonstrate once treatment is underway.

As with many aspects of life, timing is crucial. Most of us realize that the moment when the path of another person's life intersects with ours can be decisive. Anyone who has attempted to convince a junior high school student who stutters to enroll in treatment knows that some people do not want our help—or at least they do not want it when we want to provide it. The moments when people choose to come to us for help can provide insight into their motivation and readiness for change. Where they are in the process of change is critical for successful intervention. Investigations into the process of assisted and self-directed change suggest that a person's location on a continuum from self-reevaluation and contemplation of change to action and maintenance of change is a powerful factor in predicting a successful treatment outcome (DiClemente, 1993; Prochaska, DiClemente, & Norcross, 1992).[3] It is often informative to ask the speaker questions such as: "Why are you here today and not six months ago? Why today and not next year? What is it that prompted you to ask for help at this time?"

The answers to such questions are important in the overall determination of motivation and especially the client's readiness for change. Sometimes people refer themselves for treatment because they realize that their speech is preventing them from career advancement. They may seek our assistance when they are facing a major speaking event such as a presentation or a ceremony in which they must take part. On a more basic level, speakers sometimes come to us as they are about to experience landmark events during their life cycle. It is at such transitional periods or "nodes" in a person's life that self-awareness and introspection may be heightened and when significant decision making and restructuring take place (Kimmel, 1974; Sheehy, 1974; Valiant, 1977). During these periods, people are frequently more likely to assume increased responsibility for their lives and begin postponed but necessary journeys. Although transitional periods occur throughout life, one major period for people who stutter is likely to be when they are in their early twenties (Plexico, Manning, & DiLollo, 2005). During this decade, people are likely to complete formal schooling, change their living status and location, enter or leave military service, initiate careers, and get married and have children. It may be that missing the opportunity to obtain effective assistance at this stage of their lives will result in decades of less-than-satisfactory communication and quality of life. Plexico and Manning (2008a) found that it was not until the completion of college that the majority of their participants began to see their stuttering as a hindrance. The prospects of employment often served as a primary impetus for change. For example, two participants stated:

> I didn't like it [stuttering] before. I didn't like that I stuttered. But it didn't really have an impact on what happened in my life. But then once I got out there [in the work force] it felt to me like it was having an impact. I wasn't getting an equal chance for a job because of it. For the first time my stuttering was a hindrance to me advancing in life. So I needed to do something to fix that or at least get to a point where it wasn't a problem. (Bob)

---

[3] See Chapter 6 for a discussion of therapeutic stages of change.

> I know that I can make progress and that I'm the only one holding myself back. [I] won't be thirty and still working . . . at a place where I'm not challenged and I don't have to talk. I don't want that. (Sarah)

Opportunities for reassessment and change may also occur during middle age, when people sometimes take the opportunity to do something about a problem that they have put into the background for much of their lives. As Newgarten indicates, middle age is characterized by "self-awareness," "heightened introspection," and "restructuring of experience" (cited in Kimmel, 1974, p. 58). Moreover, as Sheehy (1974) suggests, midlife is often characterized by a reexamination, whereby a person questions many views of self and others. At this time, he or she is more likely to readjust old responses to lifelong problems (Sheehy, 1974; Vailant, 1977). Of course, adopting new approaches to old problems is possible at any time during the life cycle, but it seems to be most frequent during the decades of the forties and fifties. It could be that if individuals in that age range are interested in treatment, significant progress can result. Or, it may be that individuals are more likely to employ self-directed change, possibly with the support of a self-help group, rather than seek formal treatment (especially if past treatment has not been helpful).

Unfortunately, there is little information available about older individuals who stutter (Manning & Shirkey, 1981). Katz, Lincoln, and McCabe (2006) analyzed 10-minute speech samples of 12 male and 4 females over the age of 55 (mean age of 70.4 years) who had stuttered since childhood. Analysis of conversational speech, reading, and telephone conversations with a stranger indicated frequencies of stuttering similar to those of younger speakers. Although there are exceptions, Manning and Monte (1981) suggest that few people who stutter beyond the age of 50 desire treatment. Manning, Dailey, and Wallace (1984) found evidence indicating that, in most instances, these people have learned to adjust to their problem and, although the problem does not appear to diminish in terms of traditional measures of severity, it represents less of a handicap for older speakers. The authors obtained the attitude and personality characteristics of 29 adults who stuttered, ranging in age from 52 to 82. Although these speakers scored approximately the same as young adults who stutter on scales assessing approach and performance speaking behaviors, the large majority of the older individuals who stuttered perceived their stuttering as less handicapping now than they did when they were young adults. While a few subjects indicated the desire for treatment, most responded by indicating that stuttering had become less of a problem with increased age. In view of the volumes written on the topic of stuttering, the lack of knowledge concerning the nature of stuttering in older speakers is unfortunate. It would seem that in order to completely understand the nature of this communication problem, it is necessary to appreciate the development of the disorder throughout the life cycle. Qualitative studies such as those conducted with younger speakers (Corcoran & Stewart, 1998; Anderson & Felsenfeld, 2003; Plexico et al., 2005) may provide insight about the nature and effectiveness of the coping process concerning stuttering in the later years of life.

The Cost of Treatment

The cost of treatment is a major consideration for nearly every client. The cost for individual treatment sessions varies widely, according to many factors such as location. Of course, university-related clinic services are typically less expensive and private therapy with professional clinicians somewhat more expensive. If the client is attending more than one individual or group session per week, the cost can quickly become prohibitive for many people.

People who stutter often experience rapid change during an intensive, residential treatment program, and one reason for this may be the motivation required to enroll. Not only does the cost of these programs represent a reasonably large financial commitment but the person also must often make significant social, educational, or vocational adjustments in order to attend. If someone is determined enough to use vacation time, spend a portion of their savings, or temporarily move some or all of their family to the location of an intensive treatment program for several weeks, it is probably a good indication that the person is highly motivated.

Some adults who stutter (and parents of children who stutter) simply cannot afford professional help unless the services are covered by insurance, which is not typically the case for fluency disorders. Treatment, especially for adolescents and adults who stutter, may require several weeks or months for successful change. Whether the treatment program is an intensive program lasting several weeks or a less intensive program where the speaker attends once or twice a week, the total cost can easily approach or go beyond several hundreds or even thousands of dollars. While this is a significant amount of money by any standard, the impact of successful treatment on the lives of the client can be momentous, even life-altering. It is interesting to note that some people (and insurance companies or state agencies) are willing to spend thousands of dollars on various assistive devices that may or may not provide increased fluency. Likewise, people who routinely choose to spend significant amounts of money for a wide variety of digital and electronic devices (or purchase expensive items such as cars every few years) are often less willing to make an investment in their— or their childrens'—ability to communicate.

The Initial Meeting

Just as the initial evaluation session provides the first opportunity for the clinician to find out about the person who has come to us for assistance, it is also the client's first opportunity to find out about the clinician. As discussed throughout the text (particularly in Chapter 6), the quality of the therapeutic alliance will be a major factor in determining how treatment will proceed or whether it will take place at all. With this in mind it is worthwhile to consider the messages we would like the speaker to take home with them. Although there are many important concepts we would like to provide, we also need to be aware that it is all too easy to overload the individual with information. Perhaps the most basic messages we can communicate at the outset include:

- You are not alone, for there are millions of other people who stutter and are facing many of the same problems as you when trying to communicate.

- With determination and persistence on your part, you will be able to employ a variety of strategies and techniques that will enable you to improve your fluency and the quality of your life.

- Along with a dedicated clinician and the support of others, you will be able increase your ability, confidence, and enjoyment when communicating with others.

These most basic concepts will be elaborated as we begin to know the speaker and more fully understand their story. How the individual tells his or her story and the themes that become apparent will provide important information about the person and their response to the problem. The quantitative and qualitative techniques described in this chapter will help to identify these themes. The individual may already have some insight about the therapeutic process for it is not uncommon for older individuals to have experienced previous treatment and know something about basic terminology concerning stuttering. Of course, there are also individuals who have had a less than satisfactory therapy experience and are skeptical of our ability to provide effective help. Some people may express their justifiable anger because of the less than competent assistance they feel they have received. Others will know absolutely nothing about the nature of stuttering and, depending on their cultural background and educational experience, bring with them numerous myths that have been associated with stuttering. While some people have a degree of inquisitiveness and openness about themselves and their stuttering, the narratives of others are pervaded by embarrassment and shame. Our task at the outset is to find out where they are on their journey of understanding their situation and their willingness to enter into the work of developing alternative ways of coping.

Based on a phenomenological analysis of in-depth narratives of adults who stutter, Plexico et al., (2005) provides a description of the "essential structure" of the stuttering experience:

> The experience of stuttering may be characterized by a story dominated by struggle and suffering. Struggling to cope with the difficulties posed by the problem of stuttering, persons who stutter tend to lead a restrictive lifestyle

dominated by attempts to avoid stuttering and to avoid revealing their stuttering to the world. These struggles, along with negative reactions from a variety of listeners, including family members, and failure associated with inadequate therapy can lead to emotions of helplessness, anxiety, low self worth, embarrassment, and disapproval and an overall life tenor of suffering. (Plexico, Manning, & DiLollo, 2005, p.16)

Generally both the surface and the deep structure of stuttering are more elaborated in adolescent and adult speakers. However, even during the early years of stuttering, some young children will display well-developed tension (sound prolongations and body movements) and fragmentation (within-word fluency breaks), as well as both awareness and negative attitudes about speaking typically associated with advanced or established stuttering (Schwartz & Conture, 1988; Vanryckeghem, Brutten, & Hernandez, 2005; Yairi, 1997). Usually, however, older speakers show much greater complexity of behavior and exhibit greater anxiety and fear. Adolescents and adults have attempted to cope with and adjust to the problem for years and the features of their stuttering, especially those having to do with avoidance and concealment, tend to be sophisticated and complex.

Two Principles of Assessment

Although the assessment process will often be comprehensive and multilayered, it is useful to realize that much of what is done during both the assessment and the treatment of stuttering can be reduced to two basic principles. Often, during both assessment and treatment, we find ourselves returning to these principles, particularly when we are uncertain of our next step. First, and perhaps most importantly, the more an individual who stutters alters the choices and narrows the options that are available in life, the greater the influence and handicapping effects of stuttering are likely to be. Assessment must focus on determining the extent of such altered decision making in all its forms. In turn, many treatment goals will focus on increasing the person's ability to make choices based on information beyond the fact that stuttering is a possibility. Later in this chapter we will describe the rationale for asking the speaker to respond to the question "What do you do *because* you stutter?" The speaker's answers to this question will provide a preliminary indication of how the possibility of stuttering impacts his or her decision making. As the members of the National Stuttering Association proclaim in the title of their newsletter *Letting GO*, the person who stutters must learn to "let go" and live life as it can best be lived rather than basing decisions on the fact that, among many other important characteristics, he or she happens to be someone who stutters.

The second basic principle of assessment has to do with the various forms of effort and struggle behavior. Everything else being equal, the more a speaker reacts to his or her stuttering by trying to prevent it from occurring or by struggling through a moment of stuttering, the greater the impact of the problem. In this case, the question we might ask is "What does the speaker do *when* he or she stutters?" The clinician can determine how and to what degree the speaker is closing down or restricting the speech production system, especially the vocal tract. What is the speaker doing with the source of energy in the respiratory system and the vocal tract resonator/filter that prevents these systems from being used efficiently? How is the speaker inhibiting normal voicing and articulation? What is the speaker doing to prohibit the transition from one sound or syllable to another? What is the speaker doing to keep from speaking (or stuttering) easily, openly, and smoothly? Much of what influences the clinician's determination of the speaker's stuttering severity and subsequent treatment decisions can be based on these two principles: (1) To what degree is the person using open decision making about communicating? and (2) To what degree is the person attempting to speak with an open and flexible vocal tract?

Estimating Severity

Assessing the severity of stuttering is not as straightforward as determining the frequency or even the form of the stuttering events. The frequency of the surface features may or may not correspond to the level of the person's problem. Regardless of the frequency and form of the stuttering, people's responses to the problem—what they tells themselves about their situation—is a critical indicator of severity (Emerick, 1988). Clearly, the severity of the problem is much greater than the features that reside on the surface. As we explained in Chapter 2, the revised ICF framework as described by Yaruss and Quesal (2004) recognizes that all disabilities involve more than the observable behaviors and includes the many disadvantages the person experiences as he or she attempts to achieve life goals. The problem involves not only the obvious features of stuttering but also the personal and environmental influences as well as the individual's response to his or her circumstances. We have seen many people who would be judged as having a severe fluency problem based on the nature of the surface features. They have frequent moments of stuttering accompanied by obvious tension and struggle behavior. However, it is as though they are not inclined to be disadvantaged or handicapped by stuttering. They make all or the majority of their decisions based on information apart from the possibility of stuttering. It is probable that most people who respond to their stuttering in this fashion never ask or seek our help. At the other extreme, we have seen adults who stutter only infrequently, with relatively little tension or obvious struggle. Their stuttering moments are exceedingly brief—hardly noticed by their listeners. Nevertheless, they are devastated by these experiences. Even though, by any objective or external standard the problem seems a minor one, the fact that they are a person who stutters is a prominent theme in their current life story. They have a difficult time tolerating the moments when they lose control of their speech, however infrequent or brief they may be. These two divergent examples of how speakers respond to stuttering are, of course, endpoints of a continuum, with most speakers falling somewhere between these extremes. A primary task for the clinician is to help the client map both the surface behaviors of stuttering as well as the intrinsic features of the problem.

The field of counseling also faces a similar dilemma for assigning a severity level to a client's problem. Mehrabian and Reed (1969) suggest the following formula for determining severity:

$$\text{Severity} = \text{Distress} \times \text{Uncontrollability} \times \text{Frequency.}$$

This formula may be particularly appropriate for assessing the severity of stuttering, because the formula factors in the speaker's reaction in terms of the affective and cognitive features of the problem. In addition, frequency of stuttering, while often a major contributor to severity, is not the only factor. Note that the multiplication signs imply that even low levels of distress or lack of control can promptly contribute to the effective severity of the stuttering problem, thereby preventing the client from fully taking part in life.

Mapping the Surface Features

The surface features of adults who stutter are relatively easy to determine, for these are the features that can be seen and heard as well as audio and video recorded. Speakers who have been stuttering for some time may be unaware of many obvious behaviors that have become incorporated into their stuttering.

Clinical **Insight**

Daniel Goleman's review of the literature on stress and health in his 2006 book *Social Intelligence* describes the effect of perceived stress on the sympathetic nervous system (SNS) and the hypothalamic-pituitary-adrenal (HPA) connections. Threatening reactions by others elicit an HPA response that produces the highest levels of cortisol (the stress hormone) of all laboratory conditions. The key factor in eliciting such high levels of stress appears to be the "judgmental scrutiny [which] delivers a particularly strong—and lingering—dose of shame" (p. 231). Furthermore, stress is further increased when the distress was not random but intended and when the person feels they are helpless to respond to the situation.

For such people, responding to the question "What do you do *when* you stutter?" will take some exploration. Some speakers may need to become desensitized to stuttering by observing stuttering behaviors in other speakers (or the clinician as he or she voluntarily produces various stuttering form types). At the most basic level, there are three basic categories of surface features—frequency, tension, and duration.

Frequency

The frequency of fluency breaks is often one of the most obvious aspects of the problem and to some degree impacts the perception of severity, particularly by the listener. Although the frequency of the fluency breaks is an aspect of the problem that is relatively easy to tabulate, it is also a feature that can be the most deceiving. For some speakers, particularly very young speakers, the frequency of fluency breaks provides a reasonable way to conceptualize severity. For other speakers, however, tabulating the frequency of stuttering events may fail to indicate the essence of the stuttering experience. But we will also have people who come to us who have other requests, as described by Jezer (1997):

> Speaking slowly and with great expression she told how she grew from a "shy, lonely, isolated little girl who never fit in" into a confident woman who was not afraid to speak in public. "We all know what stuttering is," she said, "and the blocking is only a very, very minor part. Stuttering is the isolation, pain, fear, and low self-esteem that must be relieved. And when they are relieved, I will be cured of my stuttering. (Jezer, p. 242)

As Brundage, Bothe, Lengeling, and Evans (2006) point out, many researchers and clinicians agree that reliable and valid tabulation of stuttering frequency is an important part of assessment and outcome measurement. The most common way to tabulate the frequency of stuttering is to determine the percentage of stuttered syllables (%SS) or stuttered words (%SW). Counts can be obtained by shadowing the syllable production of the speaker and indicating those syllables on which stuttering occurs. Stuttered syllables can be indicated with a keyboard or by hand by marking dots and dashes for fluent and stuttered syllables, respectively. Tabulating the frequency of stuttered syllables is thought to be a reasonable approach indicating fluency because it is generally agreed that the timing of speech movements is closely related to syllable-sized (as opposed to word-based) units (Allen, 1975; Starkweather, 1987; Stetson, 1951).

Nevertheless, a number of studies have pointed out difficulties in obtaining reliable frequency counts, particularly across clinics (Kully & Boberg, 1988; Ham, 1989; Ingham & Cordes, 1992). Rather than counting specific stuttering events or focusing on the particular form of stuttering taking place, some have advocated time-interval judgments whereby observers indicate whether or not stuttering has taken place during short (e.g., 5 seconds) intervals. This procedure is found to result in increased inter- and intra-judge consistency and greater accuracy for inexperienced observers (Cordes & Ingham, 1994, 1996; Ingham, Cordes, & Gow, 1993). Brundage et al. (2006) investigated the ability of 41 university students with relatively little experience observing stuttering and 31 speech-language pathologists (averaging 11.1 years of clinical experience) to identify the presence of stuttering during an audiovisual presentation of 216 five-second intervals. The judgments by both groups were then contrasted to those of 10 highly experienced observers. Both students and clinicians demonstrated relatively high levels of agreement (average of 88.5% and 87.4%, respectively), results that coincided with several earlier investigations of student raters. However, although students accurately identified 98% of the intervals determined to be nonstuttered, they only identified 37.5% of the intervals determined to be stuttered by experienced judges. Similarly, the clinicians accurately identified 94.1% of the intervals determined to be nonstuttered but only 51.6% of the intervals determined to be stuttered by the experienced judges. The authors point out that greater familiarity with the speakers as well as speaker input about the occurrence of normal or stuttered fluency breaks may increase accuracy. The results of these and earlier investigations indicate the necessity of training students and clinicians in the accurate identification of both stuttered and nonstuttered events.

Although it is advisable to tabulate %SS or %SW during both conversational speech and reading activities, it is good to remember that these values tend to be highly variable for a speaker, depending on the speaking situation and the reading material. Speakers who are adept at avoiding and substituting words may have a greater frequency of stuttering when reading aloud because they are less able to avoid or substitute sounds and words. For these speakers, conversely, conversational speech provides the opportunity to alter words, sometimes possibly yielding a smaller %SS value than would otherwise be the case.

Although the frequency of fluency breaks is often positively correlated with other estimates of stuttering severity, it is important to appreciate that the frequency of these breaks also may be negatively related to the actual severity of the problem. That is, speakers who are adept at substituting words or circumlocuting portions of sentences may have a severe problem but overt stuttering will be infrequent. Although the individual may not be seen or heard as a person who stutters, their manner of communication may convey other perceptions. As one adult client who was extremely good at hiding his stuttering by circumventing speaking situations and avoiding and substituting words said, "People never knew that I was stuttering. They just thought that I was weird."

Cooper (1985) has referred to the hazards of viewing stuttering primarily in terms of the number of fluency breaks as the "frequency fallacy." Persons who stutter and who choose not to raise their hand in the classroom in spite of knowing the answer, not to ask for directions or assistance, not to order a particular item in a restaurant, not to use their spouse's name during introductions, not to make or answer a telephone call (especially in a crowded room), or not to use a paging or intercom system at the office, are severely impacted by their stuttering. Unlike the tree falling in the forest, there is no sound. Nevertheless, such choices are examples of profound stuttering events. These events are insidious because they nearly always have a subtle—but powerful—influence on the person's quality of life.

Although it is not surprising that individuals who stutter are likely to hide their stuttering from everyday listeners, some may be surprised to find that it is not unusual for speakers to do the same when interacting with their clinician. This may result from the speaker's desire to please the clinician, particularly if the clinician overemphasizes or places a high value on the achievement of fluency as the ultimate or only goal of therapy. In other instances, a speaker who has yet to become desensitized to the experience of stuttering may take the easier path of avoidance. As Sarah, a women in her mid-twenties, describes:

> When I was in therapy in junior high I would substitute and I would not stutter and she would think that I was making progress, but I was hiding it the whole time. I don't know why I would hide it from the speech pathologist, you know. But it was just that I was ashamed of it, so any chance I could dodge a block I took it. So she thought I was making so much progress.

Clinical Decision-Making

There are occasions during the assessment of adolescents and adults when little, if any, overt stuttering will occur. This may be the result of the speaker being able to temporarily will himself to override (or possibly avoid) moments of stuttering. This atypical level of fluency may simply be the result of the speaker's having a particularly fluent day. When this occurs during an evaluation we have often thought (and on occasions expressed to the speaker) how this situation is similar to taking your car in to a mechanic only to find that it has stopped making that funny sound. Some clients, in frustration, will plead for the clinician to understand that despite the fact that they are speaking fluently at the moment, they really do stutter. An appreciation by the clinician for this situation can show the client your understanding about the nature of stuttering. The clinician can acknowledge the variability of stuttering and that often, especially where stuttering is permitted or even encouraged, stuttering is less likely to occur. Furthermore, a thorough diagnostic interview will confirm patterns of behavior and decision making that are consistent with what is known about people who stutter. If the clinician is interested in obtaining examples of overt stuttering, all that is usually necessary is to have the client make telephone calls or speak to strangers in or outside of the building.

Tension and Duration

The tension and duration of observable stuttering are closely related and therefore discussed here together. Generally, the greater the tension or effort associated with a moment of stuttering, the longer the duration of the event. Some speakers exhibit muscular tension throughout their entire body both during and in anticipation of stuttering. Even when the speaker exhibits a relatively low frequency of stuttering, if any one of the events lasts for several seconds and is associated with considerable muscular tension, the ability of the person to communicate is severely compromised. With high levels of tension, particularly if it is focused at a specific point in the vocal tract such as the lips, tongue, or velum, a tremor is likely to occur. Tremors are the rapid involuntary oscillatory movement of muscles of the neck and head—considerably faster than a voluntary movement. The effect is often dramatic and contributes to the cosmetic abnormality of the problem.

Another concept related to tension and one that is helpful to consider is the degree to which a word is fragmented. As described in Chapter 2, fragmentation of the word—particularly a monosyllabic word—is a fundamental feature of nonfluent speech. Bloodstein (1993) describes stuttering in its most basic form as "speech transformed by tension and fragmentation." As Bloodstein points out, the fragmentation of movement tends to occur prior to—or early in the performance of—a difficult motor task. Nearly all fragmentation during stuttering occurs during the initiation of a word or a syntactic unit of a sentence or phrase. Speakers who stutter appear to be doing, to a more extreme degree, what nonstuttering speakers do.

With greater levels of tension there is also the possibility of a stuttering "block" whereby the vocal tract becomes occluded and both airflow and voicing cease. Closure often occurs at the level of the vocal folds (a natural point of stricture), but obstruction may also occur at any supraglottal point, during, for example, the production of plosive sounds. A good way for the clinician to interpret what is taking place is to consider what is physically occurring in the vocal tract in terms of the source-filter model of speech production (Fant, 1960; Kent, 1997; Kent & Read, 1992; Pickett, 1980). That is, the clinician asks him- or herself: "What is the speaker doing to disrupt the source of energy, the air supply from the lungs? How is the speaker preventing the modulation of the air flow at the level of the vocal folds? How is the person constricting or occluding his or her vocal tract so as to adversely affect the resonant characteristics of this system?" A basic understanding of the anatomy and physiology, as well as the acoustics, of the speech production system enables the clinician to appreciate what the speaker is doing to make the process of moving from one speech segment to another so difficult.

It is also important for the person who stutters to understand the structure and function of the speech production system. Most individuals are not even vaguely aware of how speech is produced, and it will be useful for the clinician to provide the speaker with some understanding about the basic anatomical and physiological aspects of speech production. By doing so, speech production becomes less of a mystery, and the speaker can begin to monitor what he is doing to make speaking so difficult and to make better decisions about using the system more effectively. The speaker comes to realize that he or she is not as helpless as he or she may feel in the midst of a moment of stuttering. In addition, by understanding the nature of this system, he or she is able to develop a heightened sense of proprioceptive feedback concerning the respiratory, phonatory, and articulatory integration necessary for fluent speech production. As he or she begins to develop this understanding and, quite literally, a feel for what he or she is doing (or not doing) with his or her system, he or she can begin making decisions that will make the process of speaking (and stuttering) easier and smoother.

Measurement of tension has been accomplished using a variety of techniques, including galvanic skin response (GSR), electroencephalography (EEG), and—most often—electromyography (EMG) (Van Riper, 1982). Most clinicians are not likely to have access to such equipment. Fortunately, however, it is not usually necessary to have a high level of precision when measuring tension in the clinical setting. The experienced clinician is able to identify the sites and the degree of tension with reasonably good consistency. Because tension and duration are often closely related, easily made measures of duration can yield an indication of the tension that is occurring. As with tension, measures of duration, such as spectrographic or waveform analysis—while helpful—are not usually necessary for clinical evaluation. The degree of tension and the duration of the fluency breaks also may be reflected in the rate of speech in words or syllables per minute, with lower rates indicating greater severity.

Clinical Insight

Bob Quesal (2006) provides an effective metaphor for understanding the tension associated with communication when you are a person who stutters. Just as it is natural for a person walking on an icy sidewalk to exercise caution and experience some tension, communicating with a faulty speech production results in the speaker putting forth greater effort, resulting in heightened tension. As with stuttering, you never know for sure when you might slip and fall. When a fall occurs you are unsure if you will be hurt and to what degree the reactions of others will cause embarrassment. As a result of the constant tension and the efforts to prevent a fall—especially during more extreme conditions—walking becomes even more difficult.

When determining the severity of stuttering, no single measure will provide the broad-based assessment necessary to capture the complex nature of the problem. The tabulation of the most prominent behaviors, as well as frequency, tension, and duration, is a good start but only a beginning. The degree of abnormality shown by the person as he or she struggles is indicated by both verbal and physical movements prior to and during a fluency break. As we discussed in Chapter 3, the multifactorial-dynamic model proposed by Smith (1990, 1999) and Smith and Kelly (1997) indicates that the stuttering event extends well beyond the most obvious features of the disfluency. Furthermore, the behaviors associated with stuttering, and especially those at the extreme of the person's inventory of overt behaviors, may only be apparent during the more difficult speaking situations. Any coping behavior that at one time or another has enabled the speaker to escape from a stuttering moment, including extreme or even bizarre movements of arms, hands, legs, or torso, may be incorporated into a coping response. Virtually nothing should be a surprise to the experienced clinician, and the presence of these behaviors should be part of the overall determination of severity.

Subtle Surface Features

There are surface features of stuttering that, although they are observable, are often extremely subtle, so much so that it may take even an experienced clinician some time to detect them. We may think of these as surface features that are closely associated with the cognitive decision-making process that speakers use to cope with stuttering.

Avoidance

To the degree that a person who stutters successfully uses avoidance behaviors, he or she can give the appearance of a person with a mild—even nonexistent—fluency problem. If the speaker is unable to use avoidance behaviors successfully, he or she will provide the listener with a portrait of greater severity. Speakers who are especially adept at avoidance behavior have been referred to as covert (Starkweather, 1987) or internalized stutterers (Douglass & Quarrington, 1952). Although it has been suggested that these clients are relatively rare, we have seen many people who are so adept at avoidance techniques that few people with whom they come into contact suspect they are a person who stutters. Because patterns of avoidance are undetectable and, in many cases, socially acceptable, some individuals are able to successfully hide the overt nature of their problem.

For many reasons, avoidance of feared stimuli associated with past fluency failure—the people, sounds, words, time pressure and environments—is a natural but unproductive strategy for people who stutter. The core issue is

Clinical Decision-Making

Avoidance behavior can be insidious, often difficult to identify and especially resistant to change. People who show a high degree of avoidance behavior, if they initiate treatment at all, often find treatment difficult until they begin to become desensitized to stuttering. They may resist any suggestion to "touch" stuttering and activities that require them to approach stuttering, such as stuttering on purpose. They recoil against techniques that ask them to stay with and vary the ways they stutter. They are likely to resist revealing to others that they are attending treatment or telling anyone about their therapy activities or goals. Because patterns of avoidance are often so subtle, and because they are such an effective way of covering up the stuttering behavior, clients want to hold on to these highly self-reinforcing techniques. Once identified, avoidance behavior in all of its forms is a crucial target both during and following treatment. Unless clients understand the many hazards associated with avoidance, this response to the anticipation of stuttering is likely to persist. As clients achieve the ability to shape the features of their stuttering and use fluency-enhancing or modification techniques as described in later chapters, avoidance tends to lose its usefulness and appeal.

that avoidance dramatically reduces participation in daily activities and choices. On many occasions, avoidance can negatively impact the person's lifestyle more than the actual stuttering. For some people, switching to another word often results in stuttering on the new word. It is not surprising that speakers can be highly resistant to letting go of what has become a primary survival response. It takes time and energy for the client to successfully change his response to feared stimuli. It takes effort to scan ahead for these stimuli, and it takes even more effort to elude or respond to them as they come along. Some clients come to us feeling tired and frustrated by the ordeal. These people often show obvious relief when we suggest that they "give themselves permission to stutter."

Substitution

Substitutions of words are a most obvious form of avoidance. In this case, another word is substituted for the feared sound or word, often with a slight change in the meaning of the sentence. Sometimes the meaning changes only a little (dog/poodle, X-ray/radiology, or white/vanilla). Sometimes it changes a lot (tea/coffee, no/yes, a grade of C/A). At the very least, substitution often results in an utterance that is less precise or appropriate given the context of the communication. To the unsophisticated listener, nothing abnormal has occurred when the speaker adeptly substitutes one word or idea for another—but

Clinical Insight

As a young man in college, on those occasions when someone would ask me where my hometown was, I would do nearly anything to avoid saying the name "Williamsport." Instead, I would often say, "Well, I'm from a small town in Pennsylvania." If they inquired further, as of course they often did, I would say, "Well, it's in central Pennsylvania" or "It's a city about 85 miles north of Harrisburg." "Lock Haven?" they would respond. And I would say, "Well, it's a little east of Lock Haven." "Bloomsburg?" they would query. And I would respond, "No, it's actually west of Bloomsburg." Sometimes we would go on for awhile, gradually narrowing down the possibilities, until they were able to correctly guess the name of the city. I would do whatever it took, including acting as though I had no idea where I lived, in order to hide my stuttering. During these exchanges I certainly appeared to be, at the very least, a little strange or, at most, not very bright. I frequently did the same thing when asked about such things as the schools I attended, the names of my teachers or classes, or my street address. The problems presented by stuttering went far beyond my speech. Stuttering was a way of making choices and a way of living in ways that I thought were necessary to survive socially.

again, the speaker has experienced stuttering. It appears to be a good prognostic sign when the substitution of words is frustrating to the speaker. When this is the case the speaker may be more inclined to reduce their habitual avoidance of feared words and make the effort to select words that coincide with their intent. Some of the most frustrated (and sometimes depressed) individuals are those who are extremely eloquent as indicated by their writing and their periods of fluent speech but are unable to speak with the same precision and eloquence when avoiding or substituting words.

Postponement

As the person who stutters chooses to approach a feared word there is often a moment of hesitation, similar to one's preparation for leaping over an obstacle. Sometimes the hesitation is subtle, taking the form of a slight pause. The speaker may be considering alternative words or thinking of different ways to structure or restructure the sentence in order to avoid using the feared word. Other times, particularly before uttering words that previously resulted in stuttering, the speaker will use a series of sounds (e.g., "ah") or words (e.g., "you know, let me see") into the flow of speech to postpone or assist in the initiation of the word. Postponements are most likely to occur with words that cannot be easily avoided, such as names, addresses, schools, or places of employment (although it is not unusual for speakers to avoid or substitute even these words, as described in the previous Clinical Insight text box.

Listening to speakers who make frequent use of postponements can be extremely difficult, even unpleasant. These extra sounds and words, while maintaining a continuous flow of sound, severely disrupt the flow of information. These postponements are justifiably called "junk words" for they can litter the speech of people who are using them to the point that listeners, if given the option, will flee. Often, as a result of treatment, clients are able to decrease the use of such postponements and starters, greatly increasing the flow of information and effectiveness of their communication. Even if the speaker makes no change in the frequency of stuttering, the perceptual effect of a decrease in the use of these distracting junk sounds and words is one of enormous improvement.

The Speaker's Self-Assessment

The perceptions of speakers about themselves and their circumstances are likely to be one of the most important aspects of any assessment process, particularly for the adolescent or adult. One of the simplest, yet potentially most useful procedures for obtaining the initial perspective of clients and their stuttering is to have them respond to a series of questions designed to survey the range of their stuttering.

Clinical **Insight**

For this author as a young adult, the often subtle aspects of avoidance, substitution, and postponement were some of the most frustrating aspects of stuttering. I would say things less precisely than I was capable of, and often my meaning was distorted. Sometimes my listener could sense that the words did not exactly match the situation or my affect. In addition, I eventually realized how my thought process was inhibited when speaking. When writing, I enjoyed the challenge of finding and using just the right word to convey my meaning. However, when I spoke, I was often limiting my choices. For many years I had things to say, yet I refused to try. On a more basic level, I had things to say and I didn't even know it. I later realized that it was much like entering words on a computer screen and not knowing what you think until you write it. The new sentences result in ideas that, in turn, lead to new thoughts that you wouldn't have had otherwise. I realized that for many years, the same thing was happening when I spoke. Not only was I screening out many feared sounds and words, I was discarding current thoughts and future ideas. As my speech became ever more spontaneous so did my thoughts, and I found myself having ideas that I had not been able to reach before.

These questions provide an opportunity to sample behavior and to assess individuals' understanding of their stuttering. The process easily leads to a brief period of trial therapy, often an important aspect of the assessment process.

In preparation for asking the questions, the clinician draws a simple scale with equal-appearing intervals (Figure 4-1), with 0 off the scale to the left representing "no stuttering," 1 representing "mild stuttering," and so on to 8 at the right representing "severe stuttering." We place the scale in front of the person and ask him or her to indicate the point on the scale that best represents his or her overall, or average, stuttering. Once this point is identified, the clinician (or preferably the speaker) can place an "A" or "Average" at that location. The act of giving speakers the pencil and placing the scale in front of them is a first step toward assigning them responsibility for their speech. It may well be the first time the speaker has directly addressed his or her stuttering in a concrete and objective manner.

Once the client marks the point on the scale associated with what he or she perceives as his or her average level of severity, the clinician asks him or her to indicate the point on the scale that best represents the sample of speech that we are hearing at the moment. Although these points may be identical, often they are not. For example, Silverman, (1975) found that older children and adults judged the severity of their stuttering differently in a clinical environment than in daily beyond-treatment situations. By asking these two questions, the clinician is able to demonstrate an understanding of the variable nature of stuttering and that the behavior observed during the evaluation does not always represent the true nature and scope of the problem.

The clinician can then ask the client to indicate the extent of his or her stuttering behavior. How far toward either end of the scale does his or her stuttering range? What point on the scale indicates the quality of his or her speech in the best of speaking situations? For some speakers, this point represents no stuttering at all, a zero (0) on the scale. The speaker is then asked to indicate the point on the other end of the scale that represents his or her speech in his or her most difficult or feared speaking situations.

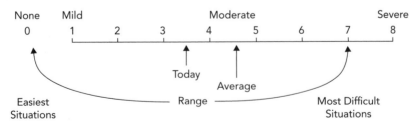

Figure 4-1 Equal-interval scale for determining the current, average, and range of stuttering behavior during the assessment of adolescents and adults.

Once he or she has identified a range of behavior, the clinician is able to make some observations about the person's speech and begin a short period of trial therapy. It will be possible for the clinician to determine, for example, whether his or her view of the surface features of the speaker's stuttering coincides with his or her own perception of severity. If it does not, and if the client perceives his or her stuttering very differently to the clinician, it may indicate that some time should be spent during treatment explaining the nature of stuttering and putting the client's stuttering into a broader perspective. Most individuals who stutter, unless they have attended group therapy or are a member of a stuttering support group, have not had the opportunity to observe a wide range of (particularly severe) stuttering behavior.

Assuming that the speaker has indicated a range of severity on the scale, the clinician can inform him or her that, in many ways at least, his or her stuttering is typical behavior for people who have this problem. That is, because of the variability and the nature of his or her stuttering, he or she is not likely to be stuttering as the result of some neurological or deep-seated psychological problem. Of course, before issuing such a statement, the person's case history should be reviewed and the speaker's overall response to the examiner's evaluations should be considered (see Chapter 10). However, by explaining this to the client, the clinician provides an important service to someone who, for many years, may have regarded him- or herself as being far from normal physically or emotionally. Depending on what he or she may have read or been told about stuttering as a physical or psychological/emotional problem, the person may have concerns about these issues.

Next, the clinician can conduct some brief trial therapy by asking the person to stutter along with the clinician. This is likely to be the first time the speaker has been invited to purposely enter into this fearful behavior. The very act of asking the client to willingly stutter demonstrates an assertive, investigative, and alternative attitude on the part of the clinician. It models a willingness to lead the way that can be highly motivating to clients. It also provides the first opportunity to explore and vary a behavior that for too long has seemed fearful and uncontrollable. Although the speaker is likely to have provided an example of stuttering at the outset of the evaluation, we would also like to have an understanding of the person's mild stuttering. Many clients will initially respond to the request "Show me what your mild stuttering looks and sounds like" by describing what they do when they stutter. Rather than a description of it, we want an example of the behavior they are concerned about and would rather avoid. Can the speaker willingly produce this behavior? Finally, can the person demonstrate, perhaps on his own or following our lead, examples of more moderate or possibly severe examples of his or her stuttering? If at any point in the procedure the person finds it difficult to voluntarily produce stuttering, the process can be facilitated by the clinician providing examples for the client to imitate.

Both participants can then produce the examples together, followed by the client doing it on his own. If, during this short period of trial therapy speakers are able to become somewhat desensitized to their stuttering, it can be useful to ask them to replicate their stuttering to the point that voluntary stuttering changes to real, "out-of-control" stuttering. The physical and emotional features that distinguish both voluntary and real stuttering provide a starting point for experimenting with techniques that allow the speaker to achieve both variation and modification of behavior that was previously thought by the speaker to be out of his or her control.

The degree to which the person can follow the clinician in experimenting with his or her stuttering tells us much about the person's levels of anxiety and motivation. These activities provide a preliminary indication of how much effort and time may be required for the person to approach, become desensitized to, and eventually manipulate his or her stuttering behavior. Can the person correctly identify occurrences and types of stuttering? Can he or she discriminate between the physical and emotional characteristics of real versus voluntary stuttering? Is he or she willing to venture with us across the threshold of control to see that that he or she is able to survive a deliberate moment of real stuttering? On the other hand, if the person is unable or unwilling to follow us in our attempts to experiment and vary his or her stuttering in this fashion, the process of treatment is likely to be more arduous. These relatively simple activities provide valuable information about the nature of stuttering, as well as the person who stutters.

Discovering the Intrinsic Features

Because of their very nature, the intrinsic or covert responses of the person to the experience of stuttering are somewhat more difficult to discover and quantify than the surface or overt speech characteristics. Because surface behaviors are more obvious, there is a tendency to spend the majority of the assessment time on these features. As suggested earlier, one of the ways to begin discovering intrinsic features is to ask the person "What do you do *because* you stutter?" That is, what choices do you make—what do you do or not do—because of the *possibility* of stuttering?

Identifying Speaker Loss of Control

Although we have discussed (see Chapter 2) the idea that the speaker's loss of control during stuttering distinguishes the experience from the fluency disruptions of typically fluent speakers, we further elaborate on this experience here in order to assist clinicians in both understanding and therefore identifying this important feature during the assessment process. These comments are also

Clinical **Insight**

We have used two procedures to help students to at least determine their level of anxiety about stuttering and self-efficacy regarding conducting treatment for individuals who stutter. The students listen to a series of audio and video examples of progressively more severe examples of stuttering by adult speakers, and using a 1–10 scale where they self-indicate less-to-more anxiety, students rate their levels of anxiety as each sample is presented both at the outset and at the end of the semester. For several reasons, including a variety of class activities as well as the student's clinical experiences, self-ratings of anxiety routinely show consistent decreases, particularly with regard to speakers who are stuttering more severely. We also ask students to fill out a self-efficacy scale composed of 100 progressively more difficult clinical situations that they are likely to encounter when working with children or adults who stutter (Rudolf, Manning, & Sewell, 1983). Students' overall scores typically show large increases, indicating greater self-efficacy for entering into and conducting a wide variety of treatment activities.

provided so that the nonstuttering clinician can establish some connection with the person who stutters. Although normally fluent speakers rarely experience a profound loss of control while speaking, everyone has had a similar experience during an athletic or physical activity. There is an instant when you perceive that you are not in control of your body, a fleeting moment when you realize that you have lost your balance. It is at this moment that you recognize that you are helpless and are unable to determine the consequences of your experience. There is, at this moment, a level of anxiety and even fear. Such an experience is more likely to occur if you are taking part in activities that require a degree of precision, timing, and balance. Activities such as skiing, skating, paddling a canoe or kayak, and wind surfing are good examples. However, it is also possible to encounter similar situations during more common activities such as riding a bike, climbing stairs, walking, running, or even driving a car. For the nonstuttering clinician who is able to be genuine and open, these experiences provide an opportunity to connect to the person who stutters and demonstrate his or her understanding about this core aspect of the stuttering experience.

Another common example for adults is the feeling you have when sliding out of control in your car through an icy intersection. During these moments one can approach the level of fear and helplessness that occurs for a person who stutters during a moment of stuttering. This loss of control can be both profound and discrete. It has been suggested that it is measurable (Moore & Erkins, 1990), at least by the person doing the stuttering. Whether a clinician

Clinical Insight

When taking a class on stuttering, students are often asked to take the part of a person who stutters in a series of daily speaking situations. On occasion, students completing this assignment report that they experience a distinct feeling of losing control as they are in the midst of stuttering. They describe having a feeling where, at least for a moment, they were uncertain about whether they would be able to stop voluntarily stuttering and continue on with what they intend to say. The experience is always described as unexpected and frightening. It can also provide some insight about why people who stutter, when they find themselves in such a condition, reflexively grasp for avoidance and escape behaviors (as irrational as they may appear to the observer) that have helped them cope with the situation in the past.

can identify such a loss of control in another speaker has yet to be demonstrated empirically. Nevertheless, over the years authors have suggested that it is possible for experienced clinicians who become calibrated to their clients to be able to accurately identify such moments (Bloodstein & Shogun, 1972; Cooper, 1968; Manning & Shrum, 1973). In discussing the difficulty of identifying successful avoidance behavior by people who stutter, Starkweather (1987) makes an important point that is pertinent to this discussion. He argues that although we may not have the means to apply rigorously scientific study to what we consider to be the essential features of an event, it should not preclude our study of those features. "Our first duty as scientists is to be true to the validity of the phenomenon being observed. If we lack the means to examine it objectively, we cannot assume or pretend that it doesn't exist" (p. 122).

It will usually take several sessions before the clinician will become calibrated to a new client and be able to recognize and verify the occurrence of some of these features. As we become attuned to the speaker we can begin to identify the three levels of fluency discussed earlier in this chapter: stuttered, unstable, and fluent. These levels of fluency tend to reflect the degree of control by the speaker. By pantomiming—imitating his or her speech production with our own mouths—we can begin to distinguish when the speaker is at each level of control. We can begin to sense when he or she is experiencing some lack of control over his or her fluency and identify those moments when stuttering does not quite reach the surface.

On other occasions, during what may initially appear to be seemingly fluent portions of speech, the person is, at best, on the edge of control. As discussed earlier, in order to prevent overt stuttering, the speaker may substitute and rearrange words. Although he or she may be producing "nonstuttered" speech, the speaker is not in control and is far from producing the effortless, smooth, and continuous speech that characterizes authentic fluency. It may also be that the perceptual effects of unstable speech also indicate a lack of sponta- neity and naturalness. The experienced listener—especially one who is familiar with how the speaker is capable of expressing himself in terms of rate, tempo, and syntax—can detect this loss of control. The clinician may be able to sense the brief pauses or slightly sticky moments present in the unstable speech. There may be a slight hesitation prior to the onset of a word or a momentary prolon- gation or stickiness during the initial portion of a word or a retreating back to an earlier portion of the sentence. The speaker may slightly constrict the vocal tract, minimally slow articulatory movements, and use somewhat more effort to produce a word. The client selects a word that is close to—but does not quite provide—the meaning the clinician has learned to anticipate. The client's body language (flaring of the nostrils, momentary loss of eye contact, and rapid eyelid movements) may indicate a brief moment of fear during the production of a word that is not smoothly produced. Without having awareness of this and by not responding to these cues the clinician may believe that he or she is reinforcing fluent speech when, in reality, unstable speech, avoidance, and word substitutions are being rewarded. Of course, one of the best ways to identify or confirm these unstable events is to ask the speaker.

It may be that many of the characteristic differences that have been noted in the acoustics of the "nonstuttered" speech of people who stutter reflect this lack of control. Over the years many researchers have observed a number of differences in the "fluent" speech of stutterers of various ages, including brief pauses (Love & Jefress, 1971), centralized formant frequencies (Klich & May, 1982), fundamental frequency variations (Healey, 1982), vocal shim- mer (Bamberg, Hanley, & Hillenbrand, 1990; Hall & Yairi, 1992; Newman, Harris, & Hilton, 1989), voice reaction times (Cross, Shadden, & Luper, 1979; Reich, Till, & Goldsmith, 1981), voice onset, initiation, and termina- tion times (Adams & Hayden, 1976; Agnello, 1975; Hillman & Gilbert, 1977; Starkweather, Hirschmann, & Tannenbaum, 1976) vocal tract instability as indicated by second formant frequency fluctuation compared to the control group of nonstuttering speakers (Robb, Blomgren & Chen, 1998). These acoustic characteristics may reflect brief moments where control was lost and unstable speech occurred. If investigators, rather than considering only the extremes of stuttered or nonstuttered speech, were to consider as a third cate- gory, the nature of this perceptually unstable speech, these acoustic measures may yield even more distinctive results.

There is another important aspect of the relationship between control and fluency. Just as a stuttering speaker may feel wildly out of control as he or she circumvents possible stuttering moments and manages to sound fluent, it is also possible for him or her to speak in an overtly stuttered manner and be in complete control. In other words, the clinician can show him or her that it is possible to stutter on purpose in an open, effortless fashion while being completely in charge of his or her speech mechanism. Being able to purposely and realistically stutter with complete control helps the speaker to break the remarkably strong link between the stuttering and helplessness. The speaker begins to consider, often for the first time, that it is possible to stutter and not be helpless. It is even possible to stutter and not to be anxious or afraid. As we will describe in more detail in subsequent chapters, it is possible to stutter in a different, easier, and more fluent manner.

Cognitive and Affective Factors

Closely related to the sensation of losing control of one's ability to speak are the related cognitive and affective features of stuttering. In an often-cited investigation, Corcoran and Stewart (1998) conducted one of the first qualitative studies of the experience of stuttering. The goal of their investigation was to discover consistent themes for eight adults (five men and three women ranging in age from 25 to 50 years.) with a history of stuttering. The authors obtained narratives from the participants that were analyzed qualitatively in order to describe the core experiences of stuttering for the participants. The primary theme that Corcoran and Stewart noted was one of suffering that included elements of helplessness, shame, fear, and avoidance. Helplessness resulted from both the involuntary nature of their stuttering and the general lack of control in their lives. Participants described their core experience as a sense that their stuttering was beyond their control. Participants described shame and stigma that were experienced to a degree that other aspects of their selves were obscured or discounted. Because of the lack of an accepted explanation for stuttering, they tended to assign blame to themselves for their stuttering and the fact that they seemed to be unable to do anything about it. The feelings of helplessness and shame and fear of the stuttering experience in general and of listener reactions in particular was also a common theme. Lastly, concealment and avoidance of even the possibility of stuttering was a consistent pattern that often resulted in a dramatically constricted lifestyle. The authors propose that the clinician is the major agent for assisting clients to transform the meaning of their stuttering, which, in turn, will provide both a reduction in suffering and facilitate the modification of overt behaviors. The processes of understanding the client's story and allowing the client to begin to consider alternate views about the experience of stuttering can begin during the initial diagnostic interview. Subsequent investigations by Crichton-Smith (2002), Anderson-Felsenfeld (2003), and Plexico et al. (2005) have confirmed and elaborated these findings during the early or pretreatment stages of stuttering. In each of these investigations, individuals who stutter consistently describe themes of suffering, struggle, and restriction across many aspects of their lives. From the speaker's perspective the impact of stuttering is represented by these intrinsic features as much or more than it is by the more obvious surface behaviors, such as the frequency of their stuttering.

Related to these affective and cognitive issues is the suspicion that people who stutter are more anxious that those who do not. Most adults who stutter do not show levels of anxiety that are clinically different from speakers who do not stutter. Molt and Guilford (1979) and Miller and Watson (1992) found no differences between adults who stutter and a group of controls on either state or trait anxiety. Craig and Hancock (1995) did find that adults who experienced self-defined relapse were three times more likely to indicate higher trait anxiety levels. In commenting on the results of pharmacological treatment for stuttering, Bothe et al. (2007) commented that the lack of effectiveness for the use of anxiolytics (medications used for the treatment of anxiety) for the treatment of stuttering indicates "that stuttering is neither inextricably nor functionally related to anxiety" (Bothe et al. 2007, p. 9).

Assessing the Speaker's Decision Making

As a result of the cognitive and affective coping responses, speakers frequently make many of their daily decisions based on the possibility as well as the reality of stuttering. We want to examine the many examples of a speaker's narrowing of options that typically result from attempts to avoid stuttering. As with detecting loss of control, it will take several treatment sessions to become calibrated to the person's lifestyle and manner of expressing him- or herself before the clinician can begin to appreciate the client's decision-making paradigm (Hayhow & Levy, 1989). The person who stutters, even after becoming aware of these choices, is not likely to associate some of them with the stuttering. Many or all of these choices become a way of understanding oneself. The client may indicate that "this is just the way I am. I'm basically a shy person. I don't want to take part in class or speak in front of groups. I don't like to use the phone. I'd rather mind my own business and would prefer not to introduce myself to strangers." Indeed, some or all these things may be true, for not everyone who is free from stuttering is a highly verbal or interactive person. But more frequently, for the person who stutters, many of these choices are informed by the probability of stuttering.

As the clinician is able to provide security and insight about the problem, the speaker is apt to become increasingly introspective about their patterns of responding to stuttering. It does little good at this point to ask the client to stop making what we see as poor choices, for these old responses are strong. Early on, the primary goal is to help the person to identify and acknowledge these choices, particularly those that foster denial or avoidance of stuttering. As people come to understand a wider range of options, they can begin to experiment with alternative choices in an ever-increasing range of communication situations. It is important to note, however, that as avoidance behaviors decrease there is the possibility that the frequency of stuttering will increase. As the speaker is beginning to achieve progress in becoming more assertive and participating in daily communication situations, the overt features of the problem may become more apparent. Because the client is now taking part in speaking situations that he or she previously avoided (e.g., asking a question in class or the office, using the telephone, expressing an opinion during a discussion), there are more opportunities for stuttering to reach the surface. The choices the person is making are far better but, for the moment at least, listeners may hear more stuttering. Consequently, in this instance at least, an increase in the frequency of stuttering can be appropriately interpreted as a sign of progress in treatment.

Formal Measures of Severity

Certainly many speakers who stutter exhibit some common patterns of behavior and reactions to stuttering but, as we indicated at the outset of this chapter, there can also be highly variable (and, on occasion, unusual) responses. There are many assessment devices that the clinician may use to obtain indications about the nature and severity of stuttering. In the following section we will describe some of the assessment instruments that we have found to be particularly useful. Importantly, many emphasize self-evaluation by the speaker (see Ingham & Cordes, 1997), particularly for indicating the intrinsic features of stuttering.

Locus of Control of Behavior (LCB)

The LCB scale, a 17-item Likert-type scale (Figure 4-2) developed by Craig, Franklin, and Andrews (1984), is designed to indicate the degree to which a person perceives daily occurrences of stuttering to be a consequence of his or her own behavior. This scaling procedure is designed to indicate the ability of a person to take responsibility for maintaining new or desired behaviors. Subjects are asked to indicate their agreement or disagreement to each of the 17 statements about their personal beliefs using a six-point bipolar Likert-type scale. The scores of the 17 statements are summed to yield a total LCB score, with items 1, 5, 7, 8, 13, and 16 scored in reverse order (e.g., a score of 4 is converted to a 1 and vice versa). Higher scores on this scale indicate a perception of external control or *externality*—the self perception that their behavior is determined by forces beyond their control), while lower scores indicate the perception of greater internal control or *internality*—the self-perception that they are able to determine their own behavior).

Since all forms of intervention for stuttering promote the speaker's assumption of increased responsibility for changing his or her circumstances, the locus

LCB SCALE

Name: Age: Date:

Directions: Below are a number of statements about how various topics affect your personal beliefs. There are no right or wrong answers. For every item there are a large number of people who agree and disagree. Could you please put in the appropriate bracket the choice you believe to be true. Answer all of the questions.

0	1	2	3	4	5
Strongly disagree	Generally disagree	Somewhat disagree	Somewhat agree	Generally agree	Strongly agree

1. I can anticipate difficulties and take action to avoid them.   ( )
2. A great deal of what happens to me is probably just a matter of chance.   ( )
3. Everyone knows that luck or chance determines one's future.   ( )
4. I can control my problem(s) only if I have outside support.   ( )
5. When I make plans, I am almost certain that I can make them work.   ( )
6. My problem(s) will dominate me all my life.   ( )
7. My mistakes and problems are my responsibility to deal with.   ( )
8. Becoming a success is a matter of hard work; luck has little or nothing to do with it.   ( )
9. My life is controlled by outside actions and events.   ( )
10. People are victims of circumstances beyond their control.   ( )
11. To continually manage my problems I need professional help.   ( )
12. When I am under stress, the tightness in my muscles is due to things outside my control.   ( )
13. I believe a person can really be the master of his fate.   ( )
14. It is impossible to control my irregular and fast breathing when I am having difficulties.   ( )
15. I understand why my problem(s) varies so much from, one occasion to the next   ( )
16. I am confident of being able to deal successfully with future problems.   ( )
17. In my case, maintaining control over my problem(s) is mostly due to luck.   ( )

Figure 4-2 Locus of Control of Behavior Scale. From Craig, A., Franklin, J., & Andrews, G. (1984). A scale to measure locus of control of behavior, *British Journal of Medical Psychology, 57,* 173–180. Reprinted with permission.

of control concept is intuitively appealing. Craig, Franklin, and Andrews (1984) administered the LCB to two groups of nonstuttering adults, 123 university students (mean score 28.3) and 53 nurses (mean score of 27.9). Both groups scored significantly lower (p < .05) compared to a group of 70 adults who were awaiting treatment for stuttering (mean score of 31.0). Craig et al. (1984) also noted that a reduced LCB score (greater internality) during treatment was predictive of fluency maintenance following treatment whereas an increase (or no change) in the LCB score was predictive of relapse 10 months after treatment. The scale was found to have acceptable internal consistency (alpha of 0.79) and scores were not influenced by age, gender, or social desirability of responses. One-week test-retest reliability with 25 nonstuttering adults resulted in a Pearson correlation of 0.90. A six-month test-retest reliability of 0.73 was found for 25 adults awaiting treatment.

We have found that scores for adults who would be regarded as severely stuttering often have LCB scores as high as 44 to 55. Nonstuttering speakers generally score in the high teens to low twenties. Craig and Andrews (1985) found that changes in LCB scores successfully predicted the outcome in 15 of 17 participants 10 months following treatment. However, (DiNil & Kroll, 1995) found LCB scores to be unrelated to a speaker's fluency and possibly influenced by whether or not increased assertiveness and responsibility are a focus of treatment (Ladouceur, Caron, & Caron, 1989). An example of progressive improvement (decreases) in LCB scores for an adult with severe stuttering can be found in Chapter 11.

Stuttering Severity Instrument for Children and Adults (SSI-4)

A frequently used instrument for determining stuttering severity, the SSI was originally developed in 1972 by Glyndon Riley for determining stuttering severity for both children and adults. The most recent (fourth edition) of this scale (SSI-4; Riley, 2009) is similar to the third edition (SSI-3; Riley, 1994) (see Figure 4-3). However, with the newest edition several additional features have been included to provide a more comprehensive perspective of stuttering severity. For example, it is recommended that the clinician (a) obtain speaking samples beyond the clinic environment, (b) acquire speech samples during a variety of telephone conversations, (c) use a 9-point naturalness rating scale, and (d) obtain self-reports of severity, locus of control, and avoidance of stuttering. These self-report processes are mentioned in the following sections describing the Clinical use of Self-Reports (CUSR) and the Subjective Screening of Stuttering: research edition (SSS-R). In addition, a computerized scoring system (CSSS-2) is available through the publisher.

When being administered the SSI-4, speakers who can read are asked to (1) describe their job or school and (2) read a short passage (passages are provided). Nonreaders are given a picture task to which they respond. Scoring is accomplished across three areas. The frequency of the fluency breaks tabulated

SSI-3

Stuttering Severity Instrument–3

TEST RECORD AND FREQUENCY COMPUTATION FORM

Identifying Information

Name _____

Sex   M   F   Grade _____   Age _____

Date _____   Date of Birth _____

School _____

Examiner _____

Preschool ___   School Age ___   Adult ___   Reader ___   Nonreader ___

FREQUENCY Use Readers Table or Nonreaders Table not both.

READERS TABLE				NONREADERS TABLE	
1. Speaking Task		2. Reading Task		3. Speaking Task	
Percentage	Task Score	Percentage	Task Score	Percentage	Task Score
1	2	1	2	1	4
2	3			2	6
3	4	2	4	3	8
4–5	5	3–4	5	4–5	10
6–7	6	5–7	6	6–7	12
8–11	7	8–12	7	8–11	14
12–21	8	13–20	8	12–21	16
22 & up	9	21 & up	9	22 & up	18

Frequency Score (use 1 + 2 or 3) [   ]

DURATION

Average length of three longest stuttering events timed to the nearest 1/10th second		Scale Score
Fleeting	(.5 sec or less)	2
Half-second	(.5– .9 sec)	4
1 full second	(1.0– 1.9 secs)	6
2 seconds	(2.0– 2.9 secs)	8
3 seconds	(3.0– 4.9 secs)	10
5 seconds	(5.0– 9.9 secs)	12
10 seconds	(10.0– 29.9 secs)	14
30 seconds	(30.0– 59.9 secs)	16
1 minute	(60 secs or more)	18

Duration Score (2 – 18) [   ]

PHYSICAL CONCOMITANTS

Evaluating Scale
0 = none
1 = not noticeable unless looking for it
2 = barely noticeable to casual observer
3 = distracting
4 = very distracting
5 = severe and painful-looking

DISTRACTING SOUNDS	Noisy breathing, whistling, sniffing, blowing, clicking sounds	0 1 2 3 4 5
FACIAL GRIMACES	Jaw jerking, tongue protruding, lip pressing, jaw muscles tense	0 1 2 3 4 5
HEAD MOVEMENTS	Back, forward, turning away, poor eye contact, constant looking around	0 1 2 3 4 5
MOVEMENTS OF THE EXTREMITIES	Arm and hand movement, hands about face, torso movement, leg movements, foot-tapping or swinging	0 1 2 3 4 5

Physical Concomitants Score [   ]

TOTAL OVERALL SCORE

Frequency _____ + Duration _____ + Physical Concomitants _____ = [   ]

Percentile _____

Severity _____

(continues)

Figure 4-3 The Stuttering Severity Instrument-3 (SSI-3). From *Stuttering Severity Instrument for Children and Adults—Third Edition (Test Record and Frequency Computation Form)*, pp. 1–2 by G. D. Riley, 1994, Austin, TX: PRO-ED. Copyright 1994 by PRO-ED. Reprinted with permission.

TABLE 2
Percentile and Severity Equivalents of SSI-3 Total Overall Scores for
Preschool Children (N = 72)

Total Overall Score	Percentile	Severity
0– 8	1– 4	Very Mild
9–10	5–11	
11–12	12–23	Mild
13–16	24–40	
17–23	41–60	Moderate
24–26	61–67	
27–28	78–88	Severe
29–31	89–95	
32 and up	96–99	Very Severe

TABLE 3
Percentile and Severity Equivalents of SSI-3 Total Overall Scores for
School-Age Children (N = 139)

Total Overall Score	Percentile	Severity
6– 8	1– 4	Very Mild
9–10	5–11	
11–15	12–23	Mild
16–20	24–40	
21–23	41–60	Moderate
24–27	61–77	
28–31	78–88	Severe
32–35	89–95	
36 and up	96–99	Very Severe

TABLE 4
Percentile and Severity Equivalents of SSI-3 Total Overall Scores for
Adults (N = 60)

Total Overall Score	Percentile	Severity
10–12	1– 4	Very Mild
13–17	5–11	
18–20	12–23	Mild
21–24	24–40	
25–27	41–60	Moderate
28–31	61–67	
32–34	78–88	Severe
35–36	89–95	
37–46	96–99	Very Severe

Figure 4-3 Continued.

and the percentage of stuttering are converted to a task score (range, 2–18). The duration of the three longest stuttering moments (fleeting to more than 60 seconds) is tabulated and converted to a scale score (range, 2–18). Last, physical concomitants across four categories are rated on a 0–5 scale (0 = none, 5 = severe and painful looking) and totaled (range, 0–20). The total overall score is computed by adding the scores for the three areas. Percentile and severity equivalents are provided for preschool children, school-age children, and adults. The scale is commonly used because it can be used with virtually all age ranges and is easily and quickly administered and scored.

Overall average intra-examiner percentages of agreement for determining frequency and duration of stuttering averaged 85.9% (range 71.4% – 92.9) and 93.9% (range 68.0% – 100%), respectively (Riley, 1994). With practice, most clinicians are able to achieve a minimum of 85% self-agreement. Average inter-examiner agreement ranged from 82.9% (physical concomitants) to 91.0% (frequency). Experienced members of the research team that developed the SSI-3 were able to achieve an average of 95% intra-examiner agreement and 89.6% inter-examiner agreement. The SSI-3 overall score was correlated with stuttering frequency ($p < .01$) for preschool (.830), school-age (.795), and adult speakers (.741). In addition Yaruss and Conture (1992) found a correlation of .72 between the research version of the SSI-3 and the Stuttering Prediction Instrument (SPI) (Riley, 1981), which includes parent's reports of their child's stuttering and reactions.

Subjective Screening of Stuttering Severity (SSS)

While the SSI provides an indication of the speaker's overt stuttering features, Riley and Riley argue that the speaker's perception of his or her problem is at least as, and often more, important, than the frequency, duration, and struggle behaviors associated with stuttering. Although it is sometimes the case that ratings of overt stuttering by the clinician may coincide with the self-perceptions of severity by the speaker, it is not uncommon for this not to be the case. Furthermore, while reductions of overt stuttering behaviors are clearly an important goal of treatment, for many speakers, an internal locus of control and the freedom to communicate without avoidance are critical goals. The authors provide a convincing argument that the most important opinion concerning the speaker's ability to communicate is that of the speaker.

Over the last 35 years J. Riley has developed questions to help her understand the attitudes and feelings of people who stutter. Chapter 4 of the manual for the SSI-4 (Riley, 2009) Clinical Use of Self-Reports (CUSR), outlines 16 questions to improve the communication between the speaker and the clinician. Three areas of the speaker's self-reported response to stuttering are covered by the CUSR: l. perceived stuttering severity, 2. level of internal or external locus of control (effort to speak without stuttering), and 3. word or situation avoidance. Each item is self-rated for the experience of several speaking audiences such as a close friend, an authority figure, speaking to someone on the telephone, and others. Each item is rated on a 9-point semantic differential scale where 1 represents a normal speaking experience (target level) and 9 the most severe stuttering experience. Speakers use a series of 9-point scales to self-rate their perception of their stuttering experience by responding to the 16 questions. The selected item or items are rated in conversation with the clinician. The CUSR does not provide a standardized way to convert the item scores into subtest scores, rather each item serves to measure a specific attitude or feeling. In this regard, each item is similar to those on the naturalness scale.

Each answer selected by the client provides an opportunity to explore an area that may need to be changed and which can become a therapy goal or objective. A change in rating from 8 to 6, for example, can communicate progress before it is obvious to the client. The examples that follow describe the use of three of the CUSR questions in therapy.

Item 1. How would you score your speech with the following audiences? (Severity)

A given client may score the speech as a 2 with a friend, a 6 with a stranger, and an 8 on the telephone. This awareness of variations in fluency during different speaking situations provides the clinician an opportunity to explore in depth what this variation in fluency means to the speaker and how to facilitate similar fluency with difficult audiences.

Item 4. How often do you change your words when you think you may stutter? (Avoidance)

This question provides a way to monitor the person who stutters' use of word or sound avoidance. Everyday listeners cannot usually observe that a person is avoiding except that they may notice the sentence sounds awkward. Treatment may require that the client and clinician become aware of avoidance and work toward modifying the behavior. Reduction in the score on this item indicates that avoidance of words and/or sounds is occurring less often.

Item 6. How much energy do you expend on how to speak rather than what to say? (Locus of control)

People who stutter often show emotion when faced with this question because they often expend so much energy trying to keep from stuttering or trying to cover it up that they do not realize that others may not notice or care if they stutter. They may even pass up or withdraw from a conversation because of the energy required to participate. When the clinician demonstrates an empathetic appreciation of the pain experienced by the person who stutters, the therapeutic relationship is enhanced. As the person shifts attention toward what is being said and away from the stuttering, the rating of this item should come down.

Four years of clinical trials by Riley et al. (2004) resulted in a research version (Figure 4-4) that includes 8 items within 3 subtests providing screening information about the speaker's self-perceived stuttering severity (2 items), level of internal/external locus of control (3 items), and word or situation avoidance (3 items). Each item is rated on a 9-point semantic differential scale where 1 represents a normal speaking experience (target level) and 9 the most severe. All items are self-rated for the experience of speaking to each of three audiences: a close friend (these ratings are used for comparison but are not included in the scoring), an authority figure, and use of the telephone. Test-retest agreement was obtained with 16 adults. Pearson product correlations for the 3 subtests were 0.90 (severity), 0.93 (locus of control), and 0.79 (avoidance). Individual subtests correlated well with the total SSS scores (0.92 for perceived severity, 0.92 for locus of control, 0.95 for avoidance).

The protocol for the research edition of the SSS (Figure 4-4), which is given using pencil and paper rather than interview, can be used to obtain numerical scores. It has been used in several studies of the effects of medications on stuttering. Scores for the eight items described above and for the three speaking situations are used to compute a subtest score for Severity, Locus of Control, and Avoidance,

J. Riley et al. (2004) describe how comparisons of the speaker's self-report responses to the above questions can be interpreted. For example, using one question having to do with *severity* may result in a low rating by the clinician on the SSI-4 in combination with a high rating by the speaker on the SSS-R. Such a discrepancy may indicate that even minimal stuttering is extremely painful to the speaker and that the person would benefit from activities involving desensitization to stuttering. A low SSS-R score in contrast to a high SSI-4 score may indicate denial, lack of awareness, or possibly some of the characteristics of cluttering (see Chapter 10).

Revised Communication Attitude Inventory (S-24)

The S-24 is an easy-to-administer 24-item inventory that continues to be used in many clinical studies (Figure 4-5). The S-24 was modified by Andrews and Cutler (1974) from the original 39-item Erickson S-Scale (1969). Clients respond to a series of 24 true-false statements according to whether or not the statements are characteristic of themselves. Designed for use with older adolescents and adults, the total score is obtained by tabulating one point for each item that is answered as a person who stutters would respond. Higher scores indicate a negative attitude about communicating. Individuals who stutter average a total of 19.22 (*SD* = 5.38) items scored in this manner, while nonstuttering individuals average a total score of 9.14 (*SD* = 4.24). Andrews and Cutler did

Subjective Stuttering Scales—research edition

Client _____ Case #_____ Sampled @_____ Date_____

1. How would you score your fluency during the session today?

    Relatively fluent   1 2 3 4 5 6 7 8 9   Severe stuttering

2. How would you score your speech with the following audiences during
    the last week?

	Relatively fluent							Severe stuttering	
Close friend	1	2	3	4	5	6	7	8	9
Authority figure	1	2	3	4	5	6	7	8	9
Telephone	1	2	3	4	5	6	7	8	9

3. How much time during conversation during the last week did you
    think about stuttering with the following audiences?

	Never							Constantly	
Close friend	1	2	3	4	5	6	7	8	9
Authority figure	1	2	3	4	5	6	7	8	9
Telephone	1	2	3	4	5	6	7	8	9

4. How often did you change words during the last week when you
    thought you might get stuck, with the following audiences?

	Never							Always	
Close friend	1	2	3	4	5	6	7	8	9
Authority figure	1	2	3	4	5	6	7	8	9
Telephone	1	2	3	4	5	6	7	8	9

5. To what extent did you feel internally hurried during conversation this
    past week with the following audiences?

	Never							Always	
Close friend	1	2	3	4	5	6	7	8	9
Authority figure	1	2	3	4	5	6	7	8	9
Telephone	1	2	3	4	5	6	7	8	9

(continues)

Figure 4-4   The research edition of the Subjective Screening of Stuttering Severity
(SSS). Reprinted from *Journal of Fluency Disorders*, 29/1, Riley, J., Riley, G., &
McGuire, G., Subjective Screening of Stuttering severity, locus of control and avoidance:
research edition., 51–62, 2004, with permission from Elsevier.

6. How much energy did you expend this week on how you speak rather than on what you wanted to say with the following audiences?

    0%   100%

    Close friend   1 2 3 4 5 6 7 8 9
    Authority figure   1 2 3 4 5 6 7 8 9
    Telephone   1 2 3 4 5 6 7 8 9

7. During the past week how often did you refrain from a conversation because of fear of stuttering with the following audiences?

    Seldom   Frequently

    Close friend   1 2 3 4 5 6 7 8 9
    Authority figure   1 2 3 4 5 6 7 8 9
    Telephone   1 2 3 4 5 6 7 8 9

8. During the past week how much choice did you feel you had to take part in a conversation with the following audiences?

    A great deal   Very little

    Close friend   1 2 3 4 5 6 7 8 9
    Authority figure   1 2 3 4 5 6 7 8 9
    Telephone   1 2 3 4 5 6 7 8 9

Figure 4-4 Continued.

Subjective Screening of Stuttering—research edition

SCORING FORM

Client _____ Case # _____ Sampled @ _____ Date _____

Stuttering Severity Subtest

1. (1-9)   _____   Severity total (3 – 27) _____   Other Measures

2. CF (1-9) [_____]*   _____
   AF (1-9) _____   _____
   TE (1-9) _____   _____

Locus of Control Subtest

3. CF (1-9) [_____]   Locus of control total (6 – 54) _____
   AF (1-9) _____
   TE (1-9) _____

5. CF (1-9) [_____]
   AF (1-9) _____
   TE (1-9) _____

6. CF (1-9) [_____]
   AF (1-9) _____
   TE (1-9) _____

Avoidance

4. CF (1-9) [_____]   Avoidance total (6 – 54) _____
   AF (1-9) _____
   TE (1-9) _____

7. CF (1-9) [_____]
   AF (1-9) _____
   TE (1-9) _____

8. CF (1-9) [_____]
   AF (1-9) _____
   TE (1-9) _____

Total score: Severity____+ Locus of Control____+ Avoidance____= Total____

* Scores with a close friend are not used to calculate the total scores.

Figure 4-4 Continued.

Modified Erickson Scale of Communication Attitudes (S-24)

Name: _____   Date: _____   Score: _____

Directions: Mark the "true" column with a check (✓) for each statement that is true or mostly true for you and mark the "false" column with a check (✓) for each statement which is false or not usually true for you.

	TRUE	FALSE
1. I usually feel that I am making a favorable impression when I talk.	_____	_____
2. I find it easy to talk with almost anyone.	_____	_____
3. I find it very easy to look at my audience while speaking to a group.	_____	_____
4. A person who is my teacher or my boss is hard to talk to.	_____	_____
5. Even the idea of giving a talk in public makes me afraid.	_____	_____
6. Some words are harder than others for me to say.	_____	_____
7. I forget all about myself shortly after I begin a speech.	_____	_____
8. I am a good mixer.	_____	_____
9. People sometimes seem uncomfortable when I am talking to them.	_____	_____

	TRUE	FALSE
10. I dislike introducing one person to another.	_____	_____
11. I often ask questions in group discussions.	_____	_____
12. I find it easy to keep control of my voice when speaking.	_____	_____
13. I do not mind speaking before a group.	_____	_____
14. I do not talk well enough to do the kind of work I'd really like to do.	_____	_____
15. My speaking voice is rather pleasant and easy to listen to.	_____	_____
16. I am sometimes embarrassed by the way I talk.	_____	_____

(continues)

Figure 4-5 Revised Communication Attitude Inventory (S-24). Andrews, G., and Cutler, J. (1974). Stuttering therapy: The relation between changes in symptom level and attitudes. *Journal of Speech and Hearing Disorders, 39*, pp. 312–319. Copyright 1974, American Speech-Language-Hearing Association. Reprinted with permission.

	TRUE	FALSE
17. I face most speaking situations with complete confidence.	___	___
18. There are few people I can talk with easily.	___	___
19. I talk better than I write.	___	___
20. I often feel nervous while talking.	___	___
21. I find it hard to make conversation when I meet new people.	___	___
22. I feel pretty confident about my speaking ability.	___	___
23. I wish that I could say things as clearly as others do.	___	___
24. Even though I knew the right answer, I have often failed to give it because I was afraid to speak out.	___	___

I. Answers

Score 1 point for each answer that matches this:

1. False	7. False	13. False	19. False
2. False	8. False	14. True	20. True
3. False	9. True	15. False	21. True
4. True	10. True	16. True	22. False
5. True	11. False	17. False	23. True
6. True	12. False	18. True	24. True

II. Adult Norms

	Mean	Range
Stutterers	19.22	9-24
Nonstutters	9.14	1-21

Figure 4-5 Continued.

not specify the reliability and validity processes but indicated that item analysis resulted in the deletion of items that resulted in poor test-retest reliability and validity. Mean scores on the S-24 discriminated between 36 individuals who stuttered and a control group of 25 fluent speakers, and pre-post treatment differences for the individuals who stuttered were significant.

Perceptions of Stuttering Inventory (PSI)

The PSI, developed by Woolf (1967), is designed to determine the speaker's self-rating of avoidance, struggle, and expectancy (of stuttering) for older adolescents and adults. The person responds to each of 60 statements according to whether or not he or she feels they are "characteristic of me." Statements that the person feels are not characteristic are left unmarked. Examples of inventory items include "Avoiding talking to people in authority" (avoidance), "Having extra and unnecessary facial movement" (struggle), and "Adding an extra sound in order to get started" (expectancy).

Self-Efficacy Scaling for Adult Stutterers (SESAS)

Based on the work of Bandura (1977) with perceptual self-efficacy scaling, the Self-Efficacy Scale for Adult Stutterers (SESAS) (Ornstein & Manning, 1985) is designed to measure a speaker's confidence for entering into and achieving fluency in speaking situations beyond the treatment environment (Figure 4-6). The first section of the scale (SESAS approach) asks speakers to indicate the likelihood that they could enter into each of 50 specific speaking situations by using a decile scale from 10 to 100 (higher scores indicate greater confidence). The speaking situations are ordered in a hierarchy, from easy to more difficult. Speaker responses are averaged over the 50 situations to obtain the SESAS approach score. The second section of the scale again asks the speaker to consider the same 50 speaking situations, this time indicating their confidence for maintaining a client-selected "level of fluency" (SESAS performance). Speaker responses are averaged over the 50 speaking situations to obtain the SESAS performance score. Ornstein and Manning (1985) found that the SESAS total score correlated with the Erickson Scale of Communication Attitudes (Erickson, 1969) at −0.71 (sign in the expected direction) and with the Perceptions of Stuttering Inventory (Woolf, 1967) at −0.52 (sign in the expected direction). In addition, test-retest reliability for the SESAS for 10 of the experimental subjects averaged +0.95 and +0.84 for the SESAS approach and performance scales, respectively.

Ornstein and Manning (1985) found that 20 adults who stuttered (mean age 26.11 years; range of 18-44 years) scored significantly lower ($p < .05$) on both the approach (mean = 66.2) and performance (mean = 55.8) portions of the SESAS than did a matched group of nonstuttering speakers. Interestingly, the mean scores of fluent speakers (94.2 and 98.0 for the approach and performance scales, respectively) indicated that they were less confident about approaching situations than about speaking fluently once they were in the situations. Conversely, the speakers who stuttered were more confident about approaching speaking situations than about maintaining fluency once they entered the situation.

A validation study by Saltuklaroglu and Kully (1998) provided both criterion and construct validity for the approach portion of the SESAS. Moderate but significant correlations between SESAS approach scores and %SS (−0.305) and global severity ratings (−0.279) were obtained for 160 adolescent and adult subjects (age range 14–74 years) prior to formal treatment. The somewhat modified scale (42 versus 50 speaking situations) resulted in a mean approach score of 53.8. The 20 subjects in the Ornstein and Manning (1985) study had received

A SELF-EFFICACY SCALE FOR ADULT STUTTERERS
(SESAS)

Name _____ Date _____

Date of Birth _____ Gender _____ Race _____

Occupation _____

Years in School _____ Months in Therapy _____

You will be presented with two lists of 50 speaking situations which
commonly occur. While you may not typically find yourself in each of these
speaking situations, indicate how you believe you would perform in each
situation. Please answer all questions. For the first set of 50 questions
ask yourself whether or not you would enter each situation. Under the
column CAN DO, check the situations you expect you would enter if you
were asked to do them now. Then, for the situations you check under
the column CAN DO, mark in the column CONFIDENCE how confident
you are that you would enter each particular situation. Rate your degree
of confidence by recording one of the following numbers from 10 to 100
using the scale below.

10	20	30	40	50	60	70	80	90	100
QUITE				MODERATELY					VERY
UNCERTAIN				CERTAIN					CERTAIN

To familiarize yourself with the rating form note the following example:

Situation	CAN DO	CONFIDENCE
1. Lift a 25 pound box above your head	__X__	100
2. Lift a 35 pound box above your head	__X__	90
3. Lift a 50 pound box above your head	__X__	80
4. Lift a 65 pound box above your head	__X__	70
5. Lift a 80 pound box above your head	__X__	50
6. Lift a 100 pound box above your head	__X__	30
7. Lift a 200 pound box above your head	_____	_____

(continues)

Figure 4-6   The Self-Efficacy Scale for Adults who Stutter. From: Ornstein, A., &
Manning, W. (1985). Self-efficacy scaling by adult stutterers. *Journal of Communication
Disorders, 18,* 313–320. Reprinted with permission.

Now complete the following example to practice using the rating scale.

Situation	CAN DO	CONFIDENCE
1. High jump 1 foot	_____	_____
2. High jump 2 feet	_____	_____
3. High jump 3 feet	_____	_____
4. High jump 4 feet	_____	_____
5. High jump 5 feet	_____	_____
6. High jump 6 feet	_____	_____

APPROACH ATTITUDE:

If you are sure that you understand the task, please complete the following list of 50 situations by (1) checking whether you feel you would enter each situation and (2) your confidence in that belief. Please make these judgements honestly with respect to your present ability, not according to what you want to do or think you should do. Rate your degree of confidence by recording one of the following numbers from 10 to 100 using the scale below. If you do not feel that you would enter a situation, do not mark that item.

10	20	30	40	50	60	70	80	90	100
QUITE				MODERATELY					VERY
UNCERTAIN				CERTAIN					CERTAIN

WOULD YOU. . .:	CAN DO	CONFIDENCE
1. Talk with a family member during a meal.	_____	_____
2. Request help in an uncrowded department store.	_____	_____
3. Talk to a close friend while walking down the street.	_____	_____
4. Talk to a family member on the phone.	_____	_____
5. Talk with your clinician while standing in line for a movie.	_____	_____
6. Talk to a fellow worker that you meet in a store.	_____	_____
7. Call up a friend on the phone.	_____	_____
8. Order food at McDonald's when there are no other customers.	_____	_____
9. Talk with your physician in a store.	_____	_____
10. Answer the phone at home.	_____	_____
11. Talk with a fellow worker at work.	_____	_____

Figure 4-6   Continued.

WOULD YOU. . .: (continued)	CAN DO	CONFIDENCE
12. Ask a friend to drive you to the airport.	_____	_____
13. Talk to a telephone operator on the phone.	_____	_____
14. Introduce two friends at a shopping mall.	_____	_____
15. Talk with your boss at a social gathering.	_____	_____
16. Ask a policeman for directions.	_____	_____
17. Call a member of the opposite sex on the phone.	_____	_____
18. Talk to a group of friends in a noisy bar or restaurant.	_____	_____
19. Talk with your instructor after class.	_____	_____
20. Make a long distance phone call.	_____	_____
21. Tell a joke in front of five people.	_____	_____
22. Answer questions during a group discussion.	_____	_____
23. Call the information operator on the phone.	_____	_____
24. Approach your boss and initiate a conversation at work.	_____	_____
25. Initiate a conversation with a stranger of the opposite sex at a party.	_____	_____
26. Answer a phone in a crowded room.	_____	_____
27. Ask questions during a group discussion.	_____	_____
28. Order food from your car through a speaker at McDonald's.	_____	_____
29. Make a phone call to say that you will be late.	_____	_____
30. Introduce yourself to a stranger.	_____	_____
31. Order a drink from a bartender at a noisy, crowded bar.	_____	_____
32. Talk to your boss on the phone.	_____	_____
33. Get in a long line at McDonald's to order food.	_____	_____
34. Request help in a crowded department store when all the salespeople seem busy.	_____	_____
35. Telephone your clinician to cancel a therapy session.	_____	_____
36. Introduce yourself to a group of strangers.	_____	_____

Figure 4-6 Continued.

WOULD YOU. . .: (continued)	CAN DO	CONFIDENCE
37. Volunteer to present a talk on your work or hobby to a group of 20 school-age children.	_____	_____
38. Talk to your boss at work about a work-related error that you have made.	_____	_____
39. Ask for directions over the phone.	_____	_____
40. Order food in a restaurant when the waitress is obviously in a hurry.	_____	_____
41. Initiate a conversation with the person sitting next to you on an airplane.	_____	_____
42. Give an important 30-minute presentation at work or school.	_____	_____
43. Volunteer to present a talk on your work or hobby to a group of 25 adults.	_____	_____
44. Order a pizza over the phone.	_____	_____
45. Ask for a raise at work.	_____	_____
46. Complain about the lack of service to your waiter/waitress.	_____	_____
47. Call a stranger on the phone to tell him or her about a meeting.	_____	_____
48. Volunteer to go on a T.V. or radio talk show.	_____	_____
49. Order exactly what you want in a restaurant even though you might stutter on the words.	_____	_____
50. Call up the telephone company to question a bill.	_____	_____

FLUENCY PERFORMANCE:

For the second set of 50 questions ask yourself whether or not you could achieve fluent speech in each situation. Please define fluency as speech that would be so fluent in a given situation that, in your opinion, a listener would not recognize that you had a history of stuttering. Again, under the column marked CAN DO, place a check if you believe you could achieve fluency in that situation. Then mark in the column CONFIDENCE, how confident you are that you could achieve fluency. Please make these judgements honestly with respect to your present ability and not according to how you would like to perform or think that you should perform. Rate your degree of confidence by recording one of the following numbers from 10 to 100 using the scale below. If you do not believe that you can achieve fluent speech in a given situation, do not mark that item.

Figure 4-6 Continued.

| 10 | 20 | 30 | 40 | 50 | 60 | 70 | 80 | 90 | 100 |

QUITE
UNCERTAIN

MODERATELY
CERTAIN

VERY
CERTAIN

If you are sure that you understand the task, please complete the following list of 50 situations by (1) indicating whether you feel you could achieve your fluency level in each situation and (2) your confidence in that belief. COULD YOU ACHIEVE YOUR FLUENCY LEVEL WHILE. . .:

COULD YOU. . .:	CAN DO	CONFIDENCE
1. Talk with a family member during a meal.	_____	_____
2. Request help in an uncrowded department store.	_____	_____
3. Talk to a close friend while walking down the street.	_____	_____
4. Talk to a family member on the phone.	_____	_____
5. Talk with your clinician while standing in line for a movie.	_____	_____
6. Talk to a fellow worker that you meet in a store.	_____	_____
7. Call up a friend on the phone.	_____	_____
8. Order food at McDonald's when there are no other customers.	_____	_____
9. Talk with your physician in a store.	_____	_____
10. Answer the phone at home.	_____	_____
11. Talk with a fellow worker at work.	_____	_____
12. Ask a friend to drive you to the airport.	_____	_____
13. Talk to a telephone operator on the phone.	_____	_____
14. Introduce two friends at a shopping mall.	_____	_____
15. Talk with your boss at a social gathering.	_____	_____
16. Ask a policeman for directions.	_____	_____
17. Call a member of the opposite sex on the phone.	_____	_____
18. Talk to a group of friends in a noisy bar or restaurant.	_____	_____
19. Talk with your instructor after class.	_____	_____
20. Make a long distance phone call.	_____	_____

Figure 4-6 Continued.

COULD YOU. . .: (Continued)	<u>CAN DO</u>	<u>CONFIDENCE</u>
21. Tell a joke in front of five people.	_____	_____
22. Answer questions during a group discussion.	_____	_____
23. Call the information operator on the phone.	_____	_____
24. Approach your boss and initiate a conversation at work.	_____	_____
25. Initiate a conversation with a stranger of the opposite sex at a party.	_____	_____
26. Answer a phone in a crowded room.	_____	_____
27. Ask questions during a group discussion.	_____	_____
28. Order food from your car through a speaker at McDonald's.	_____	_____
29. Make a phone call to say that you will be late.	_____	_____
30. Introduce yourself to a stranger.	_____	_____
31. Order a drink from a bartender at a noisy, crowded bar.	_____	_____
32. Talk to your boss on the phone.	_____	_____
33. Get in a long line at McDonald's to order food.	_____	_____
34. Request help in a crowded department store when all the salespeople seem busy.	_____	_____
35. Telephone your clinician to cancel a therapy session.	_____	_____
36. Introduce yourself to a group of strangers.	_____	_____
37. Volunteer to present a talk on your work or hobby to a group of 20 school-age children.	_____	_____
38. Talk to your boss at work about a work-related error that you have made.	_____	_____
39. Ask for directions over the phone.	_____	_____
40. Order food in a restaurant when the waitress is obviously in a hurry.	_____	_____
41. Initiate a conversation with the person sitting next to you on an airplane.	_____	_____
42. Give an important 30-minute presentation at work or school.	_____	_____

Figure 4-6   Continued.

COULD YOU. . .: (Continued)	<u>CAN DO</u>	<u>CONFIDENCE</u>
43. Volunteer to present a talk on your work or hobby to a group of 25 adults.	_____	_____
44. Order a pizza over the phone.	_____	_____
45. Ask for a raise at work.	_____	_____
46. Complain about the lack of service to your waiter/waitress.	_____	_____
47. Call a stranger on the phone to tell him or her about a meeting.	_____	_____
48. Volunteer to go on a T.V. or radio talk show.	_____	_____
49. Order exactly what you want in a restaurant even though you might stutter on the words.	_____	_____
50. Call up the telephone company to question a bill.	_____	_____

Figure 4-6   Continued.

an average of 9.4 months of treatment and averaged 66.2. Pearson correlations of SESAS approach items showed significant relationships for all items and the total SESAS score, indicating that all items were a representative measure of speaking situations, a finding that strengthened the construct validity of the measure. Finally, factor analysis identified five underlying constructs contained in the scale: 1. speaking to multiple listeners, 2. speaking to one familiar listener, 3. speaking to one unfamiliar listener, 4. speaking to an important listener, and 5. speaking situations in social settings.

Subsequent investigation (Manning, Perkins, Winn, & Coles, 1984) indicated that during treatment, adults who stutter demonstrate increasingly higher scores. In addition, the speakers began to normalize their approach and performance scores, in the sense that performance scores were slightly greater than approach scores. Several investigators have reported increases in SESAS scores as a result of treatment (Blood, 1995; Hillis, 1993; Manning, Perkins, Winn, & Cole, 1984; Langevin & Kully, 2003, Langevin, et al., 2006). In some cases, adults who consider themselves recovered from stuttering have recorded SESAS scores that exceed those of nonstuttering adults (Hillis & Manning, 1996).

The SEA-Scale: Self-Efficacy for Adolescents Scale

Developed by Manning (1994), the SEA-Scale: Self-Efficacy for Adolescents, also based on the work of Bandura and his colleagues, is designed for older school-age children and adolescents (Figure 4-7). Clients are asked to assign a whole number value (1 to 10) to indicate their confidence for entering into and speaking in each of 100 progressively more difficult communication situations (higher scores indicate greater confidence). The procedure allows clients and clinicians to obtain a total average score for all 100 speaking situations and to map the speaker's predicted performance in 13 categories (Watson, 1988) of beyond-therapy speaking situations appropriate for younger speakers. The SEA-Scale was normed on 40 adolescent children who stuttered and a matched group of fluent children. The overall alpha level for the entire scale was 0.98, with subscale alphas ranging from 0.74 to 0.94. The children who stuttered scored significantly ($p < .001$) lower (mean = 7.21; SD = 1.8) than a matched group of fluent speakers (mean = 8.65; SD = 1.2).

Bray et al. (2003) investigated the relationship of self-efficacy to verbal fluency, academic self-efficacy, and depression for 21 adolescents who stuttered (13–19 years old) and a group of 21 adolescents matched for gender, age, grades, and academic achievement. The authors hypothesized that differences in each of these measures would be found between the two groups of speakers. The authors adapted the 100-item SEA-Scale as described above and created an abbreviated 39-item version of SEA-Scale, finding a Cronbach's coefficient alpha of .98 for the abbreviated version. The results of a discriminant function analysis indicat-

SELF-EFFICACY FOR ADOLESCENTS SCALE:
(SEA-Scale)

Name _____   Date _____

Date of Birth _____   Gender _____

Grade _____   Months in Treatment _____

Clinician _____   School _____

Instructions

You are asked to consider a list of 100 speaking situations. Even though you may not typically find yourself in some of these situations, indicate how confident you are about entering into and speaking in each situation by placing one of the following numbers after each situation.

1	2	3	4	5	6	7	8	9	10
No Way, I would be too uptight to speak	I would be very un-comfortable speaking	Unsure				I would be somewhat comfortable speaking	No Problem, I would be confident speaking		

(continues)

Figure 4-7   The Self-Efficacy Scale for Adolescents Scale (SEA-Scale).

EXAMPLE:

SITUATION	CONFIDENCE
1. Lift a 5 pound box above your head.	10
2. Lift a 15 pound box above your head.	9
3. Lift a 25 pound box above your head.	7
4. Lift a 40 pound box above your head.	6
5. Lift a 50 pound box above your head.	1
6. Lift a 80 pound box above your head.	___

Please complete the following practice items:

PRACTICE:

SITUATION	CONFIDENCE
1. Jump over a fence 1 foot high.	___
2. Jump over a fence 2 feet high.	___
3. Jump over a fence 3 feet high.	___
4. Jump over a fence 4 feet high.	___
5. Jump over a fence 5 feet high.	___
6. Jump over a fence 6 feet high.	___

If you are sure that you understand what you are to do, please respond to the following 100 speaking situations by indicating your degree of confidence in your ability to enter into and speak in that situation. When ranking your confidence use a number from 1 to 10. If you do not feel that you can do a particular speaking task, do not enter a number.

SITUATION	CONFIDENCE
1. Talking with a parent about a movie you recently saw together.	___
2. Talking to a brother or sister at the dinner table.	___
3. Talking with a brother or sister about what TV program you would like to watch.	___
4. Talking with three friends your own age during lunch at school about a movie.	___
5. Asking a friend to come to your house after school.	___
6. Asking a parent if a friend can spend the night at your house.	___
7. Arguing with a brother or sister.	___
8. Asking a parent if you can spend the night at a friend's house.	___

Figure 4-7 Continued.

SITUATION	CONFIDENCE
9. Asking a friend to help you with your homework after school.	____
10. Talking with a group of friends as you have lunch at school.	____
11. Talking about your homework to the people who go with you to school.	____
12. Asking a parent for permission to study with a friend.	____
13. Asking a parent for permission to go to see a movie with friends.	____
14. Asking a friend to come to your birthday party.	____
15. Talking with three friends at school about a new student in your class.	____
16. Talking with a group of classmates during a meeting at school.	____
17. Telling a new friend the names and ages of your brothers or sisters.	____
18. Giving your locker number to a teacher.	____
19. Telling a parent that you do not deserve to be grounded.	____
20. Giving your place and date of birth to an official of your school.	____
21. Calling your best friend on the telephone just to talk.	____
22. Asking a parent for permission to stay out one hour later than usual.	____
23. Telling your teacher at school your name and address.	____
24. Talking with a grandparent on the telephone.	____
25. Explaining how to play a new game to a group of friends.	____
26. Talking with two new people in your class who just began attending your school.	____
27. Talking on the telephone with a classmate about your homework assignment.	____
28. Telling your parent the allowance you are given is not enough.	____
29. Asking a librarian for help in finding a book.	____

Figure 4-7 Continued.

SITUATION	CONFIDENCE

30. Asking a sales clerk about the cost of an item in a store. ____

31. Telling a police officer your home address. ____

32. Telling one of your classmates that he or she picked up your pencil by mistake. ____

33. Asking a sales clerk if a particular item is in stock. ____

34. Calling a store clerk to see what time the store opens. ____

35. Arguing with a friend about who gets to go first in a game. ____

36. Calling a theater to see when a movie starts. ____

37. Talking to other students at a new school. ____

38. Talking on the telephone with relatives who live in another city. ____

39. Arguing with a friend about who gets the last piece of candy. ____

40. Arguing with two friends about which movie you should see. ____

41. Taking a telephone message for a brother or sister. ____

42. Talking with a group of four new students in your class the first week of school. ____

43. Arguing with another student because you let a friend cut in line in front of you. ____

44. Telling a parent that you have to stay after school because you were disruptive in class. ____

45. Asking a stranger where the nearest telephone is located. ____

46. Confronting someone who cuts in front of you in line. ____

47. Raising your hand and asking your teacher for permission to leave the room. ____

48. Arguing with an older, larger, friend about who gets the last coke. ____

49. Arguing with a friend about a boy/girl that you both like. ____

Figure 4-7 Continued.

SITUATION	CONFIDENCE
50. Answering a question in class.	___
51. Asking a question in class.	___
52. Raising your hand in order to give an answer before the teacher calls on someone else.	___
53. Telling the teacher you were not the one who was talking in class	___
54. Introducing yourself to a group of new students at your school.	___
55. Asking someone in a group of five people the correct time.	___
56. Asking a coach of a sports team at school how to join the team.	___
57. Beginning a conversation with a group of three strangers at a party.	___
58. Going to a fast food restaurant with your family and ordering a sandwich.	___
59. Introducing yourself to a group of five students at a new school.	___
60. Telling a parent that you just broke your neighbor's window with a ball.	___
61. Accusing a friend because you believe he or she copied your homework.	___
62. Asking a stranger for directions to get to a restaurant.	___
63. Taking your turn ordering when you are having dinner in a restaurant with your family.	___
64. Telling a group of friends that you will not smoke with them.	___
65. Telling your teacher you do not understand an assignment.	___
66. Talking on the phone with a teacher about attending a class party.	___
67. Answering the telephone at a friend's house.	___
68. Telling a friend that he or she tore a pair of jeans they borrowed from you.	___

Figure 4-7   Continued.

	SITUATION	CONFIDENCE

69. Asking for directions from someone who is in a hurry. ___

70. Telling an usher at a movie theater that you are old enough to see a particular movie. ___

71. Asking your classroom teacher to move your desk to the front of the classroom. ___

72. Talking on the telephone with a classmate of the opposite sex. ___

73. Questioning a teacher about letting the same student always be first in line. ___

74. Telling a parent about a bad report card. ___

75. Introducing yourself to a new teacher. ___

76. Talking to a teacher about something that is bothering you. ___

77. Going to a party when the only person you know is the one giving the party. ___

78. Explaining to a teacher why you are late to class. ___

79. Giving directions to a group of adults who are driving by your home in a car. ___

80. Explaining to a teacher why you were absent from school. ___

81. Asking an adult if this is the house where your friend lives. ___

82. Ordering something at a fast food restaurant when they are very busy. ___

83. Telling a joke to group of friends at a party. ___

84. Leaving a message on someone's telephone answering machine. ___

85. Walking door to door and asking unfamiliar neighbors to buy items you are selling. ___

86. Reading aloud to a group of seven classmates. ___

87. Explaining to the school principal why you are in the hall during a class. ___

Figure 4-7 Continued.

SITUATION	CONFIDENCE
88. Asking a girl/boy to dance at a school party.	____
89. Taking part in a spelling contest.	____
90. Explaining to your school principal why you were sent to the school office.	____
91. Reading a paragraph from a book to the people in your class at school.	____
92. Introducing a speaker to a club or religious group.	____
93. Asking a person in your school to go with you to a school dance.	____
94. Giving a book report in front of the class.	____
95. Reading aloud to a group of seven adults.	____
96. Reciting a poem in your English class.	____
97. Being videotaped when giving a report to your history class.	____
98. Taking a speaking part in a school play.	____
99. Making a five-minute speech in a school assembly.	____
100. Reading an announcement to everyone in your school over the intercom.	____
OVERALL AVERAGE:	____

Note: The overall SEA-Scale score is obtained by averaging the scores for all 100 items. Items not checked are scored as a zero.

Clinical Notes:

Figure 4-7   Continued.

Sub-scale items and Alpha scores

Overall Alpha = 0.98

SUBSCALE 1   **Telephone Conversations**
10 Items: 21 24 27 34 36 38 41 67 72 84   Alpha = 0.88

SUBSCALE 2   **Argument or Conflict with a Friend or Family Member**
13 Items: 7 19 35 39 40 44 48 49 60 61   Alpha = 0.85
64 68 74

SUBSCALE 3   **Argument or Conflict with a Stranger**
4 Items: 32 43 46 90   Alpha = 0.73

SUBSCALE 4   **One-to-One Conversation with a Family Member**   Alpha = 0.88
3 Items: 1 2 3

SUBSCALE 5   **One-to-One Conversation with an Authority Figure**   Alpha = 0.86
7 Items: 31 66 75 76 80 81 87

SUBSCALE 6   **Group Conversation with a Known Group (Informal)**   Alpha = 0.85
7 Items: 4 10 11 15 16 25 83

SUBSCALE 7   **Group Conversation with an Unknown Group (Formal)**   Alpha = 0.91
8 Items: 26 37 42 54 57 59 77 79

SUBSCALE 8   **Formal Presentation**
11 Items: 86 89 91 92 94 95 96 97 98   Alpha = 0.94
99 100

SUBSCALE 9   **Questioning a Friend/Family Member for Information/Action**   Alpha = 0.83
9 Items: 5 6 8 9 12 13 14 22 28

SUBSCALE 10   **Questioning a Stranger for Information or Action**
8 Items: 29 30 33 45 55 62 88 93   Alpha = 0.82

SUBSCALE 11   **Questioning an Authority Figure for Information or Action**
10 Items: 47 51 53 56 65 70 71 73 78 85   Alpha = 0.89

SUBSCALE 12   **Situations Involving Time Constraints**
4 Items: 52 63 69 82   Alpha = 0.84

SUBSCALE 13   **Situations Involving Memorized or Unchangeable Content**
6 Items: 17 18 20 23 50 58   Alpha = 0.80

Figure 4-7   Continued.

ed that speech self-efficacy in the form of the modified SEA-Scale was the only significant variable ($F_{(1, 40)} = 23.2$, $p < .01$) in the equation accounting for 61% of the variance in group status. A second discriminant function analysis that excluded the nonsignificant variables resulted in a single discriminant function that correctly classified 81% of the participants into their groups. The authors suggest that not only are adolescents able to use self-efficacy scaling as a measure of their confidence for verbal fluency but also that such change, in and of itself, is a viable target of treatment.

Adult Behavior Assessment Battery (BAB)

Recommending that the assessment of a fluency problem should be multidimensional and go beyond the molar count of stuttering moments, Brutten and Vanryckeghem and their associates have created several self-report measures designed for Adults (Brutten, 1973, 1975; Brutten & Vanryckeghem, 2003). A parallel series of measures has also been designed for preschool and school-age children (Brutten & Vanryckeghem, 2003b, 2007; Vanryckeghem & Brutten, 2007) (See Chapter 5). Both the adult and child forms of the BAB are designed to provide the clinician with an "evidence-based approach to diagnostic and therapeutic decision making." The Behavior Assessment Battery has been translated into 15 languages with norms established for different countries. The adult portion of the BAB includes three subscales as described in the following sections.

Speech Situation Checklist — Emotional Reaction (SSC-ER)

As with the earlier versions of the BAB, the current updated form of the Speech Situations Checklist (SSC) has two components. The first component provides a way to identify the adult speaker's emotional reactions (anxiety, concern, worry) about entering situation-specific communication situations. Speakers respond to the question "Are you anxious, concerned, or worried about your speech when you are entering . . . ?" that includes 51 communication situations (e.g., talking on the telephone, giving your name, ordering in a restaurant, talking with a sales clerk)[4]. Speakers are asked to indicate their emotional response to each situation by using a 5-point Likert-type scale ranging from 1 (not anxious) to 5 (very anxious). The ratings are totaled and compared with the norms that are provided. The Cronbach alpha measure of reliability for the SSC-ER is .98 for PWS and .96 for people who do not stutter (Brutten & Vanryckeghem, 2003a). Ezrati-Vinacour & Levin (2004) found a .96 Cronbach alpha reliability, indicating a "high level of internal consistency" (p. 141).

Speech Situation Checklist — Speech Disruption (SSC-SD)

Adults also independently respond to the same 51 communication situations by indicating the extent of speech disruption (part-word repetitions and audible or

---

[4]For additional examples of communication situations see Bakker, K. (1995). Two supplemental scoring procedures for diagnostic evaluations with the Speech Situation Checklist. *Journal of Fluency Disorders, 20,* 117–126.

silent prolongations) that they are likely to experience in each situation. This time the adult speaker rates the extent of his or her speech disruption they are likely to experience in each of the 51 speaking situations, making use of a second Likert-type scale from 1 (no disruption) to 5 (great disruption). Bakker (1995) found that the two components of the SSC were able to significantly ($p < .00001$) discriminate adults who stutter from those who do not. The Cronbach alpha measure of reliability for the SSC-SD is .97 for both PWS and PWNS.

The Behavior Checklist (BCL)

The BCL provides a way for adults who stutter to indicate their avoidance and escape behaviors (e.g., substituting one word for another, pausing before trying to say a feared word, avoiding eye contact) that he or she typically uses when anticipating or experiencing a moment of stuttering. Respondents first check whether or not they use a particular coping behavior and then indicate on a 5-point Likert-type scale the frequency with which they use a particular behavior (1 = very infrequently to 5 = very frequently). Investigations with the adult BCL indicate that adults who stutter are likely to employ significantly more ($p = .000$) of these behaviors than those who do not stutter (Vanryckeghem, Brutten, Uddin, & Van Borsel, 2004). Current research with the adult *BCL* indicates that Cronbach alpha measures are similar to those found for the children's version (.88 for CWS and .91 for CWNS).

✳ *Overall Assessment of the Speaker's Experience of Stuttering (OASES)*

Developed by Yaruss & Quesal (2006), the OASES is designed to obtain information about the totality of the stuttering experience as delineated by the World Health Organization's most recent *International Classification of Functioning, Disability, and Health* (ICF; WHO, 2001). Following the development and testing of several preliminary versions to establish validity and reliability (N = 173, adults ages 18 to 70), test-retest reliability of the final version was provided by 14 adults (mean age 45.4, SD = 9.26 years). Participants' scores on individual items were identical for 77.7% of the 1,399 responses and within plus-or-minus 1 for 98.5% of all responses. Pearson product-moment correlations for two administrations of the test were .90 to .97.

Available in both English and Spanish versions, the OASES can be completed in less than 20 minutes. The broad impact of stuttering is assessed across four major sections. Section I (*General Information*) contains 20 items indicating the speaker's self-assessment of his or her impairment as well as the speaker's knowledge about stuttering and stuttering therapy. Section II (*Reactions to Stuttering*) contains 30 items providing information concerning the speaker's affective, behavioral, and cognitive reactions to stuttering. Section III (*Communication in Daily Situations*) contains 25 items about the difficulty the speaker experiences when communicating in important speaking situations. Section IV (*Quality of Life*) contains 25 items providing information about the overall impact of stuttering on the speaker's quality of life. Overall, the various items provide the clinician with information about such factors as how much stuttering interferes with the speaker's communication, relationships, sense of confidence, and well-being. The client responds to the individual items using a Likert-type scale from 1–5, and the scores are then totaled for each of the four sections and the test as a whole. The points for each of the four sections (and overall) are totaled and divided by the number of items completed, resulting in impact scores. Impact ratings across five levels of severity are then determined based on the impact scores: Mild (1:00–1.49), Mild/Moderate (1.50–2.24), Moderate (2.25–2.99), Moderate/Severe (3.00–3.74), and Severe (3.75–5.00). The authors are currently in the process of completing versions designed for school-age children (the OASES-S, ages 7–12), and teenagers (The OASES-T, ages 13–17).

The Wright and Ayre Stuttering Self-Rating Profile (WASSP)

Also based on the World Health Organization's ICF model and similar in many ways to the OASES, the WASSP (Figure 4-9) is intended primarily as an efficient but comprehensive device for identifying behavioral and attitudinal features of stuttering for adolescents and adults (Ayre & Wright, 2000, 2008). Speakers are asked to respond to a series of 24 items, which are grouped into five sections: Stuttering behaviors (8 items), Thoughts about stuttering (3 items), Feelings about stuttering (5 items), Avoidance due to stuttering (4 items), and Disadvantage due to stuttering (4 items). Self-ratings are indicated by the respondent circling a number on a 7-point Likert-type scale that best describes their self-perceived severity (1 = none, 7 = very severe). The results can be indicated using a summary profile whereby two ratings (e.g., pre- and post-treatment) scores for each item can be graphically displayed according to perceived severity. Forms are provided for including summary comments by the clinician regarding client changes relating to each of the five sections on the Response Sheet and future treatment goals. Reliability was indicated by 32 individuals who stuttered but who were not presently receiving treatment. Testing over three administrations indicated consistent results for the five subscales with all Pearson product moment correlations above 0.80 (range 0.80–.95). Item analysis indicating the degree of association of each item with the five sub-scales indicated correlations ranging from 0.6–0.95 ($p < 0.005$) that met a predetermined level of agreement (0.65). Finally, Cronbach's alpha coefficients for each of the subscales were above 0.78, with the majority greater than 0.90. Content validity was determined by continuous feedback from clinicians and clients during the development of pilot versions of the

Overall Assessment of the Speaker's Experience of Stuttering (OASES)

Name: Sample   Age: XX   Sex: [M] F   Date: 2005

Instructions. This test consists of four sections that examine different aspects of your experience of stuttering. Please complete each item by circling the appropriate number. If an item does not apply to you, leave it blank and move on to the next item.

Section I: General Information

A. General information about your speech.	Always	Frequently	Sometimes	Rarely	Never
1. How often are you able to speak fluently?	1	2	3	[4]	5
2. How often does your speech *sound* "natural" to you (i.e., like the speech of other people)?	1	2	[3]	4	5
3. How consistently are you able to maintain fluency from day to day?	1	2	3	[4]	5
4. How often do you use techniques, strategies, or tools you learned in speech therapy?	1	2	3	4	[5]
5. How often do you say exactly what you want to say even if you think you might stutter?	1	2	3	[4]	5

(continues)

Figure 4-8 Sample Form for the OASES. Reprinted from *Journal of Fluency Disorders*, 31/2, Yaruss, J. S. & Quesal, R., Overall Assessment of the Speaker's Experience of Stuttering (OASES): Documenting multiple outcomes in stuttering treatment, 90–115, 2006, with permission from Elsevier.

B. How <u>knowledgeable</u> are you about . . .?	Extremely	Very	Somewhat	A Little	Not At All
1. Stuttering in general	1	2	3	[4]	5
2. Factors that affect stuttering	1	2	3	[4]	5
3. What happens with your speech when you stutter	1	2	3	4	[5]
4. Treatment options for people who stutter	1	2	3	[4]	5
5. Self-help or support groups for people who stutter	1	2	3	[4]	5

C. Overall, how do you <u>feel</u> about . . .?	Very Positively	Somewhat Positively	Neutral	Somewhat Negatively	Very Negatively
1. Your speaking ability	1	2	3	[4]	5
2. Your ability to communicate (i.e., to get your message across regardless of your fluency)	1	2	[3]	4	5
3. The way you sound when you speak	1	2	3	[4]	5
4. Techniques for speaking fluently (e.g., techniques learned in therapy)	1	2	3	[4]	5

Figure 4-8   Continued.

C. Overall, how do you <u>feel</u> about . . . ?	Very Positively	Somewhat Positively	Neutral	Somewhat Negatively	Very Negatively
5. Your ability to use techniques you learned in speech therapy	1	2	3	[4]	5
6. Being a person who stutters	1	2	3	4	[5]
7. The speech therapy program you attended most recently	1	2	[3]	4	5
8. Being identified by other people as a stutterer/person who stutters	1	2	3	[4]	5
9. Variations in your speech fluency in different situations	1	[2]	3	4	5
10. Self-help or support groups for people who stutter	1	[2]	3	4	5

Figure 4-8   Continued.

Section II: Your Reactions to Stuttering

A. When you think about your stuttering, how often do you feel . . .? *(Note: please complete both columns in this section)*					
	Never	Rarely	Sometimes	Often	Always
1. helpless	1	2	[3]	4	5
2. angry	1	2	3	[4]	5
3. ashamed	1	2	3	4	[5]
4. lonely	1	2	[3]	4	5
5. anxious	1	2	3	[4]	5
6. depressed	1	2	[3]	4	5
7. defensive	1	2	3	[4]	5
8. embarrassed	1	2	3	4	[5]
9. guilty	1	2	3	[4]	5
10. frustrated	1	2	3	4	[5]

B. How often do you . . .?	Never	Rarely	Sometimes	Frequently	Always
1. Experience physical tension when stuttering	[1]	2	3	4	5
2. Experience physical tension when speaking fluently	[1]	2	3	4	5
3. Exhibit eye blinks, facial grimaces, arm movements, etc. when stuttering	1	2	[3]	4	5
4. Break eye contact or avoid looking at your listener	1	2	3	4	[5]

Figure 4-8   Continued.

B. How often do you . . .?	Never	Rarely	Sometimes	Frequently	Always
5. Avoid speaking in certain situations or to certain people	1	2	3	[4]	5
6. Leave a situation because you think you might stutter	1	2	3	[4]	5
7. Not say what you want to say (e.g., avoid or substitute words, refuse to answer questions, order something you do not want because it is easier to say)	1	2	3	[4]	5
8. Use filler words or starters (e.g., "um," clearing throat), or change something about your speech (e.g., use an accent) to be more fluent. (Note: this does not refer to techniques you may have learned in therapy.)	1	2	3	4	[5]
9. Experience a period of increased stuttering just after you stutter on a word	1	2	3	[4]	5
10. Let somebody else speak for you	1	2	[3]	4	5

Figure 4-8 Continued.

C. To what extent do you agree or disagree with the following statements.	Strongly Disagree	Somewhat Disagree	Neutral	Somewhat Agree	Strongly Agree
1. I think about my stuttering nearly all the time.	1	2	3	4	[5]
2. People's opinions about me are based primarily on how I speak.	1	2	3	[4]	5
3. If I did not stutter, I would be better able to achieve my goals in life.	1	2	3	4	[5]
4. I do not want people to know that I stutter.	1	2	3	[4]	5
5. When I am stuttering, there is nothing I can do about it.	1	2	3	[4]	5
6. People should do everything they can do to keep themselves from stuttering.	1	2	3	[4]	5

Figure 4-8   Continued.

C. To what extent do you agree or disagree with the following statements.	Strongly Disagree	Somewhat Disagree	Neutral	Somewhat Agree	Strongly Agree
7. People who stutter should not take jobs that require a lot of speaking.	1	2	3	4	5
8. I do not speak as well as most other people.	1	2	3	4	5
9. I cannot accept the fuel that I stutter.	1	2	3	4	5
10. I do not have confidence in my abilities as a speaker.	1	2	3	4	5

Figure 4-8 Continued.

Section III: Communication in Daily Situations
(In this section, indicate how much <u>difficulty</u> YOU experience in these situations, <u>not</u> how fluent you are.)

A. How *difficult* is it for you to communicate in the following general situations?	Not at all Difficult	Not Very Difficult	Somewhat Difficult	Very Difficult	Extremely Difficult
1. Talking with another person "one-on-one"	1	2	3	☐4	5
2. Talking while under time pressure	1	2	☐3	4	5
3. Talking in front of a small group of people	1	2	☐3	4	5
4. Talking in front of a large group of people	1	2	3	☐4	5
5. Talking with people you *do* know well (e.g., friends)	1	☐2	3	4	5
6. Talking with people you *do not* know well (e.g., strangers)	1	2	3	4	☐5
7. Talking on the telephone in general	1	2	☐3	4	5

Figure 4-8 Continued.

A. How *difficult* is it for you to communicate in the following general situations?	Not at all Difficult	Not Very Difficult	Somewhat Difficult	Very Difficult	Extremely Difficult
8. Initiating conversations with other people (e.g., introducing yourself)	1	2	3	[4]	5
9. Continuing to speak regardless of how your listener responds to you	1	2	3	[4]	5
10. Standing up for yourself verbally (e.g., defending your opinion, challenging someone who cuts in line in front of you)	1	[2]	3	4	5

Figure 4-8   Continued.

B. How *difficult* is it for you to communicate in the following situations at work?	Not at all Difficult	Not Very Difficult	Somewhat Difficult	Very Difficult	Extremely Difficult
1. Using the telephone at work	1	2	3	4	5
2. Giving oral presentations or speaking in front of other people at work	1	2	3	4	5
3. Talking with co-workers or other people you work with (e.g., participating in meetings)	1	2	3	4	5
4. Talking with customers or clients	1	2	3	4	5
5. Talking with your supervisor or boss	1	2	3	4	5

Figure 4-8   Continued.

C. How *difficult* is it for you to communicate in the following social situations?	Not at all Difficult	Not Very Difficult	Somewhat Difficult	Very Difficult	Extremely Difficult
1. Participating in social events (e.g., making "small talk" at parties)	1	2	3	4	5
2. Telling stories or jokes	1	2	3	4	5
3. Asking for information (e.g., asking for directions or other people's opinions)	1	2	3	4	5
4. Ordering food in a restaurant	1	2	3	4	5
5. Ordering food at a drive-thru	1	2	3	4	5

Figure 4-8   Continued.

D. How *difficult* is it for you to communicate in the following situations at home?	Not at all Difficult	Not Very Difficult	Somewhat Difficult	Very Difficult	Extremely Difficult
1. Using the telephone at home	1	[2]	3	4	5
2. Talking to your spouse / significant other	1	[2]	3	4	5
3. Talking to your children	1	2	3	4	5
4. Talking to members of your extended family	1	[2]	3	4	5
5. Taking part in family discussions	1	2	[3]	4	5

Section IV: Quality of Life

A. How much is your overall quality of life negatively affected by...?	Stuttering *negatively affects my quality of life . . .*				
	Not At All	A Little	Some	A Lot	Completely
1. Your stuttering	1	2	3	[4]	5
2. Your reactions to your stuttering	1	2	3	[4]	5
3. Other people's reactions to your stuttering	1	2	[3]	4	5

Figure 4-8 Continued.

B. Overall, how much does stuttering *interfere with your satisfaction* with communication . . .?	Stuttering *interferes* with my communication satisfaction . . .				
	Not At All	A Little	Some	A Lot	Completely
1. In general	1	2	3	[4]	5
2. At work	1	2	[3]	4	5
3. In social situations	1	2	3	[4]	5
4. At home	1	[2]	3	4	5

C. Overall, how much does stuttering *interfere* with your . . .?	Stuttering *interferes* with my relationships . . .				
	Not At All	A Little	Some	A Lot	Completely
1. Relationships with family	[1]	2	3	4	5
2. Relationships with friends	1	[2]	3	4	5
3. Relationships with other people	1	2	[3]	4	5
4. Intimate relationships	1	2	[3]	4	5
5. Ability to function in society	1	[2]	3	4	5

Figure 4-8 Continued.

D. Overall, how much does stuttering *interfere* with your . . .?	Stuttering *interferes* with my career . . .				
	Not At All	A Little	Some	A Lot	Completely
1. Ability to do your job	☐1	2	3	4	5
2. Satisfaction with your job	1	2	3	4	5
3. Ability to advance in your career	1	2	☐3	4	5
4. Educational opportunities	1	2	☐3	4	5
5. Ability to earn as much as you feel you should	1	2	3	☐4	5

E. Overall, how much does stuttering *interfere* with your . . .?	Stuttering *interferes* with my personal life . . .				
	Not At All	A Little	Some	A Lot	Completely
1. Sense of self-worth or self-esteem	1	2	3	☐4	5
2. Overall outlook on life	1	2	3	☐4	5
3. Confidence in yourself	1	2	3	☐4	5
4. Enthusiasm for life	1	2	3	☐4	5
5. Overall health and physical well-being	1	☐2	3	4	5

Figure 4-8   Continued.

E. Overall, how much does stuttering *interfere* with your . . .?	Stuttering *interferes with my personal life* . . .				
	Not At All	A Little	Some	A Lot	Completely
6. Overall stamina or energy level	1	2	3	4	5
7. Sense of control over your life	1	2	3	4	5
8. Spiritual well-being	1	2	3	4	5

Overall Assessment of the Speaker's Experience of Stuttering (OASES)
Scoring Summary

Instructions

Calculate **Impact Scores** for each of the 4 sections on the OASES by (a) totaling the number of points in each section and (b) counting the number of items completed in each section. Multiply the number of items completed by 5 to obtain the total points *possible* for each section. The impact score for each section is equal to 100 times the points in each section divided by the total points possible for that section. (Impact scores will always range between 20 and 100.) Determine **Impact Ratings** for each section based on the impact scores in the table at the bottom of the page.

Name: **Sample**   Age: XX   Sex: M F   Date: **2005**

Section I: General Information (20 Items Total)
    Section I Points: **76**   Items Completed in Section I: **20**
    Section I Points Possible (Section I Items Completed x 5): **100**
    Section I Impact Score: 76   Impact Rating: Severe

Section II: Reactions to Stuttering (30 Items Total)
    Section II Points: **117**   Items Completed in Section II: **30**
    Section II Points Possible (Section II Items Completed x 5): **150**
    Section II Impact Score: 78   Impact Rating: Severe

Section III: Communication in Daily Situations (25 Items Total)
    Section III Points: **74**   Items Completed in Section III: **24**
    Section III Points Possible (Section III Items Completed x 5): **120**
    Section III Impact Score: 61.7   Impact Rating: Moderate-to-Severe

Figure 4-8   Continued.

Section IV: Quality of Life (25 Items Total)
Section IV Points: **70**   Items Completed in Section IV: **24**
Section IV Points Possible (Section IV Items Completed × 5): **120**
Section IV Impact Score: 58.3   Impact Rating: Moderate

TOTAL IMPACT SCORE (100 Items Total)
Total Points: **337**   Total Items Completed: **98**
(Total Points = Section I Points + Section II Points + Section III Points + Section IV Points)
(Total Items Completed! = Section I Items Completed + Section II Items Completed + Section III Items Completed + Section IV Items Completed)
Total Points Possible (Total Items Completed × 5): **490**
Total Impact Score: 68.8   Impact Rating: Moderate-to-Severe

Impact Rating	Impact Scores
Mid	20.0–29.9
Mild-to-Moderate	30.0–44.9
Moderate	45.0–59.9
Moderate-to-Severe	60.0–74.9
Severe	75.0–100

Figure 4-8   Continued.

WASSP. A new edition of the manual will be available in 2009, and a version of the WASSP intended for young adults and teenagers is in development.

The Origins and Pawns Scaling

As we have seen, clinical researchers recognize that the speaker who stutters can provide highly relevant information about the nature and impact of the problem. Some researchers have suggested that it may be more appropriate to obtain this information using a nonrestricted format by seeking responses to open-ended questions rather than asking individuals to respond to a predetermined scale or questionnaire. For example, Westbrook and Viney (1980) argue that a better way to determine the dynamic, multidimensional nature of a person's locus of control is by eliciting a spontaneously produced narrative rather than using a predetermined questionnaire. Like the Locus of Control of Behavior (LCB) described earlier, The Origins and Pawns Scales developed by Westbrook and Viney is designed to assist the clinician in extracting meaningful information from narrative responses to open-ended questions or conversations that can be recorded and transcribed. Statements made by

WASSP Summary Profile

Client John S

Speech and Language Therapist (SLT) Louise W

Dates: Time 1   06/25/08   Time 2   08/20/08

This profile aims to record how the person who stutters perceives his or her stutter at the beginning and the end of a block of speech and language therapy. It is one way of measuring change and planning future management.

BRIEF INSTRUCTIONS

Materials

Each block of therapy requires two *WASSP* Rating Sheets, one *WASSP* Summary Profile Folder and two highlighter pens of contrasting colors.

Before a block of therapy

The client completes a rating sheet (Time 1) using the seven point rating scale and recording any aims / expectations for the block of therapy. The SLT stores the completed rating sheet in the Summary Profile in the case notes.

At the end of a block of therapy

The client completes a second dated rating sheet (Time 2) and records his or her achievements during the block of therapy. (**NB** The second rating sheet must be completed without reference to the first. The SLT therefore reminds the client of any 'other' aspects of behaviors or feelings which he or she may have added at Time 1.)

Discussion of *WASSP* Summary profile

Ratings from Time 1 and Time 2 are transferred on to page 2 of the *WASSP* summary profile using two different colors of highlighter pen. This provides a visual representation of changes made which will be individual to each client.

Each section is reviewed and discussed with the client and any comments or explanations recorded on page 3 in the spaces provided. Sufficient time must be allowed in the final session for discussion. Discussion increases client and SLT understanding of the outcomes particularly when unexpected changes in ratings occur or ratings differ from the SLT's perception. A brief summary of progress can be recorded on page 4.

(continues)

Figure 4-9   An example of a completed WASSP Rating Sheet and Summary Profile from *The 2000 Wright and Ayre Stuttering Self-Rating Profile (WASSP)*, Wright, L., & Ayre, A., (2000). Oxon, UK: Winslow Press Ltd. Reprinted with permission.

Identification of future therapy needs

These should arise during the discussion of the summary profile and can be recorded on page 4.

Repeated administration

WASSP can be repeated at the beginning and end of a number of consecutive blocks of therapy providing a record of long-term change and evolving therapy needs.

WASSP Rating Sheet

Name John S   Date 06/25/08

Please circle: Time 1 / Time 2

Instructions: Please rate each of the following aspects of your stutter using a 7-point scale, 1 indicating 'none' and 7 indicating 'very severe.'
Place a circle round the number which you judge best describes each aspect of your stutter.

Stuttering behaviors	*None*					*Very Severe*	
Frequency of stutters	1	2	3	4	(5)	6	7
Physical struggle during stutters	1	2	3	4	(5)	6	7
Duration of stutters	1	2	3	4	(5)	6	7
Uncontrollable stutters	1	2	3	4	(5)	6	7
Urgency/fast speech rate	1	2	(3)	4	5	6	7
Associated facial/body movements	1	2	(3)	4	5	6	7
General level of physical tension	1	2	3	(4)	5	6	7
Loss of eye contact	1	2	3	4	5	6	(7)
Other (describe) *Gasping for breath*	1	2	3	4	(5)	6	7

Figure 4-9   Continued.

Thoughts about stuttering	None				Very Severe		
Negative thoughts before speaking	1	2	3	4	⑤	6	7
Negative thoughts during speaking	1	2	3	4	⑤	6	7
Negative thoughts after speaking	1	2	③	4	5	6	7

Feelings about stuttering	None				Very Severe		
Frustration	1	2	3	4	5	⑥	7
Embarrassment	1	2	③	4	5	6	7
Fear	1	2	3	4	⑤	6	7
Anger	1	2	3	4	⑤	6	7
Helplessness	1	2	3	4	5	6	⑦
Other (describe) *Panic*	1	2	3	4	⑤	6	7

Avoidance due to stuttering	None				Very Severe		
Of words	1	2	3	4	⑤	6	7
Of situations	1	2	3	4	⑤	6	7
Of talking about stuttering with others	①	2	3	4	5	6	7
Of admitting the problem to yourself	①	2	3	4	5	6	7

Disadvantage due to stuttering	None				Very Severe		
At home	1	②	3	4	5	6	7
Socially	1	2	3	④	5	6	7
Educationally *N/A*	1	2	3	4	5	6	7
At work	1	2	3	4	5	6	⑦

Time 1: Please write down any aims/expectations you have for this block of therapy

Time 2: Please summarize what you feel you have achieved during this block
Stutter less, reduces avoidance and feel more confident at work

Figure 4-9 Continued.

WASSP Summary Profile

		None						Very Severe
		1	2	3	4	5	6	7
Behaviors	Frequency of stutters	1	▓	▓	▓	▓	▓	▓	
		2	▓	▓	▓				
	Physical struggle during stutters	1	▓	▓	▓	▓			
		2	▓	▓					
	Duration of stutters	1	▓	▓	▓	▓	▓		
		2	▓	▓					
	Uncontrollable stutters	1	▓	▓	▓	▓	▓	▓	
		2	▓						
	Urgency / fast speech rate	1	▓	▓	▓				
		2	▓						
	Associated facial / body movements	1	▓	▓	▓	▓			
		2	▓						
	General level of physical tension	1	▓	▓	▓	▓	▓		
		2	▓	▓					
	Loss of eye Contact	1	▓	▓	▓	▓	▓	▓	▓
		2	▓						
	Other (describe) *Gasping for breath*	1	▓	▓	▓	▓	▓		
		2	▓						
Thoughts	Negative thoughts before speaking	1	▓	▓	▓	▓	▓		
		2	▓						
	Negative thoughts during speaking	1	▓	▓	▓	▓	▓	▓	
		2	▓	▓					
	Negative thoughts after speaking	1	▓	▓	▓				
		2	▓						

Figure 4-9   Continued.

Feelings	Frustration	1									
		2									
	Embarrassment	1									
		2									
	Fear	1									
		2									
	Anger	1									
		2									
	Helplessness	1									
		2									
	Other (describe) *Panic*	1									
		2									
Avoidance	Of words	1									
		2									
	Of situations	1									
		2									
	Of talking about stuttering with others	1									
		2									
	Of admitting your problem to yourself	1									
		2									
Disadvantage	At home	1									
		2									
	Socially	1									
		2									
	Educationally *N/A*	1									
		2									
	At work	1									
		2									

Figure 4-9 Continued.

Client / Speech & Language Therapist Comments

Behaviors	Client: Feels has skills how to stutter less and more easily if they do occur. Is able to look at people and is pleased has managed to stop the gasping noise most of the time.
	Therapist: Confirms these changes in clinic and in group in therapy and socially.
Thoughts	Client: Able to think more positively about using the technique, rather than just worrying.
Feelings	Client: Feels more able to help self now—has the tools. Still feels some embarrassment and frustration when can't use the technique fully.
Avoidance	Client: Is really pleased with less avoidance—makes a big difference to life and confidence levels.
Disadvantage	Client: Feels much more confident socially but still gets the occasional negative reaction from customers at work.

Figure 4-9 Continued.

Summary of Progress / Future Needs

Summary of progress made in this book of therapy:

Stuttering less and more easily.

Better eye contact and less gasping.

Thinking more positively and feeling less helpless.

Reduced avoidance, feels much better about stutter at work.

Any other comments:

Progress really picked up when John realized how much he needed to practice skills at home and work.

Future needs:

Continue to use the tools and to self monitor to eliminate the gasping completely.

Think more about ways to manage stuttering with customers, and how to deal with their reactions.

Figure 4-9   Continued.

the speaker that are *origin* in nature are related to an *internal locus of control.* Statements that are *pawn* in nature are related to an *external locus of control.*

Scoring is accomplished by first placing the transcribed speech into clauses and then carefully considering 10 criteria for identifying origin and pawn verbalizations. Westbrook and Viney (1980) achieved inter-rater reliability ranging from .91 to .94 for the Origin Scale and from .87 to .93 for the Pawn Scale. Validity was determined by considering the origin and pawn scores for groups of people experiencing widely varying degrees of life situations (e.g., physical, mental, and socioeconomic status). The groups differed significantly in the predicted directions for origin and pawn scores according to the degree of physical and social restrictions, measures of anxiety, sociality, and emotional status. Westbrook and Viney concluded that pawn perception is a more stable characteristic than origin perception and that both are state rather than trait variables. The results also indicated that levels of origin and pawn perception tend to be independent of each of each other.

Initial attempts to apply Westbrooks and Viney's (1980) Origins and Pawns Scale with individuals who stutter indicated significant decreases in pawn scores and significant increases in origin scores as a result of successful therapy or self-directed change (Plexico & Manning, 2004; Manning, Hodak, & Plexico, 2005). However, in each case, the authors were able to achieve less than satisfactory reliability (Cohen's kappa) for identifying origin (.58) and pawn (.74) statements. Subsequent research by Lee, Manning and Herder (2009) demonstrated considerably improved reliability (Cohen's kappa) of .92 and .85 for origin and pawn statements, respectively (see Chapter 11).

Conclusion

Because most adolescents and adults who stutter choose not to seek professional help, our understanding of the problem is determined by what is certainly a nonrepresentative and possibly biased sample of all people who stutter. From the speakers we do see, it appears that developmental stuttering is a highly variable communication problem, a fact that can provide misleading information unless the speaker is seen in a variety of speaking tasks and environments. Because of this variability, as well as the ability of some speakers to mask the overt features of their stuttering by using a variety of coping behaviors, individuals who stutter are sometimes misdiagnosed as having expressive language, social anxiety disorders, voice disorders, neurological problems (e.g., Tourette's Syndrome), or a variety of emotional problems. For many individuals who stutter, a thorough assessment is ongoing and continues well into the early stages of treatment.

The severity of stuttering is indicated by many important surface features, including the frequency, duration, and tension associated with stuttering events as well as by the more subtle features such as the quality and stability of the individual's nonstuttered speech, avoidance and substitution of words, and post-ponement and escape behaviors. These surface features, as important as they are, fall short of indicating the full impact of the problem, particularly when the experience of the speaker is considered. The detection of the person's cognitive and affective responses (e.g., shame, fear, helplessness, and loss of control) to stuttering is especially relevant to understanding how stuttering impacts the speaker's daily functioning and quality of life. Much of the impact of stuttering is manifested by these cognitive and affective features. The continued development of both quantitative and qualitative tools has enhanced the ability of the clinician to discover and track these core features of the stuttering experience.

The assessment meeting provides the opportunity to establish the nature of the journey and the therapeutic alliance of the speaker and the clinician. It also provides the first opportunity for the clinician to demonstrate his or her under-standing of stuttering. For adolescent and adult speakers, it can be helpful for understanding the individual's story to appreciate how and why they are seeking assistance at this particular moment. The initial meeting provides the clinician with the opportunity to determine the speaker's motivation and readiness for change. At the most basic level, the assessment process involves two primary issues: (1) To what extent the person is altering the choices and choosing to restrict the options that are available to them and (2) How the person is using his or her vocal apparatus in ways that prevent the production of easy, open, and smooth speech.

Many assessment devices have been created that assist the clinician in de-termining the extent of the problem for the person who stutters. It is important to consider the speaker's self-perception of their situation and, in many cases, qualitative measures of the speaker's narrative can provide valuable insight into the extent that stuttering influences the person's ability to communicate and participate in daily activities. As we will emphasize in subsequent chapters that address therapeutic procedures, the effective clinician not only tracks behavioral and cognitive change via formal assessment tools but also pays close attention to the words speakers use to describe themselves and their situation.

Topics for Discussion

1. Although stuttering behavior may be apparent for an adolescent or adult speaker, describe how a person's coping responses sometimes mask many covert stuttering behaviors.

2. Explain to a family member or a friend who knows nothing about stuttering, the nature of the cognitive and affective features of the problem.

3. Make a list of activities, people, and situations you have avoided or would like to avoid. Describe your motivation for and the impact of this coping strategy.

4. How would you go about determining a speaker's level of motivation for initiating treatment?

5. Produce a 300- to 500-word script that you can use to produce a short video recording that contains several normal and stuttered fluency breaks (moderate level of stuttering). Exchange the tape with a colleague who has made a similar tape. Practice with the tapes to establish both inter- and intra-reliability (achieving at least .80) for identifying both normal and stuttered fluency breaks.

6. Describe to a colleague the steps for taking a client through the process of self-assessment and trial therapy as described in Figure 4-1.

7. Create a list of the basic take-home messages you would like to communicate to an adolescent or adult during the initial assessment meeting.

8. Describe in your own words the two fundamental principles of assessment discussed in this chapter.

9. Prepare a description of one or more situations where you have experienced a loss of control, emphasizing the cognitive (thought processes) and affective (anxiety, fear, embarrassment) nature of the experience.

10. Ask one or more friends to describe both a positive and enjoyable experience and a negative and anxiety-producing experience. Replay each tape two to three times while listening for quality words that indicate origin or pawn statements.

Recommended Readings

Anderson, T. K. & Felsenfeld, S. (2003). A thematic analysis of late recovery from stuttering. *American Journal of Speech-Language Pathology, 12,* 243–253.

Corcoran, J. A., & Stewart, M. (1998). Stories of stuttering: A qualitative analysis of interview narratives. *Journal of Fluency Disorders, 23,* 247–264.

Finn, P. (1997). Adults recovered from stuttering without formal treatment: Perceptual assessment of speech normalcy. *Journal of Speech, Language, and Hearing Research, 40,* 821–831.

Plexico, L., Manning, W., & DiLollo, A. (2005). A phenomenological understanding of successful stuttering management, *Journal of Fluency Disorders, 30(1)* 1–22.

The Assessment Process with Young Speakers: Preschool and School-age Children

I think that inside my mouth there is something wrong with me. And that is why I'm going to speech therapy to help my speaking. I have to take my time and be brave. I think my body is ready to talk but my mouth isn't. If I take my time I think I will be all right. But it is very hard because I want to be like everybody else. It's hard being different from everyone else. I'm lucky that I have such supportive parents and friends to help me get through my problem. I've learned that real friends do listen and I love them for it.

Lester L., 10 (nearly 11), Philadelphia, PA

It's not enough to know what type of fluency problem the child has. We need to know what type of child has the problem.

Charles Van Riper (1965)

Chapter Objectives

The emphasis of this chapter concerns two primary decisions that the clinician will need to make when evaluating the possibility of stuttering in young children. Considering the suggested criteria for distinguishing unusual from usual fluency breaks described in Chapter 2, the clinician must first make a judgment about the nature of the child's fluency and whether or not it is within reasonably normal limits. Guidelines discussed earlier including the occurrence of stuttering-like disfluencies (SLDs) at a rate of more than 3 SLDs per 100 syllables, the number and rate of repetitions, the clustering of SLDs, the child's reaction to his or her fluency disruptions, and the concern of the parents will help to inform the clinician about whether the child is stuttering or not. Nevertheless, because of the variability in the fluency of young children the clinician may need to obtain samples of the child's speech in a variety of speaking conditions.

Once the clinician concludes that the child's fluency breaks are characteristic of stuttering, he or she will then need to make a second, more difficult decision: Are the stuttering like-disfluencies likely to be a temporary or a permanent characteristic of the child's speech? As Yairi and his colleagues have pointed out, remission following the onset of stuttering is generally gradual, with most children recovering within three to four years following onset. Remission from stuttering with young speakers was suggested many years ago, with estimates of this phenomenon varying widely from approximately 32% to more than 80% (Andrews & Harris, 1964; Bryngelson, 1938; Cooper, 1972; Curlee & Yairi, 1997; Kloth, Kraaimaat, Janssen, & Brutten, 1999; Panelli, McFarlane, & Shipley, 1978; Starkweather, 1987; Van Riper, 1982; Yairi & Ambrose, 1992a; Young, 1975).

Yairi and Ambrose (2005) suggest that the often-cited recovery rate of 75% for younger speakers who stutter may be an underestimate. They argue that since some children who continue to stutter show only traces of stuttering and many who recover on their own go unreported, they propose a rate of recovery that is closer to 85%. It is also noteworthy that the nature of the remission is typically complete, for once these young children recover there is little or no chance of relapse and the quality of their speech appears to be identical to normally fluent children (Finn, Ingham, Ambrose, & Yairi, 1997). In part because there are so many variables involved—not to mention that it requires the clinician to predict the future—making the decision about whether or not a young child will continue to stutter is problematic. Conture (1997) concludes that while clinicians may be reasonably good at identifying stuttering-like fluency breaks, they are not particularly good at predicting whether or not a child will continue to stutter or benefit from intervention. Given the uncertainty about the chronicity of stuttering, the clinician will need to consider a response that—depending on such factors as the child's age, length of time since onset, family history of stuttering, language and speech characteristics, cognitive development, and temperamental nature—can range from informal monitoring of the child's speech to direct therapeutic intervention.

The Importance of the Initial Meeting: Two Basic Decisions

As with older speakers it is important to realize that the initial assessment meeting with the child and the parents is the first opportunity for the clinician to show his or her understanding about both the general nature of stuttering

Clinical **Insight**

Although authors now agree that many children recover from stuttering, few have questioned whether these same speakers are more likely to begin stuttering again later in their adult years. As we described in the previous chapter, it is relatively rare to find speakers who begin to stutter as adults (see also Chapter 10). It may be, however, that some people who begin stuttering later in life are those people who stuttered as children, more or less spontaneously recovered, and later—apparently in response to one or more sources of stress—again began to experience breaks in their fluency. We have seen a few such adults with whom a reoccurrence of stuttering seems to be a central component for what originally appeared to be a "late or adult onset" of stuttering.

and the impact it can have on the child and the family. This is the first chance for the clinician to begin making the problem less mysterious, to alter some of the myths or misinformation that the family may associate with the problem, to alleviate the feelings of guilt that often accompany stuttering, and to begin to provide the parents with a sense of direction and control about the problem. As Conture (1997) suggests, the clinician's ability to orient the family to the true nature of the problem may be the main benefit that the child and the family receive from the diagnostic meeting(s). Another excellent comment by Yairi and Ambrose (2005) will echo throughout the following chapters on intervention: "It is also important for clinicians to understand, and to impart to parents, that *stuttering* is not a bad word" (p. 283).

Decision 1: Determining Whether or Not the Child is Stuttering

The variability of stuttering for older speakers described in the previous chapter is even more apparent with young children, in part because children are rapidly maturing neurologically, physiologically, emotionally, and linguistically. Although some authors have found that nonstuttering children demonstrate relatively little variability in fluency across speaking situations (Martin, Haroldson, & Kuhl, 1972a,b; Wexler, 1982), many others have noted the highly variable nature of fluency in young speakers who stutter (Bloodstein, 1995; Conture, 1990; Starkweather, 1987; Van Riper, 1982; Yaruss, 1997a). Such variability provides clinicians with both good and bad news. The good news is that it is generally easier to change behavior that is variable and relatively new, making treatment more likely to be successful (Starkweather, 1992, 1999; Starkweather, Gottwald, & Halfond, 1990). The bad news is that this same variability can make obtaining representative samples of a child's fluency more complicated than with older speakers.

The case history information that is available to the clinician prior to the first meeting with the family will often provide a variety of clues about the nature of the child and the potential for stuttering. For example, as we described in Chapter 3, it has long been recognized that stuttering tends to occur more often in some families than in others (Andrews & Harris, 1964; Bloodstein, 1995). Ambrose et al. (1993) found that for children who stutter there is a 42% chance that someone in the nuclear family also stutters and a 71% chance that there is someone in the extended family who stutters. Many other factors such as the academic performance of school-age children, estimates of self-esteem, psychosocial functioning, and family structure and history, may be influential in determining the whether or not the child is stuttering. Of course, the assessment process provides a face-to-face opportunity to obtain the characteristics of the child and the nature of the fluency breaks that are of concern to the parents.

Eliciting Fluency Breaks

Assuming that the child will cooperate, speech samples can be elicited and recorded during the initial clinical evaluation. Audio or video speech samples recorded by the parents from representative situations outside the clinic setting can also be obtained either prior to or following the evaluation and are often especially useful. A 300- to 500-word sample produced in a variety of natural settings is a reasonable goal. The frequency of SLDs can be obtained in either percent syllables stuttered (%SS) or percent words stuttered (%WS) and the types of fluency breaks analyzed.[1]

During the assessment of children, there will be occasions when the very behaviors the clinician would like to observe and evaluate are not present. Although this also may occur during the assessment of adults who stutter, it is more often the case with younger speakers. On the day and time of the evaluation, the child may fail to exhibit the behaviors that concern the parents (or teacher). On such occasions the clinician assessing the young child can introduce forms of communicative stress at various points during the assessment process. Of course, as suggested in Chapter 1, this requires a clinician who is uninhibited and unafraid of stuttering and one who understands that a momentary increase in stuttering will not only do no harm but will provide helpful information. Moreover, throughout both assessment and treatment it is constructive to communicate curiosity and interest rather than aversion about stuttered or "bumpy" speech. Minimal examples of such speech are all that are usually required in

---

[1]The frequency of %WS can be converted to %SS by multiplying %WS by 1.5 (Andrews & Ingham, 1971).

order for the clinician to obtain adequate samples. Of course, as it becomes necessary to elicit fluency breaks from children in this fashion, parents or others who may be observing the evaluation should be informed about the purpose of these activities.

There are many benign techniques the clinician may use to elicit fluency breaks in children. Essentially, what we are doing is creating a speaking situation where temporary demands are placed on the child. As the demands exceed the child's ability to produce fluent speech, fluency breaks are likely to occur. Perhaps the most subtle form of disrupting a child's fluency is for the clinician to turn away as the child is describing an event or activity. Loss of the listener's attention has long been acknowledged as an effectual technique for eliciting fluency breaks in children (Johnson, 1962; Van Riper, 1982). One of the most effective procedures is to create some form of time pressure for the child to speak. This can be accomplished by asking to child to name objects (e.g., in a book or in the room) as rapidly as possible, possibly with the aid of a stopwatch. Other, more subtle forms of time pressure may be achieved by an increase in the speech rate of the clinician or "overtalking" the child's conversational responses. The clinician also may ask the child to respond to a series of questions or ask him or her to answer somewhat abstract or difficult-to-answer queries (Guitar & Peters, 1980), such as, "How far is it from here to your home and how do you get there?" "What does your mother (or father) do when they go to work?" Depending on the age of the child, he or she could be asked to read from books that are somewhat above grade level (Blood & Hood, 1978) or asked to describe a series of pictures presented at a rapid rate, creating a degree of time pressure. Although it is not often necessary, the clinician can also interrupt the child's response prior to completion. Other listeners may be brought into the room or additional listeners can take the role of distracting or interrupting the child. Typically, only one or a few of these activities is necessary to obtain examples of fluency breaks. Obviously, these techniques must be performed with appropriate understanding and sensitivity by the clinician as well as others who are involved. It is not necessary to elicit many of these breaks and once a few examples have been obtained, the clinician can consult with the parents to determine if these behaviors are indeed the behavior they have observed and are concerned about. The clinician cannot assume that the fluency breaks that occur during the assessment are of the same form and degree that the parents have noticed before.

The importance of observing children in a variety of speaking situations was underscored by Yaruss (1997a) in a study of 45 preschool children undergoing diagnostic evaluations for stuttering. Frequency counts were obtained for both usual and stuttering-like disfluencies (SLDs) for each of the children as they took part in three to five of the following situations during the evaluation session. Reliability measures using video recordings for 15% of the speech samples indicated no significant differences and high positive correlations between the original and recalculated observations.

1. Parent–Child Interaction—The child interacts with the parents (usually the mother) while playing with figures or games.

2. Play—The child and the clinician play with objects in a natural, free-play situation.

3. Play with Pressures Imposed—The clinician gradually increases conversational pressure by asking questions, breaking eye contact, interrupting, or increasing time pressure (e.g., speaking faster).

4. Story Retell—The child retells a familiar story while using a picture book.

5. Picture Description—The child describes pictures with minimal input from the clinician.

Yaruss found that the children who stuttered showed significantly greater variability across the speaking situations than within any single situation. Children who produced a higher overall frequency of SLDs also exhibited greater variability ($r = 0.88$; $p < .001$). No significant correlation was found for the more usual fluency breaks. Finally, the "Play with Pressure" situation resulted in the greatest number of disfluencies, although this was not the case for all the participants, as many children exhibited highly individualized patterns.

Based on these results, Yaruss (1997a) suggested that sampling of a child's fluency in a single speaking situation is unlikely to result in a representative sample of behavior, particularly for children who exhibit a greater number of stuttering-like disfluencies. He also noted that approximately 19 of the children evaluated had fewer than 3% SLDs in at least one situation and that 18 of these children produced more than 10% stuttering in another situation. In other words, if the common guideline of 3% disfluencies has been used as a threshold, approximately 40% of the children would not have been correctly identified as stuttering. Of course, as Yaruss points out, a single metric of stuttering frequency would not be used alone to indicate the presence of stuttering. The results also indicate the potential problem of placing too much importance on the frequency of stuttering, especially during a single speaking situation.

In some instances, in spite of our best attempts within several speaking situations and environments, we are unable to obtain samples of the fluency breaks that are of concern to the parents. It is usually possible to reschedule another assessment during a period when the child is experiencing more difficulty, or we may observe the child in a more natural setting at home or in school. An alternative is to ask the parents to make a video of the child at home as he or she is experiencing the fluency breaks the parents are concerned about. It can also be beneficial to recommend this step prior to the assessment in order to perform a preliminary analysis of the child's speech.

The Nature of Stuttering at Onset

In describing the onset and development of stuttering in Chapter 2 we discussed the overt behaviors that tend to differentiate the fluency breaks of children who stutter (CWS) from normally fluent children (NFC). In this section we present a variety of additional characteristics that help to make this distinction. As in Chapter 2, many of the comments in this section are taken from the work of Yairi and his colleagues at the University of Illinois Stuttering Research Program as discussed in the Yairi and Ambrose text *Early Childhood Stuttering, for Clinicians by Clinicians* (2005). The highlights of their findings are briefly reviewed here.

A summary of findings by Yairi and Ambrose (2005) indicates that the disfluencies of stuttering and normally fluent children are markedly different. In contrast to the widely held view in the middle decades of the 20th century, stuttering does not appear to rise from normal disfluencies and, in many ways, is distinguishable from the common fluency breaks of young children. These authors argue that parents who believe that their child has begun stuttering are often correct. On the other hand, Yairi and Ambrose state that "if it is unclear whether the disfluency is stuttering or not, there is no objective basis for great concern at that moment" (p. 139). While children who stutter (CWS) do produce normal or typical fluency breaks, they are not prominent. While two-thirds of the disfluencies of children who stutter are composed of stuttering-like disfluencies (SLDs), two-thirds of the disfluencies of normally fluent children (NFC) are composed of normal disfluencies.

According to Yairi and Ambrose (2005), parents commonly indicate some degree of physical, emotional, and language stress associated with stuttering onset with only about 20% of onset occurring under unremarkable circumstances. Secondary characteristics are often present at onset, with about half of the CWS showing tense movements in parts of the body, especially the head, face, or neck. Following onset, relatively few children show a linear progression of more severe and complex stuttering over time. For children who have begun to stutter the rate of the repetitions is significantly faster, with shorter intervals between the repeated units than the repetitions of normally fluent children. Normally fluent children rarely, if ever, produce disrhythmic phonations.

The expressive language skills of CWS tend to be at or above norm (Yairi, Ambrose, Paden, & Throneberg, 1996), a characteristic that is often the case for children who continue to stutter as well as those whose stuttering subsides. Soon after onset of stuttering the phonological ability of CWS tend to fall behind NFC, a finding that may be compounded by the occurrence of both stuttering and disordered phonology occurring more frequently in boys. Furthermore, this difference is likely to disappear within 2 years post-onset of stuttering when the phonological development of CWS becomes similar to NFC both in order of progression and strategies. In contrast to considerable earlier research, Yairi and Ambrose and others (e.g., Miles & Bernstein Ratner, 2001) found that many young CWS have average or above-average expressive language skills. One effect of successful treatment for stuttering may be the reduction of these relatively advanced pre-treatment expressive language levels to more age-appropriate levels (Bonelli, Dixon, & Bernstein Ratner, 2000; Ratner & Guitar, 2006; Tetnowski, 1998).

Yairi and Ambrose (2005) found no clear cut differences in CWS from NFC in levels of anxiety at the outset of stuttering (although anxiety in CWS tends to increase over time) and cognitive ability was within, or even above normal limits. The speech production system of some children who stutter may be less stable and more easily perturbed, as indicated by greater shimmer, slower phone production, and slightly more limited articulatory movement than their normally fluent peers.

In order to increase diagnostic sensitivity, Yairi and Ambrose (1999; 2005) developed a single score that combines three primary dimensions of disfluent speech (frequency, type, and extent of stuttering) (see Table 5-1). Ambrose and Yairi found that the *weighted SLD* score did a better job in distinguishing stuttering from normally fluent children than a basic count of SLDs. For example, a weighted SLD of 4 or above and associated nonspeech and psychosocial characteristics (e.g., awareness, negative attitude about communicating, struggle and escape behavior) are indicative of stuttering. The weighted SLD is tabulated using the following three steps.

1. Add together the number of part-word and single-syllable word repetitions per 100 syllables (PW + SS).

2. Multiply that sum by the mean number of repetition units (RU) (Repetition units are the number of times a sound, syllable or word is repeated prior to saying the word, divided by the number of words where this occurred.)

3. Add to the above total twice the number of disrhythmic phonations (DP) (blocks and prolongations) per 100 syllables. Ambrose and Yairi explain that because disrhythmic phonations are absent or rare in fluent speakers they are a strong indicator of stuttering and are thus weighted. The resulting formula is: $[(PW + SS) \times RU] + (2 \times DP)$[2]

Conture (2001) provides a list of seven criteria to consider when making the decision whether to initiate treatment with young children. Treatment is recommended if children meet two or more of the following: (1) the frequency of disfluencies is greater than 10%, (2) sound prolongations make up more than 30% of the within-word disfluencies, (3) score of 19 or greater on the Stuttering Severity Instrument (SSI) (Riley, 1994), (4) a score of 17 or greater on the Stuttering Prediction

---

[2]See Yairi and Ambrose (2005, p. 123) for examples of the ability of clinicians to distinguish mild but obvious stuttering from normal fluency breaks using the weighted SLD.

Table 5-1   Disfluency Criteria to Diagnose Mild Stuttering.

Measure (Frequency Per 100 Syllables)	Minimum Criteria for Stuttering
Part-word repetitions (PW)	≥1.5
Single-syllable word repetitions (SS)	≥2.5
Disrhythmic phonation	≥0.5
Repetition units	≥1.5
Stuttering-like disfluency (SLD)	≥3.0
Weighted SLD	≥4.0
Repetitions (PW + SS) with 2 or more *extra* units	≥1.0

Note. The child must meet three criteria to be diagnosed with stuttering.

From *Early Childhood Stuttering* (p. 338), by E. Yairi and N. G. Ambrose, 2005, Austin, TX: PRO-ED. Copyright 2005 by PRO-ED, Inc. Reprinted with permission.

Instrument (Riley. 1981); (5) the child's stuttering is associated with eyeball movements to the side and/or eyelid blinking, (6) clusters of stuttering constitute 25% of the child's disfluencies, and (7) the child has been stuttering for 18 months or more.

Indicators of Awareness

Many years ago Johnson and his colleagues (1959) noted that young children who stutter tend to display a variety of nonspeech reactions to their stuttering, such as tense body movements. These movements have often been referred to as "secondary behaviors" or "secondary characteristics" and may provide the clinician with an indication of the child's awareness about his or her stuttering. A number of studies by Conture and his associates (Schwartz & Conture, 1988; Schwartz, Zebrowski, & Conture, 1990; Conture & Kelly, 1991), as well as studies by Yairi, Ambrose, and Niermann (1993), indicated that young children who stuttered exhibited many such behaviors—including head, eye, torso, and limb movements—during (or in anticipation of) stuttering. Children who stuttered averaged 1.48 movements during stuttered words and 0.63 movements during nonstuttered words (Conture & Kelly, 1991).

Conture (1990) suggests two categories of nonspeech behavior that should be considered: (a) body movement and tension and (b) psychosocial discomfort and concern. These coping responses are likely a result of the child's awareness that speaking is difficult as well as the recognition of unfavorable reactions by listeners. Conture and Kelly (1991) observed more nonspeech movement and tension in 30 three to seven-year-old children who stuttered than a matched group of 30 year-old fluent children during comparable fluent sections of fluent speech. Specifically, the CWS (1) showed more frequent movement of their eyeballs to the left or right, (2) blinked their eyelids, and (3) raised their upper lip. Conture and Kelly theorized that these nonverbal responses were ways of coping with listener responses to their speech difficulty. Yairi et al. (1993) found that 16 young children who were within three months of stuttering onset averaged 3.18 (range of 0.8 to 5.9) head and neck movements per moment of stuttering. During follow-up testing, the authors found that as stuttering decreased the movements decreased. The awareness of young speakers who have begun to stutter may also be reflected by pitch rise; prolongations; schwa substitutions, the substitution of the neutral schwa vowel for the appropriate vowel (Manning, Emal, & Jamison, 1975); a high rate of part-word repetitions; and cessation of airflow and voicing (Adams, 1977a; Throneberg & Yairi, 1994; Van Riper, 1982; Walle, 1975). With the presence of such behaviors, it can be assumed that the child is aware of the problem, and is searching for ways of coping. Even at a young age, the child is attempting to cope with the helplessness and loss of control inherent in the experience of stuttering.

In a classic study of this important issue, Ambrose and Yairi (1994) used a unique videotape of puppets, one of whom stuttered. Children were asked to "point to the puppet that talks the way you do" (p. 234). The researchers found that 20 children who stuttered (aged two to five years) were more likely to identify with the disfluent puppet, while normally fluent control children identified with the fluent puppet. Although the majority of the young children who stuttered were not overtly aware of their stuttering, the results indicated the presence of awareness at some level and increasing awareness with increasing age. They also noted that awareness of stuttering was not related to stuttering severity (as indicated by an 8-point stuttering severity scale).

Based on their experience with many young children, Rustin and Cook (1995) point out that some preschool children are able to be very clear about the difficulties they experience. There are ample investigations indicating that school-age children as young as six who stutter are not only aware of their stuttering but quickly develop a negative attitude toward about their speech and communicating (DeNil & Brutten, 1991; Riley & Riley, 1979; Vanryckeghem & Brutten, 1996, 1997), as well as fears and avoidance behaviors (Conture, 1990; Peters & Guitar, 1991; Williams, 1985). Vanryckeghem, Brutten, and Hernandez (2005) extended the age of this negative self-response to the experience of stuttering to preschool and kindergarten children to as young as three, approximately the time when stuttering onset is observed. Bloodstein (1960) observed that parents reported that their children experienced consistent difficulty producing specific sounds or words as early as 2.5 years. Vanryckeghem et al. studied 45 children (ages 3–6) who stuttered and a matched group of 64 normally fluent children. The children's responses to a 12-item self-report measure, the Communication Attitude Test for Preschool and Kindergarten Children who Stutter (the KiddyCAT), resulted in significantly more negative scores for the stuttering children (mean score 4.36, SD = 2.78) than their normally fluent peers (mean score 1.79, SD = 1.78) ($P <$ .000, effect size = 1.14). No significant differences were found for age (3–4 vs. 5–6) or gender.

Although the use of projective drawings has received limited attention, some clinicians (e.g., Chemla and Reardon, 2001) have found that drawings by children clearly reflect their interpretation of their circumstances and their perceived ability to communicate, including their frustration and anxiety about speaking. Compared to young children (ages 5–10 years) who stutter (CWS), DeVore, Nandur, and Manning (1984) found that children who did not stutter (CWNS) drew significantly larger drawings that were placed nearer the center of the page. As a result of a 12-week program of individual therapy, the children who stuttered show significant changes in position and size of their drawings. They created larger drawings and placed them nearer to the center of the page and the figures were more likely to extend to all four quadrants of the sheet rather than in only the lower left quadrant. Post-treatment there were no significant differences in the drawings by the CWS and the CWNS, and the A-19 Attitude Scale (Guitar & Grims, 1977) indicated no significant differences between the two groups of children.

When children reach school age and begin to experience the social penalties that are likely to occur around their speech difficulties (if they have not already occurred), they quickly become acutely aware of their stuttering. Depending on such factors as the nature and severity of the child's stuttering and the support from his or her family, teachers, and friends, the child's reactions to his or her fluency problem can vary widely. Some children are able to adjust and to some extent counter the negative effects of stuttering by developing their academic, social, and athletic talents and abilities. In rare instances, a child who stutters may aggressively respond to his or her situation by developing speaking skills and engaging in activities such as acting or debating. Others may be devastated by their inability to achieve fluency and withdraw into a restrictive lifestyle, as described by Alan Rabinowitz:

> At some point in my childhood, maybe the first time I tried to speak and the only sound out of my mouth was an unintelligible stutter, I lost the ability to laugh, even to smile, without conscious thought or effort. I was judged by my words or, rather by my inability to produce them in the way that others did. From then on, I learned to trust no one and to speak only when absolutely necessary. As far as I was concerned, trusting led to betrayal and pain, and speaking was an unbearable horror. Words were my enemy. (Rabinowitz, 2001, p. 189)

Personality Characteristics

Early theories often attributed the onset of stuttering to personality characteristics and unconscious conflicts over unsatisfied needs or neurotic parental personalities (see chapter 3). Although a common view held by several authors in the early and middle years of the 20th century, little data were found to support the idea that children who stuttered, or their parents, displayed basic emotional maladjustments. However, some of the more current models of stuttering onset and development (Conture, 2001; Riley & Riley, 2000; Smith & Kelly, 1997), as well as several investigations into the temperamental characteristics of children who stutter (Anderson, Pellowski, Conture, & Kelly, 2003; Embrechts, Ebbin, Franke, & van de Poel, 2000; Ezrati-Vinacour, Plazky, & Yairi, 2001; Glasner, 1949; Vanryckeghem & Brutten, 1997; Wakaba, 1998), indicate that many children who stutter tend to be more sensitive, inhibited, and reactive than their nonstuttering peers. As discussed briefly in Chapter 2, there is convincing research indicating that some children are more likely than others to be upset by changes in routine or inhibited with strangers (Calkins and Fox, 1994 and Kagan et al., 1987). It is also possible that such children have a low tolerance for their own disfluent speech. While it is entirely possible that living with a problem such as stuttering results in older speakers being particularly sensitive to the plights of others, the results of these investigations indicate that some of these characteristics are present at birth and may exacerbate the effect of disfluent speech and contribute to the possibility of chronicity. Yairi and Ambrose (2005), for example, suggest that such personality and temperamental factors may play a role in determining speech fluency for some subtypes of individuals who stutter. They conclude that it is difficult to determine if the relationship of these perceived characteristics of young children who stutter are the result of inherent biological and personality characteristics, a consequence of early self-awareness of stuttering, or an interaction of several influences.

On a related topic, research concerning anxiety in children who stutter began to occur in the 1990s. Two types of anxiety have been identified and have been the focus of this research. Trait anxiety (indicated as A-Trait) is said to indicate a person's general level of anxiety. Evidence of trait anxiety is obtained by having the individual respond to self-report scales containing questions about how he or she generally feels (e.g., I feel happy "hardly ever, sometimes, or often"). Measures of state anxiety (indicated as A-State) are said to indicate a person's anxiety as he or she reacts to specific situational stimuli. A frequently used measure of anxiety is the State-Trait Anxiety Inventory for Children (STAIC) developed by Spielberger, Edwards, Luschene, Montuori, and Platzek (1972). Scores on both the State and Trait subscales of the STAIC range from 20 to 60, with higher scores representing greater anxiety. Using the STAIC, Craig and Hancock (1996) found no significant differences between 96 (untreated) children who stuttered and 104 children who did not stutter (age range of 9–14 years). This was the case for both State and Trait subscales. In addition, the authors found no significant association between stuttering frequency and state anxiety. Likewise, Yairi and Ambrose (2005), using the *Revised Children's Manifest Anxiety Scale* (RCMAS; Reynolds & Richmond, 1994), found no clear indications of higher anxiety on any of the subscales during the early stages of stuttering, but did note that anxiety tends to increase with time.

Participation of the Parents in Assessment

In the sections of this book where we discuss the importance of counseling (Chapter 7) and the treatment of young children (Chapter 9), the importance of parent participation in the therapeutic process is emphasized. Unfortunately, in some cases parent involvement during assessment and especially treatment will be nonexistent. The motivation for initiating treatment may be minimal if the family physician or friends and family members suggest that the problem will be likely to go away by itself (Ramig, 1993c). In contrast to Rustin, who is reluctant to recommend treatment without parent involvement (1987; Rustin & Cook, 1995), Ramig contends that even in cases where parents cannot or will not become involved in treatment, the clinician should enroll the child. In our experience, while some children may benefit from increased understanding about the nature of their problem and some practice with basic therapeutic techniques, real long-term changes are less likely to occur without the involvement of at least one dedicated parent.

Rustin and Cook (1995) provide several questions the clinician can use to discover the nature of the family and of parent–child interaction. Though the questions themselves are important, the most important facet of the interview process is the clinician's style and ability to be flexible and creative as he or she interacts with the parents. As Caruso (1988) describes, the intent is to follow the parent's lead, all the while probing for areas of interest and concern. As Rustin and Cook indicate:

> In the interview, we learn about the rules and regulations in the child's life, the parents' attitudes toward child rearing, pertinent issues within the parental relationship, the problem-solving strategies employed, and the place the disfluency problem holds within the family. The interview is structured in such a way that the basic and noncontentious case details are gathered in the early stages of the process, with a gradual move toward more sensitive and emotional material as it progresses. (1995, p. 129)

Educational Impact

For some children the academic impact of stuttering is obvious. Teachers may recognize that a child will consistently refuse to participate in class discussions, consistently avoid oral presentations, or not respond to questions. Most experienced clinicians have heard many descriptions from school-age children and college students who coped with their stuttering by being absent on the first day of class to avoid the usual round of introductions. Later in the semester they may have feigned an illness on the day of a scheduled oral presentation. Often the coping strategies are much more subtle, as when a student pretends not to know the answer to a question or intentionally responds incorrectly in order to minimize verbal participation (Gregory, 2004). In many such cases the teacher is unlikely to be aware that the motivation for a student's response is the possibility of stuttering and may consider the student to be shy, aloof, withdrawn, or anxious. In other instances, the child may be classified as a "slow learner," and in some instances, placed in a class for such students. Because children who stutter are adept at hiding, they are less likely to be identified by teachers and clinicians than, for example, children with a variety of other communication problems.

For other children, particularly those who appear to be succeeding academically, school administrators may take the stance that the child is not experiencing any adverse effects as a result of his or her stuttering. However, as Ribbler (2006) counsels, a full appreciation of the multidimensional nature of the stuttering

Clinical Insight

Several years ago I worked with a college student who described a pattern of avoidance and word substitution. He was the starting running back for a highly ranked Division 1 football team. He had always been a good student and had received an academic, rather than a football, scholarship to the university. During a group meeting, he described a speaking event that took place when he was in junior high school. Rob had completed a class quiz, which was then graded by a student in the adjoining aisle. His paper was returned, and he saw that he had received a score of 95. The teacher went up and down the rows of desks, asking each student in turn to report his or her grade. When it was his turn, Rob stood and attempted to say "ninety-five." After enduring a speech block for several moments, he decided he would be less likely to stutter if he said "eighty-five." Also experiencing a block as he attempted to say that number he quickly decided to say "seventy-five" and this time he was successful! The teacher recorded the grade and Rob sat down. No one in the room, including the teacher, suspected he had stuttered. But of course, Rob had experienced a profound moment of stuttering.

experience suggests several ways in which such children are likely to experience limitations (Table 5-2). Ribbler points out the wide variety of adverse educational effects that children who stutter are likely to face, both within and beyond the communication domain. Even for the child who is able to achieve grades that are at or above the level of his or her peers, the child's awareness of his or her stuttering and the possibility of social penalty is likely to influence his or her choices across a broad range of areas, including academic competency, academic

Table 5-2 Domains and potential adverse effects on education.

Domains	Adverse Effect on Education
Academics and Learning	Decreased participation in classroom lectures. Difficulties giving oral presentations. Trouble reading aloud. Reluctant to ask teacher questions for clarification of work. Courses and career paths may be selected that require the least amount of verbal communication skills.
Socio-Emotional Functioning	Difficulties establishing and maintaining interpersonal relationships. Trouble introducing oneself. Decreased ability to verbally negotiate teasing and bullying situations. Student may resort to physical/aggressive ways of coping or show withdrawal behaviors by avoiding interaction with peers. Absenteeism due to anxiety about stuttering in class. Reluctance to speak to adults in authority.
Independent Functioning	May avoid asking for directions when maneuvering around school or campus. Difficulty seeking help and explaining conflicts in stressful and/or emergency situations. Embarrassed to clarify information about assignment deadlines so work may be turned in late.
Communication	Stuttering can distract from intended message. Decreased ability to express opinion and ideas in a classroom discussion. Difficulties talking on the phone with peers to discuss homework and group projects.

From Ribbler, N. (2006, February) When a student stutters: Identifying the adverse educational impact. *Perspectives on Fluency Disorders, 16(1),* 16–17. Rockville, MD: American Speech-Language-Hearing Association.

learning, and social-emotional and independent functioning, any of which can prevent the child from realizing his or her full potential. Such children are apt to experience more difficulty establishing interpersonal relationships, joining conversations, introducing themselves, and initiating friendships. Some children who stutter will choose not to talk at lunch, recess, or field trips. As Ribbler describes, many children who stutter are less likely to use the telephone to help clarify assignments, discuss upcoming quizzes or tests, and join others in preparing school projects.

Finally, there is the potential for an adverse impact on the social aspects of the academic experience, including quality of life issues. Students who stutter may be less able function independently and problem solve a variety of circumstances, including obtaining help or assistance from teacher or peers. Something as seemingly simple as asking for directions to find a classroom or dormitory may be a major challenge, even for a college student. The lack of social interaction and associated information about school relationships and activities decrease the speaker's participation and awareness. Some students who stutter are unwilling to participate or play positions on athletic teams if they are required to deliver plays from the sidelines or assume leadership roles.

The potential for adverse educational impact due to a child's stuttering is not necessarily indicated by passing grades or the ability of the child to score within the normal range on standardized tests. As with anyone, the point is whether or not the child will have the opportunity to reach his or her potential. What choices is the child likely to be making that will limit his or her participation within each of the domains described by Ribbler? It may be that such choices are more likely indicated using qualitative measures such as self-generated oral or written narratives by the child.

Based on the information described in the above section, the following box summarizes the speech and nonspeech characteristics that are likely to occur with children who stutter.

Speech and Nonspeech Characteristics of Children Who Stutter

Occurrence of stuttering in nuclear or extended family
Parents identify child as stuttering
Weighted SLD score of 4 or greater
SLDs increase when communicating under pressure
SLDs accompanied by tense movements of head, face, and neck
Behavioral or formal indicators of negative psychosocial reactions to stuttering
The child self-restricts communication and social interaction
The child is easily upset by changes in routine or inhibited with strangers

Decision 2: Determining the Course of Stuttering

Once it is determined that a young speaker's fluency breaks are unusual or abnormal, the next clinical decision is whether this pattern is likely to continue and develop into a chronic problem. As Yairi and Ambrose (2005) comment, ". . . as stuttering continues, the difficulty lies not in correct diagnosis of stuttering, but in correct diagnosis of its recovery" (p. 139). Although the nature of the fluency breaks (particularly SLDs) are important to consider, there are several factors that appear to influence whether the child is likely to continue stuttering.

The clinician will also need to consider a related decision about the extent and nature of the intervention that may be appropriate for the child and his family. This will involve factoring in the history of stuttering in the child's family, the response of the child to his or her speech problem, and the willingness of the parent(s) to support and become actively involved in the therapeutic process. Because of the large proportion of children in which stuttering will likely subside, the reasonably good probability that treatment will be successful with young children and the likelihood that treatment will be more demanding for adolescents and adults, the issue has been hotly debated (Curlee & Yairi, 1997). Although the decision is a difficult one an informed and wise decision at this point is critical.

The longitudinal data of Yairi and Ambrose (2005) indicate that there is no one factor that can be used to predict the course of stuttering and that the best we can do is determine those factors that are most likely to *suggest* the chances of recovery or persistence. However, there are several trends that have obvious clinical utility and allow the clinician to make informed predictions. Yairi and Ambrose (2005) indicate that a strong family history is one of the most reliable predictors of persistence. As described in Chapter 3, although we are currently uncertain about what is being transmitted, there appears to be a strong genetic component for both recovery and persistence of stuttering. Children who come from families where one or more members stutter are less likely to recover; where stuttering has persisted for family members the child is more likely to follow the same pattern. And although the outcome is far from certain, the majority of the time children are more likely to recover if the family member who has stuttered has recovered.

Gender is also a relatively strong indicator of the course of stuttering in that females are more likely to recover and males are more likely to continue stuttering once they begin. Yairi and Ambrose (2005, p. 298) provide incidence figures indicating that for a boy, the risk of persistent stuttering is 1.5% and the risk of recovered stuttering is 5.3%, with a total risk of 6.8%. For a girl, the risk of persistent stuttering is 0.5% and the risk of recovered stuttering is 2.7% with a total risk of 3.2%. In addition, Yairi and Ambrose (2005) point out that recovery is more likely to take place sooner for girls than for boys. Whereas girls are more likely to recover within a year after the onset of stuttering boys may take several years to recover. For girls, a pattern of stuttering for 12 months without improvement suggests the possibility of chronicity. Furthermore, those children who recovered early and maintained fluency for at least 12 months did not relapse.

Another trend that appears to be strongly predictive of recovery or persistence is the pattern of SLDs during the first year following onset (Figure 5-1). In contrast to the more traditional view of gradually increasing stuttering severity described at the outset of this chapter, in the majority of early childhood cases, stuttering starts out being readily obvious and after continuing for several weeks or months, gradually decreases. Yairi and Ambrose suggest that although a child may continue to stutter for several months, a downward pattern in the number of SLDs during the first year is a strong sign of eventual recovery. Particularly for children who are going to recover, the frequency of SLDs and overall severity of stuttering is likely to decrease during the first six months following onset and nearly always begins to subside by the end of the first year. Although the overall level of severity at the outset is unrelated to whether the young child will persist or recover from stuttering, Yairi and Ambrose indicate that continued severity is a primary indication for concern. That is, when children continue to maintain a stable or escalating level of SLDs during the first year following onset,

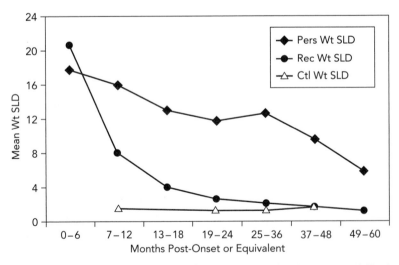

Figure 5-1 Mean weighted (Wt) SLD for persistent (Pers), recovered (Rec), and control (Ctl) groups over time. From *Early Childhood Stuttering* (p. 177), by E. Yairi and N. G. Ambrose, 2005, Austin, TX: PRO-ED. Copyright 2005 by PRO-ED, Inc. Reprinted with permission.

persistence of stuttering is more likely. That is, a stable or inclining pattern of SLDs is indicative of persistent stuttering.

In a related issue, for many children, the ratings of SLDs and stuttering severity by both the parents and clinicians also begin to decrease during the first year following onset. These findings indicate that parental judgment of their child's speech difficulty should be considered a fundamental part of a diagnosis of stuttering (Conture & Caruso, 1987; Onslow, 1992; Riley & Riley, 1983) for, as presented in Figure 5-2, parental and clinician ratings tend to coincide rather closely (Yairi & Ambrose, 2005).

Yairi and Ambrose (2005) also noted that longer strings of part-word repetitions (more than three but often much longer) were found to indicate persistence of stuttering. Conversely, recovery was indicated by a gradual decrease in the number of repetitions. In contrast to some suggestions in the literature, Yairi and Ambrose did not find the duration of individual stuttering events to be predictive of persistent stuttering. In fact, children who recovered showed an *increase* in the silent intervals between repetition units such that the resulting iterations were slower in tempo. Yairi and Ambrose interpreted this as a normalization process that clinicians can perceptually distinguish without the use of sophisticated measuring equipment. Finally, Yairi and Ambrose found that although at the outset of stuttering there were no differences in the occurrences of head and facial movements for children who recovered or were persistent, a decline in secondary characteristics was predictive of recovery.

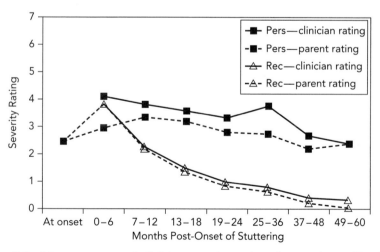

Figure 5-2   Mean parent and clinician severity ratings for persistent (Pers) and recovered (Rec) children over time. *Note.* From *Early Childhood Stuttering* (p. 184), by E. Yairi and N. G. Ambrose, 2005, Austin, TX: PRO-ED. Copyright 2005 by PRO-ED, Inc. Reprinted with permission.

Yairi and Ambrose (2005) also report a tendency for children who begin stuttering somewhat later (35 months rather than the typical onset of 33 months) to persist in stuttering. This factor may interact with the possibility that somewhat older children are more likely to be aware of the stuttering closer to the time of onset and may react to the unfavorable responses of others as they experience the effects of socialization during the early preschool years. A related factor is the duration of the child's stuttering following onset. As indicated earlier, Yairi and Ambrose found that a history of stuttering lasting beyond one year indicates the likelihood of persistence, particularly for females. Nevertheless, natural recovery can occur three years following onset with some children taking as long as four years to recover. Given that the most common age of onset is 33 months (2 years, 9 months), the data from Yairi and Ambrose indicate that some children are still likely to recover through six or seven years of age. Although, as we have seen, awareness by the child as well as negative affective reactions can occur shortly following onset, the older the child and the longer he or she experiences the frustration and communicative effort associated with stuttering, the more affective and cognitive coping responses will come into play.

It is important to note that expressive language skills are *not* predictive of recovery and, as indicated earlier, Yairi and Ambrose (2005) found that both persistent and recovered groups of CWS display expressive language ability at or above normative expectations. These findings are similar to those of Kloth et al. (1998) who, in a prospective study, found that children at risk for stuttering (as indicated by a parental history of stuttering) and who subsequently stuttered or were fluent followed the same patterns of articulatory rate and linguistic development. Yairi and Ambrose point out, however, that most language measures are general and suggest that a more detailed analysis of language skills may help to predict chronicity. Yairi and Ambrose point out that their results provide initial empirical validation for the idea that "Many young children who begin stuttering seem to have language abilities that exceed their capabilities for fluent production of speech" (p. 251). However, these findings do not support reducing the child's language stimulation or suggest that adults simplify their language when working with children who stutter (Bonelli, et al., 2000). Although at the outset of stuttering children who continue to stutter tend to be slower in phonological development, phonological skills alone are insufficient to predict the course of stuttering.

Yairi and Ambrose did not design their longitudinal studies to directly consider the predictive value of concomitant learning and language-speech problems often present in children who stutter. They do agree with others that the presence of other problems is likely to degrade a child's ability to communicate, decreasing the possibility of remission. This may be an important consideration given that Blood and Seider (1981) found that 68% of 1,060 children being treated for stuttering in elementary schools had other speech, language, hearing, or learning problems, with articulation disorders the most often reported. Just how these other communication problems influence the possibility of natural remission, the likelihood of successful treatment and the possibility of relapse following treatment is unclear.

One possibility for this type of interaction of speech and language domains is suggested by two investigations of the same children by Watkins, Ehud, and Ambrose (1999) and Paden, Yairi, and Ambrose (1999). Watkins et al. conducted an extensive evaluation of the expressive language abilities of 84 preschool children close the onset of their stuttering. Both the children who recovered from stuttering (N = 62) and the children who persisted in stuttering (N = 22) were found to have similar expressive language abilities. Overall, and regardless of whether or not the children recovered, language abilities were near or above normative expectations. However, the extent of the children's language abilities varied according to age. Advanced language abilities were especially the case for those children who experienced an early onset of stuttering and therefore entered the study in the youngest age group (2–3 years of age). These children were found to consistently demonstrate language skills that were well above age expectations, often meeting expectations for children a full year older. This was true for these younger children whether they recovered or not.

On the other hand, the children who experienced a later onset of stuttering and entered the study at 4–5 years of age *and* persisted in stuttering tended to show language skills that were slightly (but not significantly) below their peers of the same age who recovered. This finding, along with the results of the investigation of the same children by Paden, Yairi, and Ambrose (1999) indicated that, regardless of age, all of the children who persisted in stuttering also scored lower on virtually every measure of phonological ability than the children who would recover. This combination of results led Watkins et al. to suggest, as Ratner (1997) had previously done, the possibility of an asynchronous or out-of-phase pattern of development, particularly for children who start to stutter prior to age three. Based on the combined results of the investigations, Watkins et al. suggested the possibility of "developmental tradeoffs operating such that advanced proficiency in one domain requires sacrifice of performance in another domain" (p. 1133). The results of investigations by Watkins et al. (1999) and Paden et al. (1999) suggest a combination of language and phonological variables that may inform the possibility of stuttering onset and remission. That is, while precocious language may be a risk factor for stuttering for children with early onset, these children are also more likely to recover than children with somewhat later onset (and more age-appropriate language skills). On the other hand, the presence of a phonology–language gap may suggest the possibility of stuttering chronicity.

Clinical **Decision-Making**

A telephone call or e-mail contact from a parent who is concerned about the onset of stuttering behavior in their child is a common occurrence for the clinician specializing in stuttering. Although the factors and trends described in this chapter are always considered, some period of informed observation is usually a reasonable course of action. The following two e-mail messages from a concerned mother provide a common example.

To begin with, the comments are especially interesting because the mother was a speech-language pathologist. Although she had relatively little experience with childhood fluency problems, she was able to provide an informed description about other related characteristics of her son's speech and language. Following the first e-mail message I suggested that the mother obtain video examples of her son's fluency in a variety of speaking situations. I also assured her that, particularly with her experience, she was unlikely to complicate the problem as long as she (and her husband) responded in a natural way typical for any situation where their child was having a problem and was frustrated. As is often the case, the parents were extremely appreciative of the information and support and expressed a great decrease in their anxiety about the situation.

The first message received during the first week of November:

Alan is 2.5 years old and his brother is 10 months old. He has had what I considered "normal disfluencies" for the past 3–4 months or so. It was not something I was concerned about. His language skills are very good, and I attributed the disfluencies to rapidly emerging language. Around 2–3 weeks ago, the stuttering really began to increase, both in number of occurrences and in severity. Within the past week it has become very concerning, not only to myself, but to other family members and his preschool teachers. Where he typically might repeat some initial sounds 3–4 times, he is now repeating up to 20 times, and now there are secondary behaviors—eye closing, grimacing. The prolongations are longer. A few times in the last few days he has sighed and just given up trying to get the message out. At these times when his awareness and frustration were evident, I acknowledged that "your words seem to be getting a little stuck" and offered reassurance that everyone has trouble with this from time to time. This did seem to make him feel better.

The disfluency is worse in the first hour or so he is awake, and again at the end of the day, so fatigue does seem to be a factor. But it happens throughout the day, too. It happens not only when he is trying to express something a little more complicated or abstract (as was the case for the past few months) but also on very simple, straightforward messages. We have had nothing out of the ordinary happening at home. I cannot think of any new stressor. We are modeling slow speech and trying to make communication as well as other activities as unhurried as possible. We make eye contact when he gets really stuck, and try not to show any distress. My ultra laid back husband is worried . . . "It's getting

(continues)

worse each day!" His language and articulation are good. My father had a first cousin who "stuttered badly" but was "cured when he joined the army" and presumably had therapy for the first time (otherwise no family history).

The second message, received the second week of December:

Hi! I was just thinking this week that I wanted to e-mail you. We never got Alan's disfluencies recorded because they abruptly stopped! I don't know what happened, but we are so thankful that he is having an easier time talking! I know he may start having difficulty again, and if he does I will get back in touch with you. For now, though, things are going really well.

Thanks again for your help, enjoy your Holidays!

The following Table (5-3) summarizes the indicators of remission (green flags) and persistence (red flags) based largely on the work of Yairi and Ambrose (2005). Indicators are listed in the probable order of their predictive ability.

Table 5-3   Indicators of recovery from (green flags) and persistent (red flags) stuttering based on Yairi and Ambrose (2005) and others.

Indicators of Remission–Green Flags	Indicators of Persistence–Red Flags
No relatives who stutter	Family history of persistent stuttering
Relatives who stuttered and recovered	Relatives continue to stutter
Female	Male
Decreasing pattern of SLDs within one year of onset	Stable or increasing number of SLDs within one year of onset
Decreasing severity ratings by clinicians and parents	Stable or increasing severity ratings by clinicians and parents
Child is stuttering but is within one year of onset	Child is stuttering more than one year following onset (especially females)
Deceasing secondary movements (e.g., head and eye movements)	Stable or increasing occurrence of secondary movements
Many (>3) part-word repetitions	Few repetitions
Slower rate of repetitions	Rapid rate of repetitions
Few reactions to stuttering by child or parents	Strong reactions to stuttering by child or parents
No concomitant learning or communication problems	Concomitant learning or communication problems
Early onset of stuttering (age 2–3 years) and precious expressive language	Later onset of stuttering (age 3–4 years) and delays in phonological development

Despite the valuable longitudinal information provided by Yairi and Ambrose as well as others, predicting the course of stuttering for young children is far from certain. Clinicians will want to develop and communicate to parents the possible indicators of remission and persistence discussed in this section and their philosophy concerning intervention. Given the high recovery rate of stuttering for young children, therapy may simply facilitate what may be a natural process of recovery. Nonetheless, the clinician will want to consider the concern of parents as well as the child's struggle to speak. The experience can be a painful one for the parents and other members of the extended family. The child may indicate obvious frustration in his or her efforts to communicate, sometimes refusing to speak at all. Even without the presence of some or many of the red flags indicated above, a brief period of therapy may be a reasonable choice, particularly if this is the desire of the parents.

Guidelines for Intervention

Zebrowski (1997) pointed out that although we may discover many characteristics that appear to be related to the chronicity of stuttering, each child who comes to us for an evaluation is unique. Zebrowski suggests that, based on the likelihood of children recovering without therapy, the clinician many want to consider one of several "decision streams" according to the characteristics of the child and the family. As shown in Figure 5-3[3], children are placed in one of four streams based on the time interval since onset. Stream I contains five characteristics, Streams II and III contain seven characteristics and Stream IV contains four characteristics. The clinician's decision (Plans A–E) are based on characteristics that have been identified in the literature—particularly those described by Yairi and his colleagues earlier in this chapter. Points are assigned when children possess the characteristics listed within each stream. For example, children who have been stuttering for fewer than six months are placed in Stream I. Children demonstrating all of the five characteristics associated with this stream are assigned a score of five points, and the clinician would respond with Plan A as described below. Children with a score of 4 or less would undergo Plan B.

---

[3]With the permission of the original author (Zebrowski) this figure has been modified from the original published in 1997. Given the current information concerning the expressive language abilities of children who stutter, the word *language* has been deleted from the final bullet in each of the four streams.

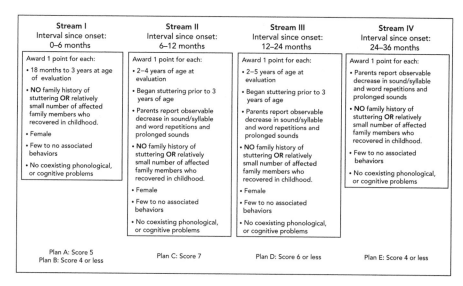

Stream I Interval since onset: 0–6 months	Stream II Interval since onset: 6–12 months	Stream III Interval since onset: 12–24 months	Stream IV Interval since onset: 24–36 months
Award 1 point for each: • 18 months to 3 years at age of evaluation • **NO** family history of stuttering **OR** relatively small number of affected family members who recovered in childhood. • Female • Few to no associated behaviors • No coexisting phonological, or cognitive problems	Award 1 point for each: • 2–4 years of age at evaluation • Began stuttering prior to 3 years of age • Parents report observable decrease in sound/syllable and word repetitions and prolonged sounds • **NO** family history of stuttering **OR** relatively small number of affected family members who recovered in childhood. • Female • Few to no associated behaviors • No coexisting phonological, or cognitive problems	Award 1 point for each: • 2–5 years of age at evaluation • Began stuttering prior to 3 years of age • Parents report observable decrease in sound/syllable and word repetitions and prolonged sounds • **NO** family history of stuttering **OR** relatively small number of affected family members who recovered in childhood. • Female • Few to no associated behaviors • No coexisting phonological, or cognitive problems	Award 1 point for each: • Parents report observable decrease in sound/syllable and word repetitions and prolonged sounds • **NO** family history of stuttering **OR** relatively small number of affected family members who recovered in childhood. • Few to no associated behaviors • No coexisting phonological, or cognitive problems
Plan A: Score 5 Plan B: Score 4 or less	Plan C: Score 7	Plan D: Score 6 or less	Plan E: Score 4 or less

Figure 5-3   Decision streams for intervention Modified from Zebrowski, P. M. Assisting young children who stutter and their families: Defining the role of the speech-language pathologist. First published in: *American Journal of Speech-Language Pathology, 6(2)*, 19–28. Reprinted with permission.

Plan A: (Stream I for children who have all five recovery characteristics)

Children with all five recovery characteristics have a high probability of recovery. Treatment consists of information sharing and bibliotherapy. The clinician provides parents with information about (1) normal speech and language development, (2) their child's speech and language relative to a normally fluent child, (3) information about what we do and do not know about causal factors for stuttering in children, and (4) the prognosis for recovery for their child given the information accumulated at that point. In addition, parents are provided with reading material. Clinicians are available for monthly contact with the parents via telephone or e-mail to further explain the information and answer questions. Parents can monitor changes in frequency or type of fluency breaks. Particular attention is given to whether there is a gradual decrease in the repetitions of stuttering-like disfluencies (SLDs). If there is a stable or increasing pattern of SLDs, a follow-up visit is indicated.

Plan B: (Stream I for children who have four of five recovery characteristics)

Children with four of the five recovery characteristics also have a high probability of recovery. Treatment consists of all the components of Plan A, with the addition of language intervention, phonological intervention, or both, if appropriate for the child. The degree of intervention will vary depending on the child's age and the severity of the problem(s). In addition, family members with a positive history of stuttering are provided with counseling, given the likelihood of greater concern about their child.

Plan C: (Stream II and III for children with a score of seven recovery characteristics)

Recovery is less likely for the child who has been stuttering longer. These children began stuttering before the age of three and have been doing so for six months to two years. If these children are female, have no family history or a family history of recovery, have few or no associated behaviors or concomitant problems, and demonstrate a decrease in symptomatology, they are more likely to recover. As the child continues to stutter two years post-onset (particularly if the child is female), recovery becomes less likely. Treatment consists of all the components of Plan B with the addition of counseling for parents about ways to indirectly enhance the fluency of their child by practicing such activities as speech-rate reduction, longer turn-switching pause durations, and avoiding interrupting. Children could also enroll the child in a parent–child group designed to facilitate fluency.

Plan D: (Stream II and III for children with a score of six or fewer recovery characteristics)

This plan contains all the components of Plan C that are applicable plus monthly visits to the clinic or the parent's home for monitoring. Taped speech samples are analyzed for the quality of the child's fluency (SLDs, speed of repetitions, and reactions of the child as well as associated behaviors). In addition, during the visits to the clinic or the home, parents can be counseled about the possibility that their child may not recover from stuttering and the possibilities for more direct intervention.

Plan E: (Stream IV for children with a score of four or fewer recovery characteristics)

These children have been stuttering from two to three years post-onset and are the least likely to recover. Treatment consists of all the factors included in the above plans plus direct intervention according to treatment protocols described in this and other texts.

Using At-Risk Registers

For decades, parents of children who stutter have been told to take a wait-and-*see* approach in the hope that the problem would go away. Such advice is a common response of pediatricians (Yairi & Carrico, 1992). Another possibility is more of a wait-and-*watch* strategy using an "at-risk" register (Adams, 1977b; Onslow, 1992) for reducing the occurrence of the false positive (a normally speaking child is incorrectly identified as a child who stutters) and the false negative (a child who stutters is incorrectly identified as a child who does not stutter). A false positive would result in a child receiving unnecessary assistance in producing fluent speech. Of course, a false negative identification would be a more serious error in that a child who may benefit from treatment fails to receive assistance, especially considering the evidence that treatment for more advanced stuttering is considerably more time-consuming and prone to failure and relapse than treatment closer to onset (Bloodstein & Bernstein Ratner, 2008; Conture, 1996; Costello, 1983; Onslow, 1992). Thus, as Onslow recommends, the process leading to negative identification should be conservative, while the process resulting in positive identification should be relatively liberal. It has been suggested that the negative identification of communication disorders may result in the inefficient use of health care services (Andrews, 1984, Curlee & Yairi, 1997). However, Onslow comments that this view is not held for other communication disorders and questions both the logic and the ethics of a decision process that could result in the withholding of treatment from young children who stutter. Onslow also suggests that because of the difficulties in treating cases of advanced stuttering, accurate early identification may actually improve the overall efficiency of service delivery.

Onslow's at-risk register is composed of both negative and positive identification components. When stuttering is suspected, the parents bring the child to a clinic for a formal evaluation. The parents are requested to bring audio- or videotapes of their child's speech made in a natural environment, indicating the fluency characteristics of concern. The identification of a problem is based on the perception of stuttering by the clinician(s) and the parents. If a parent considers that a child is stuttering (an important factor, according to Yairi and Ambrose, 2005) but the clinician fails to perceive stuttered speech in the clinic or in the recording, the child is listed in the at-risk register. In the case where a clinician perceives stuttered speech but an parent does not, positive identification occurs if a second clinician perceives stuttered speech. If the second clinician does not perceive stuttered speech, then the child is placed in an at-risk register.

Those children listed in the at-risk register are observed on a regular basis for a period of months or years. Onslow suggests that ongoing evaluations can take a variety of forms, including telephone conversations, face-to-face interviews with parents, or questionnaires mailed to the home. Another tactic is to have the parents periodically call the clinic and respond to a series of questions that might indicate forms of speech fragmentation, tension, or struggle. Those children who pass the ongoing evaluations will continue being included on the register until a negative identification is made. How long this process should continue is a good question, but based on Bloodstein's (1987) literature review, Onslow suggests a possible upper limit of 12 years. A child is moved to the positive identification component if at any point a parent becomes concerned, and a formal evaluation is again scheduled.

The use of an at-risk strategy places no pressure on the clinician to make either a positive or a negative identification. If there is uncertainty concerning the diagnosis, the child is listed on the register and, if necessary, will remain there until a decision is made. The clinician should not necessarily feel pressured to make a decision concerning intervention, for as Curlee and Yairi (1997) explain, no evidence is available that indicates that postponing treatment for a year or more results in poorer treatment outcomes. However, if the clinician is in doubt and there are several factors suggesting the persistence of stuttering, a period of trial therapy may be the best decision. Curlee (2007) recommends that when faced with such a dilemma it is often best to support the parents' choice of whether or not to initiate treatment.

The Component Model: A Comprehensive Diagnostic Approach

Because the component model by Glyndon and Jeanna Riley (1979, 1984, 2000) represents a comprehensive approach for the assessment of children who stutter, a summary of this model is presented here. Similar in many ways to the demands and capacities model (Adams, 1990; Gottwald, 1999; Gottwald & Starkweather, 1999; Starkweather, 1987; Starkweather & Gottwald, 1990) described in Chapter 3, it provides greater detail for clinicians who would like to consider factors that, based on the many years of clinical research by the Rileys, inform the clinician concerning the course of stuttering in young children.

The model is based on the premise that the onset of stuttering is related to a "vulnerable system" in a young child. Those components of the child's system that contribute to the vulnerability of the child's speech production are identified. Treatment, as we will describe in Chapter 9, emphasizes improving the child's areas of vulnerability and reducing those components that are stressing the child's system, followed by procedures for enhancing the child's fluency.

The approach for assessing children who may be in the early stages of stuttering evolved from Riley and Riley's clinical observations of subgroups of children based on risk factors for stuttering onset and development. Using a correlation approach and the results of diagnostic information from 54 children, they developed an assessment model that included what they determined to be the most salient components. Of the nine components included in their original model (1984), five were found to be most common among children who stuttered: Attending Disorders, Auditory Processing Disorders, Sentence Formulation Disorders, Oral Motor Discoordination, and High Self-Expectations. Children were defined as being disordered if they scored in excess of the normal expectations for performance on a standardized measure of each component.

The revised component model (RCM) (2000) includes three generic factors with associated subcategories:

I. Physical Attributes

    A. Attending Disorders

    B. Speech Motor Coordination

II. Temperamental Factors

    A. High Self-Expectations

    B. Overly Sensitive

III. Listener Reactions

    A. Disruptive Communication Environment

    B. Secondary Gains

    C. Teasing/Bullying

The factor of Physical Attributes is subdivided into components of Attending Disorders and Speech Motor Coordination. Attending Disorders were identified by using the Poor Impulse Control Scale (e.g., cannot control self, is impulsive) and Poor Attention Scale (e.g., easily distracted, cannot finish things) of the Burks Behavior Rating Scales (BBRS; Burks, 1976), the Hyperactivity Index from the Conner's Parent Rating Scale (Conners, 1998) and the clinician's judgment that the child has a reduced attention span and was distractible. The Rileys found that 36% of the children in the original study (1979) presented with either severe (20%) or moderate (16%) attending disorders. Subsequent research (2000) found that 26% of the 50 CWS were found to have severe (18%) or moderate

(8%) attending disorders. Speech motor control problems were identified using the Oral Motor Assessment Scale (OMAS; Riley & Riley, 1985). This measure determines—among other areas—the child's accuracy of voicing coarticulatory movements between syllables, and rate, including diadochokinetic rate for syllable production. In the original study, 69% of the CWS indicated oral motor disorders (36% severe and 33% moderate), and 33% had moderate or severe articulation disorders. The more recent (2000) sample of 50 children yielded 68% of the CWS with speech motor difficulties (50% severe and 18% moderate), compared to levels in the non-CWS population of 2% severe and 8% moderate. Moderate or severe articulation or phonological disorders occurred in 50% of the more recent sample.

The next generic category of Temperamental Factors includes the components of High Self-Expectations and Overly Sensitive. Overly high self-expectations were determined by parent report (e.g., the child appears perfectionistic, is cautious, and has a low threshold for frustration), clinician observation, and the child's performance on three subtests of the BBRS: Excessive Anxiety Scale (e.g., appears tense, worries too much) and Excessive Self-Blame (e.g., blames self if things go wrong, upset if makes a mistake). The Overly Sensitive components are determined by scores on the Excessive Suffering subtest of the BBRS. In 1979, the authors found that 89% of the children assessed had abnormally high self-expectations; the more recent study indicated that 70% of the CWS had either severe (13%) or moderate (57%) levels of unusually high expectations.

The Overly Sensitive component is reflective of children who appear to overly react to their environment. The Excessive Suffering Scale of the BBRS (e.g., feelings easily hurt, appears unhappy) is used along with parent reports and clinician judgment of the child's tendency to be easily upset, shy, or withdrawn to determine whether children are unusually sensitive. This component was not measured in the earlier model (1979), but this component occurred in 73% of the 50 children most recently studied (30% severe, 43% moderate).[4]

The final factor is termed Listener Reactions and is described by three components: Disruptive Communication Environment, Secondary Gains, and Teasing/Bullying. Disruptive Communication Environment is determined by parent reports that the child has a difficult time obtaining the parent's attention, family members tend to rush the child's speech, the existence of interruption by the family members and teasing about the child's speech, and observations of critical or negative comments about the child's speech.

---

[4]These findings parallel those described by several clinical researchers in Chapter 3.

This component occurred in 53% of the children in the 1979 sample and 61% of the families in the more recent sample (32% severe, 29% moderate).

Secondary Gains indicate that the child is able to manipulate family members as a result of his or stuttered speech (e.g., obtaining special privileges, not being told "no" due to fear of placing stress on the child, ability to dominate family conversations). This form of manipulative behavior was found in 25% of the 1979 sample and 35% in the more recent sample (9% severe, 26% moderate).

The final component of this factor is Teasing and Bullying and is identified by both parent and child report concerning the amount and type of these negative reactions that the child has experienced. Children in the most recent sample were found to have experienced these listener responses in 31% of the cases (9% severe, 22% moderate).

Examples of Assessment Measures

There are many inventories, scales, and procedures that have been developed for evaluating the quality of both the surface as well as the associated cognitive and affective features of stuttering. These measures are helpful for obtaining both data-based and criterion-referenced information for assessing fluency disorders. Although the descriptions, situations, and categories associated with any single measure do not always coincide within a particular child, these measures can provide helpful information that often proves useful for determining possible treatment strategies and indicating therapeutic progress. Of course, assessment must go beyond formal procedures and include daily observation of the child's ongoing cognitive change and behavioral adaptation to the therapy process. The data obtained by using assessment protocols are no substitute for the clinician's ongoing observation of the child's response in naturalistic settings.

Cooper Chronicity Prediction Checklist

In order to assist clinicians in determining the likelihood that a child's stuttering will persist, Cooper (1973) developed the *Chronicity Prediction Checklist* (Figure 5-4). This checklist is scored on the basis of the number of "yes" responses to questions concerning the historical, attitudinal, and behavioral aspects of stuttering in children. Based on the findings of McLelland and Cooper (1978), 2 to 6 "yes" responses are indicative of possible recovery, 7 to 15 "yes" responses indicate the need for continued monitoring of the child, and 16 to 27 "yes" responses are predictive of chronicity. Many of the items assume that the greater the degree of both tension and fragmentation (Bloodstein, 1960, 1987; Schwartz, Zebrowski, & Conture, 1990), the less likely the child will recover from stuttering.

The Cooper Chronicity Prediction Checklist

Instructions: To be completed for children ages three to eight. Answers to questions require the assistance of the child's parents. Each item should be explained and discussed with the parents. Place a check (✔) on the appropriate blank.

		Yes	No	Unknown
I.	Historical Indicators of Chronicity			
1.	Is there a history of chronic stuttering in the family?	____	____	____
2.	Is the severity (frequency, duration, consistency) of the disfluencies increasing?	____	____	____
3.	Did the disfluencies begin with blockings rather than with easy repetitions?	____	____	____
4.	Have the child's disfluencies persisted since being observed (as opposed to being episodic with long periods of normal fluency)?	____	____	____
5.	Has the child been disfluent for two or more years?	____	____	____
II.	Attitudinal Indicators of Chronicity			
1.	Does the child perceive himself or herself to be disfluent?	____	____	____
2.	Does the child experience communicative fear because of the disfluencies?	____	____	____
3.	Does the child believe the disfluency problem to be getting worse?	____	____	____
4.	Does the child avoid speaking situations?	____	____	____
5.	Does the child express anger or frustration because of the disfluencies?	____	____	____

(continues)

Figure 5-4 Stuttering Chronicity Prediction Checklist. From *Cooper Personalized Fluency Control Therapy for Children—Clinician's Manual, 3rd Ed.* (p. 156), by E. B. Cooper and C. S. Cooper, 2003, Austin, TX: PRO-ED. Copyright 2003 by PRO-ED, Inc. Reprinted with permission.

	Yes	No	Unknown

III. Behavioral Indicators of Chronicity

1. Do sound prolongations or hesitations occur among the disfluencies? ____ ____ ____

2. Are the repetitions more frequently whole word or phrase repetitions rather than part-word repetitions? ____ ____ ____

3. Are part-word repetitions accompanied by visible tension or stress? ____ ____ ____

4. Do part-word repetitions occur more than three times on the same word? ____ ____ ____

5. Is the rapidity of the syllable repetitions faster than normal? ____ ____ ____

6. Is the schwa vowel inappropriately inserted in the syllable repetition? ____ ____ ____

7. Is the air flow during repetitions often interrupted? ____ ____ ____

8. Do prolongations last longer than one second? ____ ____ ____

9. Do prolongations occur on more than one word in a hundred during periods of disfluency? ____ ____ ____

10. Are prolongations uneven or interrupted as opposed to being smooth? ____ ____ ____

11. Is there observable tension during prolongation? ____ ____ ____

12. Are the terminations of the prolongations sudden as opposed to being gradual? ____ ____ ____

13. During prolongations of voiced sounds is the airflow interrupted? ____ ____ ____

14. Are the silent pauses prior to the speech attempt unusually long? ____ ____ ____

15. Are the inflection patterns restricted and monotone? ____ ____ ____

16. Is there loss of eye contact during the moment of disfluency? ____ ____ ____

17. Are there observable and/or distracting extraneous facial or body movements during the moment of disfluency? ____ ____ ____

Total "Yes" Responses ____

Figure 5-4 Continued.

Instructions: Place a check on the appropriate blank.

Predictive of Recovery: 0–6   ____
Requiring Vigilance: 7–15   ____
Predictive of Chronicity: 16–27   ____

Caution: The categorization of scores used on this checklist is based on an interpretation of data reported by McClelland and Cooper (*Journal of Fluency Disorders*, 1978) and on clinical observation. It is not based on longitudinal studies. Judgments as to probable stuttering chronicity should not be based solely on the scoring of this checklist.

Figure 5-4 Continued.

Stuttering Prediction Instrument

The *Stuttering Prediction Instrument for Young Children* (SPI) (Riley, 1981) was also developed in order to determine the likelihood of chronicity (Figure 5-5). As with the *Chronicity Prediction Checklist*, stuttering events of longer duration are associated with chronicity, an association that Yairi and Ambrose (2005) failed to support in their research. This is likely related to the fact that these two instruments were not developed for use with children near the onset of stuttering, the population studied by Yairi and Ambrose. These two procedures may be useful adjuncts to the diagnostic procedure with young children, but to date there have been no longitudinal investigations using these instruments.

A-19 Scale

Another scale designed for use with young children is the A-19 Scale for Children Who Stutter (Guitar & Grims, 1977) (Figure 5-6). Guitar and his colleagues have found that once a secure and trusting relationship between clinician and child is established, this 19-item scale helps to distinguish between children who stutter and those who do not. Once the clinician is assured that the child understands the task, the scale is administered by the clinician, who asks the child a series of questions concerning speech and related general attitude. One point is assigned for each question that is answered as a child who stutters might respond. The authors found that the average (and standard deviation) scores of 28 kindergarten through fourth-grade children who stuttered was 9.07 (2.44), while a matched group of nonstuttering children averaged 8.17 (1.80) on the A-19.

Behavior Assessment Battery (BAB)

As part of the Behavior Assessment Battery (BAB) described in Chapter 4, Brutten and Vanryckeghem also developed a series of assessment measures for

Stuttering Prediction Instrument
For Young Children
by Glyndon D. Riley, Ph. D.

TEST FORM

NAME _____   SEX M F   GRADE _____

SCHOOL _____   DATE OF BIRTH _____

EXAMINER _____   DATE _____ AGE _____

SECTION I: HISTORY

BACKGROUND

1. When did your child first exhibit disfluencies? _____

    What were the related circumstances? _____

    _____

2. Is the severity of the stuttering increasing? _____

    Is the severity of the stuttering decreasing? _____

3. Does the stuttering come and go? _____

    Is today's speech more or less disfluent than usual
    or is it about average? _____

FAMILY HISTORY OF STUTTERING

4. Have any family members ever stuttered?

    a. The biological father?   Yes _____   No _____
        From age ____ to age ____
    b. The biological mother?   Yes _____   No _____
        From age ____ to age ____
    c. Any biological siblings?   Yes _____   No _____
        From age ____ to age ____
    d. Any other relatives?
        Grandfather   Yes _____   No _____
        Grandmother   Yes _____   No _____
        Aunt   Yes _____   No _____
        Uncle   Yes _____   No _____
        Cousin   Yes _____   No _____
        Other _____

(continues)

Figure 5-5   *The Stuttering Prediction Inventory for Young Children*, Glyndon
D. Riley. Austin, TX: PRO-ED. Reprinted with Permission.

SECTION II: REACTIONS

5. Does the child's disfluency make you feel:

   a. Unconcerned   (Score 0)
   b. Concerned   (Score 1)
   c. Very concerned   (Score 2)   Score [   ]

6. Has your child been teased about his stuttering?

   a. never observed   (Score 0)
   b. observed to a mild degree (Score 1)
   c. observed to a moderate or
      severe degree   (Score 2)   Score [   ]

7. Does your child get frustrated when he cannot get the word out? (e.g., cries, stamps foot, hits himself, or asks, "Why can't I talk right?")

   a. never observed   (Score 0)
   b. observed to a mild degree (Score 1)
   c. observed to a moderate or
      severe degree   (Score 2)   Score [   ]

8. Does your child sometimes change a word because of a fear of stuttering?

   a. never observed   (Score 0)
   b. observed to a mild degree (Score 1)
   c. observed to a moderate or
      severe degree   (Score 2)   Score [   ]

9. Does your child avoid some situations because of a fear of stuttering?

   a. never observed   (Score 0)
   b. observed to a mild degree (Score 1)
   c. observed to a moderate or
      severe degree   (Score 2)   Score [   ]

10. Are there any observable and/or distracting extraneous facial or bodily movements during stuttering?

   a. never observed   (Score 0)
   b. observed to a mild degree (Score 1)
   c. observed to a moderate or
      severe degree   (Score 2)   Score [   ]

                              Subtotal Score [   ]

Figure 5-5 Continued.

SECTION III: PART-WORD REPETITIONS

number: <u>none</u>   <u>1-3</u>   <u>4 or more</u>

score: 0   1   3   Score [   ]

Transcribe the most severe abnormalities ____ ____ ____ ____

Abnormality of repeated syllables <u>normal</u> <u>mild</u> <u>mod</u> <u>sev.</u>

(e.g., schwa, tension, abruptness)   0   1   2   4

                                                Score [   ]

                             Subtotal Score [   ]

SECTION IV: PROLONGATIONS

Record only the highest score obtained, i.e., A or B or C but *not* the total.

A. Vowel Prolongations

      duration: <u>less than 1.5 secs.</u>   <u>1.5-2 secs.</u>   <u>2-4 secs.</u>   <u>4 secs. +</u>

      score: 0   2   4   6

B. Phonatory Arrest

      duration: <u>none</u>   <u>.51 secs.</u>   <u>1-3 secs.</u>   <u>3 secs. +</u>

      score: 0   4   8   12

C. Articulatory Posturing

      duration: <u>none</u>   <u>.51 secs.</u>   <u>1-3 secs.</u>   <u>3 secs. +</u>

      score: 0   4   8   12

                             Subtotal score [   ]

SECTION V: FREQUENCY

percentage: 0   1   2-3   4   5-6   7-9   10-14   15-28   29 +

score: 0   2   3   4   5   6   7   8   9

                             Subtotal Score [   ]

Add subtotal scores for sections II-V to arrive at the total score.

                             Total Score [   ]

Figure 5-5 Continued.

SECTION VI
TABLE IV

Distribution of *SPI* scores for 85 children ages 3-8 who stutter.

Stanine	Total Score	Percentile	Severity
1	10-11	0-4	Very mild
2	12-13	5-11	Mild
3	14-17	12-23	
4	18-19	24-40	
5	20-24	41-60	Moderate
6	25-28	61-77	
7	29-30	78-89	Severe
8	31-35	90-96	
9	36-37	97-100	Very Severe

Median = 21; Mean = 22.2; SD = 7.01

SECTION VII
TABLE V

Distribution of *SPI* scores for 17 children whose disfluencies had not become chronic.

Stanine	Total Score	Percentile	Severity
1	0-1	0-4	
2	2	5-11	
3	3-4	12-23	
4	5	24-40	Sub-clinical
5	6	41-60	
6	7-8	61-77	
7	9	78-89	
8	10	90-96	Very Mild
9	11-13	97-100	Mild

Median = 6; Mean = 6.17; SD = 3.13

Figure 5-5 Continued.

A-19 Scale for Children Who Stutter

Susan Andre and Barry Guitar
University of Vermont

Establish rapport with the child, and make sure that he or she is physically comfortable before beginning administration. Explain the task to the child and make sure he or she understands what is required. Some simple directions might be used:

> I am going to ask you some questions. Listen carefully and then tell me what you think: Yes or No. There is no right or wrong answer. I just want to know what you think.

To begin the scale, ask the questions in a natural manner. Do not urge the child to respond before he or she is ready, and repeat the question if the child did not hear it or you feel that he or she did not understand it. Do not re-word the question unless you feel it is absolutely necessary, and then write the question you asked under that item.

Circle the answer that corresponds to the child's response. Be accepting of the child's response because there is no right or wrong answer. If all the child will say is "I don't know" even after prompting, record that response next to the question.

For the younger children (kindergarten and first grade), it might be necessary to give a few simple examples to ensure comprehension of the required task:

> a. Are you a boy?   Yes   No
> b. Do you have black hair?   Yes   No

Similar, obvious questions may be inserted, if necessary, to reassure the examiner that the child is <u>actively</u> cooperating at all times. Adequately praise the child for listening and assure him or her that a good job is being done.

It is important to be familiar with the questions so that they can be read in a natural manner.

The child is given 1 point for each answer that matches those given below. The higher a child's score, the more probable it is that he or she has developed negative attitudes toward communication. In our study, the mean score of the K through 4th grade stutterers (N = 28) was 9.07 (S.D. = 2.44), and for the 28 matched controls, it was 8.17 (S.D. = 1.80).

(continues)

Figure 5-6   A-19 Scale. Reprinted with permission from Susan Andre and Barry Guitar.

Score 1 point for each answer that matches these:

1. Yes	11. No
2. Yes	12. No
3. No	13. Yes
4. No	14. Yes
5. No	15. Yes
6. Yes	16. No
7. No	17. No
8. Yes	18. Yes
9. Yes	19. Yes
10. No	

A-19 SCALE

Name _____   Date _____

1. Is it best to keep your mouth shut when you are in trouble?	Yes	No
2. When the teacher calls on you, do you get nervous?	Yes	No
3. Do you ask a lot of questions in class?	Yes	No
4. Do you like to talk on the phone?	Yes	No
5. If you did not know a person, would you tell your name?	Yes	No
6. Is it hard to talk to your teacher?	Yes	No
7. Would you go up to a new boy or girl in your class?	Yes	No
8. Is it hard to keep control of your voice when talking?	Yes	No
9. Even when you know the right answer, are you afraid to say it?	Yes	No
10. Do you like to tell other children what to do?	Yes	No
11. Is it fun to talk to your dad?	Yes	No
12. Do you like to tell stories to your classmates?	Yes	No
13. Do you wish you could say things as clearly as the other kids do?	Yes	No

Figure 5-6 Continued.

14. Would you rather look at a comic book than talk to a friend?   Yes   No

15. Are you upset when someone interrupts you?   Yes   No

16. When you want to say something, do you just say it?   Yes   No

17. Is talking to your friends more fun than playing by yourself?   Yes   No

18. Are you sometimes unhappy?   Yes   No

19. Are you a little afraid to talk on the phone?   Yes   No

Figure 5-6 Continued.

preschool, kindergarten, (Vanryckeghem & Brutten, 2007) and school-age children (Brutten & Vanryckeghem, 2003b, 2007). Four self-report measures are designed for school-age children and include the Communication Attitude Test (CAT), the Speech Situation Checklist – Emotional Reaction (SSC-ER), the Speech Situation Checklist – Speech Disruption (SSC-SD) and the Behavior Checklist (BCL). The Communication Attitude Test for preschool and kindergarten children who stutter (KiddyCAT) is a measure intended for preschool and kindergarten children.

Communication Attitude Test (CAT)

The original version of the CAT was developed by Brutten (Brutten & Dunham, 1989) and revised by DeNil & Brutten (1991) and Vanryckeghem & Brutten (1997). This self-administered measure asks the child to indicate a "true" or "false" response to a series of statements (e.g., I like the way I talk, I don't talk like other children, Kids make fun of the way I talk). One point is scored for each response that corresponds to the way a child who stutters is apt to respond. The CAT significantly ($p = .000$) differentiates children who stutter (CWS) from those who do not (effect size is 1.82) and has both good test-retest reliability (.83) (Vanryckeghem & Brutten, 1992) and internal reliability (Cronbach alpha for CWS and CWNS was .90 and .84, respectively) (Brutten & Vanryckeghem, 2007). The measure also appears to have good content and criterion-related validity for indicating a child's negative belief system about their speech compared to children who are fluent. The current updated version of the CAT (Brutten & Vanryckeghem, 2007) has 33 true-false items; two of the original 35 items were removed due to the lack of a significant correlation with the test's total score.

Speech Situation Checklist – Emotional Reaction (SSC-ER)

As with the adult version, this checklist has two components. The first portion determines a child's situation-specific emotional reactions (fear, anxiety, worry, concern) to 55 communication situations (e.g., giving your name, raising your hand to talk in class, talking on the telephone, reading aloud from a book). Children are asked to indicate their emotional response to each situation using a 5-point Likert-type scale ranging from 1 (not afraid) to 5 (very much afraid). The child's ratings are totaled and contrasted with the norms provided in order to determine the how the scores compare to children who do or do not stutter.

Speech Situation Checklist – Speech Disruption (SSC-SD)

Children are also independently asked to respond to the same 55 communication situations as on the SSC-ER by indicating the amount of speech disruption (part-word repetitions, sound prolongations) they experience. In the SSC-SD, the children also indicate their perceived degree of speech disruption on a second 5-point Likert-type scale ranging from 1 (no trouble) to 5 (very much trouble). The authors suggest that the clinician develop therapy targets that focus on those speaking situations the child rates as 3, 4, or 5 in order to highlight sounds and words, interpersonal situations, and school experiences that are especially difficult. The ER and SD components of the SSC have shown high internal reliability with Cronbach alpha correlation coefficients of .95 or higher (Brutten & Vanryckeghem, 2007). The two sections of the SSC also correlate with each other (.78). Content validity is indicated by a representative sample of the variety of speaking situations that young children are likely to experience. On both sections of the SSC, children who stutter score statistically significantly higher than those who do not ($p = .000$). The effect size for the SSC-ER and SSC-SD was .76 and .75, respectively.

Behavior Checklist (BCL)

This checklist provides a way for the child to identify his or her style of coping with sounds, words, and situations by using avoidance and escape behaviors. The child is asked to indicate "yes" or "no" as to whether or not they use each of the 50 behaviors described by the clinician "to help the sounds or words come out." The list of behaviors include categories of body movements (e.g., closing your eyes), breathing (e.g., letting some air out before starting to speak) or speech-specific behaviors (e.g., changing sounds or words). The 50 behaviors were derived by accumulating avoidance and escape behaviors reported by a large and diverse group of children who stutter. The total number of behaviors reported by a child is contrasted with the normative data provided for CWS and CWNS. Investigations with the BCL indicate that CWS use significantly

(p =.000) more of these behaviors than CWNS (Brutten & Vanryckeghem, 2003b, 2007; Vanryckeghem & Herder, 2004). This difference is reflected in an effect size of .94. Cronbach alpha reliability coefficients for the BCL are .88 and .91 for CWS and CWNS, respectively (Brutten & Vanryckeghem, 2007).

Communication Attitude Test for Preschool and Kindergarten Children who Stutter (KiddyCAT)

Intended for use with children between the ages of three and six, the KiddyCAT was originally developed by Vanryckeghem and colleagues (Vanryckeghem & Brutten, 2007; Vanryckeghem, Brutten, & Hernandez, 2005). The brief and easily administered measure provides a way for the preschool child to respond to 12 statements verbally presented by the clinician (e.g., Do you think that you talk right? Is talking hard for you? Do mom and dad like the way you talk?). Children with a negative attitude about speaking are likely to answer six of the statements with a "yes" response and six with a "no," resulting in a possible score range of 0–12. The mode, median, and mean scores for children who do not stutter (CWNS) was 0, 1, and 1.79, respectively and mode, median and mean scores for children who stutter (CWS) was 5, 5, and 4.36, respectively. No significant effects were found for gender (Vanryckeghem et al., 2005). The KiddyCAT was found to have good internal reliability (Cronbach alpha = .75 for CWS and .72 for CWNS). Vanryckeghem et al. found that preschoolers (3- and 4-year-olds) and kindergartners (5- and 6-year-olds) who stutter are significantly more likely to report a negative attitude toward speech than their nonstuttering peers (p < 0.000). An effect size of 1.44 indicated that 92% of the scores of the CWNS fell below the average CWS.

Finally, as indicated in Chapter 4, the creators of the Overall Assessment of the Speaker's Experience of Stuttering (OASES) (Yaruss & Quesal) are currently completing versions of the OASES for school age children (the OASES-S, ages 7–12).

The Responsibilities of the IEP Team

Following the guidelines mandated by the Individuals with Disabilities Education Act (IDEA), clinicians working in a school setting are required to work with a multidisciplinary team to develop an assessment plan for each child for whom intervention is desired. Based on the knowledge gathered from case history information, formal assessment measures, and observation of the child's speech and interactive behavior in a variety of communication situations, it is first necessary to document that the child meets the state and local eligibility criteria. Unfortunately, eligibility guidelines are often considered only in terms of academic achievement (grades), a restrictive and often prejudicial perspective

(Ramig & Dodge, 2005).[5] It is important to emphasize that the clinician should take the widest possible perspective, which includes the areas of academic competency, academic learning, and social-emotional and independent functioning as described earlier by Ribbler (2006). Ramig and Dodge recommend that the clinician go well beyond a detailed documentation of the child's overt stuttering behavior (both in frequency and form) by also documenting and explaining the occurrence of coping behaviors, which often result in a far greater impact on social interaction and restricted participation (e.g., avoidance or changing of words or communication situations, escape or struggle behaviors that draw attention to the speaker and invite teasing and bullying by others). Even when the child does make a choice to participate, the child's response is apt to give the listener the impression that the child is uncertain as he or she hesitates, carefully scans ahead for feared words, or selects syntax that is less appropriate and eloquent that it would otherwise be. As Ramig and Dodge explain, such coping responses often prevent others from observing the child's real personality and emotions when communicating.

Once the child is qualified to receive intervention, the clinician will then participate with the multidisciplinary team in the development of an Individualized Education Program (IEP) designed to address the variety of ways that the child can be assisted in achieving his or her educational potential. As Ramig and Dodge (2005) note, it will usually be necessary to argue for specific intervention beyond what would be available as a result of the opportunities afforded by the general education program. The individualized program must include measurable goals and short-term objectives for each of the objectives broadly related to all aspects of the child's educational program. Narrow goals that focus on high levels of fluency, although often part of an IEP, are far too restrictive and sometimes counterproductive. In some instances such goals may set up the child (and the IEP team) for failure. It is better to view the process of therapeutic change for these young speakers as one of ever-more successful management of stuttering, often providing supportive counseling to reduce the shame and avoidance that can continue formally (or informally) through the upper grades.

Most people, including educators, have no idea of the depth and breadth of the impact that stuttering can have on the restrictive decision making that is a basic part of the coping responses by people who stutter. The challenge for the clinician is to make this clear to all concerned and to document the educational impact of these decisions. Ramig and Dodge (2005) suggest that the various versions of the OASES, particularly the OASES-S, which are based on the World Health Organization's International Classification of Function, Disability and Health described in Chapter 2, may of particular help to the

---

[5]Ramig and Dodge (2005) point out that children who clutter (which often accompanies stuttering) are sometimes more likely to qualify for services due to the possibility of associated learning disabilities.

Sample IEP Goal

Sample Short-Term Objective
Will increase use of noticeable prolonged onsets to at least three per day when participating in class (or another situation, such as a reading group).

Method of Measurement
Teacher observation of general behavior; SLP observation and report; student report.

Schedule for Achieving Objective
Beginning date: January 12th
Target completion date: May 25th

Levels of Progress and Date
In this case, care must be taken to eliminate online verbal prompts or cues that may interfere with communication and undermine the child's willingness to perform the speech modifications. The danger here is that classmates may pick up on these verbal commands and use them to ridicule or try to gain control over the child when he is stuttering outside the classroom. Instead, prompts and cues can consist of offline reminders made by the teacher or by the SLP. In some cases, the student and teacher or SLP may want to develop a discreet nonverbal signaling system.

Objective Will Be Completed or Continued
By setting stepwise, achievable objectives, the IEP can provide the child and SLP with a way of measuring progress through recovery. The recovery path for stuttering is different and in many cases somewhat slower than for other challenges and this must be acknowledged. Continuing an objective for several semesters would not be unusual for stuttering therapy transfer and this should not be seen as negative or a failure.

Figure 5-7   IEP goal and short-term objectives for a child who stutters. From Ramig and Dodge (2005). *The Child and Adolescent Stuttering Resource Guide.* Clifton Park, NY: Thomson Delmar Learning.

clinician for documenting the many levels of impairments to education that the child is likely to face. Ramig and Dodge (2005) also provide a list of short-term instructional objectives for a child who stutters, along with a sample IEP goal (Figure 5-7) for these objectives. The instructional objectives to be addressed in the IEP goal include:

- Use of fluency-enhancing behaviors such as continuous voicing or gentle onset in specified situations

- Use of stuttering modification techniques such as initial sound stretches, pullouts, and cancellations in specified situations

- Reduced frequency of use of a secondary stuttering behavior
- Reduced use of a stuttering avoidance technique, such as interjections, word avoidance, pretending not to know an answer, or avoiding speech
- Measured stuttering severity in a therapy setting/class participation, such as asking questions and volunteering to answer questions posed by the teacher
- Participation in groups and extracurricular activities that require various speaking skills, such as music groups, choirs, sports, crafts, chess clubs, writing clubs, stage set preparation, and management groups
- Participation in activities that require speech, such as debating clubs or drama groups

Conclusion

In recent years a number of important research findings have emerged that have expanded our understanding about the onset and development of early stuttering. These studies have shown that, in contrast to our understanding only a few decades ago, the fluency breaks of young children who stutter are distinctly different from those who are fluent, a distinction that is most clearly indicated by the occurrence of SLDs (part-word repetitions, single-syllable word repetitions, and disrhythmic phonations). Furthermore, stuttering does *not* appear to evolve from normal fluency breaks and become progressively more severe, a view that very likely continues to be held by some clinicians. In fact, particularly considering the remission of stuttering for the large majority of children who initially experience stuttering, the overall pattern of stuttering severity shows a decreasing, rather than an increasing, curve.

Of the two primary decisions the clinician must make during the assessment process, determining whether or not a child's disfluencies are typical of stuttering is not especially difficult. In fact, it seems that parents are more accurate than some clinicians have given them credit for in identifying stuttering behavior in their children. Accordingly, parents play an essential role in the assessment process, providing historical, developmental, and psychosocial information about their child. Because fluency is often highly variable for young children, clinicians may need to obtain examples of speech in a variety of conditions and, on some occasions, employ tactics that are likely to introduce a moderate level of stress (e.g., time pressure) in order to elicit from the child the fluency characteristics of concern. The presence of many factors, including the occurrence of SLDs and the child's behavioral and psychosocial response to their difficulties in producing fluent speech, provide important indicators.

The clinician's ability to predict whether or not a child who begins to stutter will continue to do so is usually more challenging. Fortunately, the most recent data from several researchers, including Yairi and Ambrose (2005) and their associates at the University of Illinois Stuttering Research Program, are providing information to help clinicians forecast the future course of stuttering. Although there are a number of factors to consider—the child's gender, patterns of familial stuttering, the inclination of SLDs during the months following onset—the decision to intervene can be made with greater confidence than was possible only a few years ago. Future longitudinal and especially prospective investigations should further increase the accuracy of this decision. The improving ability to predict the likely persistence of a young child's stuttering will allow for early intervention before stuttering develops to the point where a successful therapeutic outcome becomes less likely.

The assessment of stuttering is best considered from a multifactorial perspective such as Riley and Riley's (2000) revised component model. This model assumes that a vulnerable speech production system is influenced by several components that place a young speaker at risk for fluency disruption. Assessment consists of identifying those components that contribute to the vulnerability of a child's speech production system as well as developing those components that will facilitate the production of fluent speech. Such an approach to assessment allows clinicians to formulate a comprehensive treatment strategy by adjusting the components that are beneficial to a particular child.

It is especially important to reemphasize that the initial assessment meeting with the clinician is often the first opportunity for the parents to acquire the information, support, and therapeutic options for their child. The depth and quality of the clinician's understanding and experience will set the stage for how the parents choose to respond to the problem. Whatever the parent's decision, it is the clinician's opportunity to provide basic take-home messages so that the parents are better able to begin coping with their circumstances and make the best possible choices. Suggested take-home messages can include concepts such as:

- Stuttering is no one's fault
- Parent involvement and support are essential for therapeutic success
- Good treatment is likely to result in therapeutic success
- Although stuttering is not a frequently occurring problem, there are many other children and families in a similar situation
- There are support groups that can be extremely helpful for children and their parents

Topics for Discussion

1. Describe several activities that would be likely to elicit fluency breaks in the speech of a young child.
2. What are both verbal and nonverbal behaviors indicating that young children are aware that they are having a difficult time communicating?

3. How might you respond to a parent who asks, "How long will it take to cure my child's stuttering?"

4. What are the "red and green flags" that indicate the likelihood of remission or recovery from stuttering for young children?

5. How closely does the Rileys' revised component model compare with the capacities and demands model described in Chapter 3?

6. Depending on the age of a child, which combination of the assessment measures and procedures described in this chapter do you feel provides the best picture of a child's affective and cognitive response to the stuttering experience?

7. What are your views concerning the efficacy and the ethical issues associated with using "at-risk" registers?

8. Describe the procedures and measures you would use to answer the two major clinical decisions discussed in this chapter.

9. With one student taking the part of the clinician and one or two others the part(s) of the parent(s), role play a discussion of the emotions a parent is likely to experience following their child's diagnosis of stuttering (see Chapter 7).

Recommended Readings

Strategies for Developing Individualized Education Programs, Chapter 4 (pp. 31–37) in Ramig, P. R., & Dodge, D. M. (2005). *The child and adolescent stuttering treatment and activity resource guide.* Clifton Park, NY: Thomson Delmar Learning.

Chapter 5, Development of Stuttering, In Yairi, E., & Ambrose, N. G. (2005). *Early Childhood Stuttering, For Clinicians by Clinicians*, Austin, TX: PRO-ED.

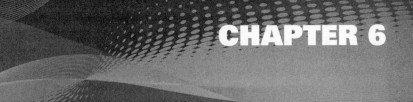

CHAPTER 6

Facilitating the Therapeutic Process

Luterman (2001) In practice, I think successful clinicians are eclectic in that they can and do mix their views and are always evaluating which particular view is most useful in facilitating a therapeutic goal that fits the client context.

David Luterman, Counseling Persons with Communication Disorders and their Families (2001; p. 9)

Parachutes reduce the risk of injury after gravitational challenge, but their effectiveness has not been proved with randomized controlled trials.

Gordon C. S. Smith & Jill P. Pell, British Medical Journal, (2003, p. 1460)

Chapter Objectives

The primary purpose of this chapter is to consider some of the underlying features of therapeutic change. How is it that some people are more adept at coping with and altering their situation? Why is it that some people respond better than others to identical treatment protocols? What factors play a role in our ability to facilitate change in the individuals who come to us for help? In a search for answers we will consider information from a variety of fields, including our own. The literature suggests that there are several levels of change and many ways to conceive of the process and the stages of change. We will consider some primary goals of successful intervention for those who stutter and highlight some potential obstacles that may impede progress. We will also discuss the important issue of evidence-based practice and offer alternative ways of conceptualizing the factors that appear to account for a successful therapeutic outcome. This chapter is intended as a prerequisite to Chapters 7 and 8, where we will discuss additional principles of change and describe specific techniques of intervention for assisting those who stutter.

The Nature of Change

On the surface of therapeutic success for individuals who stutter are the more apparent behavioral changes associated with increased speech fluency. By instruction and modeling we propose the techniques that are known to provide speakers with new ways of using their speech production system. This is an obvious response to the problem of stuttering, for as Yairi and Ambrose (2005) state: "Speech disfluency lies at the core of the disorder of stuttering. . . . disfluency is the essence of the disorder in its widely understood conventional sense" (p. 137). In addition, however, we also want people who come to us for help to develop new ways of considering themselves and their choices about communicating. In the previous chapter we noted some of the important affective and cognitive aspects of the stuttering experience that often impact even the youngest of speakers. Even during the early years, the experience of stuttering often goes far beyond the overt surface features as children recognize and react with frustration and struggle as they try to cope with their inability to speak. For many of these children, modeling of fluency-enhancing techniques by the clinician along with guidance and support by the parents can result in a relatively brief and successful intervention. As children begin formal schooling and experience the effects of socialization, there is the increasing possibility of a negative self-interpretation associated with disfluent speech. Children may begin to define themselves as someone who stutters, and certainly for adolescents and adults, the process of therapeutic change becomes considerably more elaborate. As we will describe, change for these older speakers is often more strenuous and is perhaps best thought of as a process that occurs in stages. It is usually possible to assign a beginning to the change process, but—in most cases–there is not necessarily a clear end stage, because the adult speaker will continue to evolve for years both as a person and a speaker.

As clinicians we often have a vision of what our client can accomplish. We quite naturally assume the role of pushing and prodding in order to nudge a person in directions we believe that he or she is capable of going. However, using a wonderful phrase, Zinker (1977, p. 23) advises that we cannot "push the river" in the creative process of therapy. As much as we would like to, we cannot "fix" the client and we cannot make the client do what he is not yet ready to do. This means that for many clients who stutter, we cannot pour fluency into a vessel that is not ready or capable of holding it. We can lead our younger clients toward fluency by modeling techniques such as easy and slow speech, and many times they will follow. For younger speakers, particularly preschool and early school-age children, change, malleability, and growth are natural. For most adolescents and adults who have been stuttering for many years, we are facing a multilayered and complex problem that will usually defy simplistic solutions. This is why we include both this and the following chapter on counseling as it relates to fluency therapy. As clinicians we are a vital part of the therapeutic process as we help to prepare the client for change. And when the client is ready, change will begin. With another colorful phrase, Zinker (1977) suggests that much of therapy involves our role in "priming the canvas" (p. 24). And, we might add, based on our upcoming comments in Chapter 8, "so that people can paint their own picture."

Hopefully, the reader of this chapter will see how information on the change process folds into the description of clinician characteristics found in Chapter 1, the principles of counseling found in Chapter 7, and the treatment approaches to be discussed in subsequent chapters. It should become clear that comprehensive treatment for adolescents and adults involves more than simply "fixing the stuttering" and making people fluent. The process of change for individuals who stutter is much bigger and far more exciting than the technical components of fluency. In many ways we are "people-making" and enabling them to live life in a broader and deeper manner as we help them to become "unstuck," not only from their speech but from a life of restricted decision making. In that sense doing therapy is, as Zinker suggests, like making art, and the medium is a human life (p. 37). For example, experienced clinicians do not work on fluency techniques in one session and the next day focus only on a speaker's cognitive or emotional characteristics such as negative and positive self-talk; it is all the same process.

The Likelihood of Successful Change

Successful treatment for stuttering and related fluency disorders must take place with an understanding on the part of the clinician that he or she is attempting to help people who have a multifaceted problem. As we have discussed, the problem is multifaceted because it involves many layers, including—but not limited to—the quantity and quality of a person's speech. If the person has been stuttering for many years, patterns of behavior and thinking become established. Helping people to move from their current state of speaking, thinking, and functioning with a communication problem that impacts virtually all aspects of life is no simple process. It should not be surprising, therefore, that stuttering, particularly for adults, is a communication problem that may take time—often years—to change (Manning, 1991b).

However, it is also important to appreciate that stuttering is probably no more enigmatic than many other problems that humans can have. Andrews, Guitar, and Howie (1980) comment that stuttering, although complex, is reasonably well understood and not so terribly difficult to treat. Using meta-analysis, these authors compared the results of 42 treatment investigations and found treatment for stuttering to be effective and the results stable over time. Craig et al.'s (1995) 12-month post-treatment outcome data on children who were treated for stuttering with a smooth speech procedure indicated that 70% of the children maintained fluency levels of less that 2% syllables stuttered (%SS). In addition, Howie, Tanner, and Andrews (1981) followed 36 adults for up to 18 months post-treatment and found that adult clients have a 70% chance of gaining substantially improved speech as well as increased speaking confidence. Indeed, some adults who have experienced successful treatment for stuttering are able to achieve high levels of spontaneous fluency. Some speakers, even those who have experienced moderate to severe stuttering in their earlier years, are able, as adults, to score higher than nonstuttering peers on measures of approach behavior in difficult speaking situations (Hillis & Manning, 1996). As a result of treatment, they are likely to have learned much about the speech mechanism and the nature of speech and language. They are likely to have gained considerable experience when speaking in a large variety of individual and group situations. They may have taken an active role in a self-help organization. If clients continue expanding these experiences following treatment, it is not surprising that some of them are able to become better-than-average speakers.

Another note of optimism is that working with children and adults who stutter can be enormously enjoyable. As described in Chapter 1, as the client grows, often the clinician grows as well, for the most effective clinicians are always learning. They are making real-time decisions about the needs of the client as these needs become apparent. Thus, although the treatment process for fluency disorders can be complex and even messy, it can also be dynamic and exciting.

If it is done well, fluency treatment can result in degrees of positive change in the speaker's perspective of the problem, level of fluency, and—in many cases—improvement in such areas as his or her relationships, problem-solving ability, self-esteem, assertiveness, and overall approach to life. It is also important to appreciate that the process of growth goes well beyond specific techniques and behavioral changes. Therapy involves helping to create a better future in addition to much-improved communication for the person we are helping. Important cognitive and affective changes occur across the client's whole life experience. Just as most athletic activities are much more than the sum of many individual skills, the process of treatment is much more than the application of techniques to be mastered. In fact, as we will see in succeeding chapters, it has frequently been argued that the consequences of overemphasizing therapeutic microskills rather than a holistic approach lead to ineffective treatment.

Matching Treatment to Client Stages of Change

Prochaska, DiClemente, and Norcross (1992) propose that individuals go through several stages as they change. Although their work generally focused on individuals with addictive behavior, their ideas have many applications to the treatment of other human conditions, including stuttering. Their stage model of change can be summarized as follows:

1. Change is cyclical through the stages.
2. There is a common set of processes that facilitate change.
3. It is possible to integrate the stages and processes of change.

Stages of Change

The success of treatment is closely tied to the ability of an experienced clinician to determine a client's readiness for change and to select treatment processes and techniques accordingly. Thus the utility of the techniques depends on the clinician's ability to apply the right therapeutic technique(s) at the right time. The first part of the model suggested by Prohaska et al. (1992) is composed of the five stages of change (Precontemplation, Contemplation, Preparation, Action, and Maintenance).

In the initial stage, *precontemplation,* the person is generally unaware of the problem and does not recognize the need for change. Awareness often develops gradually, along with a desire for change; however, at this stage the person has no intention of doing something about his or her situation in the immediate future (i.e., the next six months). When the issue comes to his or her attention, the individual may become defensive or deny that a problem exists, and he or she generally feels that the situation is under control.

It is important to appreciate that relatively few people who have a chronic or long-standing problem are actually ready to make changes. Summary data obtained on smoking cessation by Prochaska et al. (1992) illustrates this point. They noted that 50–60% of smokers are in the precontemplation stage and 30–40% in the succeeding contemplation stage. Only 10–14% of this population can be categorized as being in the action stage. A key implication of this stage model is that people in different stages of change need to be matched with different treatment processes, or change will be less likely to occur.

As awareness of the problem increases, the individual begins to actively consider the possibility of change (i.e., during the next six months). As yet, there is no formal plan, but the person begins seeking information about the problem. This *contemplation* stage may extend for years as the person weighs the pros and cons of his or her situation and the time, effort, and money it will take to change, as well as the likelihood of success.

As people move closer to the point of taking action about their situations (i.e., within the next few weeks), they reach the *preparation* stage by beginning to identify goals and priorities and may begin to make some small (although not necessarily effective) changes. They are, nevertheless, moving in a new direction by making decisions in terms of specific goals. At this stage they are likely to seek information by reading, speaking with others, and searching on the Internet.

As individuals reach the *action* stage they begin to modify specific behaviors, their environment, or both. A key aspect of this stage is that people begin to use newly acquired skills to achieve specific goals. Importantly, these changes are apt to receive recognition and possibly support by others.

In the *maintenance* stage, people begin to stabilize their behavioral and cognitive changes in order to prevent relapse or regression. This critical part of the process involves altering of well-established behaviors, attitudes, and cognitions lasting from six months to an undetermined period of time. A marker of this final stage is the appearance of new and more effective behaviors and choices in daily situations beyond the treatment environment.

It is likely that the vast majority of all people who stutter are in the precontemplation stage. Those who seek our assistance are most likely in the preparation or action stages. Of course, our understanding of the person's stage of change will influence how we respond to those seeking out help. The situation for preschool and most school-age children (and to some degree adolescents) is somewhat different because they are more likely to be brought to us by their parents or referred by other professionals such as classroom teachers, physicians, or relatives. Depending on the age and maturity of the child, he or she will have varying degrees of awareness of their stuttering as well as varying degrees of motivation for taking part in treatment. Few of these younger individuals are likely to be in the action stage of change.

Floyd, Zebrowski, and Flamme (2007) found support for the stages of change model for determining a speaker's readiness for change with 44 adolescents and adults who stuttered (mean age of 34.9; range 16–61 years). Using a modification of the Stages of Change Questionnaire[1] (McConnaughy, Prochaska & Velicer, 1983), the researchers found that confirmatory and exploratory factor analysis of participant responses indicated that the cognitive, affective, and behavioral factors that characterize stuttering discriminate stages of change for individuals moving through treatment. Of the 32 items on the questionnaire, 26 items were significantly related to their hypothesized stage. Floyd et al. also found some support for the additive nature of the stages (people moving through the stages in sequence) in that the contemplation and action stages were positively correlated

---

[1]The Stages of Change Questionnaire is also referred to as the University of Rhode Island Change Assessment (URICA). For a review of the development and reliability of the original as well as the modified scale, see Floyd, Zebrowski, & Flamme (2007).

with their adjacent stages (action and maintenance, respectively). A goodness-of-fit test indicated that although the interpretive questionnaire structure that was used fit the data, it was not a perfect fit. The authors suggested that the questionnaire may be able to better discriminate between stages of change with the inclusion of items that provided a more sensitive indication of the unique characteristics of the stuttering experience. Future research with a larger and more diverse population of participants who are in differing stages of change should improve the ability of the test to determine where speakers are in the process of therapeutic and self-directed change.

The Cyclical Nature of Change

An important feature of the change model proposed by Prochaska, DiClemente, and Norcross (1992) concerns the cyclical nature of the process. Prochaska et al. found that people often move from the action stage into maintenance and then back to precontemplation. As clients learn from their mistakes, they again advance to the next stage of change. Furthermore, relapse at any point in the change process is the rule rather than the exception, although in some cases, particularly if the circumstances are relatively uncomplicated, the process may indeed be thought of as a straight, smooth trajectory from beginning to end. Linear models of human adaptation to the loss of a loved one (e.g., Kübler-Ross, 1969) imply that people work through the various stages of grief, eventually reaching a stage called "acceptance." However, anyone who has worked through the arduous process of mastering a complicated athletic activity, obtaining an advanced degree, adjusting to a new city, or the loss of a relationship or a job, knows that the process of change is not usually linear. The process often requires a revisiting the various stages of change, stages that you thought (and hoped) you were finished with. Things are never quite "back to normal" as a result of major change and, in some ways, the process continues for the rest of your life. This cyclical view of change also closely corresponds to findings by Neimeyer (2000) in his investigations about grief and loss.

Processes of Change

Based on a comparative analysis of 29 major psychotherapeutic approaches DiClemente (1993) described 10 categories of processes and associated techniques that facilitate change. These techniques are common to many therapeutic protocols (DiClemente, 1993; Prochaska, DiClemente, & Norcross, 1992).[2]

---

[2]The concept that there are common techniques or factors that are effective across a wide variety of therapeutic approaches is a particularly important one that will discuss later in this chapter.

1. Consciousness-raising helps individuals to increase information about themselves and their situation and employs techniques such as observation, confrontation, interpretation, and bibliotherapy (reading educational materials addressing the problem).

2. Self-reevaluation processes help individuals to assess how they feel and think about themselves with respect to their problem by using techniques of value clarification, imagery, and challenging beliefs and expectations.

3. Self-liberation processes help people to select goals, increase their belief in their ability to change, and commit to taking action. Techniques include decision-making therapy and developing resolutions.

4. Counter-conditioning activities enable individuals to substitute alternatives for the anxiety associated with their condition and may be accomplished by techniques of relaxation, desensitization, assertion, and positive self-statements.

5. Stimulus-control processes help people to respond to aversive stimuli using techniques of restructuring the environment, avoiding high-risk cues, and fading/desensitization.

6. Reinforcement management helps people to reward themselves or create rewards from others using contingency contracts and overt and covert reinforcement for self-reward.

7. Helping relationships enable individuals to be open and trusting about problems with others who are supportive through the development of therapeutic alliances, increased social support, and association with support groups.

8. Emotional arousal and dramatic relief helps people to confront, experience, and express feelings about their problems and develop insight concerning possible solutions. Techniques involve role-playing and group therapy.

9. Environmental reevaluation helps individuals to assess how their problem impacts their personal and physical environment using techniques of empathy training and journaling.

10. Social liberation helps people to advocate for the rights and involvement of others by joining support groups and empowering policy changes.

Matching Stages and Processes

The third, and most important, feature of Prohaska et al's (1992) stage model of change is the application of the various therapeutic processes during the appropriate stage of the client's process of change. Prochaska et al. (1992) propose that mismatches in stage and process by clinicians often prevent or impede successful change by clients. This commonly occurs, for example, when clinicians select processes associated with the contemplation stage (e.g., consciousness-raising, self-evaluation) at a time when a client is ready to move into the action stage. Becoming more aware and gaining insight alone do not bring about behavioral change, so these are not likely to be efficient processes at this stage of change. Such mismatches may explain some of the criticisms directed at counseling and non-directive approaches for changing behaviors. Another common mismatch is using action-oriented processes (e.g., behavioral changes, desensitization, assertiveness training) with clients who are in the contemplation or preparation stages of change. Accordingly, attempts to modify behaviors in the absence of a client's awareness and understanding of his or her situation have been a frequent criticism of radical behaviorism. In addition, behavioral changes achieved in the absence of insight are likely to be temporary, according to Prochaska et al. (1992).

Prochaska and DiClemente (1986) also propose five *levels of change* from least to most complex (symptom, maladaptive cognitions, current interpersonal conflicts, family/system conflicts, and interpersonal conflicts). Therapy typically begins at the lowest level (symptom) with modification of the symptoms that drove the individual to seek assistance. For this reason (and because the person is highly aware of the problem at this level), change tends to occur rapidly. Addressing the more complex levels of the problem, which focus on the less obvious cognitive and relational levels, typically require longer and generally more complex therapy. Because the various levels or layers of the problem are closely interrelated, the clinician will frequently work at several levels of change according to the client's perspective and objectives of the therapeutic journey.

Turnbull (2000) illustrates how the clinician's understanding of the levels of change and the client's location within the sequence of stages can inform the use of appropriate therapeutic processes for individuals who stutter. For example, individuals who are in the *precontemplation* stage and who are resigned to the inertia of their situation may benefit from an effective emphatic response on the part of the clinician, who has the ability to instill hope through reflective listening, (e.g., paraphrasing of the client's comments to check for understanding) the consideration of alternative responses, and the careful use of paradox (e.g., purposefully engaging in the behavior or thought processes the individual wants to stop). Providing people who may feel that they are being pushed or coerced with a broader view of their situation (including the realistic option of not taking part in therapy—at least for the moment) may provide a glimmer of hope that they may not always have to endure their current circumstances and that there is the possibility of change. The effective clinician can communicate the understanding that, aside from the obvious investment of time and money, the possibility of therapy may present a genuine threat to the speaker. As Turnbull points out, facing up to a problem they have not previously acknowledged, the unknown demands of therapy, the loss of control, and the possibility of failure represent enormous risks to some individuals.

However, for clients who are in the *action* stage, the clinician is likely to assume the role of a consultant fostering greater autonomy on the part of the client. Group therapy and enlisting the support of others to support and document behavioral and cognitive changes are often especially helpful at this stage. Turnbull (2000) also suggests the therapeutic activities of self-liberation (role-playing and self-characterization), counter-conditioning (desensitization and assertiveness training), stimulus control (self-acknowledgement of stuttering and informing others about desired responses), and contingency management (creating rewards for successful change). See Turnbull (2000) for examples of what are likely to be the most useful therapeutic procedures for individuals at other stages of change.

Obstacles to Creating and Maintaining Change

For all the positive features of treatment, both for the client as well as the clinician, the process is often difficult. It is difficult for many reasons, but most often because it requires persistence and discipline. Over the years the speaker may have learned many inefficient and maladaptive coping behaviors that tend to call attention to the fact that he or she is stuck. Patterns of denial, fear, shame, and avoidance are powerful and complex. Some ways of thinking and living that have become habitual will need to be altered. At times it can be difficult to separate the individual from the influence of stuttering. That is, the clinician (as well as the speaker) may not always know to what extent patterns of avoidance, perceived helplessness, missed opportunities, and unused potential are the consequences or the cause of stuttering.

It can be a daunting task to help another person work toward constructive change, and often we are faced with our lack of power to make things happen (as much as we would like to, we cannot "push the river"). Clinicians who are new to the task of helping people who stutter need to appreciate the difficulty of what we are asking the speaker to do. We are asking our clients to put themselves at risk and enter into anxiety-producing tasks and speaking situations. Especially for adolescents and adults, treatment is far more than demonstrating and practicing techniques that decrease stuttering and enhance fluency. With timing that may be uncertain, we try to assist them to understand, monitor, and eventually change the many levels of their stuttering experience in increasingly challenging communicative circumstances.

Successful intervention requires continued commitment and determination by the client. Because success is neither linear nor consistent, the journey can be frustrating. Although Peck (1978) is reflecting on the nature of psychotherapy in his book *The Road Less Traveled*, his comments apply to any treatment that requires behavioral as well as cognitive change. He suggests that of the choices one may have in dealing with a problem, treatment is usually the most difficult path.

This is so, he argues, because each of us is always working against entropy: the tendency for things—including the process of therapeutic change—to fall apart. Peck sees entropy manifested as laziness and indicates that as many as 9 out of 10 patients who begin psychotherapy (or other therapies) stop long before the clinician believes that the process has been completed. Sometimes, after the client experiences success and a corresponding lessening of the problem, the cost-benefit ratio decreases and the person finds that additional change is no longer worth the effort; the price for continued change is too high.

It is also worth noting that there are some influential forces against which the clinician and the client must work during treatment. For example, there are old, comfortable ways of interpreting the problem and oneself. There may be a period of holding on to the old, established and comfortable perceptions of the speaker's relationship with stuttering (DiLollo, Neimeyer & Manning, 2002; Emerick, 1988; Fransella, 1972; Fransella & Dalton, 1990; Hayhow & Levy, 1989). This is more likely, of course, with adults. We show them new ways of viewing themselves and the problem that, although often attractive, also suggest that the old view of life may be in error. Many authors (e.g., Egan, 2007; Luterman, 2001; Peck, 1978) acknowledge that giving up the old way of doing things, particularly the loss of the old belief system, will be difficult. New insights about the shortcomings of the old system of beliefs can be a blow to a client's self-esteem. Kuhlman (1984) suggests that a "mourning process" may be necessary. This is not necessarily a major problem during treatment, but it is likely to occur to some degree and thus create some resistance to change.

Egan (2007) also describes what he terms the "shadow side" of change. He suggests that even as we respond to a person's request to change, what is in many cases, a limited lifestyle, we are precipitating a degree of disequilibrium or disorganization in the person's life. We are asking those we are trying to help to give up patterns of functioning that have been useful in helping them to survive in a fluent world. In a variety of ways, we are asking people to "let go" of highly refined strategies for coping with their problem. It should not be surprising that, for some people, the possibility of losing these strategies can create a crisis. Understanding such idiopathic responses as a natural part of the change process is one characteristic of the experienced (and wise) clinician.

Starkweather (1999) also discusses the various forms of denial that people who stutter may use as a means of survival. Starkweather points out that denial is often difficult to detect, even for adults. Clients may deny that many of their decisions and their behaviors are a function of stuttering. Crowe (1977b) cites Kübler-Ross (1969) in suggesting that an individual's tendency to rely on denial as a defense against life's pressures increases the possibility of this response to an illness or disability. As Crowe points out, although clinicians should understand that denial is a natural reaction to unwanted situations, denial should gradually lessen to the point that the client is able to move forward and approach the problem. If denial does not lessen, it could be a function of the clinician moving too quickly into action-oriented processes when the client is still in the contemplation or preparation stage of change.

Some people will show a reluctance to get started, or once the process is started, they tire of the discipline and persistence necessary for completing the tasks they have agreed to do. Egan (2007) also describes several reasons why clients fail to change. He suggests that much of the art in helping people change has to do with overcoming these forms of reluctance without pushing our clients too much and turning reluctance into resistance. Some clients have acquired a passive lifestyle and clinicians, beyond listening and understanding, must act as agents of change to help their clients take responsibility for their own change. Sometimes a client's inability to change presents as "learned helplessness," and a clinician may find ways of increasing the person's resourcefulness for changing specific aspects of one's life. These clients may also be minimally depressed. Their self-talk, what they tell themselves about themselves and about their stuttering, may provide a window for understanding their view of their situation.

Because it often requires time and effort to change behaviors and belief systems developed over many years, some people will choose not to change. They may begin to understand some of the basic characteristics of their speaking problem and develop a good idea of what it will take to change their situation. For some, this understanding and acceptance of their situation may be enough. It may be that, quite literally, the cost in terms of time, effort, or money is not worth it. As Egan (2007) states, they feel that "The price of more effective living is too high" (p. 355).

Perhaps the most important ingredient for success, as it is with many things, is that of persistence. Many of us have had the experience during our freshman year of college of looking around the room at the faces and being told that many of these people would not be there by the senior year. There is no shortage of these occurrences throughout life (including, as many readers will appreciate, the first several months of graduate school). Many factors, including innate intelligence, talent, and good fortune, play a major role in the achievement of success. However, the most critical factor is usually persistence.

Leading from Behind

Conducting treatment with fluency disorders is similar to many other relationships, both therapeutic and otherwise. Certainly, as clinicians we must have a clear direction where treatment is heading. However, it is also true that if we too closely direct the direction and pace of the therapeutic process we may narrow the possibilities for change and growth. Unquestionably, the clinician must have an overall plan and a direction for treatment and must be familiar with many associated treatment techniques. However, we cannot control all aspects of the other person and make him or her into our own image; the journey is theirs. Our goal is to help the speaker to self-manage his or her situation, and we can assist in that process. However, sometimes it is clear that we have to lead from behind, following clients where they need to go and helping them to get there. We can assist them in developing new views of themselves and new options concerning their fluency. With the right timing in response to changes by clients, we can help them to make better choices and thereby decrease the problem. We can also acknowledge that while we provide direction, insight, and information, the person who must ultimately take the lead in successfully managing the problem is the client. The clinician must know the choices that are available in terms of overall treatment strategies and associated applications. However, the mark of an experienced clinician is not in knowing what strategies or techniques to use. Every clinician should have that information. The mark of an effective clinician is reflected in his or her clinical insight about why and when to employ them.

Clinical Insight

It's good to have a guide when you are entering new and possibly scary territory for the first time. The experienced guide has taken the journey many times before and knows both the obstacles and rewards of the various trails. In many cases, especially at the outset of the journey, the guide is apt to lead and set the pace. The guide will select the trail and the direction based on his or her knowledge of the conditions and the person who has requested guidance. Experienced guides also sometimes have the client take the lead even on trails the guide suspects may not be ideal under the circumstances. On occasion, it may be best to have the client take trails of their choosing and expend some time and energy on what turns out to be the wrong choice. There may be lessons to be learned from the experience. The wisdom of such guides is indicated by their ability to "lead from behind" rather than continually dictating the direction and pace of the journey.

Goals of Treatment

One of the first objectives during the initial treatment sessions is to demonstrate our sense of direction to the client by providing a map of the journey. For excellent examples of pretreatment orientation statements see Cooper, 1985; Guitar, 2006; and Maxwell, 1982. It is important for the client to have a clear understanding of the treatment process, and success may be more likely to occur if both the client and the clinician share a similar view (Ahn & Wampold, 2001).

Clinical **Decision-Making**

By all accounts, Dean Williams was the embodiment of the expert clinician. His description of one of his "clinical failures" provides a comment on the principle of following the client's lead in the clinical process. Upon analysis of this case, Dean felt that this person was "helpable" but that he was unable to help her (Susan) because of his own errors in judgment. Dean's description of one such error:

> Unfortunately, I began therapy with the preconceived idea of what it was I wanted her to accomplish. There was no attempt to first find out what she considered to be her problems and then to begin at this point. In other words, I did not bother to listen to what she was trying to tell me. I was too busy explaining the "stuttering problem" and the therapy procedures she was to follow. (p. 131)

Source: Williams, D. E. (1995). A clinical failure: *Susan (pp. 130-131). In Stuttering: Successes and failures in therapy.* Memphis: Stuttering Foundation. See also, *The Genius of Dean Williams* (2004) (pp 71–76). Memphis: The Stuttering Foundation.

At the outset of treatment the client's concept of his or her fluency disorder itself is apt to be unclear. The clinician who is able to help the client decrease the mystery and understand what is known about the stuttering experience provides a valuable service to the speaker. Before speakers can begin to accurately monitor and self-manage themselves and their speech, they must begin to appreciate the nature of the problem in general and the dynamics of their own specific response to their situation.

Although we will discuss the goals of therapeutic change in more detail in Chapter 8, it is worth considering three primary objectives when working with a person, regardless of age, who stutters. We would like to help them (1) increase their level of fluency, (2) improve their ability to communicate, and (3) develop greater autonomy. While each of these objectives is important and, of course, highly related to the others, we can conceptualize them as being progressively more basic for long-term success, as expressed in Figure 6-1. That is, although a clear goal of therapy for fluency problems is to assist the speaker in increasing his or her level of fluency, a more central goal is to help the speaker to develop his or her ability to communicate more effectively—perhaps by reducing the avoidance of feared words, producing easier and less effortful stuttering, maintaining appropriate eye contact and turn taking. Most basic,

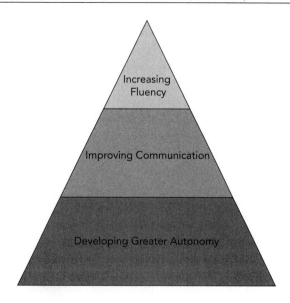

Figure 6-1   Three primary therapeutic objectives for assisting individuals who stutter.

however, is the clinician's ability to foster the speaker's development of an autonomous, agentic lifestyle, a therapeutic objective that will be discussed in Chapter 8.

Levels of Fluency

Speakers who are regarded as normally fluent demonstrate a wide range of fluency across different situations. As discussed in Chapter 3, this range of fluency is greater in speakers who stutter. When considering the goals of treatment, authors have found it useful to distinguish at least three levels of fluency (see Guitar, 2006).

Spontaneous fluency can be thought of as ideal, normal speech. The speech is smooth and may contain only sporadic fluency breaks, which are primarily a function of formulating language and speech. Speech flows easily with little apparent effort, and virtually no attention is paid to how the speech is produced and fluency is achieved. Speakers, as well as the listener, are able to attend to the message, and the speaker's fluency does not detract from the information being delivered. It is important to recognize that, following successful treatment, people who have stuttered for many years are sometimes able to achieve this level of spontaneous fluency in all speaking situations.

Controlled fluency is normal or nearly normal speech production, but with the price of increased effort on the part of the speaker. Although the speaker must attend to his manner of speaking in order to achieve and maintain fluency, the speech moves forward with few, if any, obvious fluency breaks. There is a price to be paid in the form of vigilance and self-management of those fluency breaks. This management, to the degree that it is perceived by the listener, may detract somewhat from the message. On occasions, the method and the message of speaking may carry nearly equal weight. Depending on the ability of the speaker to apply techniques that facilitate the smooth coordination of respiration, phonation, and articulation, this type of fluency may be perceived as unstable speech. In many ways, this type of fluency is similar to that of a normal speaker who is placed in a speaking situation that contains a high level of communicative or emotional stress.

Acceptable fluency takes the level of self-monitoring and self-management of the speaker to another stage. Now the effort to manage fluency is increased, and the techniques being used to change the form of the stuttering may become more prominent than the content of the message. The speaker may be producing less than ideal fluency but still, speech that is much preferred to the client's old automatic, reflexive form of stuttering. Although stuttering is taking place, because these events are undergoing modification or smoothing it is possible for the speaker and the listener to achieve a good level of communication.

The Importance of Modeling

Although modeling of both attitudes and techniques by the clinician and others is discussed throughout this text we will take a moment to emphasize this important aspect of the change process. Modeling of different ways of considering stuttering attitudes and behaviors can have a profound impact for some speakers. Examples of alternative and possibly better ways of doing and thinking about things can be modeled by the clinician as well as other people in the client's environment. If we want our clients to give themselves permission to take risks and experiment with new ways of doing things, modeling is a good way to demonstrate this. Observing people as they successfully perform athletic, singing, writing, or speaking activities can be a critical and motivating influence for those who desire to perform these activities. The experience often helps to increase the observer's self-expectations and willingness to invest the effort to undertake difficult tasks. Our expectation of our client's ability to change is confirmed by our willingness to lead the way by challenging ourselves and changing aspects of our own lives. Our modeling of attitudes and behaviors can provide a way to challenge, disrupt, and eventually alter the client's current belief system and behaviors. Furthermore, as discussed in Chapter 1, in order to provide a helpful model, the clinician will need to completely understand the stuttering experience and become desensitized to playing the role of a person who stutters.

Variables in Choosing a Treatment

There are several basic treatment considerations that are influenced by such things as the clinical setting and the client's needs and capabilities. These characteristics require the clinician to make decisions about the form that treatment will take. In some instances, the choices are already made for the clinician and the client according to the nature of the treatment setting or the options that are available because of such issues as time and expense (Starkweather, St. Louis, Blood, Peters, & Westbrook, 1994).

The Timing and Duration of Treatment

There is considerable variation here, ranging from intensive, residential programs lasting six or more hours each day for one or more weeks to treatment in public schools, which may take place as little as one hour or less each week. Generally, adolescents and adults who have been stuttering for years require a longer time in treatment; preschool speakers often make faster progress and require a shorter time. Less intensive treatment disrupts the client's everyday life less, but changes may come slower and the client may become discouraged. On the other hand, intensive treatment, particularly in settings apart from the speaker's daily environment, often results in more rapid change (Prins, 1970) but with possible problems in transferring the gains to the speaker's more typical surroundings. The duration of treatment also can be influenced by such factors as the complexity of the fluency disorder, other coexisting communication problems, and the person's motivation. For adult speakers, formal treatment lasting one year with at least one individual and one group meeting each week has been suggested as a minimum requirement for success (Maxwell, 1982; Van Riper, 1973).

The Complexity of Treatment

A client's degree of handicap across the social, educational, and vocational aspects of his or her life will be a major factor in determining the course and length of intervention. Children and adults who come to us with a variety of linguistic, learning, social, emotional, and family issues are usually more likely to also have greater difficulty with the process of therapeutic change. On the other hand, those children with few other problems and qualities such as high self-esteem, good academic performance, high levels of family support, social and athletic skills, generally are more likely to achieve success in therapy. Furthermore, the client's personality and emotional characteristics such as defensive behaviors, coping strategies, resistance to change, anxiety, inhibited behavior, depression or even—on occasion—alcohol or chemical dependence can also increase the length and complexity of treatment. In such instances, treatment may require the use of many strategies and techniques as well as other professional clinicians in areas such as counseling, psychology, or psychiatry.

The Cost and Treatment Setting

This important aspect of treatment also varies widely. Undoubtedly many individuals do not seek treatment due to the cost. Because of the typical length of treatment and the lack of reimbursement by insurance companies, the cost of successful treatment can quickly become prohibitive for many people. Fees for diagnosis and treatment are generally lower in academic programs but scheduling and quality of service can sometimes be secondary to the academic and clinical training requirements of the program (semester breaks, changes in the consistency or availability of student clinicians). The level of service can also be compromised somewhat in public or private school settings, where availability of specialists, scheduling, and caseload requirements may vary widely.

The treatment that is provided is often determined in large measure by the setting. In this regard, St. Louis and Westbrook (1987) provide an insightful comment explaining that the choice of treatment may not always be made with the client as the primary consideration. It seems plausible that typical delivery models for stuttering therapy evolved as much to suit clinicians' tastes; administrators' desires; school, university, or hospital schedules; or physicians' prescriptions as they did to provide the maximum benefit to stutterers (p. 250).

The treatment strategies and techniques the clinician selects may or may not coincide with the available environment. That is, the clinician may want to schedule the client for several sessions each week, but multiple sessions may not be possible due to the logistics of the client's work schedule and distance from the treatment center. The clinician may consider parent participation to be critical for success, but the parents may be employed in one or more jobs and unable or unwilling to attend treatment sessions. Individual treatment may be necessary, yet the caseload in the clinical facility (particularly in the public schools) may only allow for group treatment, sometimes including children who possess a variety of other communication problems.

In addition, the opportunity for monitored practice outside the clinic or school setting is essential. Often, however, because of logistic, legal, insurance, or time constraints, the clinician may be unable to go with the child or adult to more realistic speaking situations in offices, restaurants, or shopping malls. This is an important feature, for as the *Guidelines for Practice in Stuttering Treatment* (American Speech-Language-Hearing Association, 1995) suggest, treatment settings that fail to create such experiences also may fail to provide realistic indications of change or progress. At the very least, the clinician should create opportunities to monitor the client's performance in the form of direct observation, interviews with the client following practice sessions, or monitoring with audio or video recordings of speech samples obtained beyond the treatment environment.

Reflections on Evidence-Based Practice

In recent years our field, along with many other health and behavioral sciences, began to embrace the concept of evidence-based practice (EBP). This means that as clinicians we should be able to provide evidence that the treatment protocols and associated techniques we select truly make a difference to the people we intend to help. Of course, the people we are helping would like to know this also, as do parents, spouses, and certainly the agencies that are financially supporting the treatment. It is this latter group of funding agencies that has driven this process as much as anyone. When considering the many implications of EBP it is necessary to appreciate some important differences between the goals and procedures that are followed by clinical researchers and practicing clinicians.

One of the regularly cited articles on the topic of evidenced-based practice is that of Sackett, Strauss, Richardson, Rosenberg, & Hayes (2000), who described it as "the conscientious, explicit, and judicious use of current best evidence in making decisions about the care of individual patients (p. 1). The practice also incorporates "the integration of best research evidence with clinical experience and patient values" (p.1). A position statement by the American Speech-Language-Hearing Association (ASHA) indicates a nearly identical description when they state: "The term *evidence-based practice* refers to an approach in which current, high-quality research evidence is integrated with practitioner expertise and client preferences and values into the process of making clinical decisions" (2005, p. 1).

In order to demonstrate the often subtle cause-and-effect relationships of our clinical procedures, considerable rigor and control is exercised by clinical researchers. Participants are included (or excluded) with the goal of maximizing the homogeneity of those participating in the investigation. Individuals with co-occurring conditions are typically excluded because that could make the results difficult to interpret. Specific protocols are followed and treatment techniques are prescribed. Typically the protocols are manualized in order to assure adherence to the associated therapeutic ingredients and maintain control of possible contaminating factors. Ideally, as in randomized controlled trials (RCT) (or meta-analysis of several RCTs), participants are randomly assigned to the groups. The results of rigorous testing during these well-controlled conditions are designed to lead to outcomes demonstrating the *efficacy* of treatment protocols.

Clinical **Decision-Making**

In an effort to consider the relative strength or weakness of the evidence supporting a diagnostic or intervention procedure, ASHA (see Mullen, 2007) introduced the concept of *levels of evidence* (LOE). This approach emphasizes the context of the clinical question being studied as well as the quality of the investigation rather than placing the primary emphasis on the type of research design. Evidence-based practice traditionally has been informed by the medical model, which specified between-group designs with large numbers of randomly selected participants. However, if the purpose of the research is to understand the richness of an individual's cognitive and behavioral response to a situation (e.g., ability to cope with a problem, response to therapeutic intervention), single-subject designs may be more appropriate than RCTs or meta-analysis of RCTs. Furthermore, regardless of the research design, a determination of the quality of the investigation is essential. Depending on the purpose and stage of the research (exploratory, efficacy, effectiveness) the quality of an investigation can be determined by such factors as study design, blinding of the assessors, random sampling of participants, equivalence of participants at the outset of the investigation, reliability and validity of outcomes, statistical significance, reporting of effect size and confidence intervals, and intention-to-treat data (to what extent individuals choose to take part in and continue in the treatment).

There are often gaps between the various theoretical models and the treatment protocols and techniques we employ with the people we see on a daily basis. Few of the techniques that are used by highly qualified clinicians have received empirical validation in forms that we desire. But while we wait for that level of evidence it is good to recognize that the call for EBP has already resulted in some interesting findings that suggest alternative ways of considering therapeutic change.

Practicing clinicians also want to demonstrate that what they are doing on a daily basis to assist their clients is likely to be helpful and result in successful therapeutic outcomes. However, clinicians see their clients under circumstances that are far less ideal and less well-controlled than those found in research laboratories. Professional clinicians are responding to individuals who have not been randomly assigned to various treatment protocols. Clinicians are likely to be helping people who are highly heterogeneous and present with a variety of other, sometimes related, communication problems. There are likely to be uncontrolled (and often unknown) environmental factors that may be impacting the influence of the treatment procedures being implemented. The results of these clinical investigations are intended to lead to outcomes demonstrating the *effectiveness* of treatment protocols.

Clinical **Decision-Making**

Assigning clients into different forms of treatment and then asking which program might, by some criteria, be the best one may be the wrong question. In many ways such a question is analogous to questions about which car, religion, or political party is the best. In 1992, Prochaska and DiClemente referred to research in behavioral therapy that attempted to determine which treatment is best for a particular problem as "horse race research." In some cases a particular approach won, while in other investigations other methods finished first. Most cases, however, produced "a disappointing abundance of ties" (p. 204). In addition, they propose that one of the major research issues for the future is how those interested in modifying human behavior can more effectively match treatment strategies and techniques to people. Thus, a better question to ask is, "What behavioral processes are best for whom, and when?"

The Medical Model

Evidenced-based clinical practice is based on the medical model, which stipulates that there are specific ingredients which account for and are necessary for the remediation of a medical disorder. Because of the specificity of the (theoretically effective) ingredients that are administered to the experimental group(s) of participants (vs. the theoretically inert placebo administered to the control participants), the researchers or their assistants follow procedural manuals in order to assure adherence to the treatment protocols. Although this model has obviously resulted in important, often critical, advances in the development of medications and procedures in the field of medicine, this model (and associated research protocols) may not be the best, or certainly is not the only, model for explaining the ability of humans to change as a function of treatment (or on their own beyond the scope of formal treatment).

It has also been suggested that the traditional medical model has other disadvantages for conceptualizing the human change process. For example, the model has been described as an illness-based model that too easily dichotomizes individuals as being either normal or abnormal (Raskin & Lewandowski, 2000). It also tends to situate the person administering the treatment as an extraspective observer of objective medical "facts." In addition, the medical model of disability tends to foster a disease-entity approach that all too easily pathologizes people and casts them in a passive role, with the inference that experts are needed to cure them (Monk, Winslade, Crocket, & Epston, 1997). Finally, others suggest that the medical model of mental health, along with the *Diagnostic and Statistical Manual of Mental Disorders* (DSM-IV) of the American Psychiatric Association (APA) (American Psychiatric Association, 2000) fosters the use of terms that, while we are accustomed to using them, may not provide the most accurate or facilitative view of the person we are attempting to help (e.g., disorder, pathology, symptoms, patient, recovery, cure) (Monk, et al., 1997; Raskin & Lewandowski, 2000).[3]

The Development of the Common Factors Model

Fortunately, many of the questions about EBP that we currently face in our field have been considered by other fields of allied health and behavioral science. For example, there are many similarities between psychotherapeutic and counseling approaches and treatments for stuttering. As Zebrowski (2006) points out, both approaches attempt to change a client's behavior primarily through nonmedical, nonsurgical, or nonpharmacological means. Clearly, psychotherapy and counseling may be considerably more complex than treatment for stuttering, for as Wampold (2005) explains, these fields are represented by more than 250 distinct psychotherapeutic approaches and more than 10,000 books describing forms of interventions. In addition, researchers and clinicians in psychotherapy and counseling must deal with a wide variety of problems (e.g., depression, anxiety, phobias, anger management). Nonetheless, the primary goal of Wampold and his associates (Ahn & Wampold, 2001; Mondin, Moody, Stich, Benson, and Ahn, 1997; Wampold, 2005) was to develop an overriding theory (a metatheory) which best accounts for treatment outcomes across many of the more prominent treatment approaches. Wampold and his colleagues used the statistical techniques of meta-analysis and *hierarchical linear modeling* (HLM). This combination of procedures allowed researchers to determine the factors that account for the variance in treatment outcomes. Using these procedures, they were able to determine effect sizes—an index of how much the dependent variable (treatment outcome) can be controlled, predicted, or explained by an independent variable such as the type of treatment administered. When they considered the issue of *absolute efficacy* (whether or not individuals received treatment) they found that effect sizes averaged .80. This large effect size (particularly for the social sciences) observed across studies using many different treatment approaches indicated that treatment was remarkably efficacious. When they considered the issue of *relative efficacy* (where all individuals received treatment) across different treatments they found that effect sizes reached a maximum of .20, a difference that is considered inconsequential both clinically and theoretically.

The fact that Wampold and his associates observed consistently uniform efficacy across treatments suggested that the specific ingredients associated with the various treatments were not responsible for treatment benefits. In fact, they calculated that specific treatment ingredients (a central part of the medical model)

---

[3]The reader may have already become aware of the infrequent use of these terms throughout the book.

Clinical **Insight**

Placebo effects have long been considered unwanted and confounding influences during the process of medical intervention. When controlled trials are conducted, the experimental participants receive the true or active medication and the control participants receive the inactive substitute. The success of the active intervention is determined by comparing the response of the people who receive the medication to those who receive the placebo. More recently, however, researchers are finding that placebos are not necessarily inactive. For example, Jerome Groopman, in his 2003 book *The Anatomy of Hope*, describes the biological effects of a person's emotions. Just as with negative emotions such as anxiety and fear, there are physical consequences associated with positive emotions such as hope. Groopman provides convincing research linking a person's beliefs and expectations (key aspects of hope) with the release or inhibition of chemicals within the body. Groopman provides fascinating medical examples of this mind–body connection and how emotions directly influence the status of tissues and organs, including the autonomic nervous system. In fact, the environmental cues provided by the physician or counselor as part of the ritual of professional interaction help to reinforce the client's expectation of benefit from the medicine or technique. To the extent that people believe that they are being helped they are likely to experience decreased levels of anxiety and despair. Groopman describes how the "spark of hope" can break the cycle of pain and hopelessness and set off a chain reaction that facilitates healing. It is likely that such mind–body connections play an active role during intervention for cognitive and behavioral concerns. As we understand more about and appreciate the true nature of placebo effects it may be that we will begin to consider some of them as an important part of comprehensive therapeutic and self-directed change. Considering placebo effects in this way may indicate that good intervention is even more effective than we previously realized.

accounted for only 1% of the variance in outcomes. In addition, placebo effects (containing some but not all factors common to many treatments) accounted for 4% of the variability in outcome. A particularly interesting outcome of their investigations of relative efficacy across treatments indicated that the use of treatment manuals did not result in increased benefits. To the contrary, there were indications that strict adherence to a treatment protocol may have detrimental effects, as it tends to suppress the effect of clinician competence; training therapists to adhere to a manual can result in deteriorating interpersonal relations between the therapist and the client.

Although specific techniques were not associated with successful treatment, Wampold et al. did identify several factors that are common across the variety of treatment approaches, factors that do much better in accounting for the variance in treatment outcome. Among the common factors that they found to contribute to a successful therapeutic outcome were (a) the nature of the working alliance of the client and the clinician accounting for 5%, (b) clinician allegiance (adherence) to the treatment protocol accounting for 10%, and (c) the quality of the clinician accounting for 22%. This last factor, the quality (effectiveness) of the clinician has consistently been found to account for the greatest outcome variance (Ahn & Wampold, 2001,; Kim, Wampold, & Bolt, 2006; Wampold, 2001; Wampold, Mondin, Moody, Stich, Benson, K. & Ahn, 1997). In fact, Ahn & Wampold (2001) have suggested that people seeking help would be well-advised to search for particular clinicians rather than particular treatments. Keep in mind that, of course, a higher degree of expertise on the part of the clinician plays a large role in the important factors of the clinician allegiance and the working alliance between the client and clinician. Based on these common factors that were identified across treatment approaches, the authors proposed what they termed the common factors model[4] of psychotherapy, which stipulates that there are a common set of factors across treatments that result in a successful treatment outcome. It is interesting to note that the existence of such common factors had been predicted as early as 1936 by Rosenzweig in his classic article titled *Some implicit common factors in diverse methods of psychotherapy*. The presence of such factors was confirmed by the work of Smith and Glass (1977) in the first meta-analysis of the effectiveness of different forms of therapy approaches.

Herder, Howard, Nye, and Vanryckeghem (2006) also found similar results in a meta-analysis of behavioral treatment for stuttering. From a total of 1,798 manuscripts identified through electronic and hand searches, 12 articles met the inclusion criteria, which included random assignment of participants to an experimental and a control (or comparison/alternative treatment) condition prior to intervention. Herder et al. found an overall (absolute efficacy) effect size of 0.91 in favor of the participants who received treatment. Analysis of the studies that compared one treatment group to another indicated an effect size of 0.21, indicating that no one treatment demonstrated a significant effect over another. It is interesting to note that, independent of the work of Wampold and his colleagues, Herder et al. came to the conclusion that "the critical element(s) for successful intervention might not lie with the intervention itself" (p. 70) but in the common element(s) found in many treatment approaches. Like Wampold and his colleagues, they further suggested that the knowledge and skills of the clinician who is providing the treatment may be a critical element influencing the success of treatment.

There are some additional, appealing aspects of the common factors model of therapeutic change that are also worth considering; for example, it is less dogmatic than the medical model in that it allows for eclecticism as long as there is

---

[4]This model is also termed the contextual or component model.

a rationale that underlies treatment and that rationale is cogent, coherent, and theoretically based. Furthermore, the model emphasizes the therapeutic context and the meaning attributed to the healing process by the participants, rather than the specific ingredients of the treatment.

This discussion is not intended to suggest that the medical model is not useful in many ways, both in general and in the area of fluency and fluency disorders in particular. However, a hallmark of the scientific approach is being open to alternative explanations. To date, most of our investigations about *why* people stutter have been informed by the modern Western medical models of human health and development. It has been commonly assumed that, as a profession, we should follow this same (medical) model in our approach to understanding and treating stuttering. Certainly this model has proven useful, and currently important progress is being made in areas such as genetics and neuroimaging. It may be, however, that our investigations about *how to help people* who stutter are less well informed by the medical model, and perhaps there are other ways of considering how it is that humans are able to successfully cope and respond to therapeutic intervention.

Authors have been responding to the need for obtaining evidence to support our diagnostic and treatment decisions. However, individuals in a number of fields have pointed out that good evidence does not have to come in the form of randomized controlled trials (RCTs). Ratner (2005) explains the limitations of RCTs for our field. The control groups called for during RCTs are a particular problem, not only because of the ethical issues of withholding treatment from individuals who would likely benefit from assistance but also because it is not possible to "wash out" the effect of learning as a result of previous treatment(s). Withdrawing treatment from people who have experienced it is not likely to undo the learning and cognitive changes that have taken place. And, as mentioned earlier, the positive placebo effects experienced by individuals who are selected for a control group may well result in some improvement, moderating the true effects of the treatment. In addition, there is the possibility for EBP to provide compelling but superficial evidence for selected "brands" of treatments. It is also possible that an overemphasis on EBP may result in the endorsement of questionable treatments that do not make use of conceptually or empirically sound principles of change. This is more likely to occur with "brands" of treatment, in which a group of individuals is involved in training and franchising (Ratner, 2005).

Ratner (2005) makes the essential point that our choice should not be between treatment protocols that advocates indicate have received the necessary levels of empirical support and what these same authors deem as nonefficacious treatments. This, however, is the only choice that is sometimes offered. As Sackett et al. (2000) cautioned at the outset of their article on evidenced-based practice, we need to be careful not be "tyrannized by evidence . . . for even excellent evidence may be inapplicable and inappropriate for an individual patient" (p.1).

More to the point, we need to be careful of those who would choose to use EBP as a "club" to force others to use particular treatment protocols, especially while discrediting what others are doing. In fact, some treatments that may be found to be efficacious may be also be unacceptable to people for a variety of reasons. It is not unusual, for example, for autonomous people to decline participation at the outset. Others fail to comply with the protocol or withdraw from the study. Researchers who are conducting efficacy or effectiveness studies should not exclude participants who were in some way noncompliant with the treatment protocol—although they often do (Hollis & Campbell, 1999). Excluding individuals who are noncompliant risks biasing the results in favor of the treatment. (LaValley, 2003) explains how intention-to-treat analysis (ITT) shows that those who are compliant with a treatment protocol (regardless of the treatment) often have better outcomes than those who are noncompliant. In fact, this is also the case for those receiving a placebo (Coronary Drug Project Research Group, 1980).

Finally, as Ratner (2005) points out, we should not confuse the concept "currently without substantial evidence" with the concept "without substantial value." As Westen and Morrison (2001) state: "To infer that one treatment is more efficacious than another because one has been subjected to empirical scrutiny using a particular set of procedures and the other . . . has not is a logical error" (p. 878). In other words, we need to be careful to distinguish the notion of empirically *unvalidated* from empirically *invalidated* treatments. Furthermore, as several authors (Ratner, 2005; Westen & Morrison, 2001; Siegel, 1993; Zebrowski, 2006) have pointed out, it is not enough to show that a treatment "works." We also need to understand the underlying principles that enable us to understand *why* it works. As Ratner suggests, people are not likely to use a program if it does not make sense to them, no matter how many RCTs have been conducted. Only by understanding what principles and cause-and-effect relationships are operating can the clinician adjust a treatment protocol when necessary to the unique characteristics of his or her clients.

Fortunately, investigators are beginning to find evidence for the usefulness of the common factors model in comparing the effectiveness of empirically informed treatments of stuttering. Following earlier reports of similar results for three treatment protocols during three-month treatment programs and up to one year post-treatment (Craig et al., 1996.), Hancock et al. (1998) conducted a two-to-six year follow-up of 62 children ages 11–18 who had received one of the three stuttering treatments used in the study (intensive smooth speech, parent-home smooth speech, and intensive electromyography feedback). Using several indicators of stuttering behavior, speech naturalness, communication attitudes, and anxiety, the authors found no differences in long-term effectiveness between the three programs. More recently, in a small randomized controlled trial, Franken, Van der Schalk, & Boelens (2005) compared the Lidcombe Program and the demands and capacities protocol. Again, stuttering frequencies and severity ratings significantly decreased and were similar for the children in both programs. Likewise, Huinck and Peters (2004) compared the outcome of three treatment programs for adults—two intensive programs (one focusing on fluency shaping and one on stuttering modification) and a third highly individualized treatment program. Subjective and objective post-treatment and follow-up measures both one and two years later demonstrated dramatic improvement for all programs with only subtle differences between programs long term. All programs resulted in substantial improvements in fluency and self-concept, lowered anxiety, and speech motor control. The previously-described investigation by Herder et al. (2006) also provides support for the equivalence of empirically-informed behavioral treatments for stuttering.

Options for the Clinician

Given this information concerning evidenced-based practice, what is a clinician to do when faced with the obvious need for evidence to support his or her clinical decisions? Some of the possible responses are informed by our comments in Chapter 1 about the characteristics of effective clinicians and the development of expertise. The common factors model also provides some good news. The research consistently indicates that the clinician is the most important factor in accounting for therapeutic success, much more so than the specific techniques associated with any particular treatment protocol. Of course, this also places considerable responsibility on the clinician to develop a high level of competency by continuing to be a student of the field and continuing to refine his or her understanding and skills. Indeed, as Brown (2006) suggests, clinicians have an ethical responsibility to assess and improve their personal effectiveness; they cannot rely on treatments alone.

In addition, the theoretical perspectives found in Chapter 3 suggest ways of considering the various aspects of the medical and common factors models for informing our clinical decisions. That is, clinicians can consider different theoretical perspectives as they become calibrated to each individual and appreciate how the phenomenon of stuttering is manifested in each individual. Clinicians can identify the principles (rather than discrete rules) of change that they find to be most useful to them in facilitating change in their clients. As a result of a continuing awareness of the literature in the field, astute clinicians will be able to select and adapt protocols and procedures that are empirically informed, if not always empirically validated. In other words, they can use a wide variety of well-documented procedures that have been shown to be valid and reliable in clinical practice (many of which are described in the succeeding chapters) and which therefore provide evidence of successful therapeutic change, regardless of whether the procedure has been through an RCT.

Clinicians can appreciate that there are many ways of knowing and there are many scientific procedures that help us to understand. Rather than asking whether one treatment is somehow better than another we should be asking why it is that certain intervention strategies appear to work better with particular clients. Based on the available research, it is likely that, regardless of the particular treatment approach, factors such as the *working alliance* between the client and the clinician and *clinician allegiance* to the treatment protocol are important. As the common factors model suggests, clinicians need to have *allegiance* to the program they are using, a belief that it will be effective, and be willing to work the program in a persistent and confident manner. In addition, the program's philosophy should be congruent with the clinician's view of therapeutic change. As the common factors model also indicates, the process of therapeutic change is likely to be more successful if the client and clinician experience a therapeutic *alliance* that reflects a similar theoretical and practical perspective about thenature of the journey.

Furthermore, we as clinicians can model a scientific approach to the process of cognitive and behavioral change as we encourage our clients to consider alternative interpretations of their relationship with stuttering and explore new narratives about themselves and their possibilities for communicating. We can model curiosity rather than anxiety or fear about the experience of stuttering. We can show them how to explore cause-and-effect relationships that make stuttering less mysterious. We can support our clients as they take risks and conduct their own experiments with themselves and their speaking abilities.

Finally, but crucially, we can be cautious of dogma and especially intolerant when we read and hear the "rhetoric of pseudoscience," where proponents of various models of stuttering and treatment protocols use the name of science as a means to debase one another (see Kitrzinger, 1990; Raskin and Lewandowski, 2000). As clinicians and as researchers we should be good scientists, which at the heart of it, means being exceedingly curious about what may be going on and at the same time being open to alternative explanations for what we find. We can recognize that there are many procedures and techniques that our clients can use to achieve success even if we did not create them or do not particularly agree with some of them.

Conclusion

Drawing upon the ideas from several fields, we have attempted to organize the factors that may be of assistance to people who desire to alter their response to the circumstances presented by their stuttering. Beyond the obvious surface features of fluency and stuttering, there are also other important and interesting levels of the phenomena that require our consideration. A successful therapy outcome necessitates our understanding of the nature of change, a process that is exciting both because it is a creative undertaking and because it is unique to each person we are attempting to help.

Therapeutic change is characteristically cyclical rather than linear. In addition, our position as a clinician will fluctuate from that of a leader to a follower as we assist individuals in considering the possibilities for change. The process is sometimes far from tidy and there may be obstacles along the way. We are likely to be asking our clients to consider fearful experiences and to take on challenges they have denied or avoided for years. Decisions by the client to engage in or continue with treatment are influenced by many critical factors, including the readiness of the person seeking help, the availability of assistance, the requirements of treatment, and the cost in terms of time, effort, and money.

We have reflected upon the call for evidenced-based research in our field and offered some alternative interpretations of this important concept. We have suggested that along with the important contributions of the medical model there are other ways of conceptualizing therapeutic (and extra-therapeutic) change. We have argued that the common factors model provides an alternative way of considering the human change process and the critical factors that inform our clinical decision making. The factors of clinician expertise, the clinical alliance of the clinician and the client, and the clinician's allegiance to the chosen treatment protocol are critical and influential factors across treatment approaches that are empirically driven. Researchers are beginning to find evidence supporting the significance of these common factors across empirically informed treatments in the field of fluency disorders. The clinical decisions of proficient and expert clinicians are apt to be guided by theoretically motivated as well as empirically informed and validated information. Beginning in Chapter 8, we will discuss a variety of strategies and associated techniques that focus more specifically on changing the levels of the stuttering experience. The authors of a recent comprehensive review of many treatment approaches concluded by saying,

> . . . we are comfortable in saying that there are a large number of reasonably well-tested therapies for stuttering that have the good potential to help a large number of individuals. Some will work better for some than for others, and some clients may establish a better therapeutic alliance with some clinicians than others. In all this variety, there is continued hope for most people who stutter. (Bloodstein & Bernstein Ratner, 2008, p. 389)

Topics for Discussion

1. How did you "prepare your canvas" in anticipation of a major change in your life?

2. What are the three basic assumptions of Prochaska et al.'s change model?

3. Considering Prochask et al.'s model, explain some possible mismatches between *stages* and *processes* of therapeutic change.

4. Recall your coping response to a difficult or threatening experience and consider to what extent you responded in either a stepwise or cyclical manner.

5. Write down (for your eyes only) examples of various forms of denial that you have employed as a coping response about a difficult problem or relationship.

6. To what degree do you believe that fluent speech is a necessary and sufficient indicator of successful therapeutic change?

7. How might you respond to a new adult PWS who, at the outset of therapy, asks you, "What are my chances of success?"

8. Explain some of the barriers to initiating and maintaining change. What does Egan mean by the "shadow side" of change?

9. Distinguish between research intended to demonstrate treatment *efficacy* and research intended to demonstrate treatment *effectiveness*.

10. Compare and contrast the basic tenets of the medical model and the common factors model of therapeutic change.

Recommended Readings

Bernstein Ratner, N. (2005). Evidenced-based practice in stuttering: Some questions to consider. *Journal of Fluency Disorders, 30(1),* 163–188.

Journal of Fluency Disorders, (2003). Special Section, Evidence-Based treatment of stuttering: a series of 5 manuscripts, *28(3),* 197–258.

Zebrowski, P. M. (2007). Treatment factors that influence therapy outcomes for children who stutter. In E. Conture & R. Curlee, *Stuttering and Related Disorders of Fluency.* (3rd Edition, pp. 23–38). New York: Thieme Medical Publishers, Inc.

CHAPTER 7

Counseling and People Who Stutter

All clinicians should also train themselves in the subtle skills that enable them to sense the hidden feelings of their clients. These are not to be found in textbooks or classrooms. They must be mastered in the situations of intimate human encounter. Some of my students and clients have felt that I had an uncanny ability to read their thoughts—and at times I have indeed experienced something akin to clairvoyance—but only after I had observed and identified closely with the person long enough. . . . It is the result of very careful observation, uninhibited inference making, and the calculation of probabilities. It comes through empathy. (pp. 107–108)

Charles Van Riper (1979). A career in speech pathology.
Englewood Cliffs, NJ: Prentice-Hall

At a certain point in this self-generated event, the client experiences an Aha! He says, "Now I understand how I am," or "Yes, that's how I feel," or "Now I know what I need to do, how I need to act to get what I want in this situation." He is his own teacher. (p. 125)

Joseph Zinker (1977). The Creative Process in Gestalt
Therapy. New York: Random House.

Chapter Objectives

In this chapter we contend that, for many people who stutter, counseling is an integral part of the therapeutic change process. While this is more likely to be the case for individuals who have been stuttering for several years, it also true for many younger school-age children and their parents. This chapter also describes the reluctance of many clinicians to deal with the emotions that accompany the serious communication problem presented by stuttering and argues, as others have done, that speech-language pathologists who specialize in stuttering are the professionals who are best prepared to provide counseling. Along with describing the philosophies associated with common counseling approaches, the chapter highlights ways of conceptualizing counseling that are considered to be less (e.g., use of techniques and dispensing of information) and more (e.g., empathetic listening and understanding) effective. A concluding section describes the importance of the therapeutic alliance and the responsibilities of both the speaker and the clinician within the process of change.

The Reluctance to Confront Emotional Issues

There is a notable history of counseling in our field in general and in the area of fluency disorders in particular. The increase during the late 1990s of the number of texts on stuttering that have included information on counseling indicates an increased appreciation of this aspect of treatment (e.g., Bloom & Cooperman, 1999; Crowe, 1997; Manning, 1996; Shapiro, 1999). We will also suggest that because the relationship of the client and the clinician is at the center of the change process, counseling activities are taking place (either directly or indirectly) regardless of the treatment protocol.

It is not uncommon for clinicians to indicate their reluctance to confront aspects of treatment beyond those that they see as directly related to modifying fluency (e.g., Cooper & Cooper, 1985a, 1996; Kelly et al., 1997). Problems associated with bullying, low self-esteem, patterns of avoidance, frustration, and depression may seem mysterious and are too often seen as the responsibility of other professionals. Certainly there is cause for concern that so few students receive adequate preparation for how to respond to these and other issues. McCarthy, Culpepper, and Lucks (1986) found that only one third of the programs in communication disorders require a course in counseling. These authors noted that only 12% of clinicians who responded to their survey felt that they were adequately prepared to counsel their clients. According to Luterman (2001), far too many clinicians, although knowledgeable about many aspects of their field, are clinically and interpersonally inept. The most recent information indicates a continued lack of academic preparation in counseling for speech-language pathologists (Flasher & Fogle, 2004).

It is understandable that students are apt to feel uncomfortable taking on the role of a counselor. After all, most students are likely to be in their early twenties, and it is appropriate that they enter into counseling activities with caution or apprehension about counseling adults and parents who have considerably more life experience than they have acquired. Still, while new clinicians can appreciate that they are not an expert in all areas, they are in the process of becoming an expert in communication disorders. Gregory states it nicely: "Because we are the specialists in communication disorders, no one else can counsel in this area as well as we. The first requisite of counseling is to understand the nature of the problem, and no other professional group knows as much about stuttering as speech-language pathologists" (1995, p. 198).

Crowe (1997a) provides a definition of counseling that is helpful for our purposes. He cites Hinsie and Campbell (1970) who differentiate counseling and psychotherapy. Counseling is seen as a type of psychotherapy for the purpose of support or (re)education for behavioral problems *not* associated with mental illness. As Crowe explains, counseling is intended for assisting those people with less severe interpersonal (as opposed to intrapersonal) problems. Psychotherapy, on the other hand, is intended for persons with mental illness related to basic problems in personality development and personal adjustment. Although communication disorders often result in serious problems on many levels, in most cases we are not working with people who have chronic life-adjustment problems. David Luterman (2001), a person who for years has taken the lead in conceptualizing our intervention for communication problems as a humanistic and psychosocial process, also agrees with this view by indicating that our clients are experiencing a normal reaction to a very difficult problem.

In many ways our training teaches us to emulate a medical model of objective detachment when making clinical decisions based on the evidence that is available. Our spontaneous or learned detachment may provide us with a coping response that allows us to function on a daily basis, for it is possible to be overwhelmed by the work load and the misfortune that we see. We may risk taking the thoughts of our client's misery home with us to cloud our already hectic and sometimes challenging lives. As Prizant comments in the Preface of David Luterman's (2001) text, "The ultimate risk is to care too much about our life's work and the persons who receive our services. But with these risks comes the greatest reward — the sense that working with clients with communication disorders and their families is an integrated part of our lives and part of our human growth and development, rather than simply a vocation that pays the bills" (p. xi).

In the previous editions of this text we focused on the work of two individuals: Gerard Egan and the many editions of his text *The Skilled Helper* and David Luterman's *Counseling Person's with Communication Disorders and their Families*. Any clinician who is serious about acquiring a philosophical and functional understanding about counseling individuals with communication programs should have a copy of David Luterman's fourth edition (2001) on their shelf. Many of the ideas in this chapter are gleaned from the most recent editions of these two texts and we will introduce additional points of view by other authors who also offer helpful suggestions. For example, we will provide information from postmodern writers who employ a constructivist-narrative approach. Although each of these authors provides somewhat different approaches, the reader will find some reassurance by noting many points of intersection among the various counseling philosophies. The primary goal of this chapter is to introduce a variety of counseling approaches so that the reader may develop his or her own philosophy concerning the ability of humans to change their circumstances, particularly as applied to stuttering.

As Van Riper suggests at the outset of this chapter, the clinician needs to possess an empathetic and insightful understanding of the person and his or her situation. Clinicians are likely to be successful as counselors to the extent that they possess a philosophy about the therapeutic process that underlies their clinical strategies and moment-by-moment clinical responses. It is essential that this philosophy incorporate the optimistic belief that the person and the families they are assisting are capable of finding new, more effective ways of coping with their situation. This philosophy is found in every source cited throughout this chapter.

The Necessity of Counseling

Should speech-language pathologists be dealing with counseling issues or should emotions and cognitive change be left to the professions of psychology, psychiatry, or counseling? If we find ourselves working with clients who have chronic life-adjustment problems, referral to other professionals is the most likely choice. However, the vast majority of the people who come to us are ordinary people experiencing a normal reaction to a communication disorder (Luterman, 2001). As Luterman indicates, such people are generally experiencing normal emotions of stress and anxiety in the face of a serious problem. Actually, if our goal is provide truly comprehensive treatment, we have no choice but to provide counseling to them and their families. Behavioral change in the absence of cognitive restructuring is a recipe for relapse.

As described in the previous chapter, the success rates in the field of counseling have more to do with the wisdom of therapist and the therapeutic alliance than any particular treatment protocol (e.g., Egan, 2007; Wampold, 2001). When reading through the current literature in counseling, the word that comes up more than any other is *relationship,* more recently termed the *therapeutic alliance.* As Backus proposed in 1957, the learning and the substance of what goes on in the therapeutic relationship between the client and clinician are more essential than the techniques or materials. In a review of research findings, Goleman (1985) found that the best predictor of success in the helping process (a better predictor than the therapy used, the attributes of the clinician, or the problems of the client) is the quality of the relationship between the client and the clinician. Patterson (1985) stated that counseling not only involves the relationship; it is the relationship.

As a participant in the therapeutic alliance, the clinician plays a pivotal role. In order to be an effective counselor, the clinician must be well-trained and clever. However, the clinician must also be wise. As Egan (2007) states, we clinicians must understand the limitations of our profession, the shortcomings of the treatment strategies and techniques, and the strengths and weaknesses of both the clients and ourselves. We must recognize that the dogma of treatment approaches and book learning can filter and, on occasion, bias what we would otherwise understand about the person we are trying to help. Egan also cautions that learning must be sifted through experience in order for the person to be wise. As difficult as it may be, we must often accept ambiguity and uncertainty as we work with others to alter their situation. Portions of the information we use to make many of our choices tends to be incorrect, incomplete, and distorted by our emotions. Although this collection of uncertain information may be complex and even confusing at times, as Egan (2007) suggests, it also reflects the richness of the human condition.

When considering the healing potential of an effective therapeutic alliance, the importance of an effective clinician is clear. In fact one of the most interesting (and perhaps threatening) aspects of much of the literature in counseling is that the focus is less on the client than on the emotional health of the clinician. We need to ask ourselves, to what degree we are able to provide the client with a "clean bandage" for their wounds. Rather than focusing our diagnostic and therapeutic efforts solely on our client, we may, at least occasionally, consider the status of our own cognitive and emotional health. For example, as a part of his rational emotive behavioral therapy (REBT), Ellis (1977) provides a list of irrational ideas to which many of us readily adhere:

- It is a dire necessity for an adult human to be loved or approved of by virtually every "significant other" in his community.

- A person should be thoroughly competent, adequate, and successful in all possible respects if he is to consider himself worthwhile, and he is utterly worthless if he is incompetent in any way.

- Certain people can be labeled bad, wicked, or villainous, and they deserve severe blame or punishment for their sins.

- It is awful or catastrophic when things are not the way an individual would very much like them to be.

- Human unhappiness is externally caused, and individuals have little or no ability to control their sorrows and disturbances.

- If something is or may be dangerous or fearsome, one should be terribly concerned about it and should keep dwelling on the possibility of its occurrence.
- It is easier to avoid certain life difficulties and self-responsibilities than to face them.
- An individual should be dependent on others and needs someone stronger than himself on whom to rely.
- A person's past history is an all-important determinant of his present behavior, and because something once strongly affected his life, it should continue to do so.
- An individual should become quite upset over other people's problems and disturbances.
- There is invariably a correct, precise, and perfect solution to human problems, and it is catastrophic if this perfect solution is not found.

In order for us to become the best possible clinicians it will be necessary that we not only continue to grow professionally but that we consider such ways of thinking in ourselves. As Egan argues, in order to move from "smart to wise" we must recognize the shadow side of ourselves (e.g., tendencies to be selfish, lazy, or even predatory) as well as the messiness of the helping process (e.g., misuse of models and techniques, receiving payment for treatment although it is ineffective, not always giving your best effort during treatment). These issues are rarely discussed, but as Egan suggests, "If helpers don't know what's in the shadows, they are naïve" (1998, p. 19).

How to "Do Counseling"

Telling someone how to conduct counseling is like telling someone how to have a relationship. How you do it "depends." It depends on the people who are involved and on the issue that brought the person to counseling to begin with. Because counseling is typically client-centered it also depends on the characteristics of the client, and each client is unique. It is also difficult to offer a prescriptive sequence of activities telling someone how to counsel because counseling is a hands-on, dynamic experience rather than an academic exercise.

It is difficult for the clinician to know what to do at a given moment during treatment until a relationship is established. As suggested by Van Riper at the outset of this chapter, even for a clinician with great expertise, establishing a meaningful therapeutic alliance normally takes more than one or two sessions. Before the clinician can make accurate and reasonable clinical decisions, she needs to find out how motivated the client is. She must understand his story and begin to appreciate his situation in order to develop some level of empathy

Clinical Decision-Making

A few years ago I had the opportunity to read through a manual that was on display at a national professional meeting of speech-language pathologists. Because the focus of the manual was on counseling people who stutter and their families, it caught my eye. On the first few pages of the manual the authors promised that upon reading this manual, the reader would know exactly what to say to parents who are concerned about their young stuttering child, exactly how to respond to the spouse and family of an adult who stutters, and exactly how to counsel an adolescent or adult who stutters. No doubt the manual gave some common responses to the questions that parents and clients typically ask and provided the clinician a measure of help. However, as we mentioned in Chapter 1, following a preprogrammed approach does not facilitate a dynamic, client-based approach for dealing with the many layers of stuttering. Although a counseling manual may provide a measure of comfort to the novice clinician, it also manifests a technical approach to counseling rather than the dynamic nature of a professional, therapeutic interaction. As pointed out by Wampold and his colleagues in the previous chapter, exacting adherence to a manual can detract from the spontaneity and elaboration of the therapeutic alliance.

for the person. She needs to have a sense about his personality before she will be able to perceptively probe and challenge him. She needs to develop a sense of how tough he is likely to be when he attempts to use his behavioral techniques amid the pressures of communication situations beyond the treatment environment.

Ways of Conceptualizing Counseling

It is important to appreciate that, for most people, counseling is an everyday experience. Indeed, we counsel others in an informal manner as we help our family, friends, and colleagues deal with daily problems. Egan provides a particularly useful suggestion when he states that the goal of professional counseling falls somewhere on a continuum between telling people what to do and leaving them to their own devices. The ideal location on the continuum is a point where we are able to help people make their own decisions and act on them (Egan, 2007).

One helpful way to characterize professional counseling is to say that the primary focus is on the person and the secondary focus is on the problems. Along with the problems the individual may be facing are the many emotions associated with them. Another issue in counseling that especially applies to clients with communication disorders is the concept of missed opportunities. These may not be directly tied to a decreased ability to communicate *per se*, but have to do with situations of daily living that the client suspects could be handled better. In many instances, counselors are asked to help with both issues: specific problems and missed opportunities.

Another useful way to consider the nature of counseling is to think in terms of "stuckness." People go to counseling because they are stuck (Ivey, 1983; cited in Egan, 1990, p. 270). Often, along with being stuck, clients feel helpless to do anything constructive about their situation. As Ivey (1983) submits, it is the responsibility of the counselor to get them unstuck. Often there is no clear or distinct way to accomplish this. It takes experience and wisdom on the part of the clinician to assist the client to move from the stuck and helpless feelings to better ways of dealing with the situation. However, as Ivey (1983) indicates, it is not an easy task to describe the "possible self" one can imagine and become.

At its most basic level, counseling requires the clinician to respond with nonjudgmental respect for a client's unique differences and a willingness to listen instead of prescribe. Often we do not have to say anything and people will provide us with quality words and subtle meanings if we are willing to become calibrated to them. Luterman (2001) describes the nature of *empathetic* (Rogers, 1951), or *reflective,* listening, which involves valuing what clients are telling us along with viewing them as people who possess the wisdom to make decisions for themselves. As the therapeutic alliance develops, simply sharing silence can send a powerful message of understanding and support.

Common Misconceptions

A good way to develop some insight into the nature of counseling is to consider some of the common misconceptions about the process. Understanding what not to do as a counselor can be as useful as appreciating what you can do. For example, it is commonly thought that a primary goal of counseling is to make people feel better. As Luterman suggests, we may try to accomplish that by distraction, humor, or emphasizing the cognitive, rather than the emotional nature of the problem. Although people may value and appreciate the many changes they are able to achieve as a result of their counseling experience, counseling sessions and the resulting insights and necessary actions are not necessarily pain free. As Peck (1978) states in the first sentence of his book, *The Road Less Traveled,* "Life is difficult" (p. 15). It is normal and acceptable for people to feel sad when undesirable or bad things happen to them. The problem and the pain associated with the problem may not go away (as with the loss of a loved one or the realization of a son's or daughter's speech, language, or hearing problem). However, with successful counseling the client should be better able to manage the situation (Egan, 1990). As Egan states: "Helpers are effective to the degree that their clients, through client–helper interactions, are in a better position to manage their problem situations and develop the unused resources and opportunities of their lives more effectively" (1990, p. 5). Luterman (2001) expresses much the same view in suggesting that the primary purpose of counseling is to enable clients to separate their feelings from their nonproductive, self-defeating behavior.

Furthermore, it is not the task of the clinician to "rescue" clients (Luterman, 2001) by solving the problem for them. Although it is possible, particularly with young children, to alleviate all of the features of stuttering, in the case of some adolescents and adults, we are less likely to "solve" or "cure" the problem. As discussed in the previous chapter, adopting a medical model that focuses on diagnosing and curing the speaker's cognitive and behavioral responses to stuttering is not always the best way to conceptualize the process of therapeutic change. Accordingly, counseling is less about doing something to clients than it is about a collaborative process between the people involved. More importantly, rescuing people enables them to continue in the patterns they have established and negates their ability to problem-solve and grow on their own. As Egan (1990) suggests, in many ways counselors stimulate clients to provide services to themselves, helping them to have "more degrees of freedom" in making choices in their lives (Egan, 1990, p. 6). We will take this approach in the following chapter as we describe the successful management of stuttering with adolescents and adults. Fortunately, it is not necessary to eradicate the last vestige of stuttering in order for individuals who stutter to achieve success.

Although the counseling process is often referred to as "taking therapy," change is facilitated at many levels. In order to be effective, the counselor must help the client translate his or her choices into action. As Egan explains, thinking and talking—even clear, creative, healthy thinking and talking—will not change anything. It is the speaker taking action that will result in more effective living. As Egan consistently indicates, counseling is not about talking, it is about acting. Contemplating the situation is fine, but too much thinking can paralyze a person ("too much analysis leads to paralysis!"). When counselors fail, Egan suggests, they most often do so by not helping their clients to act, for counseling can too easily become a process of too much talking and too little action. Most of us know people who frequently talk about losing weight, running a marathon, taking a trip, or writing a manuscript and yet never get around to actually doing any of those things. Wonderful things often take place during the treatment or counseling session, but this is of little consequence if the person takes no action, especially in situations beyond the treatment setting.

The counselor plays a critical role by providing the security, insight and empathy necessary for the client to explore new possibilities and take risks. The support of the counselor makes it possible for the client to move into a future of his own creation. The security provided by a trusting therapeutic alliance is understandably an essential part of a successful therapeutic process. As Egan eloquently states, at the conclusion of successful counseling the clinician may be able to say about the client:

> Because I trusted him, he trusts himself more; because I cared for him, he is now more capable of caring for himself; because I invited him to challenge himself and because I took the risk of challenging him, he is now better able to challenge himself. Because of the way I related to him, he now relates better both to himself and to others. Because I respected his inner resources, he is now more likely to tap these resources. (Egan, 1990, p. 59)

To many clinicians, counseling means giving information and advice, often from a detached stance. However, as Luterman cautions, counseling by informing or persuading are seductive models. It presents the view that "I as a professional have all of this information and experience. You as clients are ignorant of so many things that you need to know; therefore, I can make a better decision for you than you can for yourself" (2001, p. 3). It is easy to see how this philosophy by a clinician can create a dependent, perhaps fanatical client who may adopt a dogmatic approach for managing their problem. Such an approach is not only likely to result in the clinician "playing the role" of a counselor or clinician, but over time, it results in the job becoming a bore for the clinician and contributes to burnout.

Luterman (2001) suggests that a better approach is learning how to relate to our clients. By listening and valuing the client's story, we allow more affect to enter into the relationship. If we are able to view the other person as possessing

Clinical Insight

Goleman (2006) in his 2006 book *Social Intelligence* describes how a secure relationship does more than insulate a person from threat. He summarizes research documenting the importance of a secure and synchronous relationship from the moment a person is born. From the outset, the interactive nature of protoconversations between a mother and their infant helps to create the mental scaffolding for subsequent conversations and "the inner conversation we call thinking" (p. 164). Children who experience this synchrony with a responsive and empathetic parent find it to be pleasurable, in part because of the activation of oxytocin and endorphins, pleasure-inducing neurotransmitters. The nature of the parent-child relationship plays a major role in the development of optimally functioning individuals and determines how the child will interact with others (e.g., " . . . well-empathized children tend to become secure; anxious parenting produces anxious children; and aloof parents produce avoidant children, who withdraw from emotion and from people" (Goleman, 2001, p. 165).

Clinical **Insight**

Responding to the inquiry "How do you do counseling?" reminds me of questions I am sometimes asked when giving workshops on fluency disorders. Invariably someone in the audience will ask me how I would respond to one of his or her clients during a particular treatment situation. When that happened early in my career, I immediately became role-bound. I felt that I had to assume the role of the expert clinician who had come from another city with answers to all of the questions I would receive. For years I tirelessly tried to provide a worthy list of suggestions. On occasion, clinicians would later report that they found my suggestions to be helpful and sometimes they would let me know that the "techniques didn't work."

Now, rather than responding to such questions with ideas that may or may not work I immediately respond to such questions by sincerely saying, "You know, I have absolutely no idea!" My response often elicits a puzzled look from some in the audience and, of course, for the moment at least, I come across as something less than an expert (a liberating feeling!). The point I want to make with the audience is that there are many reasonable techniques that may or may not work depending on many factors. I am unable to know the likelihood of success of any technique until I spend time with the speaker and begin to comprehend how determined and resilient the person may be. I need to understand the speaker's history of success and failure in communicating within the context of the educational, vocational, and social aspects of their life. I need to appreciate the level of support the person is likely to have from his family and friends. I need to determine how willing the person is to experiment with different techniques and the extent of their persistence in applying the techniques across a range of speaking situations. For these reasons and more, because I know absolutely nothing about the child or adult being referred to, I don't believe that it's my role to suggest specific techniques. That adventure is the responsibility of the clinician and the speaker as they journey together.

the inherent wisdom to ultimately make good decisions for him- or herself, we are less likely to take a role of lecturer, providing information that we assume will be helpful to this person. By listening and valuing, however, the counselor is more apt to assign the responsibility for change and action to the client. This strategy also increases the client's locus of control, as well as his or her options.

Emotions Encountered During Treatment

As Prizant (2001) points out, coping with the anxiety and emotions of our clients is often the most challenging issue for clinicians and students, resulting in the greatest degree of discomfort and anxiety. The anxiety and emotions associated with the communication problem may cause greater stress on the speaker than the problem itself. The requirements of the therapeutic process therapy can result in clinicians experiencing their own emotions of grief, anger, guilt, and joy as eloquently described by Luterman (2001, pp. 64–65).

Emotions are brought to the treatment session not only, of course, by the client, but also by parents, spouses, and the clinician. Some clinicians tend to believe their clients are fragile and expresses concern that openly and directly discussing stuttering and associated emotions will result in increased stuttering (Cooper and Cooper, 1985b, 1992). As a result the clinician may tend to be careful about revealing his or her own feelings. In nearly all cases individuals who stutter are impressed with genuine honesty on the part of the clinician. Most clients are strong and resilient enough that they are able to tolerate a truthful, if frank, comment by a clinician. Any increase in stuttering by the client as a result of such honesty is rare, temporary, and of little consequence. In some instances, as we explain in subsequent chapters, an increase in stuttering may even be advantageous.

According to Luterman (2001), an underlying principle when counseling is that emotions are neither good nor bad; they just are. Emotions of the client, and on occasion, those of the clinician, need to be acknowledged and accepted rather than judged. This, of course, is not necessarily an easy thing to do. There is often deep pain in those involved in a communication disorder (Luterman, 2001) and in many cases, that pain is not going to go away. It is appropriate to acknowledge it for what it is—a normal reaction to an unwanted situation. In any case, as Luterman points out, it is always a mistake in any relationship to tell people that they should not feel a particular way.

There are several sources of emotions during treatment. The emotions of everyone who may be involved in the treatment process—including the client, the clinician, parents, spouses, siblings, and friends—all come into play. Luterman (2001) describes several of these emotions and indicates that they are universal and not disorder-specific.

1. **Grief**: Grief may be more likely to be associated with a communication problem if there is a relatively sudden onset, such as with a stroke or traumatic brain injury. However, grief also exists for other problems, including fluency disorders. As explained in the previous chapter, clients and parents are unlikely to move through Kübler-Ross's stages of grief—denial, anger, bargaining, depression, and acceptance—in a stepwise fashion. As Luterman (2001) suggests, the process is likely to be cyclical without set boundaries separating the stages. Participants will often find themselves revisiting stages they have experienced before. By recognizing and confronting grief and loss, one is able to slowly appreciate the joy of accomplishments and success that are nonetheless available.

2. **Inadequacy:** There is frustration in being unable to "fix" a problem; clinicians as well as parents feel a great desire to help the person with an obvious problem. However, Luterman (2001) calls attention to what he terms the "Annie Sullivan syndrome" (referring to the teacher, counselor, and caretaker of Helen Keller). Danger lies in rescuing the client. There is a profound difference between empowering the client or the parents to manage the problem themselves and taking charge of the situation (and the client). As in many forms of instruction, including parenting, the ultimate goal for the clinician is for the person being counseled to achieve independence. Clinicians need to be aware of their own need to be needed, and clients must be aware that their situation is their responsibility.

3. **Anger:** Anger has many sources, one of which is violation of expectations. Clients, parents, and spouses have many expectations of themselves and each other. Clinicians and clients also have expectations of each other. When these expectations and hopes are not realized, anger may be the result. Communication problems typically restrict many options for the client and his or her family, which can be extremely frustrating for all involved. Moreover, as we see every day, when people are continually frustrated, anger will surface. Another source of anger is loss of control. As Luterman (2001) compassionately illustrates on several occasions throughout his book, caring for a loved one, especially a child or a spouse, who is hurting in some way makes one angry. One danger is that such anger eventually can be displaced to others or turned inward to become depression.

   One way not to be angry is not to care, to become numb. This is a well-known response of people who are unable to escape chaotic or threatening situations and is a common topic for support groups such as Al-Anon or Al-Ateen. Rather than suppressing anger, it is generally better to recognize it and understand the circumstances that led to the anger. For example, professionals have the right to be angry at clients. If the client means enough to the clinician, a behavior that provokes frustration and eventually anger—such as not completing a clinical contract—should be acknowledged. In some cases, anger can be healthy, for as Luterman (2001) points out, there is a great deal of caring and energy therein; the energy contained in anger can become the fuel for change.

4. **Guilt:** Along with anger, guilt is another common emotion experienced by families of clients. As parents verbalize their feelings about their child's stuttering, they may also experience a form of secondary guilt as they feel bad about feeling sorry or embarrassed for their child. They may express guilt for believing that they have somehow caused their child's stuttering or perhaps for having waited so long to seek help. Some of this guilt may abate as parents learn about the nature of stuttering. Luterman (2001, p. 60) points out

that parents experiencing guilt may overprotect their children or become a "super-dedicated" parent that clinicians or teachers value for their commitment and hard work on behalf of their child. However, unless the guilt is resolved it can also result in the compromising of family structure and relationships. Difficulties may also arise when the child becomes a teenager and the parents face the prospect of letting the child go to grow on his or her own. Acknowledgement and acceptance of these naturally occurring feelings during parent support-group meetings can be especially helpful in lessening guilt.

Luterman (1991) makes the observation that guilt is often a statement concerning power. It says, "I have had some power to influence or cause this bad result." Feeling guilty about something (or worrying) implies that the person can control the situation. It is a little like worrying about the weather or your safety before leaving for a trip. Obviously, it is possible to do appropriate and judicious planning for the weather or a trip, but worrying will not control the situation or save you from harm.

5. **Vulnerability**: We are all vulnerable. Luterman states, "If we live long enough something bad will happen to us, and if we don't live long enough then something bad has already happened" (2001, p. 61). Speakers who stutter can be especially vulnerable in social settings. The ability to separate the problem (stuttering) from the client's reaction to the problem (feelings of vulnerability) is one measure of progress. Fortunately, vulnerability is usually easier to deal with than guilt and can actually be a positive force. Once our vulnerable and finite nature is acknowledged and even accepted, we are free to take action to do what we can to change.

6. **Feelings of Confusion**: Communication disorders can be not only anxiety-producing, but confusing, especially for parents. It is difficult to know what to do and whom to turn to for assistance. By giving information-based counseling, the clinician can add to feelings of confusion by providing information before the client is ready to receive it. On the other hand, such information can function to establish the credibility of the clinician at the outset of treatment. In any case, confusion on the part of the client can become a motivating force for learning.

In summary, the clinician's task is not to alter but to acknowledge and accept the various emotions indicated by the client. They are, for better or worse, part of the problem and one important component of the treatment process. Although we will not always be able to make our clients feel better, we can help them by preventing the many emotional components of the problem from developing into inappropriate behaviors and secondary, negative feelings such as feeling guilty about feeling guilty or being depressed as a result of anger. Table 7-1 provides conceptualizations of counseling that are more or less constructive.

Table 7-1   Ways to Conceptualize Counseling

Counseling Can Be	Counseling is Not
Facilitating understanding and action	Making people feel better
Listening to understand the person's story	Giving information and advice
Assisting the person to take action	Rescuing the person
Successful management of the problem	Fixing the problem
Increasing choice in spite of emotions	Decreasing client emotions
The therapeutic alliance	Counseling techniques

Egan's Three-Stage Skilled-Helper Model

In the previous editions of this text we often described counseling concepts from the work of Gerard Egan. Now in its seventh edition, his text is reported to be the most widely used counseling text in the world. In this most recent edition, Egan (2007) continues to elaborate a model for helping people who have a wide variety of problems. Because only the most basic features of Egan's model are included in this chapter and because it offers guidance that is helpful for all clinicians, readers are urged to obtain the most recent edition of this text.

Egan's three-stage model presents an interactive approach for helping people to clarify their problem(s) and to systematically select a plan of action for changing their situation. As we will describe, this model is not designed to fix or solve problems but rather to help people cope with and manage their situation. Egan proposes that the two primary goals of counseling are to (a) help the person live more effectively and develop unused opportunities more fully and to (b) help clients become better at helping themselves in their everyday lives. An overview of the model is summarized in Figure 7-1.

Stage I is designed to help both the clinician and client begin to understand the current state of affairs. This is accomplished by enabling the client to tell his or her story with enough detail in order for the clinician (as well as the client) to fully understand the current scenario. Once the current problem situation is understood, the client is helped to identify "blind spots" that prevent him or her from more clearly and objectively seeing the problem as well as unused opportunities. Finally, given a possible range of behavioral and cognitive features associated with the problem, the client is helped to select the features that have a major impact on his or her current situation.

Stage II is intended to identify the preferred scenario: the things that the client wants and needs in order to live a better life. This stage is about the preferred

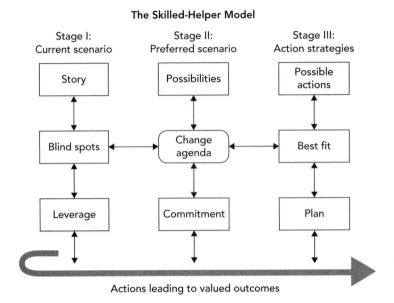

Figure 7-1 Egan's three-stage Skilled-Helper Model. From Egan, G. (2007). *The skilled helper: A problem-management approach to helping (8th edition)*, Pacific Grove, CA: Brooks/Cole Publishing Co. Reprinted with permission.

outcomes of therapy. The client's preferences are identified by helping him or her imagine the possibilities for a better future. What would a different life look like? The clinician then assists the client in developing a "change agenda" for determining realistic and challenging goals necessary for achieving the new scenario. Finally, in this stage, the clinician helps the client in developing the courage and persistence for accomplishing the work necessary for achieving the desired goals. The client considers whether or not the selected outcomes are worth the effort it will take to achieve them.

Stage III is focused on developing strategies for taking action and the activities the client will need to do to get what he or she wants. Egan points out that one reason "clients are clients is that they are not very creative in looking for ways of getting what they want" (Egan, 1998, p. 275). The clinician and the client brainstorm possible actions for achieving what the client wants. Next, the clinician helps the client to choose the best plan given the talents, resources (e.g., support groups and family members), and style of the client. It is important to remember that, in general, simpler plans are usually better. Finally, the clinician assists the client in creating a specific plan for accomplishing the goals. This final stage can be long and arduous. Clients will need guidance in formulating small steps, help in developing discipline, support when they are feeling overwhelmed, assistance in developing procedures for realistically evaluating success, insight into being flexible, and help in dealing with unanticipated problems.

The bidirectional arrows shown in Figure 7-1 indicate that although the overall direction of change generally precedes from Stage I through Stage III, there is also the likelihood of returning to a previous stage. That is, sometimes action will precede understanding, and strategies may need to be refined as the result of attempts to implement change. This, of course, is similar to the interpretation of the change process described for the cyclical nature of change described in the previous chapter. Contemplating the possibility of what things could be like (Stage II) may highlight aspects of the client's current situation (Stage I) and help to identify blind spots not yet considered.

In the final analysis, clients must act in their own behalf and choose to take action to change their situation. Thus, the "Action Arrow" begins at the outset of therapy and underlies all stages of the model. The Action Arrow also represents transition as clients move from their current state to their preferred scenario. This transition can bring with it a degree of disruption and anxiety, as clients begin to give up familiar but often dysfunctional behavior and ways of viewing themselves and their world. Lastly, the activities of the model are delivered and filtered through the developing relationship between the clinician and the client.

The primary features of Egan's model have much in common with the specifics of treatment for stuttering. Regardless of the treatment approach the clinician selects for a child, adolescent, or adult who stutters, the clinician must understand the client and his or her story. Unlike the situation in the field of counseling, we generally (but not always) know that the problem is stuttering. Nevertheless, as in Egan's Stage I, we want to begin treatment by understanding clients' history of stuttering, their awareness of their behavior, and their success or failure in negotiating within the world of fluency. It is essential to find out the motivation for why the person is coming to us for help at this time. We will want to discover possible blind spots and untapped potential the client has about his or her situation. We want to know the extent of his or her motivation for and commitment to the process of change. These concepts are also emphasized with the narrative approach to therapy described later in this chapter.

Clinicians working with people who stutter typically may not consider Stage II issues. That is, we might assume that our clients know what the preferred scenario would be—we want our clients to decrease their stuttering and begin living the life of a fluent speaker. However, as we have said, a multidimensional problem such as stuttering requires the consideration of multidimensional outcomes. At the outset of therapy, many people have a single target—they want to be fluent. They are not as likely to recognize the larger view of the stuttering phenomenon and how their relationship with stuttering is impacting their life. They often place themselves in a "me–them" dichotomy with themselves being uniquely separate from all normally fluent speakers. It is not surprising that they only want to spend time on activities that result in an immediate cessation of stuttering. On the other hand, there are many people who do not necessarily want or expect perfect fluency. Many adults who stutter do not need to achieve spontaneous levels of fluency in order to become good communicators. As we shall see in later chapters, fluency, particularly in the long term, requires many cognitive adjustments by the speaker as well as others with whom the person interacts. Different clients will select different agendas and rates of change, and not everyone will choose the same short- and long-term goals. Finally, we need to determine clients' ability to implement the activities of Stage III and be sure that they appreciate the energy and time they will need to invest in order to achieve their desired outcomes.

As we suggested earlier in this chapter, the activities of Stage III can be based on principles of change rather than the dogma of a particular stuttering treatment package. Although there are many treatment programs that provide activities and techniques that clients will find helpful, the therapeutic alliance of the client and clinician is likely to benefit from brainstorming across many programs and associated techniques. Particularly at the outset of treatment, most speakers expect the clinician to tell them what to do. However, once the therapy is underway it is reasonable and often desirable for the speaker to assume increased responsibility in formulating the direction and pace of treatment activities. Throughout the process the clinician will continue to support and guide the client both within and beyond the treatment environment.

Counseling Philosophies

As we mentioned in Chapter 1, a clinician with experience and expertise is less likely to follow a dogmatic or "one book" approach that may limit the possibility of experimental and creative ideas. Just as there is no one ideal treatment strategy for the treatment of stuttering, there is no experimental evidence supporting the superiority of any one counseling strategy (Luterman, 2001; Wampold, 2001). Often, an approach is chosen because it coincides with the personality of the clinician and his or her view of reality (Ahn & Wampold, 2001; Wampold, 2001). Webster (1966) suggested that the risk of hurting a client may be heightened by a nonaccepting and noncompassionate clinician using a prescriptive approach. For the clinician who is in doubt about what strategy to employ, Webster recommended a less direct approach, because she believes it is virtually impossible for the clinician to damage a client by listening and trying to understand what his or her world looks like. Conversely, Luterman's (2001) view is that the safest approach is not an entirely nondirective approach, because this may generate client anger when it violates expectations of what the clinician should provide. He suggests that the safest choice is a cognitive approach that advises clients to restructure their view of the situation. People can survive bad advice, he suggests, for we have been doing it for most of our lives.

Luterman (2001) describes four general approaches to counseling: behavioral, humanistic, existential, and cognitive.

Behavioral Counseling

The original and strict version of the behavioral approach held that the individual has little or no choice and that all behavior is the result of environmental reinforcements (Skinner, 1953). Because of its structure, behavioral counseling provides an appealing strategy for engineering changes in the observable behaviors of speakers, especially for new clinicians. Structure is provided by a series of steps whereby behaviors are positively or negatively reinforced (or punished) in a precise and timely manner resulting in a series of successive approximations toward the desired goal. The concrete nature of the techniques and the specific, overt criteria for moving on to the next level make it relatively easy to teach and administer. The structured nature of the behavioral approach also lends itself to the creation of programmed or manualized therapeutic programs, a major reason why such approaches have achieved more empirical support in the form of randomized controlled trials. There is no question that reinforcement schedules can have an important therapeutic impact both within and beyond the therapeutic setting. Many investigations have demonstrated that a speaker can be guided through a series of successful speaking experiences and achieve long-term success (Onslow, Packman, & Harrison, 2003). As with all approaches, this approach by itself has some limitations, particularly in attending to the often critical issues such as the speaker's quality of life, anxiety, and self-esteem. In addition, it is clear that our clients are able to make informed choices and take responsibility for their cognitive and behavioral responses in spite of a variety of powerful environmental influences.

Humanistic Counseling

Underlying the humanistic counseling approach developed by Carl Rogers (1951) and Abraham Maslow (1968) is the concept that humans have an innate drive toward self-actualization (e.g., "the true Buddha is within oneself"). The basic elements of this approach include the concepts of congruence (bringing into parallel the parts of the self, particularity the intellectual and emotional components), empathy, self-actualization, and unconditional positive regard for the client. The clinician's goal is to assist the person in removing the barriers to self-actualization and to help him or her to follow his or her innate drive toward growth. This form of counseling stresses the quality of the therapeutic alliance, with little emphasis on diagnosis and testing. The clinician's role is primarily one of *unconditional regard* for the client and *empathetic listening.* These qualities, when combined with the *congruence* of the counselor (the coming together of the clinician's experience of the moment, the awareness of the experience, and the genuine communication of the experience) facilitate the client's "resources for self-understanding and growth"(Luterman, 2001, p. 14). Humanistic counseling and the critical nature of the therapeutic alliance have often been advocated for clients and their families (Backus and Beasley, 1951; Cooper, 1966, 1968; Webster, 1966, 1968, 1977). However, as Luterman points out, the abstract nature of the basic concepts involved can be difficult both to teach and to understand. Furthermore, the unstructured approach places the responsibility for change almost completely on the client, and, for some clients, it is difficult to accept that the self-actualizing drive will come into effect. According to Luterman, this approach does not work well with children, severely self-involved adults, or those with limited abilities, or with novice or insecure clinicians.

Existential Counseling

The existential approach comes from the French intellectual movement of the mid-1800s and the work of the Danish philosopher Søren Kierkegaard. This view holds that many human problems are a result of anxiety due to the basic facts of our existence. That is, we must die, we have freedom to make choices, we are alone, and life is meaningless. This view is different from traditional psychoanalytic theory, where the source of anxiety results from the conflict between the *id* (the pleasure drive) and the *superego* (social restrictions). In existential theory, there is no clinical value in understanding the client's past history or behavior. For individuals whose response to life is to avoid the basic facts of human existence, there are some negative, sometimes neurotic results.

Death

Existentialists hold that anxiety resulting from our eventual death can result in the avoidance or postponement of activities or decisions. Furthermore, it can result in a decreased ability to appreciate our everyday existence. By not recognizing the boundaries of our existence, we are likely to miss the beauty of the commonplace. The greater this death anxiety, the more one is likely to experience a restricted and unfulfilled life. The recognition that nothing is permanent enables us to value what we have been given while we can. In an interesting extension of such "death awareness," Luterman explains that he clearly explains or contracts with the client about how long a counseling session will last, thereby creating an awareness that tends to mobilize both the client and the clinician. The client's knowledge of the finite nature of the session means that they are less likely to waste the available time. Without the awareness of limits, the client is more likely to delay facing difficult issues and emotions, leaving them for sometime in the future.

Responsibility

Each of us is responsible for our own actions. Whether we admit it or not, in many respects, at least, we are in charge. Because of this, the clinician should not feel sorry for the client with a problem. There is no intention to blame clients or make them feel guilty but rather a recognition that people have a choice about what to do about their situation and about what to tell themselves about their circumstances. If they choose, their problems can be approached as a series of challenges or opportunities to learn and grow. Virtually every writer in counseling agrees that the starting point of therapeutic change is the assumption of responsibility by the client and a decision to change (DiClemente, 1993). As Luterman (2001) points out, the assumption of responsibility coincides with his earlier comments that we ought not to play the role of the rescuer. To the degree that we attempt to fix or rescue clients, they will continue to feel powerless and rely on the clinician.

Loneliness

As Luterman states, "We are alone and that crushing fact is central to existential thought" (1991, p. 19). Of course, all of us are lonely at times but clients with communication disorders are apt to be uncommonly so. By confronting our loneliness, we are able to generate an unconditional regard for humanity in general.

Meaninglessness

As if loneliness were not difficult enough to face, existentialists propose that there is no intrinsic meaning to the world; the cosmos is indifferent to our circumstances. This central aspect of existential thought cannot be judged as good or bad. Nevertheless, as Luterman (2001) points out, we are able to construct our interpretation of our purpose in life. For a clinician this means that our basic task is not to judge the client but to understand his or her view of the world and to assist him or her in finding more appropriate and functional ways of managing life's circumstances.

Luterman explains that the existential approach lacks a unifying approach for confronting the various sources of anxiety. The approach offers more of a philosophy than a treatment protocol and goes beyond the accepted limits for most speech-language pathologists. Nevertheless, the concepts provided by this counseling philosophy may provide a way to understand the narratives of our clients, as well as our own.

Cognitive Counseling

This view of counseling holds that many human problems are, in many important ways, a function of how we think about the problem. The clinician helps clients to identify specific misconceptions and unrealistic expectations that underlie their situation and their behavior. This process can be highly confrontational, because the clinician challenges clients to examine the underlying irrational and inaccurate assumptions that are reflected in their language and their actions. Ellis's (1977) list of irrational thought processes presented earlier in this chapter provide good examples of inaccurate assumptions held by many of us.

There is historical precedence for cognitive approaches in the area of fluency disorders. A number of authors advocate the use of some form of cognitive restructuring as a primary or supplemental approach to treatment, particularly for adolescents and adults (Bryngelson, Chapman, & Hansen, 1944; Emerick, 1988; Johnson, 1946; Maxwell, 1982; Van Riper, 1947, 1982; Williams, 1979). Specific recommendations of several of these authors will be described in the next chapter.

Because speakers often indicate their cognitive positions through the language that they use it is important to listen closely and consider what our clients (and others) are telling us, consciously or unconsciously. As Luterman and others explain, we can listen for "quality words" such as "can't," "should," "ought," and "but," as well as the ways in which people describe themselves and their circumstances: "I'm an idiot" or "I can't speak in front of a group." The point is, the language people use informs the clinician about the speaker's cognitive state. Alternatively, choosing language that more accurately reflects the situation can inform and alter the speaker's cognitive interpretation: "I am not an idiot but in that instance I did an idiotic thing" and "Although I am anxious I am capable of speaking in front of a group." As Luterman (2001) states, "I find that when I listen to the irrational assumptions that are reflected in the language of the client, and when I gently change the language, there is often immense benefit to the client" (p. 28).

Luterman (2001) suggests that speech-language pathologists (and audiologists) unknowingly use this counseling approach as we frequently attempt to persuade our clients how they "ought" to be thinking and behaving. The problem is that a rigid cognitive approach risks such persuasion of the client to adopt what the clinician believes to be a more reality-based response to the problem. As described earlier, an approach that emphasizes the accuracy of the clinician's perceptions and authority usually results in a dependent client. Luterman (2001) also cautions that the emphasis of some cognitive therapies prevents the expression of real and natural emotions that accompany communication problems. The emotions are an important component of the problem and, as we shall see, an important aspect of the inclusive process of therapeutic change.

Postmodern Counseling

Postmodernism is best seen as a broad cultural trend in many fields, including art, architecture, law, literary criticism, and philosophy (Neimeyer and Raskin, 2000). In contrast, the modern, objectivist orientation consists of "experts" telling the client what is "real" or "true" or "healthy." For modernists there is a single, knowable reality. Disorders are viewed in terms of the degree that an individual's cognitive distortions result in a deviation from reality as defined by what is considered by society as the norm. The focus of diagnosis and intervention is on "measuring essential structures and empirically establishing the efficacy of preferred interventions designed to correct such disorders" (Neimeyer & Raskin, 2000, p. 5).

The understanding proposed by those advocating postmodern approaches may appear as shocking or blatantly wrong to those raised and schooled in the modernist tradition. The postmodern view, rather than espousing a single reality, proposes that there are multiple realities that are created by individual, social, and temporal factors. There is both the recognition and a celebration of these multiple realities according to the contextual history of a person's life. With this view, treatment is not informed by a process of discovering the truth about a person and helping that person to adjust to the norm. Rather, the therapeutic process is centered on "an exploration of how people construct truths about themselves and their relationships" (Monk et al., 1997, p. 85). This approach to how individuals come to understand their world is reflected in the constructivist view that each individual creates his or her own story based on the experiential exploration of his or her intimate attachment relationships. Individual narratives are influenced by such primary factors as culture and gender. It is within this crucible that individual identity and disorder are constructed. The implications of this perspective provide optimistic and creative possibilities for liberating the individual from what has become a limiting and oppressive story (Neimeyer & Raskin, 2000).

Personal Construct Theory

The constructivist counseling approach evolved from the work of Kelly (1955a, b) and his development of the theory of personal constructs (PCT).[1] Kelly takes a "people-as-scientists" view in which people are continuously engaged in a

[1]For a more detailed presentation of Kelly's theory as it applies to stuttering see Franscella (2003), DiLollo, Neimeyer, and Manning (2002) and Hayhow and Levy (1989).

process of creating hypotheses about their environment. As people experience life events they note recurring patterns from which they abstract the recurring themes and their contrasts. This dual process of abstracting and contrasting comes together in a process of construing that leads to our understanding and construction of meaning. This understanding, in turn, leads to the development of the person's *personal constructs*. Landfield and Leitner describe constructs as "personal dimensions of awareness anchored by contrasts in meaning" (p. 5). Constructs are subsequently organized into systems or templates that a person uses to explain and predict future events. New experiences may require the review and subsequent adjustment or alteration of one's constructs. Adjustments to the individual's system of constructs may be resisted (or not accomplished) depending on the extent of damage to the individual's existing system.

Kelly (1955) also provided "corollaries" that operationalize the system of personal constructs. The corollaries enable the individual to elaborate meaning and anticipate future events. For example, the *range corollary* indicates that a construct has a specific "range of convenience" in that it applies only to a specific set of events. The *experience corollary* states that experience is gained actively rather than passively and is made up of the successive *construing* of events, not merely the succession of events themselves. The *choice corollary* specifies that an individual will choose the construct pole that will provide him or her with greater meaning and greater possibilities for anticipating future events.

Finally, the manner in which such emotions as threat, fear, anxiety, guilt, and hostility are defined in personal construct theory are especially helpful for appreciating a PCT perspective of stuttering. *Threat* is defined as "an awareness of an imminent and comprehensive change in core structure" (Landfield & Leitner, 1980). *Fear* is defined as "the awareness of imminent *incidental* change in one's core structures" (p.12). Landfield and Leitner (1980) state that "if a person has defined his life-role in terms of sickness, the prospect of successful therapy could be traumatizing" (p.12). *Anxiety* is an awareness that the events a person is experiencing are beyond the range of convenience of the construct system. In such a case, the person has no way of understanding or predicting the course of events.[2] *Guilt*, in personal construct terms, occurs when a person acts in a way that is contradictory to his or her core role structure. For example, guilt occurs when the person does something that violates a strongly held belief about oneself as a person. *Hostility* occurs when the person is persistent in trying to validate a social prediction in the face of repeated invalidation of that prediction. Change, particularly as a result of therapy, requires a person to develop alternative constructs (reconstrue), a process that is difficult because it

---

[2] The reader may have experienced such anxiety when traveling in another country and not being able to predict events due to not knowing the language and protocols concerning social interaction, driving, and eating.

means letting go of accepted and safe views and attempting new ways of thinking and acting. As applied to people who stutter, the clinician helps the client to consider and experiment with alternative views (constructions) of themselves, their stuttering, their responsibility for their situation, and the nature of speech modification techniques. The client is taught to problem-solve as he or she considers a set of alternatives about interacting and speaking and to experiment with alternative ways of responding, including ways that may appear unique or even threatening. In the following chapter we will describe in more detail the clinical research that has helped to elaborate therapeutic change from a personal construct perspective.

The Constructivist-Narrative Approach

Although the term *narrative* is commonly used in speech-language pathology to refer to a type of discourse that has certain linguistic properties (McCabe & Bliss, 2003), in this context the term takes on a narrower focus. In this application the term narrative refers to an individual's personal story, which influences how events and experiences are interpreted, consolidates self-understanding, and guides behavior (Dilollo & Manning, 2006). Following Kelly's development of the theory of personal constructs, psychotherapeutic and counseling approaches progressed to constructivist and constructivist-narrative models of therapy (e.g., Monk, Winslade, Crocket, & Epston, 1997; Neimeyer & Raskin, 2000; Perry & Doan, 1994; White & Epston, 1990). This counseling approach shares some of the features of the humanistic approach described by Luterman (2001).

The narrative therapy model (White & Epston, 1990) has several appealing features. It provides an optimistic orientation that assumes that people are able to take action and rewrite their stories in order to alter meaning in their lives. It allows the clinician and others to view the person as a "courageous victor rather than a pathologized victim" (Monk, 1997, p. 4). The emphasis of the therapeutic interaction is on the person and his or her story rather than specific therapeutic techniques or the clinician. The process does not require that the clinician know "the way" but emphasizes the client and the client and clinician working together to discover the directions and techniques that are likely to be the most helpful for the client. It does not place the clinician in the role of an authority charged with solving people's problems (see also Leahy, 2004; Leahy & Warren, 2006). The following two paragraphs summarize the comments of several authors (particularly McKenzie & Monk, 1997; Monk, et al., 1997; Payne, 2000) concerning the essential elements of the narrative approach.

A narrative approach invites the clinician to take up an investigative, archaeological position in order to discover the partially visible and often scattered fragments of a person's story. Like the archaeologist, the clinician will need to have genuine curiosity, persistence, care, and sensitivity. Eventually, the clinician begins to assemble the fragments in order to understand the person's story and the social and cultural context in which it was formed. The clinician appreciates that he or she is in a privileged position that allows him or her to hear the person's unique and dynamic story. In keeping with a postmodern perspective, this does not imply that the clinician has a privileged access to the truth. In fact, on occasion, he or she will display a "deliberate ignorance" in order to elicit more extensive and detailed information from the person. The goal is to understand how people construct their understanding about themselves and their relationships.

As described by DiLollo, Neimeyer and Manning (2007), who first discussed the application of this approach to individuals who stutter, the clinician attempts to appreciate the nature of the person's current, problem-saturated story and the influence of the stuttering on the person's life and relationships. As the clinician begins to understand the story, he or she assists the client in deconstructing the dominant themes of the current narrative. Importantly, the speaker is seen as assuming the role of an actor rather than a passive character in the story. The clinician helps the person to externalize the problem in order to separate the person from the problem—the person is not the problem, the problem is the problem. The clinician looks for talents and abilities that may be currently veiled by the problem of stuttering and identifies story subplots that run counter to the dominant story line. These *unique outcomes* or *sparkling moments* are used to develop a new, richer, and more coherent narrative that coincides with the client's preferred story. The client's role during this process of "re–storying" is that of senior author with the clinician taking the role of co-author or perhaps editor. The new story is appended to the previous one, which remains a valued part of the person's history. Finally, the new story is anchored in the social context of the person's life, where other individuals provide a memorable history to help carry it forward into the future. The application of this approach is elaborated in the following chapter.

Perspectives on Counseling Techniques

In this section we are not presenting specific counseling techniques, for these can be found in a variety of sources, including those cited in this chapter. Moreover, the essence of counseling as well as therapy in general, is not about techniques. For example, Rogers (1980) spoke against the appalling consequences of overemphasizing microskills during counseling; to be effective, the clinician must approach counseling as a fully human endeavor. The clinician's counseling skills must become extensions of the helper's humanity, not just bits of technology. As we have indicated in our earlier discussion of expert performance (see Chapter 1) and as many experienced therapists recognize, good counseling techniques flow from the clinician's personality (Luterman, 2001). Ideally, technique becomes congruent with the personality of the clinician and blend into the treatment process. If the clinician acts mechanically, the technique is likely to fail because it will be discontinuous with the authenticity of the relationship. As Luterman explains, "Technique should not be apparent to the person being counseled or to an observer. If people know they are being counseled, you are probably doing it wrong" (Luterman, 2001, p. 89).

Silence

One of the best examples of the importance of integrating technique into the therapeutic alliance is an appreciation of silence during treatment. Silence can be embarrassing for the client as well as the clinician, and its intensity will eventually force the inexperienced clinician to become role-bound and act (Luterman, 2001). The client, meanwhile, is able to sit back and wait for the clinician to take the lead. Silence can be a powerful technique to facilitate change, for where there is silence, there is often growth. Indeed, silence can be a powerful motivator for the client to assume responsibility and to take action. As the clinician comes to appreciate how silence can serve many functions for promoting change, he or she is likely to become more comfortable with the pauses in the conversation. As Luterman states, "It often shows a fine command of language to say nothing" (2001, p. 96).

Silence is not a void, but a vital part of communication and the change process. As in Oriental ink drawings, the open spaces are an intentional and important part of the overall composition. The deepest feelings in a relationship can take place in silence, for there is companionship in thoughtful silence. When observing couples who are congruent it is possible to see that communication continues during moments of silence.

Empathy

The clinician who is able to express empathy is able to journey inside another's world. As Egan (1990) explains, "being with" the client is temporarily living another's life as a means to viewing the person without labels, interpretation, or categories. It is important to distinguish empathy from sympathy. Sympathy denotes agreement, whereas empathy denotes understanding and acceptance of the person. Rogers suggested that empathy is, in and of itself, a healing agent. "It is one of the most potent aspects of therapy, because it releases, it confirms, it brings even the most frightened client into the human race. If a person is understood, he or she belongs" (1986, p. 129).

Egan (2007) indicates that while listening to the client helps the clinician get in touch with the client's world, empathy helps the clinician to understand that world. He noted that clients rate understanding as the thing they find most helpful during counseling. Virtually all authorities agree that active listening and expressing empathy are affirming and highly therapeutic for the client. Listening with understanding allows the clinician to establish a cognitive map that describes the client's experience of himself (Zinker, 1977). It is from this map—this understanding of the person—that the clinician can begin to formulate the direction(s) of change that will assist the client through the treatment process. Although the majority of clinicians who assist individuals who stutter do not themselves stutter, it is possible for the fluent clinician to understand and to fully empathize with their clients (see Manning, 2004b). It is also good to realize that it is not always necessary to say anything in order to demonstrate empathy. Empathy is indicated by the very act of spending time with and listening to someone, as well as a glance or a touch (see also the comments in Chapter 1 by Goleman [2006] concerning empathy).

Probing and Challenging

As explained in Chapter 1, one of the responsibilities of the clinician is to challenge clients to consider alternative scenarios about their current situation and to take risks. Probing may result in the discovery of the clients' blind spots about their situation (Egan, 1990) or, alternatively, their unique abilities and potential. Egan (1990) describes probes as verbal tactics that help clients talk about themselves and define their problems in terms of specific experiences, behaviors, and feelings. The goal of probing is not to identify a single, momentous piece of information but rather to increase understanding. The speech-language pathologist assisting a person who stutters is not likely to probe as often or as deeply as the psychologist who is working with a client with a personality disorder. Nonetheless, on many occasions throughout treatment, clinicians may want to obtain more specific and better information about a client's behavior, motivation, and cognitive processes in order to help him or her make better decisions. Egan provides several recommendations concerning the quality of the clinician's probes, including the suggestions that verbal probes should just add spice to the communication process and should remain condiments, rather than the main meal. In addition, clinicians should not grill the client with too many questions, and the "questions should have teeth but not fangs."

As the clinician determines the client's strength and resilience, it is often necessary to challenging him or her with attitudes and behaviors that he or she is likely to resist. It is possible, of course, to challenge someone and still be

Clinical **Insight**

Several years ago I was working with a colleague who was both insightful and gentle. She rarely said anything negative about anyone. One day, after working with one of our young graduate students and an adult who stuttered severely, she turned to me and said something that surprised me. "You know, I don't think that some of our students have had the opportunity to suffer enough to be able to relate to our clients!" Her comment rang true, for I had experienced the same feelings about some (thankfully few) other clinicians. I have smiled over the years when students would ask questions such as "Is grief going to be on the test?" or "How much do we need to know about suffering for the final?" Of course, there are many possible explanations for why this young person had difficulty relating to the suffering her client had experienced. Whether or not this clinician had not yet suffered enough, she did not appear to have learned from whatever suffering she had experienced, or at least was not able to use her experience in relating to another person.

"for" that person. Challenging another person signifies that you take him or her seriously enough to respond when his or her choices are not in his or her best interest. It also indicates the clinician's belief in the client's potential. As Fisher and Ury (1981) suggest, it is best to be soft on the person and hard on the problem. Still, we must demonstrate to the other person our appreciation of what we are asking him or her to consider doing and express our willingness to engage in the same or equivalent risks ourselves.

Humor

As discussed in Chapter 1, humor can play an important part in a dynamic clinical relationship. Humor allows the clinician to challenge the client and to discuss things that would otherwise be risky or even taboo. Humor involves aspects of distancing oneself from a problem, conceptually shifting one's view of the situation, and mastering events and situations that were previously avoided or anxiety-producing. As Rusk (1989; cited in Egan, 1990) suggests, deliberate self-change requires a willingness to (a) stand back from yourself far enough to question your familiar beliefs and attitudes about yourself and others, and (b) persist at awkward and risky experiments designed to increase your self-respect and satisfy your needs. Not only can humor facilitate such self-change, but for the clinician, humor provides a window for viewing the cognitive changes associated with a problem.

The Therapeutic Alliance

Client Responsibilities

At the core of the helping process is the assumption by the clinician that, within reasonable limits, people are capable of making choices and controlling their destinies. But often our clients come to us with what appears to be a form of learned helplessness. As Egan (1990) suggests, many people adopt a deterministic view of life without realizing it. Of course, people are assisted in this process because many limits are imposed on us by social, political, economic, and cultural forces. Nonetheless, accepting responsibility for one's own life is at the heart of self-respect and happiness. In part because "professionals do not have access to all the relevant data," Luterman has found throughout a lifetime of successful counseling that he has "learned to trust people to make their own decisions" (2001, p. 110). Egan cites Farrelly and Brandsma (1974), who suggest assumptions about the people we are trying to assist that are both encouraging and probably accurate:

- Clients can change if they choose to do so.
- Clients have more resources for managing problems in living than most clinicians assume.
- The psychological fragility of clients is overrated both by themselves and others.
- Maladaptive attitudes and behaviors of clients can be significantly altered, no matter how severe or chronic.
- Effective challenge can provide in the client a self-annoyance that can lead to a decision to change.

The Metalinguistics of Change and the Therapeutic Discourse

Sensitivity to the language we use within the therapeutic alliance (and with others in our daily life) is critical as it indicates the reality that we create (Payne, 2000). The language our clients use to describe themselves and their experience indicates the reality of their world. This reality, of course, is influenced by many experiential factors such as culture, gender, age, and especially relationships. Although some words used by the client and the clinician may seem trivial, they often convey important distinctions. For example, Payne (2000, p. 9) cites White (1995) in suggesting that clinicians use the term *assist* rather than *help* when working with individuals, due to the subtle distinction regarding power; the term *help* implies that the helper is in the role of offering expertise to a subordinate whereas the term *assist* implies a sharing of knowledge and skills to someone who has a degree of competence. Rather than describing the people we are assisting as patients or clients it may be more appropriate to refer to them as a person, or simply to call them by name.

Leahy's (2004) suggestions concerning the therapeutic discourse by speech-language pathologists also have important implications for the therapeutic alliance. She points out the many word choices by the clinician that promote an asymmetrical interaction. For example, therapeutic discourse is often characterized by a three-step process of the clinician making a *request* (or asking a question), the person *responding*, followed by the clinician *evaluating* the person's response (RRE). When evaluating the client's response the clinician often provides markers of authority and compliance such as "mmm," "good," "right," or "OK." The clinician often follows the client's response with another request. Leahy provides several examples of the RRE pattern with discourse examples from clinicians and clients presenting with several communication problems, including fluency. Many of Leahy's suggestions are similar to Luterman's admonitions concerning the ineffectiveness of counseling based on informing or persuading.

As Leahy (2004) also points out, an asymmetrical relationship is also enhanced by the environmental context of the encounter and the framing of the participants' social and speaking roles. Leahy quotes Simmons-Mackie and Damico (1999, p. 315), who describe the "routinized therapeutic context, with its well-defined and expected roles" and "standard features which served to reinforce the underlying social contract and therapeutic goals." Most people recognize these verbal and nonverbal cues as we seek the services of, for example, a physician or a dentist. From the outset we find ourselves in a subordinate position, coming to the provider's location at the appointed time, sitting in a reception area (often for a lengthy interval), responding to a series of instructions (typically followed by additional waiting), being seen for a specific period of time, and eventually being told that we can leave.

Of course, this standardized procedure or script (see Pangos & Bliss, 1990) and the common sequence of the RRE discourse may be driven by the clinician's concept of his or her role and the pursuit of the session objectives. As Leahy points out, when demonstrating a therapy technique the clinician's role is to keep the person "on task" and "to model, monitor, encourage self-monitoring, and evaluate progress"(p. 78). This can occur, for example, when clinicians seem to be in "mad pursuit of fluency" rather than attending to the contextual characteristics of the message or the individual. Leahy suggests that this "institutional pattern" of discourse conceptualizes and promotes the client as an "error-maker." As the client assumes this role it results in limited engagement by the client and minimal exchange of information. These patterns typically promote an asymmetrical relationship, with the clinician in the authoritative role of the expert and the client in the subordinate role (Leahy, 2004).

Leahy (2004) invites the clinician to consider moving away from this style of interaction and to increase the symmetrical features of the therapeutic discourse. This is accomplished by the clinician following the speaker's lead and engaging in a socio–relational rather than an institutional frame, which focuses on the person rather than the problem. As we begin to frame the interaction in a socio–relational context, the participants are able to adjust their roles to promote the development of the speaker's communicative competence. Leahy provides examples of how the participants' roles can be negotiated in ways that elaborate the client's role as a competent communicator. The clinician can, for example, reduce his or her institutional and authoritative stance by decreasing his or her role as an evaluator and the frequent use of authoritative markers. The clinician can become sensitive in the use of pronouns (e.g., I, you, we) when requesting (rather than directing) the speaker in using behavioral techniques. The clinician can follow the conversational lead of the client and summarize the speaker's comments as a way of recognizing the speaker's contributions.

Clinician Responsibilities

This chapter began by stressing the importance of the therapeutic alliance of the client and the clinician. The characteristics of the clinician have a primary impact on the nature of that relationship. We discussed many of the characteristics of the clinician in Chapter 1 and will briefly mention here a few additional factors as they relate to this alliance. As Luterman (2001) comments, if the literature on the desirable personality characteristics of the ideal counselor were to be believed, the only people who might conceivably have a chance to qualify as clinicians would be some of the more outstanding saints. Fortunately, Egan (1990) suggests that it is neither realistic nor necessary for the effective clinician to be an entirely self-actualized person. In the final paragraph of his 2001 edition, Luterman indicates that the competent counselor does "need to be a caring individual who does not impose beliefs on others, who maintains a constant awareness of self, and who does not hide behind the artificiality of being a professional" (p. 190). He also states:

> I think the key to counseling is the congruence of the counselor. As I become more congruent, technique slips away or, more accurately, becomes incorporated into everything I do. I think the most important thing a counselor brings to the helping relationship is self. The importance of the congruent professional far exceeds the value of any diagnostic test or specific techniques in counseling. (2001, p. 190)

In a similar manner, Egan points out that for clinicians to be effective counselors, it is essential they understand themselves, including their own assumptions, beliefs, values, standards, skills, strengths, weaknesses, idiosyncrasies, style of doing things, foibles, and temptations. They need to appreciate how their characteristics will be apt to influence their interactions with their clients. To begin the process of introspection, Egan suggests counselors ask themselves the following questions (1990, p. 25):

- How did you decide to be a helper?
- Why do you want to be a helper?
- With what emotions are you comfortable?
- What emotions—in yourself or others—give you trouble?
- What are your expectations of clients?
- How will you deal with your clients' feelings toward you?
- How will you handle your feelings toward your clients?
- To what degree can you be flexible, accepting, and gentle?

As we suggested in Chapter 1, an essential characteristic of an effective clinician and counselor is the continual development of expertise. Whatever true competence may be for each professional, it is likely to be a lifelong pursuit. Competence means more than simply an academic understanding of models, strategies, and techniques. It means being able to "deliver the goods" to the people we are trying to help. All effective clinicians must continue to learn—it is basic for counseling and for life. Beyond learning, effective counselors must model many of the things they challenge their clients to do. As Egan (1990) suggests, if clinicians want their clients to act, they must be active in their own lives in regard to their own challenges. Berenson and Mitchell (1974) forcefully suggest that only those counselors who are committed to living fully themselves deserve to help others.

Being competent does not mean having solutions to all the problems that clients bring to us. Luterman (2001) stresses the importance of accepting our limitations and recognizing that particularly difficult cases will cause the icy finger of possible failure to threaten and test our confidence. Nonetheless, if the clinician is learning, if he or she is a truly responsible professional, he or she should be operating on the fringes of incompetence (Luterman, 2001). Effective counselors, clinicians, and people in general should take risks and occasionally make mistakes, or they will not grow.

At the conclusion of his 1990 edition, Egan provides a paragraph discussing the need for the counselor to go beyond the technology of helping and move toward becoming authentic. He indicates that our clinical and other life experiences can be either a teacher or a tyrant.

> Going through these experiences provides us with the opportunity to recognize and accept the shadow side of ourselves, our clients, and the world. To do so without becoming a victim is crucial but not the reward of

the experience. The events of each life need to be wrestled with, reflected on, and learned from. Only then can these events become our teacher and friend. Wrestling with our self, our colleagues, our friends, our demons, and our God will provide us both pain and comfort. It is that struggle that will help the skilled helper become the wise helper. (1990, p. 409)

Conclusion

Counseling is an essential part of the therapeutic change process for individuals who experience a communication problem and this is certainly the case for people who stutter. Unfortunately, relatively little information is provided to our students concerning the principles of counseling in many of our academic programs. The people who seek our help tend not to have serious psychological problems but normal reactions to the stress resulting from their communication problems. For some, emotions presented by the communication problems represent the most handicapping features of the problem. These natural and expected emotions should not, however, represent an intimidating aspect of therapy for the clinician. It is helpful to realize that our goal is not to "fix" these emotions but rather to help the person take action and function in spite of them.

Although there is a variety of counseling approaches, many common principles are found in each of them. Two common principles are the importance of the therapeutic alliance and the willingness of the clinician to listen carefully to the person's story in order to develop an emphatic understanding of the person and his or her situation. Such understanding allows the clinician to develop an appreciation of clients' interpretations of themselves and their situation and also the coping resources they have at their disposal. As suggested by Leahy (2004), the quality of the therapeutic alliance is likely enhanced by a therapeutic discourse that promotes a symmetrical rather than an asymmetrical (institutional or authoritative) pattern.

The particular counseling model adopted as a guide by each clinician is influenced by a variety of factors, including the individual's training, personality, and view of the world. As reflected in the various models, a basic issue is the degree to which we indirectly or directly assist our clients in making their own decisions, an issue that may vary both between and within clients. We are likely to employ counseling in some form with most of the people we see, and everyone involved, including spouses and families, is part of the therapeutic process. To the extent that we can show them that we understand their plight and assist them in developing more degrees of freedom in dealing with their problem, our clients will be moving forward. On many occasions, our ability to truly understand and to provide timely support makes more difference to our clients than we realize.

Topics for Discussion

1. Describe the characteristics of an effective therapeutic alliance and ways that the clinician can promote such a relationship with the client.

2. Describe some of Ellis's examples of "irrational thinking" that you have found yourself and others expressing.

3. Considering the emotions discussed by Luterman in this chapter, describe some of the emotions you have experienced when facing a chronic and stressful problem. How do these emotions compare with those your clients have expressed?

4. What are the primary problems with viewing counseling as a process of informing and persuading clients?

5. Describe the key components of Egan's three-stage skilled-helper model.

6. Compare the "attractor states" described by Smith's dynamic-multifactoral model in Chapter 3 with Kelly's "core constructs" in his personal construct theory.

7. Considering the counseling philosophies described by Luterman, describe why one (or more) is more appealing to you than others.

8. Describe the basic elements of the constructivist-narrative counseling approach.

9. What counseling techniques described in this chapter are you most (and least) comfortable with?

10. What is your opinion of Luterman's philosophy of limiting a counseling or therapy session to a specified and finite amount of time? How would you explain this to someone you are assisting?

Recommended Readings

Egan, G. (2002). *The skilled helper: A problem-management and opportunity development approach to helping* (7th ed.). Pacific Grove, CA: Brooks/Cole.

Leahy, M. M. (2004). Therapy talk: Analyzing therapeutic discourse. *Language, Speech and Hearing Services in Schools, 35,* 70–81.

Luterman, D. M. (2001). *Counseling persons with communication disorders and their families* (4th ed.). Austin, TX: PRO-ED.

Manning, W. (2004). "How can you understand? You don't stutter!" *Contemporary issues in Communication Science and Disorders, 31,* 58–68.

St. Louis, K. O. (2001). *Living with Stuttering: Stories, Resources, and Hope.* Morgantown, WV: Populore Publishing Company.

CHAPTER 8

Successful Management of Stuttering for Adolescents and Adults

We must do the thing we think we cannot do.

Helen Keller

Nothing in this world can take the place of persistence.
Talent will not; nothing is more common than unsuccessful people
    with talent.
Genius will not; unrewarded genius is almost a proverb.
Education will not; the world is full of educated derelicts.
Persistence and determination alone are omnipotent.
The slogan "press on" has solved and always will solve
the problems of the human race.

Calvin Coolidge

Chapter Objectives

This chapter describes a variety of treatment options intended for individuals who have stuttered for some time. The primary objective is to provide a rationale and description of the most frequently employed therapeutic models (fluency modification and stuttering modification) as well as some of the less commonly used approaches (pharmacological agents and assistive devices). In many instances clinicians will make use of more than one treatment protocol depending on the response of the speaker, often blending approaches and the associated techniques. As we discussed in Chapter 6, the issue is not that a particular approach is likely to be especially better than another. As long as the common factors that drive therapeutic change are present in a therapeutic protocol the issue is more about the ability of the clinician to determine what is likely to be most beneficial for the speaker at a particular point in time. Regardless of the therapeutic protocol, there are likely to exist a relatively few overarching basic principles that account for therapeutic success. As in the earlier chapters describing the diagnostic process, successful management of stuttering is viewed from a multidimensional perspective in that many aspects of both behavioral and cognitive/affective change are considered essential for success. The concluding portion of the chapter describes the many characteristics and advantages of group therapy.

Understanding What Informs our Treatment Decisions

To this point in the text we have developed several important themes that are essential for the successful therapeutic intervention for individuals who stutter. We have intentionally avoided the discussion of specific treatment techniques in order to first provide the principles that underlie the process of change. For example, we have argued that first and foremost it is important for the clinician to develop a thorough understanding of the stuttering experience and a speaker's successful and unsuccessful efforts to cope with his or her communication problem. Silverman puts it well when he says, "The better able you are to understand the problems your clients will encounter as they try to change, the better able you will be to help them do so" (1996, p. 170). In addition, we have suggested that as clinicians accumulate experience and continue to develop clinical expertise they are more likely to make clinical decisions based on principles rather than rules. Experts are more apt to respond in nondogmatic and creative ways in response to the dynamic characteristics of the person and the situation. We have consistently indicated that, particularly for adolescents and adults who stutter, there are several interrelated goals of treatment for stuttering. Increasing the speaker's fluency (and conversely, decreasing stuttering) is the most obvious goal. But as we indicated in Chapter 6, other, more fundamental, goals include increasing the person's ability to communicate and promoting increased autonomy. And finally, even though the experienced clinician is apt to develop an empirically informed and theoretically based sense of direction about the therapeutic journey, we have maintained that, more than anything else, both the path and the pace of treatment should be set by the individual we are trying to assist. The primary objectives of this chapter are to provide the reader with examples of treatment alternatives based both on the therapeutic philosophy of the clinician and the goals and abilities of the speaker. There are nearly infinite varieties of therapy techniques that the clinician may select, experiment with, and adapt to the therapeutic situation. People who take pride in doing a good job are constantly seeking new tools and adaptations of techniques that are useful to them and compatible with their approach to problem solving.

We begin our discussion of intervention with older speakers, adolescents, and adults who have stuttered for several years, perhaps decades. These individuals are likely to have become sophisticated travelers within the culture of stuttering. By the time we are able to connect with them they have a lengthy history of coping strategies that they have come to rely on. They have made many life choices and important decisions based on the fact that they are a person who stutters. To a greater or lesser degree they have learned how to survive, and because of the shame and stigma associated with stuttering (Bennett & Chmela, 1998; Murphy, 1999), they have learned subtle ways to hide and avoid revealing themselves as a person who stutters. It is not unusual for their fluency breaks to be so well-disguised that the surface features of stuttering behavior are sometimes unapparent, even to the sophisticated observer.

It is good to begin this chapter with a note of optimism regarding treatment for adolescents and adults who stutter, for there is more than enough literature that is confusing or not so encouraging. Because of the volume of information and the many uncertainties about the important issues of etiology, treatment, and relapse, the literature can be discouraging for clinicians interested in helping these somewhat older speakers with fluency problems. As we described in Chapter 1, it is no secret that many clinicians are unsure of the general strategies and specific techniques to employ with those who stutter. Students graduating with a master's degree are no longer required to receive specific training in fluency disorders. They are required, however, to gain experience with the continually increasing variety of concerns that define our scope of practice (e.g., language and learning disabilities, literacy, aphasia, motor-speech problems, dysphagia, neurogenics, augmentative communication, and multicultural aspects of diagnostics and treatment). Fluency disorders, an area that for many years was at the core of the academic and clinical experience of students, is often omitted from the student's program or given far less than adequate emphasis. As a result, many clinicians actively avoid—or at the very least are anxious about—the possibility of working with children and adults with fluency disorders. But as we indicate throughout this book, there are many instances of highly successful management by adolescents and adults who have stuttered. Individuals who have stuttered for years are able to achieve high levels of spontaneous fluency and communicative skill (Anderson & Felsenfeld, 2003; Finn, 1997; Plexico, Manning, & DiLollo, 2005). To be sure, some individuals continue to stutter to a degree, but are able to monitor and modify their stuttering to the point that it has little or no effect on their ability to communicate and to live a high-quality and autonomous lifestyle.

It may be helpful (as well as more realistic) for the clinician to conceptualize the therapy process for speakers who have been stuttering for several years as one of successful management rather than recovery. The term recovery implies that the primary goal of treatment is to cure the speaker and suggests that the speaker has moved from a pathologizing position to a symptom-free condition of normalcy. As we have indicated in Chapter 6, such a view reflects a medical approach to therapeutic change. An alternative understanding of therapeutic- or self-change for many individuals who stutter is one of successful management whereby the person's history of being a person who stutters is incorporated into new and more effective ways of managing stuttering.

The Goals of Therapy

Achieving Fluency

Even for the most severe clients, the quickest way to reduce the frequency of stuttering is to have the speaker use a number of fluency-enhancing techniques or electronic devices that result in nearly instantaneous fluency. It has been known for many years that immediate, if temporary, fluency can be achieved by having most speakers who stutter sing, read, or speak in unison with another person; speak in a loud or whispered voice; use a dialect or bouncy intonation; or speak while rhythmically moving a finger, arm, or leg (Bloodstein, 1949). The fluency-enhancing effects of these activities have been attributed to both the rhythmic effects (Van Riper, 1973), the modification of phonation (Wingate, 1969), and more recently, the activation of the lateral (rather than the medial) pre-motor tract, as discussed in Chapter 3 (Alm, 2004, 2006). Some of the fluency-enhancing activities can provide highly dramatic results, and such in-stantaneous improvements in fluency tend to have the effect of making anyone who uses them an "expert" in helping those who stutter. Although many early stuttering and stammering schools were based on some of these activities, the effects on the speaker's fluency are short-lived (Silverman, 1976).

Assistive Devices

Devices that alter the auditory feedback of the speaker's voice (sometimes referred to as "sidetone") have been shown to passively (vs. active behavioral techniques) enhance the fluency of some individuals who stutter. As discussed in Chapter 3, several explanations have been proposed for the fluency-enhancing effect of such altered or distorted feedback. Although the fluency-enhancing effect of several different forms of auditory feedback distortion results in imme-diate fluency for some speakers there is typically little carryover once the device is removed. The altered auditory feedback (AAF) may be achieved by masking the speaker's auditory feedback (MAF), usually with white noise; delayed audi-tory feedback (DAF) with delays of 75–100 milliseconds; and, more recently, frequency-altered feedback (FAF), which shifts the fundamental frequency of the speaker's voice up or down (for a comprehensive review of the current literature see Lincoln, Packman & Onslow, 2006). Devices that provided masking or delayed auditory feedback were popular in the 1960s through the 1980s. More recent devices are considerably more sophisticated, offering combinations of digitally controlled feedback effects, greater miniaturization, and programmable options.

A good example of a recently developed device is the SpeechEasy®. As a result of marketing and an increasing number of professional presentations and peer-reviewed publications, this device is undoubtedly the most widely known[1]. Some models of the SpeechEasy allow placement behind the speaker's ear or in the ear canal and offer programmable combinations of DAF and FAF alterations of the speaker's auditory feedback. Prior to the introduction of the SpeechEasy device in 2001, a number of laboratory studies demonstrated that combinations of DAF (often set at 20–200 milliseconds) and FAF (e.g., 500 Hz above or below the speaker's voice) often resulted in decreased stuttering (Kalinowski et al., 1993; Kalinowski et al., 1996). The authors propose that speech delay and frequency shifting of the speaker's voice creates a "choral reading effect" similar to that experienced as one reads in unison with another speaker. Group data indicated that speakers experiencing this effect produced significantly less, and in some instances no, stuttering. Stuttering was typically reduced more during reading than conversational speech tasks. However, when individual data was reported, results varied widely with some speakers showing dramatic reductions in stuttering and others showing little or no decrease in the frequency of stuttering (Armson & Stuart, 1998; Ingham, Moglia, Frank, Ingham, & Cordes, 1997). Aside from some evidence (telephone conversations) of a reduction in stuttering during telephone calls and public speaking situations (Kalinowski, Guntupalli, Steward, & Saltuklaroglu, 2004), few studies considered the effect of these devices beyond laboratory or clinic environments. O'Donnell, Armson, and Kiefte (2008) did find that five of seven adults who reduced their stuttering by at least 30% in laboratory settings also experienced reduced stuttering during daily activities (face-to-face and telephone conversations). However, only three of these five participants experienced stable amounts of stuttering reduction (less than 3 %SS) during long-term use (9–16 weeks). O'Donnell et al. pointed out the difficulty in determining the ameliorative effects of the device based on a speaker's performance in laboratory conditions.

Subsequent investigations with the actual SpeechEasy device in clinical settings found similar variability across speakers and speaking tasks (Armson & Kiefte, 2008; Merson, 2003; Molt, 2006a, 2006b; Pollard, Ramig, Ellis, & Finan, 2007). For example Armson, Kiefte, Mason, and De Croos (2006) investigated the effect of the SpeechEasy on the frequency of stuttering for

---

[1]This device is marketed and distributed by the Janus Development Group, Inc. of Greenville, North Carolina.

13 adults ages 21–54 during three speaking tasks of oral reading (two 300-syllable passages), monologue (three-minute talk about a topic of choice), and a five-minute conversation. With speakers performing each of these tasks, the experimenters tabulated percent syllables stuttered (%SS) during a baseline session; two experimental conditions (a *Device Only* condition with DAF and FAF settings set optimally for the speaker and a *Device Plus* condition, the device combined with instructions to the speakers to prolong vowels at the outset of each new breath); and a post-device condition. The 13 participants experienced reductions in stuttering ranging from 50–85% with the greatest reduction occurring during the reading condition. Relative to the baseline condition, the Device Only condition resulted in significantly fewer reductions during the reading (42%), monologue (30%), and conversation (36%). When participants were instructed to prolong vowels during the Device Plus condition, stuttering was significantly reduced by 74%, 36%, and 49%, respectively. Armson et al. (2006) noted large variations in the responses of the individual speakers to the two experimental conditions. As the group data indicated, stuttering was decreased the most for the reading task in comparison to the monologue or conversation tasks, for which speakers had to formulate speech. For 11 of the 13 participants, stuttering increased during the post-device condition. Five speakers showed modest or minimal reduction in their stuttering and the five participants who had highest levels of stuttering at the outset continued to have the highest levels in the post-device condition, a finding also noted by Van Borsel, Reunes, and Van den Berg using delayed auditory feedback (2003).

One of the more consistent and interesting findings is the discrepancy between the extent that the SpeechEasy enables speakers to reduce their stuttering and their satisfaction with the device (Ramig, et al., 2008; Pollard, Ellis, Finan, & Ramig, 2009). Though many speakers continue to stutter to varying degrees with the device in place, they indicate high levels of satisfaction and would choose to purchase the device again. Conversely, investigators have also found speakers who, despite obvious fluency enhancement when using the device, choose not to purchase it (Pollard et al., 2009 and Ramig et al. 2008). Regardless of the fluency-enhancing effect, some speakers reported that the device increased their confidence in the ability to communicate and lessened avoidance and anxiety (Cook & Smith, 2006; Molt, 2006a; O'Donnell, Armson, & Kiefte, 2008; Runyan, Runyan, & Hibbard, 2006). Ramig et al. (2008) suggest that these inconsistencies may reflect the complex and variable nature of stuttering across a variety of communicative situations.

There are several additional issues that may help to explain the lack of correspondence between the resulting fluency and the choice to use such a device. At this writing, the SpeechEasy costs $4,100 to $4,900 depending on the particular model, a cost that is comparable to (or greater than) the cost of more traditional therapy. The initial evaluation (2–3 hours) and audiological fees (a hearing evaluation and ear impression) are approximately $300 to $500 (Ramig et al., 2008). Ramig et al. also point out that although the device may be returned for a 90% refund within 60 days, the total cost to this point is likely to be approximately $1,000. For the majority of speakers, there appears to be little to no carryover of the effect without the device (Stewart, Kalinowski, Rastatter, Saltuklaroglu, & Dayalu, 2004; Molt, 2006b; Pollard et al., 2009). There are, however, indications that some speakers are able to wean themselves from the device[2] and use it only during especially difficult communication situations (Pollard et al. 2007, 2009; Ramig et al., 2008). Despite research indicating that binaural delivery of the signal is more effective than a monaural presentation (Stuart, Kalinowski, & Rastatter, 1997), the devices are normally worn monaurally. As Armson et al. (2006) noted, this monaural arrangement in daily speaking situations allows for the inclusion and distortion of background sounds in noisy environments and the speech of others as well as the speaker's unaltered speech in the other ear. Another issue is the requirement of initiating airflow and voicing during blocking (the device's feedback is voice-activated). In order to initiate the altered feedback, speakers are advised to initiate speech by producing the schwa or /m/ (Stuart et al., 2004). Such techniques are contrary to most traditional therapeutic protocols because they can easily result in undesirable associated (secondary) behaviors. Although the SpeechEasy is designed for both children and adults, clinicians prefer to fit the device with adolescents and adults (Ramig, Ellis, & Pollard, 2009) and little research has taken place with younger speakers. Howell, Sackin, & Williams (1999) found that younger speakers (9–12 years) decreased their stuttering much less than adults in response to frequency-altered feedback (approximately 3% vs. 8.5%, respectively). Because of the documented success of more traditional treatment approaches for younger children, the fitting of such devices with children is especially questionable (Lincoln et al., 2006).

Literature from The Janus Group (SpeechEasy Professional Information Packet) recommends that the SpeechEasy is most effective when used in conjunction with traditional behavioral techniques that assist the speaker in actively changing patterns of stuttering. Preliminary research supports this recommendation (Pollard et al., 2009; Molt, 2006a, 2006b). Of course, traditional therapy, particularly for adults, requires the active participation of the speaker as well as concerted effort and time to produce both cognitive and behavioral change. The less active role required by devices such as the SpeechEasy may explain their appeal to some individuals. Nevertheless, as discussed by Pollard et al. (2009) and Ramig et al., (2008), because of a variety of logistical, socioeconomic, and scheduling issues, it can be difficult for individuals to attend treatment. Even in those instances where individuals are able to obtain a SpeechEasy, professional

---

[2]See the related comments by Alan Badmington in Chapter 12.

help may not be available. Furthermore, it has been suggested that in instances where the speaker has been unable to achieve lasting benefit from other treatment methods, or for individuals with especially severe or chronic stuttering, such devices may be an important adjunct to traditional treatment (Cooper, 1986a; Merson, 2003; Ramig et al., 2008).

Perhaps the most severe criticism of the SpeechEasy is provided by Finn, Bothe, and Bramlett (2005) in suggesting that the research used to support the efficacy of the device is best considered as pseudoscience (Lilienfeld, Lynn, & Lohr, 2003).[3] In 2008 the Janus Corporation initiated a research program that provides support for investigations designed to explore the effectiveness of the SpeechEasy device.

Use of Pharmacological Agents

Researchers have also investigated the fluency-enhancing influences of pharmacological agents for adults who stutter (Bothe, Davidow, Bramlett, Franic, & Ingham, 2006; Brady, 1991; Ingham, 1984). A comprehensive review, employing trial-quality inclusion criteria, was conducted by Bothe et al. (2006), who classified a variety of agents into the following categories along with the problems the agents are intended to treat. The authors point out that none of the agents were intended to be used by individuals who stutter but rather were designed to treat a variety of psychological and medical problems that have in some way been associated with stuttering.

Anticonvulsant Agents (*carbamazepine*), used for the treatment of epilepsy, manic features of bipolar disorder.

Antidepressant Agents: Selective Serotonin Reuptake Inhibitors (*Paroxetine*), used for the treatment of depression, panic disorders, obsessive–compulsive disorders in adults, social anxiety disorder, and posttraumantic stress disorder.

Antidepressant Agents: Tricyclic Antidepressants (*Clomipramine* and *desipramine*), used for the treatment of obsessive–compulsive disorders, depression, panic disorder, and delusional disorder.

Antipsychotic Agents: Conventional (*Haloperidol*), an antipsychotic agent used for treating schizophrenia, Tourette's syndrome, severe behavioral problems, and hyperactivity in pediatric patients.

Antipsychotic Agents: Atypical (*Risperidone*), resulting in fewer side effects than conventional agents, these agents are used for treating bipolar disorder and schizopohrenia.

---

[3]Readers are directed to a lively exchange concerning the efficacy of the SpeechEasy® device in *Language, Speech, and Hearing Services in Schools, 16,* 69–83.

Cardiovascular Agents: Alpha Receptor Agonists   (*Clondine*), used for the treatment of hypertensive and migraine problems and some aspects of Tourette's syndrome.

Cardiovascular Agents: Beta-Receptor Blockers   (*Oxprenolol*), used for treating chronic angina pectoris, hypertension, post-myocardial infarction.

Cardiovacsular Agents: Calcium Channel Blockers   (*Verapamil*), used for the treatment angina, arrythmia, and hypertension.

Dopamine Antagonists   (*Pimozide*), antipsychotic agents used for treating Tourette's syndrome.

Based on their review of 31 articles published between 1970 and 2005, Bothe et al. (2006) concluded that the evidence for using these pharmacological agents was "overwhelmingly negative" (p. 348). They found few instances where the participants' stuttering was reduced below 5%. In some cases where control groups were included (e.g., Maguire et al., 2000, using risperidone) the placebo group experienced nearly the same reduction in stuttering as the experimental group. Even considering what Bothe et al. indicate are relatively lenient standards of improvement (5% stuttering or a 50% reduction in stuttering, or documented improvement in social, emotional, or cognitive variables), there were few examples of meaningful change, particularly beyond the clinic environment. Beyond the poorly demonstrated efficacy of these agents, there was considerable variability in the ability of the participants to tolerate the many dangerous and even deadly side effects (e.g., hyperglycemia, ketoacidosis, hyperosmolar coma). Finally, the authors pointed out potentially dangerous interactions between the agents and other common medications (e.g., blood pressure prescriptions). The findings of Bothe et al. (2006) coincide with a number of other authors who have concluded that there is insufficient evidence to recommend the use of currently available pharmacological agents for the treatment of individuals who stutter.

Fluency and Therapeutic Success

At the outset of treatment, fluent speech is often the primary (and frequently the only) outcome our clients ask of us. Spontaneous and natural-sounding fluency is more likely to be an achievable goal for young children. Something approaching complete fluency is also attainable for the infrequent adult who, as a result of emotional trauma, has experienced a sudden onset of stuttering in adulthood. As the underlying or associated problems are resolved, these speakers may be able to achieve their previous levels of fluency. High levels of fluency may also occur for adults after taking part in an intensive residential program. However, because of logistic or financial reasons, that is not where many clients are able to find help. In addition, the difficult transition from the focused and supportive clinical environment of an intensive program to the speaker's home and work environments often has an adverse effect on the gains made during treatment. It has been suggested that rapid and dramatic improvements that can occur in an intensive program may result in a fluent speaker who is unsure what he or she did to accomplish change (Boberg, 1986). Prins (1970) indicated that intensive residential programs may produce disfluency overkill and provide clients with the notion that stuttering will not occur as long as they follow the techniques they have begun to master. A similar comment is made by Kamhi (1982), who cautions clinicians who suggest to clients that the use of fluency-enhancing techniques will result in error-free speech on all occasions. An insightful statement is also offered by Sheehan (1980), who comments that producing stutter-free speech is no more realistic than playing error-free baseball; just because a person possesses the capacity to function in an error-free manner it does not follow that this will always be the case.

It is not surprising that the surface features of stuttering will be the first to change as a result of treatment. In fact, a speaker may show rapid improvement in his level of fluency prior to initiating treatment (Andrews & Harvey, 1981. During the initial days or weeks of treatment an improvement in fluency is likely to result simply from the speaker's acknowledgement of the problem as well as adaptation to the clinician, the treatment setting, and the client's understanding of the treatment protocol. Certainly, an increase in fluency is reflective of change; however, it does not necessarily indicate progress. That is, the increased fluency in the treatment setting may have little relationship to the client's level of fluency in his daily environment. Even complete fluency in a clinical environment can provide an unrealistic indication about the probability of such success in beyond-treatment speaking situations. It is one thing to hit 10 out of 10 shots when playing basketball alone. The real question is how many shots will be successful during competitive game conditions, when the pressure is great and there are clear penalties for failure.

With a multidimensional approach, the criterion of success in treatment is considerably broader and more inclusive of the many features of the stuttering experience than simply the number of fluency breaks expressed as a percentage of syllables or words stuttered. The descriptions provided by adult speakers who have accomplished successful management of their speech unmistakably indicate that absolute fluency is not a necessary nor sufficient criterion for therapeutic success (Anderson & Felsenfeld, 2003; Krauss-Lehrman & Reeves, 1988; Plexico et al. 2005; Reeves, 2006; St. Louis, 2006; Yaruss & Quesal, 2002; Yaruss, Quesal, & Murphy, 2002). For many adults who have stuttered since childhood, it is not unusual for some fluency breaks to occur following successful treatment. The question is not so much whether the client will stutter, especially during unique, unexpected, or especially difficult communication situations. The more fundamental question is whether or not the person will choose to enter into the situation and how he or she will manage possible stuttering events. As Van Riper often stated, the speaker may not always have much of a choice about *when* he is going to stutter, but he certainly can have a choice about *how* he is going to stutter (Van Riper, 1990).

The Primary Goal of Agency

When discussing the goals of treatment in Chapter 6, we indicated three primary goals. We suggested that when assisting people who stutter we are interested in helping speakers to increase their level of fluency, improve their ability to communicate, and develop their autonomy. Because we consider this third goal to be the most basic of all, we will briefly elaborate on this concept as we prepare to discuss the specifics of treatment. Recall also that in Chapter 7 we suggested that one of the basic goals of counseling is to help our clients in their desire to get unstuck; to free them from the disruptions in their speech and the coping responses that have restricted their quality of life. We would like them to become autonomous and to develop an agentic lifestyle. Monk et al. (1997) define agency as a lifestyle in which people become able to "act for themselves and speak on their own behalf" (p. 301). This, of course, is an especially appropriate goal for individuals who stutter. But more profoundly, with the development of agentic behavior people are able to become the originator rather than the receiver of actions. They can live an autonomous life and make choices as they desire, without the help of others, including their clinician. Furthermore, Drewery, Winslade, and Monk (2000) make the related comment that "health, in our view, has much to do with the capacity for agency and less to do with the absence of disease" (p. 256). These comments coincide with a postmodern (rather than an illness- or disease-based) model of the human change process. In addition, as we will continue to elaborate, agency, or the ability for the speaker to live life and achieve a voice in a literal as well as a metaphorical sense, is not dependent on complete fluency.

Principles of Change for Individuals who Stutter

As we indicated at the outset of this chapter, one objective is to discuss basic principles (rather than specific rules) to be considered when assisting individuals who stutter to alter their situation as it relates to fluency, communication, and agency. With this in mind, we begin to consider the principles of change that are present in a wide variety of treatment approaches and are consistently employed by experienced clinicians when assisting those who stutter. Pachankis and Goldfried (2007) suggest that principles of change are shared by all theoretical perspectives and lie "somewhere between the abstract level of theory and the more concrete level of technique" (p. 55).

A review of many current therapeutic approaches was assisted in large part by the comprehensive summary provided by Guitar in his 2006 text *Stuttering, An Integrated Approach to Its Nature and Treatment,* third edition. In addition, a review of additional manuscripts that investigated the ability of individuals to achieve successful management of their stuttering via therapeutic or self-directed change was conducted (Anderson & Felsenfeld, 2003; Conture, 2001; Finn, 1996; Onslow, Packman & Harrison, 2003; Plexico, Manning, & DiLollo, 2005; Ratner & Guitar, 2006). The principles associated with successful stuttering management also surface in detailed case histories, anecdotal reports, and presentations at professional and support-group meetings. Interestingly, many of these same principles are reflected in the insightful comments by the 14-year-old Brad Sara appearing later in this chapter. There are, of course, variations and interactions of the common themes. Nevertheless, the common factors appear consistently in many treatment protocols both within our field and other related professions (Hubble, Duncan, & Miller, 1999; Luborsky, Rosenthal, Diguer et al, 2002; Luborsky, Singer, & Luborsky, 1975; Pachankis, & Goldfried, 2007; Rosenzweig, 1936; Walmpold, 2001; Wampold & Brown, 2005). The following are four basic principles that, as clinicians, we can reflect on as we assist our clients along their journey of successful therapeutic change.

Move toward rather than away from the problem. Professionals are likely to refer to this as an approach–avoidance continuum. As most of us have experienced or at least witnessed on the news, often it is not the crime, it is the cover-up that creates the greatest problem. Whatever the nature of the problem, moving away from the situation through denial or avoidance nearly always makes the situation worse. Experienced clinicians provide innumerable examples of activities that assist children and adults who stutter to move toward the problem, become desensitized, confront the situation, and take action (e.g., Guitar, 2006; Chemla & Reardon, 2001; Murphy, Yaruss & Quesal, 2007(a, b); Reardon & Yarusss, 2004; Sheehan, 1970; Van Riper, 1973; Williams, 1971, 1983).

It is clear that the process of approaching stuttering involves the related theme of acceptance or at least acknowledgement of the situation (Plexico, Manning, & DiLollo, 2005; Sheehan & Martin, 1966, 1970; Wingate, 1964). We use the term acceptance not in a passive sense indicating that the person is resigned to his or her circumstances. Rather, we are suggesting that by accepting, or perhaps integrating, the experience of stuttering, people achieve the opportunity to become fully engaged with the problem and become desensitized to the extent that they can begin to experiment with creative and alternative responses to their situation. The process is similar to the notion of *mindfulness,* whereby the person pays attention to an experience as it occurs in the present moment, without judgment. Rather than trying to change the situation or circumstance by struggling against the experience—often

Clinical Insight

One of the common events when paddling in white water is the experience of encountering a large rock or a wave that rolls back on itself, called a hydraulic. If you are new to paddling your instinct is to struggle against the often powerful flow of the river to avoid a threatening obstacle. Of course, as a novice, you are often unable to avoid the barriers to your progress as you flow down the river. As you approach obstacles your instinct is to lean back (upstream) away from the problem. But you quickly learn that when you respond in this way you will immediately find yourself upside-down. This is where a good coach can help. With proper instruction and experience, you'll discover something that's both subtle and amazing. You learn that, rather than expending so much effort trying to elude the obstacles, you'll have much better success by actively moving toward them! For example, as you approach a rock you will notice a pillow of water recoiling off the rock that will help you to move around it. You realize that the pillow of water wasn't detectable until you allowed yourself to get close to the rock. Furthermore, if you throw your upper body *into* the rock you find increased stability and you will be able to use the rock for support. Similarly, if you lean into a hydraulic on the river or a wave on the ocean—not just tentatively reach for it with your paddle, but actively throw yourself into it with your paddle and entire upper body—you will achieve increased and dramatic stability as you use the energy of the water to support and right yourself. As you learn these techniques, paddling becomes much more dynamic and enjoyable and you begin to connect with the river. You can now begin to dramatically improve your paddling experience and enjoy the journey.

in unhelpful ways that result in increased tension and dissatisfaction—such mindfulness invites us to just be with what it is (Cheasman, 2007). Paradoxically, such a response can result in more positive and helpful changes in the experience. As Cheasman states, "It seems as though sometimes the best way of getting from A to B is to just allow ourselves to be at A!" (2007, p. 10).

Assume the responsibility for taking action. As we have suggested in earlier chapters, although specific techniques are an important part of a therapeutic program, the treatment process is far more comprehensive than any set of specific techniques. Clinicians are likely to use behavioral techniques that they have become comfortable with and that they feel have been useful to previous clients. Individuals, however, will not necessarily see these techniques in the same way. It is the speaker, who, based on such factors as his or her level of desensitization to stuttering, understanding of the technique(s) and ability in and motivation for using the techniques, will make the decision whether or not to use them, particularly in situations beyond the treatment setting.

Regardless of the treatment protocol, it is the speaker who will need to take responsibility for identifying and developing their strengths. The speaker will need to take action by learning to self-monitor his or her performance and practice the techniques in daily communication situations. The behavioral techniques are not usually difficult to master within the safety and support of the therapeutic environment. The more difficult challenge is discovering ways to motivate the speaker to diligently practice the techniques in daily speaking situations, particularly situations that provide gradually increasing levels of communicative stress. As we emphasized in Chapter 6, to the extent that individuals are able to practice beyond the treatment environment and make use of the many important extratherapeutic factors, real progress takes place (Hubble, Duncan, & Miller, 1999; Miller, Duncan, and Hubble, 1997; Lambert, 1992). Miller et al. (1997), for example, found that regardless of the therapeutic approach, participation in extratherapeutic activities and events accounted for approximately 40% of positive therapeutic outcome in psychotherapy while specific methods or techniques accounted for only 15%.

As with most forms of training or therapy, the extent to which the person practices between sessions is a major determinant of mastery. Continual practice on a daily basis will result in a level of proficiency (and eventually expertise, as described in Chapter 1) whereby the speaker becomes one with the techniques. The techniques gradually begin to feel and sound more comfortable and habitual. Rather than consciously choosing to use a technique, the speaker immediately reacts to the impending or actual disruption of fluency with the new response and moves forward with the flow of speech. Furthermore, because the person has successfully employed the technique on many occasions, a level of self-efficacy or confidence develops, which increases the likelihood of continued progress.

Restructure the cognitive view of the self and the problem. When people come to us with a history of suffering, struggle, and a restricted lifestyle where stuttering is a dominant theme, as described in Chapter 4, there is little doubt that some form of cognitive restructuring is required in order to achieve a successful therapeutic outcome. As noted throughout the previous chapters, the severity of the problem presented by stuttering is represented by these intrinsic features as much as or more than it is by the more obvious surface behaviors. Those who have studied the ability of individuals to make the transition to the successful management of stuttering have found that cognitive restructuring is an important part of the process (Anderson-Felsenfeld, 2003; Corcoran & Stewart, 1998; Crichton-Smith, 2002; Finn, 1996; Plexico et al. 2005). Such cognitive changes are especially important for long-term success. As a result of speakers' ability to reconstrue themselves and their situation, they become increasingly assertive. They are able to take risks by acknowledging their stuttering and entering into difficult speaking situations; themes associated with successful change as reported by Anderson and Felsenfeld (2003) and Plexico et al. (2005). In addition these authors found that participants indicated a reciprocal relationship in that cognitive changes facilitated the use of behavioral (speech) techniques and that the successful use of behavioral techniques led to further cognitive change.

Recruit the support of others. Closely related to the first three principles is the action required to identify individuals or groups who are able to provide mentorship and support. Mentors and support groups have been found to be important aids in the successful management of stuttering (Plexico et al. 2005; Plexico & Manning, 2007). For those who stutter, mentors may be clinicians or other people who stutter who have achieved success. Members of support groups (see Chapter 12) can provide invaluable support and understanding as the person is able to connect with others who share a similar story. Observing individuals who have achieved success on many levels can provide the encouragement to undertake a similar journey that will result in the creation of a new set of strategies for modifying the speaker's present situation. If possible, it is especially important to elicit the support and understanding of individuals who are part of the speaker's daily environment in order for them to recognize and reward the many indicators of successful change (see Chapter 11). Accordingly, as soon as possible, it is useful to have these individuals (e.g., parents, spouse, friends, coworkers) attend one or more treatment sessions so that they can appreciate what success looks and sounds like and so that they can acknowledge and verify it and help to place the changes into an historical context.

Choosing a Treatment Strategy

Depending on how one conceptualizes the treatment strategies available for assisting those who stutter, there are several options open to the clinician. Therapy approaches vary according to such factors as the therapeutic philosophy, treatment goals and associated activities, duration and intensity of the sessions, and the age of the person who is receiving assistance. Although different treatment protocols may vary in one or more of these characteristics, for the most part, the principles of change and common factors described earlier are common to each of them (see Chapter 6).

Most recent graduates of an academic program are apt to adopt the treatment protocols they were taught and are familiar with. However, as professional clinicians achieve increased levels of competency they are less likely to employ a rigid, dogmatic therapeutic approach. They begin to take greater responsibility for elaborating their clinical philosophy and adopting their clinical techniques to match their clinical style. As described in Chapter 1, experts develop a flexible and holistic approach where the focus is on the person they are helping.

Most treatment strategies for people who stutter are reasonably straightforward and easy to understand. However, it is one thing to be able to grasp

Clinical **Insight**

It is good, as I have mentioned previously, to be wary of those who intensely advocate for a particular therapeutic approach, particularly if at the same time they rage against the perceived inadequacies of others. On occasion, the literature concerning treatment strategies has taken on the flavor of the commentaries by zealous political or religious groups. In such instances, authors, who are certain of their virtue, invite the reader to take a stand concerning the treatment of this problem, offering a sure road to success to the exclusion of other possibilities. In nearly all cases, such injunctions do more harm than good. In fact, there are many therapeutic approaches that have been shown to help people who stutter. To be sure, the logic and techniques associated with most intervention strategies provide the clinician with a framework and a sense of direction about treatment. Each strategy can provide something of value for the clinician and the client, depending on such variables as the abilities and needs of the client, the stage of treatment, and the expertise of the clinician. As Bloodstein (1999) comments, "Almost any therapy has the power to eliminate stuttering in someone, sometime, someplace."

the description of a technique in a textbook and quite another to know when and how to apply the technique when responding to a particular individual during treatment. Despite what may be written in a text or treatment manual, the most appropriate clinical choice is not always obvious, even to the experienced clinician. Some experimentation may be required. Whatever the rationale and structure of the treatment program, the process of change is far more dynamic than the application of techniques. At its finest, effective intervention is the result of the clinician's astute and precise response to the person who has come for help. These responses become more likely as treatment progresses and the clinician becomes calibrated to the client. Depending on the client, the clinician may use a variety of techniques and possibly more than one overall treatment strategy. Even if a single overall strategy is used, the application will never be quite the same with each client. Our clients respond diversely to identical behavioral techniques, just as people do to identical dosages of the same medications.

When initiating treatment the first decision for the clinician is the choice of a general intervention strategy. There are many paths for the clinician to follow, each with something to offer. We will begin by simplifying the situation and discussing the most fundamental approaches: fluency modification and stuttering modification. We will also discuss a third option, a strategy of cognitive restructuring that, although sometimes used independently, is more typically combined with the first two approaches. To take the possibilities further, ASHA's Guidelines for Practice in Stuttering Treatment[4] describe a total of 10 treatment goals involving a variety of treatment choices.

The essential difference between fluency modification, stuttering modification, and cognitive reconstruction is best illustrated by considering the relative emphasis placed on the surface and intrinsic features of stuttering. Fluency modification approaches may be thought of as a form of physical therapy for the speech production system. The primary goal with this strategy is to enhance fluency by altering how the speaker uses his or her respiratory, phonatory and articulatory systems. One assumption of the fluency-modification strategy is that once the client has learned new ways of producing fluent speech, he or she will eventually show a corresponding change in the cognitive and affective features of his or her problem. Relatively little counseling in a traditional sense takes place. Fluency-modification programs tend to be highly structured and often manualized. A highly detailed description of such a program may be found in Ryan's 2001 text *Programmed Therapy for Stuttering in Children and Adults*. It is interesting to note, as have others (McFarlane & Goldberg, 1987; Ratner & Healey, 1999), that fluency-modification approaches tend to be favored by clinicians who do not have a personal history of stuttering, whereas stuttering-modification approaches tend to be the treatment of choice by clinicians who have experienced stuttering.

The stuttering-modification strategy, by nature, requires more cognitive intensity on the part of the clinician as well as the speaker. The speaker must not only evaluate and change his or her manner of speaking but must also attend to and alter his or her cognitive and attitudinal responses as well. As a result, informal counseling in some form is typically an integral part of this approach. Stuttering-modification programs are somewhat less structured and take a more eclectic view of stuttering, involving layers of behavioral and cognitive change. As a result, stuttering-modification is generally somewhat more difficult to teach and to learn, and it generally takes longer for the speaker to achieve fluency than with a fluency-modification approach. Shapiro (1999, pp. 184–191) provides a succinct description comparing the rationale, goals, and procedures for fluency- and stuttering-modification approaches.

Citing Peters and Guitar (1991), Shapiro (1999, p. 191) provides suggestions for initiating therapy with a fluency- or stuttering-modification approach.

---

[4] The Guidelines for Practice in Stuttering Treatment can be accessed via ASHA's website at http://www.asha.org/docs/html/GL1995-00048.html.

A stuttering-modification approach may be indicated if the speaker:

- hides or disguises his or her stuttering,
- avoids speaking,
- perceives personal penalty as a consequence of stuttering,
- feels poorly about self as a communicator, and
- demonstrates a more positive response to stuttering modification trial therapy.

A fluency-modification approach may be indicated if the speaker:

- stutters openly,
- does not avoid speaking,
- perceives annoyance or interference but no personal penalty from stuttering,
- feels positive about self as a communicator, and
- demonstrates a positive response to fluency shaping trial therapy.

With the third generic path, which we have termed cognitive restructuring, the cognitive and attitudinal features of the stuttering experience are the major focus of treatment. In a pure version of this approach, relatively little effort is directed toward the direct modification of speech or fluency. The primary goal is to change the way in which clients consider both themselves and their stuttering and interpret the responses of others. By decreasing avoidance behavior and becoming more assertive, the speaker is often able to make significant changes in the handicapping nature of stuttering. Rather than fighting speech blocks, the speaker is asked to stutter more openly and with less effort. Although the frequency of stuttering moments will stay the same or even increase, the quality of the fluency will improve. In addition, and most important, the quality of the client's communication style, as well as overall lifestyle, will often change for the better.

Although there are obvious differences between these three generic treatment strategies, they are far from mutually exclusive. For example, the consistent contact between the clinician and the client that is required during any treatment approach is, by nature, interpersonal and offers the likelihood of some form of supportive counseling. The very nature of a clinician working closely with an individual and guiding him or her through the many components of treatment provides the client with support and insight about the problem. Therapy, by definition, is always personal, for treatment involves one person assisting another in order to define and manage the problem (Emerick, 1988). Any systematic analysis and subsequent self-management of attitudes and speech behaviors will provide a degree of desensitization during treatment. Whether or not counseling is regarded as a basic or formal goal of treatment, in some form it is taking place if the client is being listened to, encouraged, motivated, and challenged.

In addition, during the later stages of stuttering-modification treatment, many of the fluency-initiating techniques (e.g., air flow, light articulatory contact, slow and effortless transitions from one sound or syllable to another) used during fluency modification coincide with and complement the stabilization and maintenance activities. Each strategy requires that the speaker monitor and practice techniques, first within the treatment setting and then gradually beyond the security of the clinic, in daily speaking situations. Each method places great emphasis on the client taking primary responsibility for self-management. By beginning from somewhat different perspectives, each approach can result in increased fluency, as well as increased assertiveness and risk-taking behavior. Finally, each approach can result in a significant reduction of the client's handicap associated with his or her fluency disorder.

Fluency-Modification Strategies

It is not usually difficult to invoke fluency even for individuals with the most severe stuttering. Bloodstein (1949, 1950) identified as many as 115 speaking activities or conditions where stuttering was reduced or absent. Such circumstances included activities such as speaking alone or during a relaxed state; speaking in unison with others; talking to an animal or an infant or in time to a rhythmic stimulus; singing; speaking with a dialect; talking and simultaneously writing; speaking during auditory masking or delayed auditory feedback; shadowing another speaker; or speaking in a slow, prolonged manner. These fluency-enhancing activities also increase fluency for typically fluent speakers and involve combinations of altered vocalization (Wingate, 1969), enhancement of the speaking rhythm (Van Riper, 1973), distraction, and decreased communicative stress.

Many of the basic targets for achieving fluent speech described in fluency-modification programs are analogous to the five parameters of forward-moving speech described by Dean Williams in his classic 1957 article "A point of view about 'stuttering'." Williams described the following five basic things a speaker must do in order to achieve fluent speech: (1) generate a consistent flow of air from the lungs; (2) create movement of the rib change and abdomen and articulators; (3) achieve timing and coordination for the onset and rate of movement for respiratory, phonatory, and articulatory activities; (4) initiate the onset of laryngeal movement for voicing and making the transition between voiceless to voiced sounds; and (5) produce appropriate levels of muscular tension required for moving the articulators. A basic aspect of Williams's view was that in order for those who stutter to be able to achieve fluency, speakers first must fully understand what they do to interfere with the achievement of these five parameters necessary for fluency.

Fluency-modification programs apply many of the principles discussed by Williams (1957) to help speakers make more efficient use of their speaking mechanisms. Fluency is created, often making use of slowed and prolonged speech segments to instate fluency with single words, gradually expanding to sentences and eventually conversational speech both within and beyond the clinical setting. The earliest versions of fluency-modification approaches were based on behavior-modification paradigms and typically placed little or no emphasis on the intrinsic features of the stuttering experience (Cordes & Ingham, 1998; Costello, 1983; Ingham, 1984; Perkins, 1973; Ryan, 1980, 2001; and Webster, 1974). No effort was made to deal directly with the speaker's cognitions concerning loss of control, fear, anxiety, and helplessness associated with stuttering. More recently, clinicians using a behavior modification approach have tended to broaden the focus of therapy to include cognitive and affective factors in the treatment process (e.g., Langevin, Huinck, Kully, Peters, Lomheim, & Tellers, 2006; Langevin & Kully, 2003; Langevin, Kully, & Ross-Harold, 2006).

An example of a fluency-modification program that has been used for many years is the precision fluency shaping program (PFSP) developed by Webster (1975), mentioned in Chapter 3. With this program, stuttering is viewed as a physical phenomenon, and there is usually little or no discussion concerning the emotional or affective impact on the person who stutters. The premise is that if the speaker follows the rules of speech mechanics the resulting speech will be fluent; if the rules are violated and the physical targets are not achieved, speech will not be fluent. With the assistance of a visual feedback system the client is carefully taken through five gradations of muscle movements associated with the features of each sound class (e.g., vowels, glides, fricatives, plosives). Clients are informed about the vocal tract features associated with speech and learn the specific muscle movements associated with the fluent production of each class of sounds. The initial goal of the speaker is to achieve movement targets related to respiration, phonation, speech rate, voice onset, and articulation. Once the speaker consistently achieves these targets, the responses are then gradually transferred to longer and more complex speech sequences and ultimately to conversational speech. All the while, the ability of the speaker to self-monitor the accuracy of their targets is emphasized. Transfer activities are structured such that the speaker is able to gradually progress from simple, one-message questions to complex conversational dialogues in natural settings. Clients are provided with systematic opportunities to practice new speaking skills in a wide variety of treatment and, during the final week of the program, beyond-treatment settings. Booster sessions are also provided to clients who desire them.

Bloodstein and Bernstein Ratner (2008) provide a summary of a recently developed prolonged speech program for adults at the Australian Stuttering Research Centre. Known as the Camperdown Program (named for a neighborhood in Sydney), the approach avoids the problems that clinicians encounter when instructing and evaluating speakers as they attempt to achieve the various fluency targets. As Bloodstein and Bernstein Ratner describe:

> Rather than detailed instruction in specific speech targets, participants in the program imitate a videotaped model of the desired speech pattern until clinicians agree that the speech pattern resembles that of the model. Then

participants may adjust their speech pattern in any way that they wish to eliminate stuttering during a requisite three-minute monologue. This is then followed by an intensive group practice day, in which participants also learn to monitor their speech fluency and naturalness. Fluency instatement is then followed by weekly problem-solving sessions and patients move to a Performance-Contingent Maintenance Phase after three weekly sessions in which within- and beyond-clinic fluency and naturalness measures reach a set criterion. (p. 358)

Because, as mentioned previously, fluency-modification treatments tend to be behavioral, highly structured, and sometimes manualized, they can be easier to teach than stuttering modification or—especially—cognitive restructuring strategies. However, as Conture (2001) points out, being able to modify aspects of fluent or stuttering behavior does not mean that we are necessarily changing all, or even the most critical, aspects of the problem. After many years of conducting behavioral studies in fluency disorders, Siegel (1970) provided a perceptive review of the problems and unresolved issues inherent in the behavioral-modification approach. Prins and Hubbard (1988) also pointed out some of the potential problems associated with this therapeutic strategy. Nevertheless, behavior modification protocols have provided valuable information about the efficacy of procedures that clinicians can use to modify the surface features of stuttering.[5]

Stuttering-Modification Strategies

The stuttering-modification strategy is also referred to as the traditional, Van Riperian, or nonavoidance approach. One premise of this approach is that central to the problem is the speaker's fear, avoidance, and struggle to escape from stuttering. Thus, a primary focus of stuttering-modification strategies is the reduction and management of fear, avoidance, and struggle. These goals are accomplished via a series of steps that help the speaker to understand and identify their stuttering, achieve desensitization to the stuttering experience, and gradually alter their stuttering into intentional, open, smooth, and less effortful forms. A key part of the process is the speaker's ability to replace the old, out-of-control, reflexive stuttering with the new, more desirable, "easy stuttering."[6] A common misconception of this treatment strategy is that it is designed to create "happy stutterers" who are content to stutter away merrily with no fear or avoidance. Although for some speakers such an outcome would represent a much improved

---

[5]Although the Lidcombe program for preschool children is proposed as a form of behavior therapy, as we will suggest in the following chapter, the program has many other components that likely account for its success.
[6]In spite of the oxymoronic nature of the term, this form of stuttering has been referred to as "fluent stuttering," indicating that the speaker is fully "in charge" of his or her speech.

situation, in fact, many speakers also achieve speech that is spontaneously fluent. Others, who, following therapy, may continue to produce some obvious fluency breaks, are able to successfully manage their previously uncontrolled stuttering moments and to make choices that are less influenced by the possibility of stuttering. Examples of this approach can be found in many sources, including Conture, (2001), Guitar (2006), Luper and Mulder (1964), Shapiro (1999), Sheehan (1970), Van Riper (1973), and Williams (1971, 1983, 2004).

With this approach, along with the achievement of fluency, there is also a major emphasis on the speaker's reinterpretation of themselves and the stuttering experience. Although the eventual achievement of fluency is obviously an indicator of progress, the quality of the stuttering is also of primary concern. Progress is seen and heard as the speaker begins to be able to alter high levels of tension and fragmentation of an utterance into fluency breaks characterized by less effort, improved airflow, and increased smoothness. Moments of stuttering are systematically identified and old patterns of stuttering are varied and modified into easier stuttering. The speaker eventually incorporates the new cognitive and behavioral responses to stuttering into conversational speech during treatment as well as daily speaking situations beyond the treatment environment.

In part, because the clinical alliance is a particularly important characteristic of the stuttering-modification approach, this strategy may be somewhat difficult for the new clinician to conceptualize. Observing a clinician demonstrate this approach is especially important when learning treatments that involve the important affective and cognitive features of stuttering. This approach requires the clinician to be particularly sensitive to the client's ability to move through the various stages of affective, behavioral, and cognitive change. The clinician will need to adjust the nature and timing of the activities and will be less able to "go by the book" or use a treatment manual. Although not always directly addressed, cognitive and affective changes may also occur during fluency-modification programs as clients begin to consider and construct new ways of thinking about themselves and their ability to communicate.

The stuttering-modification strategy, as described by Van Riper (1982), takes the client through the stages of Identification, Desensitization, Variation, Modification, and Stabilization.

Identification

Speakers are first asked to identify both the surface and cognitive features of their stuttering. They are asked to identify, analyze, and confront the specifics of their individual patterns of stuttering. For example, with the assistance of the clinician, clients can make a list of "things I do when I stutter" to identify the surface features of their stuttering. These are behaviors that can be observed in a mirror, recorded, and identified on video- and audiotapes. The identification

Clinical **Insight**

On the afternoon of one of our first therapy sessions, I was helping Joyce, a woman in her fifties, to identify some of the characteristic behaviors that accompanied her moments of stuttering. As we worked together to identify and experiment with the various behaviors we were seeing and hearing, I commented on a particularly severe example. With a good deal of enthusiasm I told her that what she had just done was "a really fascinating and wonderful way of stuttering." My interest and positive attitude about a behavior that had represented only embarrassment, shame, and misery for more than 50 years elicited spontaneous laughter from her and from me as well as I experienced her delight.

of features that occur frequently during treatment is often a good place to begin simply because there are multiple occurrences.

Some speakers, especially if they also have characteristics of cluttering (Chapter 10), will have difficulty identifying and monitoring overt behaviors that are obvious to the listener. They may also miss short but obvious fluency breaks. In such situations the clinician can become a "human tape recorder." Rather than recording and replaying examples of stuttering on an audio or video tape (which, while somewhat cumbersome, may also help) the clinician can replicate what the speaker does on a real-time basis. By paying close attention to the speaker, the clinician can shadow the person's fluent speech and imitate the person's fluency breaks as they occur, immediately "playing them back" to the speaker. As the clinician closely follows the speaker and accurately imitates the physical and acoustic characteristics of the fluency break, the self-monitoring skills of the speaker improve.

Another list, termed "things I do because I stutter," can include the less obvious, intrinsic features such as avoidances, anxieties, feelings of fear and helplessness, and the decisions and choices the speaker makes because of the possibility of stuttering. These choices may not be obvious and typically take longer to discover. For example, speakers may not associate many of their decisions to avoid certain words or activities with stuttering, thinking that "this is just who I am." Depending on the age and maturity of the client, there are several ways to for the clinician to describe this process, including the following:

> Our goal at the outset is to create a map of the territory we will be traveling through. At the outset of our journey we want to understand the nature of the terrain and some of our options. In order to make the trip less mysterious and frightening, we want to understand the places that are likely to be particularly difficult. We want to know what skills and strengths we can bring along with

us to help us respond to and perhaps change some of the things that we will encounter. As with any adventure, parts of the journey will be more difficult than others. But I want you to know that you are not alone and that together we will be able to make good choices. We know the direction we want to go, and there are many victories that await you along the way.

Although the clinician will obviously lead the way during the initial stages of identifying the characteristics of the speaker and his or her stuttering, it is important for the client to take the lead in developing this list. This is likely to be the first time the person has been asked to assume this level of responsibility for the behavioral and cognitive features of his or her stuttering. By writing down and analyzing these surface and intrinsic features, the client is taking the first step toward self-management. In addition (as we will discuss in greater detail in a section of this chapter titled A Constructivist-Narrative Approach), this activity provides a way for the person to begin to externalize and objectify the features of the problem.

At the outset of treatment the clinician may also ask the client to prepare an autobiography. The goal here is to understand the client's story and the influence that stuttering has played in the many facets of the person's life to this point. The assignment may also reveal something about how motivated the client is, his or her general intellectual and linguistic abilities, and his or her understanding about the nature of stuttering. After some training by the clinician, the speaker can also analyze tapes of him- or herself or other people who stutter in order to begin categorizing and understanding the different surface features of stuttering. A good place to begin is to identify examples of good stuttering, the relatively brief and effortless examples of stuttering moments that most clients produce. These forms of relatively easy stuttering provide a good example of the more fluent stuttering we would like the speaker to eventually produce and which are usually easier for the person to approach and analyze than the more effortful and complex forms of stuttering. Although we want to identify and demystify as many characteristics of the speaker's stuttering as possible, some features may not be obvious until we become calibrated to the speaker and his or her cognitive and linguistic styles.

During this initial stage of therapy the speaker is inclined to be highly motivated, for they have reached the stage where they are ready to take action about their problem. Clinicians can take this opportunity to demonstrate a genuine interest and curiosity as, along with the speaker, they begin to explore how the client manifests the problem in his or her own unique way. The clinician has the opportunity to introduce information about what stuttering is and what it is not. To the extent that the speaker is able to understand and become desensitized to the stuttering experience, this initial stage of exploration will be an exciting first step in the process of change.

Desensitization

As the speaker begins to appreciate that many of his or her responses to stuttering (or the possibility of stuttering) are understandable and natural, he or she will experience a degree of desensitization to both the overt (surface) and covert (intrinsic) features of the experience. For many people this is a critical step, because it will be difficult to critically identify, analyze, and vary behavior without achieving at least some distance and objectivity. For some clients who continue to be overwhelmed by the stuttering experience, identification and desensitization will take considerably longer. Eventually, the speaker will understand that it is possible to stay still in the midst of stuttering and to reduce their fear to a manageable level. The person will begin to realize that they are not as helpless as in the past and that they have some options. As the speaker is able to stay in the moment[7] of stuttering with some level of objectivity, the stage is set for beginning to vary the surface features of stuttering.

If the clinician has not already done so, he or she may want to consider introducing the idea of stuttering on purpose, a technique often termed voluntary, intentional, or pseudostuttering. As we indicated in Chapter 4, the speaker's response to this activity provides the clinician with a clear indication of the fear associated with the stuttering experience. Until the speaker is able to decrease excessive levels of fear to more manageable levels, he or she will have little success in the succeeding steps of treatment.

The clinician often introduces voluntary stuttering by asking the client to follow him or her in producing easy one- or two-unit repetitions and brief (1–2 second) prolongations. The clinician demonstrates to the client that it is possible to stutter and remain calm and completely in control of their speaking. Some speakers who are quite desensitized may want to experiment with more elaborate stuttering, gradually incorporating the characteristics that are typical of their stuttered speech during more severe moments, including struggle behaviors such as the blocking of airflow and voicing. Speakers can voluntarily stutter in a variety of treatment (including telephone calls) and beyond-treatment settings in order to continually desensitize themselves, acknowledge their stuttering to others, and extend their levels of assertiveness.

It is not surprising that some speakers will resist the idea of stuttering on purpose. It seems counterintuitive to perform the very behavior they have come to us to help them prevent. However, with the clinician leading the way, voluntary stuttering opens the door for the speaker to experiment with other ways of stuttering and to become continually desensitized to the stuttering moment. After fighting for so many years to keep from stuttering they can "let go" and

---

[7]Videos available from the Stuttering Foundation (# 1076, 1079, 1080) provide good examples of experienced clinicians modeling and encouraging speakers to stay in the moment of stuttering in order to experience desensitization and to vary and modify their habitual responses to stuttering.

(likely for the first time) give themselves "permission" to stutter. Many people find this to be a highly liberating experience that characteristically results in dramatically increased fluency. Perhaps most importantly, stuttering on purpose—particularly if it is done in an open and easy manner—provides a way for the speaker to break the link between the experience of stuttering and being out of control. As the speaker learns to stay in the moment of stuttering, he will gradually see that instead of being helpless, he or she has some good options available for revising his or her fluency.

Variation

As the speaker becomes able to identify specific behaviors and attitudes and to decrease his reflexive reaction of anxiety and fear associated with the anticipation or onset of stuttering, he will slowly achieve the ability to make some changes. Instead of seeing stuttering as something that feels like it is "happening to him," he begins to recognize that much of his stuttering is a result of the decisions he is making about speaking; things that he can identify and change. Coaching by the clinician during the moment of stuttering provides the speaker with a model for altering selected features of stuttering.

Of course, going from his old, reflexive, and automatic pattern of stuttering to fluent speech is an enormous leap and not one that he should be expected to accomplish early in treatment. The speaker will have a much greater chance of success if he is asked to simply alter or vary some selected features of his stuttering. A small step forward is all that is necessary—or expected—at the outset. Moreover, success is apt to be intermittent. As during the Identification stage, secondary or surface behaviors (eye blinks, junk words, postponement devices) that occur frequently, and are especially distracting or unappealing, are ideal features on which to concentrate. The speaker is not asked to stop performing these features, but rather to vary them in some preplanned and creative manner. That is, the person may select the behavior of producing a series of "ahs" prior to the utterance of a feared word. Rather than attempting to cease production of the "ah" as a postponement or timing device as he anticipates a feared word, he could begin to systematically vary the rate, intensity, number, or type of vowel segment (e.g., "eh," "oh," or "uh," instead of "ah"). As long as the speaker achieves some measure of control as evidenced by his ability to vary his old automatic utterance of "ah," a victory is achieved.

Another example might involve the slight variation of the especially difficult and scary blocks where airflow and voicing have stopped. At the initial stages of variation, a speaker may be able to move from being stuck to saying the word fluently. However, a more likely victory is for the speaker to let some air leak out in order to achieve airflow and possibly even voicing. Although some of these activities will detract from the speaker's overall fluency, the critical issue is the ability of the person to achieve a degree of control over his or her speech, a degree of control that he or she has never before experienced or appreciated. The variation of this previously uncontrolled behavior will set the stage for the client to modify his or her stuttering in more specific and refined ways.

A useful technique that has been advocated by many clinicians, including Dean Williams, has been termed "freezing." As the desensitized speaker willingly continues to stutter, the clinician explains and demonstrates how the stuttering can be systematically altered. The primary goal is to experiment and to "play" with the possibilities for stuttering in a different, easier, manner. With this coaching by the clinician the speaker continues to become desensitized and begins to recognize what he or she is doing to prevent the forward movement of speech and the transition to the next sound, syllable, or word. While following instructions by the clinician to slowly allow airflow and a gradual lessening of tension and struggle, the speaker attends to the physiological features necessary for making the transition to the next speech segment.

This form of coaching is vividly demonstrated on videos available through the Stuttering Foundation (see especially #76, Do you Stutter?: Straight Talk for Teens; #79, Therapy in Action: The School-Age Child Who Stutters; and #83, If you Stutter: Advice for Adults). Such coaching might sound something like the following, in which a client is describing a conversation with his supervisor:

Client: "I was trying to tell my su, su, su . . ."

Clinician: *(reaching quickly to touch the arm of the client)* "Good, OK get that one . . . stay with it. Keep stuttering just as you are.
Now see if you can gradually begin to slow the rate of your repetitions slightly."

Client: The client continues to repeat the syllable "su" and finds that he is able to continue stuttering while gradually slowing his rate of repetitions.

Clinician: "Now, produce the repetitions more rapidly. Now slowly again." *(Client does so.)*
"Good, now slow down again and slowly move through the word by slowly stretching out the sounds and continue."

Modification

Now that speakers have become knowledgeable about their stuttering, somewhat desensitized, and have experienced success in varying their typical pattern of stuttering, they are asked to develop more focused and specific responses. Again, the goal is to replace the habitual, reflexive and out-of-control stuttering with a new, smoother (although not necessarily fluent) utterance.

It is important for both the clinician and client to appreciate that the old behavioral (and cognitive) responses to stuttering are well-practiced and habitual.

The old patterns of speaking are also comfortable and, on many occasions, what is expected by both the speaker and the listener. The new, albeit better, ways of speaking will feel awkward and strange until they are practiced enough and begin to become habituated. Smith (1997) proposes a helpful theoretical explanation of what occurs as clinicians attempt to assist a person who has stuttered for many years. She suggests that stuttering behaviors may be best considered as hypercoordinated rather than discoordinated behaviors[8]. That is, complex systems have a tendency to self-organize and settle into a mode of behavior that is preferred over other possible modes (attractor states). The more stable the attractor state the more effort or energy is required to move the system out of that condition. The process of change may involve helping the system (or person) to reorganize in order to move from a coordinated and stable mode of functioning to a different and unstable mode. Furthermore, because many systems are likely to function in a nonlinear and dynamic manner, it is unlikely that a single approach will facilitate the transition from one mode to another. That is, the process of change goes beyond simple cause-and-effect relationships, since there are many levels of functioning and many interactions occurring in complex and dynamic systems. Finally, there are no particular end-states to be defined for such systems. Rather, the properties of a complex and dynamic system interact and combine to produce new emergent properties that are likely to be unique to each system.

What this model means for the process of therapeutic change is that established ways of thinking and behaving are usually stable. In a sense, the old behavioral and cognitive responses have built up a good deal of inertia that needs to be overcome if they are to be replaced with new and better responses. It is not surprising then that the process will often require discipline and practice in order to reorganize the system. Because people and the problem of stuttering are complex and dynamic, there is no single best strategy for assisting the person in accomplishing this reorganization. Finally, the end result of successful intervention and reorganization is not necessarily predictable or likely to be identical for every speaker. As the reader will note, many of these ideas coincide with the basic principles of change described at the outset of this chapter.

The first step in the modification techniques is called cancellation. This is sometimes referred to as a post-event modification because the speaker changes the form of the stuttering after it occurs. Immediately after a stuttered word, the speaker stops and pauses for 2–3 seconds. The brief pause highlights the stuttering and may serve as a mild form of punishment for the speaker as his or her ability to communicate is terminated. Some people (including those who stutter) are somewhat determined to complete the message and any stoppage both

---

[8]It is also reasonable to consider the speaker's cognitive/emotional response to the stuttering experience as habitual and hypercoordinated.

Clinical **Insight**

During the initial stages of acquiring a skill many of the things we are asked to do seem counter-intuitive. When we first learn to drive we are told that if the car goes into a skid that we should steer in the direction that our car is sliding. Of course, that seems nonsensical until we try it and it works! When traveling at even a moderate speed on a motorcycle, one way to turn to the *right* is to push on the *right* handgrip; when turning to the *left* you push on the *left* handgrip. It's called counter-steering, and it allows the bike to lean and move in the direction you want to go. In various forms of karate it is frequently best to step toward rather than away from your competitor. To most people, each of these choices would be the last response you would intuitively select. Similarly, to someone who has spent years hiding their stuttering, attending a support group with other people who stutter is not likely to be intuitive (Trichon & Tetnowski, 2006). Likewise, voluntarily stuttering is the last thing you would think of doing. It is counter-intuitive to stutter in the moment that you would rather avoid or escape from the experience. Many treatment techniques require a different, often unique way of talking. The new way of speaking, although it may yield much sought-after fluency, is unstable, often sounds unnatural and feels strange. Even with greater fluency, the new ways of talking are likely to be uncomfortable and different from the way of speaking that you have become used to. The new way of speaking may feel like a façade and not who you are. You feel like you are not being yourself and that adds to the anxiety when you try to communicate. However, with the courage and trust to face the very thing you wish to avoid, you may discover unexpected positive results.

increases the time pressure to communicate and creates the hurdle of having to reinitiate speech. As easy as this task may seem, many individuals who stutter have some difficulty doing this during reading and more so during conversational speech. Those speakers who have not yet achieved a reasonable degree of desensitization often find this task especially difficult. However, the activities performed during this brief period provide the foundation of the stuttering modification procedure.

As the client is able to detect his stuttering and consistently pause following the event he is asked to analyze the more obvious physiological features of his stuttering. Now, during the pause, the speaker slowly pantomimes his stuttering, examining the physical features of his behavior. As he rehearses the physical patterns that correspond to his just-stuttered speech he can begin to get a feel for his stuttering by considering such questions as "Did I cut off my airflow and voicing? How and where am I constricting my vocal tract? What are the articulatory postures, respiratory, or phonatory movements I am doing that prevent me from saying the next sound or syllable?" At the outset this process will require a few moments but, with practice, can be completed promptly. Once this analysis is accomplished, the speaker is rewarded by being able to continue with his message.

In the next step of the procedure, the clinician asks the speaker to use the pause following the stuttered word to silently pantomime a new, easy version of the stuttering. The speaker gradually includes both airflow and voicing and produces the word out loud. The speaker now reaches the final stage of this technique. Following each stuttered word, the speaker briefly pauses, quickly formulates the appropriate combinations of respiratory, articulatory, and phonatory patterns, and then produces the previously stuttered event with a slightly slower, effortless, and smooth form of "fluent stuttering." The new form of stuttering has the characteristics of fluency in terms of airflow, easy contact of the articulators, gradual and continual voicing, and smooth transitional movements to the next sounds and syllables. It is important to note once again that although the speaker could likely say the stuttered word again fluently, the purpose at this point is not to achieve fluency. The goal is to replace (or cancel) the old, habitual stuttering response with a new and easier form of stuttering. The ability to use this technique is usually facilitated in a progression of reading, monologue, and conversation, both inside and then beyond the treatment setting.

It is important to stress that the speaker is not canceling the stuttering event with the goal of achieving fluency. After all, the addition of yet another moment of fluent stuttering following a real stuttering event will result in speech that is even less fluent. The speaker is, however, breaking the link between stuttering and the experience of losing control. Rather than reflexively fleeing from the event they are now able to stay in the moment, take charge of the experience, and select a new and better response. It is important for the speaker to appreciate the sense of agency than accompanies this experience. Each moment of stuttering, while it may be undesirable, is an opportunity to take charge of the stuttering—a chance at bat. At the outset of treatment, stuttering is scoring run after run while the speaker, although catching, taking charge, and systematically modifying the stuttering, has not rounded the bases once. Once the speaker begins to take charge of the large majority of the stuttering moments (something approaching 80%), there is often an increase in the flow of fluency and, more importantly, a dramatic increase in the speaker's confidence about their ability to repair the situation.

As a result of practice and persistence, persons who stutter can succeed both within and beyond the treatment environment. As the individual gains ability and confidence, the ability to successfully repair his situation in the stream of speech increases. He begins to realize that he is not helpless. He comes to understand that it is possible for him to be able to count on and successfully use well-practiced responses to previously feared situations, to manipulate and play

Clinical **Insight**

Kayaking in white water requires a high level of balance and confidence. It is easy to lose control and find yourself under the surface of the water and in a threatening situation. Some anxiety is part of the experience. Complicating the situation is the fact that the novice tends to be rigid and inflexible. With increasing stress associated with the approach of a difficult section of the river, the likelihood of a mistake is high. Fortunately, with practice the novice becomes more proficient. Progress is seen as the paddler's strokes become more efficient and blended together. A crucial step takes place when the person learns to repair a mistake by rolling back to the surface.

Learning to roll a kayak takes considerable practice. It is best to begin in the safe environment of a pool or lake. An experienced instructor explains the rationale and details of the rolling technique, and, together, the instructor and the paddler go over the sequence of events that must take place if the roll is to be successful. The techniques are done deliberately and slowly, in a preplanned manner by setting up for the ideal roll position. The paddler learns to roll to both the left and the right, to roll with the kayak filled with water, and to roll without a paddle using only the arms and an associated hip snap. Eventually, the paddler learns to roll without first setting up in a roll position in order to approximate the unexpected situations found on the river. Finally, it is time to move from the safety of the flat water to the dynamic and unpredictable tumult of the river.

Depending on such factors as the water temperature, turbulence, and obstacles that appear in the boater's path, the first attempts of the paddler to roll in a moving stream are not likely to be successful. The likelihood of success decreases dramatically when the stresses of time pressure, distraction, and especially fear enter the picture. The paddler's initial reaction to being upside down for the first time in the river is apt to be one of fear or even panic. The techniques that worked so well in the secure environment of the pool are quickly forgotten and the first reaction of the paddler is to exit the boat and swim to the surface. The paddler comes to the realization that his techniques must be practiced to the point that they are automatic and do not require thought. If the paddler takes time to think, what he will think about is fear.

As the paddler learns to react to the situations on the river in this manner, positive things begin to occur. Confidence builds and paddling skills increase geometrically. The person becomes more flexible and begins to adopt a style of working with, rather than against, the power of the river. If a mistake is made, the person will repair it by getting back to the surface of the water and achieving control. The person will begin to experiment and play with different new techniques, intentionally entering difficult sections of the river. The paddler gradually becomes less rigid, paddling with greater flexibility. Because he is more flexible, the paddler and his boat are able to absorb the impacts that previously had such a profound influence on progress. The person gradually gains confidence in his ability to correct his mistakes and thus, is less concerned about making them. Fewer mistakes are made. It's not long before the person begins to seek out more challenging rapids to paddle and new rivers to navigate. Source: Adapted from "Paddling in Stream of Speech," *Letting GO*, National Stuttering Association, September/October, 1995.

Clinical Decision-Making

The fluency that results from the cancellation repair technique is earned fluency to be sure, but it is extremely tenuous. On occasion, especially if a speaker requires additional desensitization, a speaker will be unable to successfully cancel the stuttered word. That is, as he begins to replace the old stuttering with a smoother, controlled version of stuttering, he will lose control and revert back to his old, automatic, and helpless stuttering. If this happens, the client should attempt the cancellation of the stuttered word again until he regains control of the fluent stuttering. Success is defined by the client indicating that he is in charge of the word. The client can signal to the clinician with his finger whether he is in control of his stuttering. On occasion, it may take several cycles of losing and regaining control before he is able to be completely in charge of the stuttered word. In any case, he should not leave that word and go on to the next one until he has taken charge of that word by successfully canceling it.

with possibilities within the turmoil of the stuttering moment. Moreover, he is free to move ahead and achieve new success in increasingly more difficult speaking situations.

It may be obvious from the previous descriptions that cancellations are usually difficult to perform, particularly during the expectations and time pressure of real-life speaking situations. Listeners tend to interrupt without waiting for the speaker to go back and modify the stuttered word. Speakers, because they are concentrating so closely on how they are speaking, tend to lose their train of thought—although this will improve with practice. Most people who have undergone treatment will indicate that while they often become efficient in using cancellations in the treatment setting and outside of treatment while in the company of the clinician, they choose not to use this technique in most daily speaking situations. Nevertheless, it is an important technique to have available. The cancellation technique provides the speaker with the rationale and initial entry into a strategy for modifying the habitual stuttering the speaker had perceived as uncontrollable.

The next step in the modification of the stuttered event is the para-event modification, often called a "pullout." Now, rather than waiting until he makes it all the way through a stuttered word, the speaker will grab the word and begin to "slide out of it" by enhancing his airflow and voicing, altering his vocal tract with more appropriate articulatory postures, and generally stuttering smoothly through the word. Clients often find that this technique of pulling out of a stuttered moment is a natural progression from the cancellation technique and may begin doing this spontaneously. The pullout is less obvious than the cancellation, communication is enhanced, and listener reactions may be more favorable. Nevertheless, it is important to continue practicing the post-event or cancellation technique as there will undoubtedly be stressful speaking situations when the speaker will be unable to catch his stuttering in time to use a pullout. On these occasions the last line of defense, the final opportunity to catch and take charge of a moment of stuttering, is the cancellation technique.

The final step in the modification sequence is the pre-event modification or preparatory set. As the speaker anticipates a moment of stuttering (and chooses not to avoid it) he begins the word with a smooth form of stuttering. With the "prep set" the speaker is preplanning, rather than reacting to, his stuttering. As with the above techniques the targets incorporated in the fluency-modification strategies (full breath, air flow, gradual onset of constant phonation, and light articulatory contacts) are essential for achieving a smooth preparatory set. Furthermore, if a client's speech contains many very brief fluency breaks that he has difficulty identifying, the preparatory set provides a good way to eliminate them.

Perhaps the most difficult thing (for both the clinician and especially the person who stutters) to understand about these techniques is that the initial goal is not the production of typically fluent speech. It is, however, the long-term goal. As the speaker begins to gradually modify the form of his stuttering and achieve a measure of command over his speech production system, fluency will follow. The process requires continued desensitization and experimentation with elements of the stuttering modification techniques that are found to be helpful for a particular speaker. The techniques will need to be overlearned in increasingly more difficult speaking situations beyond the clinic environment. The speaker will need to recruit the understanding and support of others, particularly friends and coworkers, so that they can facilitate the use of these techniques in the person's daily speaking situations. Listeners will need to understand the rationale and nature of the techniques so that they can recognize and reward what may first appear to be the speaker's somewhat unusual speaking patterns.

In order to be sure that the client understands both the rationale and the steps associated with each technique, it is often effective for the clinician to ask the client to explain a technique as well as demonstrate it for the clinician. Of course, this can also be done with others present in the treatment setting or at home with a spouse or parent. Another related approach is for the clinician and client to switch roles, with the client guiding the clinician through the use of a technique. This can be enjoyable as well as instructive as the clinician makes intentional errors and feigns a misunderstanding concerning the technique or rationale for using the technique.

As we have stressed, in most cases it will take extensive and disciplined practice for the speaker to incorporate any technique into his or her habitual response during daily speaking situations. After learning a technique during a therapy session it is not unusual for some people to come to the next session and inform the clinician that they were unable to use the technique.

Client: "I tried the technique we practiced last time, and you know what? It didn't work."

Clinician: "How many times did you try it?"

Client: "Well, I attempted it yesterday, maybe ten times!"
When we get that response, maybe we should respond by saying something like:
"Well, try it *500 times* and we'll see how you're doing then!"

Listener Response to Management and Acknowledgement Techniques

Kamhi (2003) suggests that most listeners respond in a generally appropriate and well-meaning manner when they encounter individuals who stutter. Of course, how a listener responds can be influenced by how the speaker is coping with his or her stuttering. On occasion, the avoidance and struggle behavior by the speaker creates confusion or even anxiety on the part of the listener. It is not unusual for listeners to be unaware that what they are witnessing is stuttering and not some other condition. To the extent that the speaker can indicate that they are stuttering, perhaps by stuttering in a manner that most everyday listeners associate with typical stuttering behavior (repetitions of sounds or words rather than blocking or extreme struggle behavior) or by acknowledging the fact that they are stuttering, listeners are apt to be more receptive to and understanding about the situation.

Kamhi (2003) also suggests that the high cognitive load experienced by the speaker (along with the stress of the communicative interaction) often results in gaze aversion by the speaker followed by a similar response by the listener. Kamhi suggests that this is what most listeners will naturally and instinctively do rather than following the "rules" suggested by professionals and support groups (e.g., maintain eye contact, wait patiently and not complete sentences or words, pay attention to the message rather than the manner of speaking, and not show discomfort, pity, or sympathy). Everyday listeners are unaware of these rules and as Kamhi points out, clinicians should not suggest to their clients that most listeners will respond in an ideal manner.

A similar situation occurs as the speaker begins to consistently use fluency- and stuttering-modification techniques beyond the therapeutic setting. Listeners may not only fail to notice the often subtle improvements in the quality of fluency but may also sense that something is different in the nature of the stuttering. Unless they are informed, the typical listener will not appreciate that the speaker is attempting to change their stuttering into slower and easier forms or to use pullout and cancellation techniques. Unless the speaker or someone else explains what is occurring, the listener is likely to wonder if, beyond the stuttering, there is "something else wrong with this person." Manning, Burlison, and Thaxton (1999) had groups of naïve listeners use a bipolar scale, a handicap scale, and open-ended questions to evaluate an adult male who simulated mild stuttering (SSI = 17) or utilized stuttering-modification techniques (cancellations or pullouts). Listeners consistently preferred the condition where the speaker was stuttering over the condition when the speaker was stuttering and using stuttering-modification techniques. The results suggested that everyday listeners may be likely to react less favorably to a speaker with mild levels of stuttering who is modifying his stuttered speech than when the same speaker is simply stuttering.

People who stutter can lead the way in determining how listeners will react by informing their listeners. For example, Van Riper (1982) suggested that listeners are likely to think better of the speaker who acknowledges their stuttering and is able to convey to the listener that they are actively working on the problem. Many authors (Blood & Blood, 1982; Breitenfeldt & Lorenz, 1989; Collins & Blood, 1990; Hastorf, Windfogel, & Cassman, 1979; Silverman, 1988a) have suggested that acknowledgement of stuttering by the speaker may assist in improving the typically negative reaction of listeners (see Chapter 3).

By presenting listeners with videos of both an acknowledgement and a non-acknowledgement condition, Collins and Blood (1990) found support for Hasdorf et al.'s suggestion that self-acknowledgment of a problem by an individual reduced listener uncertainty and promoted a more positive reaction. Collins and Blood (1990) also observed that the speaker's acknowledgement of their stuttering was particularly effective in eliciting a more positive response from listeners when the stuttering was rated as severe rather than mild.

One the other hand, Healey, Gabel, Daniels, and Kawai (2007) found no effect for the strategy of speaker acknowledgement of their stuttering. Likert-type scale data of five personality traits (sincerity, likeability, trustworthiness, character, and emotional adjustment) indicated no differences in listener reactions to speakers who acknowledged their stuttering in one of three conditions—at the beginning, at the end, or not at all—during brief videotaped interviews. Healey et al. (2007) explained the contrasting results of their study and that of Collins and Blood (1990) in terms of a variety of differences in the research design, instructions, and stimuli conditions. For example, the listeners in the Healey et al. investigation took part in only one of the three acknowledgement conditions, while the participants in the Collins and Blood investigation observed speakers in both an acknowledgement and a non-acknowledgement condition. It appears to be that listeners are able to appreciate the potentially helpful effect of acknowledgement only when they have the opportunity to consider and contrast both conditions.

An investigation by Lee and Manning (2008) contrasting both research designs suggests that this is the case. The results indicate that unless listeners have the opportunity to directly compare both (Collins & Blood, 1990) the self-acknowledgement of stuttering with a more common stuttering-only experience (Healey et al., 2007), self-acknowledgement by the speaker is not likely to be appreciated. It may be that as naïve listeners gain even minimal experience and understanding about the speaker's situation through a forthright and nonapologetic self-acknowledgement they are better able to make an adjustment resulting in a more favorable evaluation of the speaker. The results provide support for the anchor-adjustment model proposed by MacKinnon, Hall, and MacIntyre (2007) suggesting that as listeners become more informed about the nature of stuttering they are more likely to respond to the person in a positive manner. Furthermore, it has also been suggested that a more important aspect of self-acknowledgement lies in the ability of the speaker to decrease the avoidance behavior and achieve an agentic lifestyle (Bloodstein, 1995; Sheehan, 1975; Van Riper, 1982).

Stabilization

From the outset of treatment it will be essential for the speaker to transfer his new perceptions and abilities to situations beyond the treatment setting. During the stabilization phase the speaker's performance in his daily world becomes the major focus. During this phase, the newly learned modification skills are practiced under increasingly more stressful conditions both within and beyond the treatment setting. The goal now is for the speaker to become resilient in responding to the variety of communicative pressures encountered in daily speaking situations. In order for the speaker to withstand these pressures, the various techniques must be overlearned. Unless such a level of performance is achieved the speaker will be unable to rely on his abilities when communicative demands are swift and serious. As we suggest many times throughout this text, speakers will have to practice techniques correctly hundreds or thousands of times in order to develop such a level of skill and confidence. This, of course, will take some time, but this is what is necessary for techniques to become an integral part of the person. Regardless of how many times it is done, successfully performing a technique within the safety of the clinic provides little indication about what will occur during the stressful speaking situations found in everyday life. Fortunately, as we mentioned in Chapter 2, humans have the opportunity to practice speech as much or more than any other activity.

It is also helpful for the speaker to test the new patterns of speaking and thinking in a systematic way. The clinician and client can develop and refine a continuum of easier to more difficult speaking situations. Some of the assessment devices described in Chapter 4 may be of help at this point. Of course, the ability of the person to develop expertise in monitoring and modifying stuttering will continue well beyond the period of formal treatment with the clinician. As described in more detail in Chapter 12, accomplished speakers will continually "push the envelope" and challenge themselves with new speaking adventures.

Stabilization activities also provide a good opportunity to heighten the ability of the speaker to monitor speech production via proprioception. By using devices that provide auditory masking, delayed auditory feedback (DAF), or frequency altered feedback (FAF) the speaker can learn to focus on the feel and timing of his articulatory movements. Although such devices are not essential they can be helpful in developing a heightened sense of the physical adjustments necessary for enhancing fluency.

At this time it is also useful for the clinician to assist the speaker in bringing forth and revisiting fears and anxieties associated with especially difficult speaking situations. These may be experiences of fluency failure in the past as well as current or upcoming situations. As explained in the following section, with practice, the speaker can learn to withstand the negative emotions and counter the negative self-talk that often accompany these experiences.

Cognitive Restructuring

Regardless of the overall treatment strategy, in order for the speaker to achieve success, he must eventually develop fresh ways of thinking about himself and his problem. Discovering that there are alternative ways of considering one's situation facilitates the development of an agentic lifestyle. Many authors have emphasized the merit of speakers experimenting with the role(s) they play as someone who stutters, or alternatively, as someone who is able to achieve fluency. As we described in the previous chapter, this aspect of therapeutic change is a core principle of therapeutic intervention in rational emotive behavioral therapy (REBT), personal construct therapy (PCT), and Gestalt Therapy. Each of these therapeutic approaches attempts to assist the client in experimenting with new ways of creating meaning and developing independent, problem-solving responses when communicating with others—changes that are necessary for long-term success. This aspect of treatment does not always need to be dealt with directly with all individuals in order for cognitive change to occur. For example, if the clinician targets behavioral change and the elaboration of fluency rather than cognitive change, the speaker may nevertheless experience constructive changes in his self-concept and his ability to communicate.

It is good to remember that it will take some time for the speaker to adjust to and incorporate the new behavioral and cognitive changes. As described earlier in this chapter, the new ways of speaking and thinking will sound and feel unfamiliar. Adolescents and adults who stutter have spent many years adjusting to their speech and coping with the problems presented by their attempts to communicate. Even though the speaker's new responses are desirable it will take some time to integrate these changes into everyday life, particularly during the transfer and maintenance phases of therapy. The client who retains self-defeating mental images and negative thoughts and beliefs about speech and his ability to manage it is much less apt to succeed once he is on his own.

Cognitive Restructuring with Fluency Disorders

There are a variety of cognitive therapy approaches (see Beck, 1995, 2005; Ellis, 1977; Luterman, 2001) that have been used for many human conditions including depression, anxiety, and phobias.[9] A common theme for each of these approaches is that what we tell ourselves about our situation is more important than the actual situation itself. The primary focus of therapy is to identify the unhelpful ways people interpret themselves and their situation and to consider more functional alternatives. The initial step is to identify and increase the person's awareness of their less functional but usual cognitive and emotional responses to difficult or threatening events. We have seen examples of some of the more common of these responses as proposed by Ellis (1977) in the previous chapter. Other interpretations may be even more dysfunctional, involving greater degrees of irrational and nonproductive thoughts (in the opinion of an external observer). The primary goal of therapy is to assist clients in identifying and using their resources in order to develop a broader perspective, thereby learning to approach their particular situation with more effective responses. This approach is highly individualistic in that each person will present with different problems and a unique pattern of less functional responses. Although there are many forms of cognitive therapy, rational emotive behavioral therapy (REBT) (Ellis, 1977) is one of the better known. Among the eight primary outcomes of this approach is the goal of helping the client to develop what Ellis calls "scientific thinking." In this case, the purpose is to help the person to decrease magical thinking and begin considering their situation logically and rationally in order to behave in ways that are more productive and fulfilling. The following paragraphs, although not necessarily suggested as protocols for all clinicians or clients, provide examples of the principles and techniques from the cognitive therapy approach for programs designed for individuals who stutter.

---

[9]Phobias are a persistent fear of and an unreasonable desire to avoid certain situations, objects, activities, or persons. Stuttering is not a phobia, because there are a variety of genuine negative consequences associated with stuttering, as any normally fluent speaker will appreciate when realistically assuming the role of a person who stutters.

Emerick (1988) suggests that clients who have an analytical and intro-spective orientation at the outset of treatment respond the most favorably to cognitive-restructuring approaches. According to Emerick, the cognitive aspects of treatment involve at least four main phases:

Phase 1   focuses on educating the client about the overall approach of the treatment. Suggesting to the client that he change his orientation to both himself and his problem can pose a threat to his self-integrity and equilib-rium. Threat or not, the clinician must frequently challenge the client if change is going to occur.

Phase 2   involves helping the client to identify his self-defeating patterns of thinking and to analyze his thoughts before, during, and after speaking situations in general and stuttering events in particular. He is asked to identify his mental constructs about the event, keep a log of his emotions and thoughts (sometimes called a "dysfunctional thought record"), and indicate the outcome of situations. He then categorizes his responses in terms of dependency/helplessness ("I know I will relapse when therapy is over"), irresponsibility ("I just cannot control my feelings"), dichotomizing ("There are good listeners and bad listeners"), catastrophizing ("I know I will fall apart if I am asked to introduce myself"), and fantasy ("Most of my problems would be solved if I didn't stutter").

Phase 3   is one of reality testing. The client's task is now to evaluate his mental constructs by asking (a) Does the construct deal with the reality of the situation? (b) Does this construct make unreasonable demands on me? and (c) Does the construct help me to accomplish the treatment goals? In addition, the client also contrasts possible negative imagery with positive, self-enhancing imagery. As Emerick says, "It is difficult to think of failing in a speaking situation while at the same time concentrating on positive thoughts" (1988, p. 262). The old, negative cognitions must become cues for the client to tell himself, "Stop." At this point, the clinician can role-play for the client, alternating between the negative and positive self-statements. As these concepts are introduced and practiced with several clients, this form of reality testing can be an ideal activity during group treatment sessions.

Phase 4   begins the process of having the client substitute self-enhancing language for the more habitual negative thoughts. The new, positive affir-mations may not always be completely true (e.g., "This may be a difficult situation, but I can deal with it"). Nonetheless, imagining success brings the possibility of success that much closer (Daly, 1994).

Clients can, of course, have problems with cognitive-restructuring activities, especially when they continue to view stuttering as something that happens to them rather than something they do (a fairly common perception). According to Emerick (1988), such clients have great difficulty stopping and changing the old negative cognitions. An even greater problem is posed by those clients who are unable to recognize the inaccuracy of their habitual cognitions. Some people believe that the way they are processing reality is the normal, correct, and most acceptable way. The client may agree intellectually that there are several ways to view a situation, but still privately believe that the current view they hold is the most accurate.

Another good example of a protocol that emphasizes cognitive restructuring along with a stuttering-modification approach is described by Maxwell (1982). The approach is educational rather than curative, with a primary goal of teaching the speaker better ways of successfully managing his speech. Clients typically attend the treatment program for one individual and one group session each week for approximately one-and-a-half years. Maxwell (1982) summarizes the program in the following 10 steps:

1. **Information giving:** The purpose of this stage is to provide the client with a map of the treatment process. The client also receives a verbal or written summary of the treatment plan.

2. **Cognitive appraisal:** The client summarizes, in his own words, the objectives and methods of the treatment plan and how the plan will meet his needs. In what may be an especially important feature, this process establishes a common perception of the treatment process for the client and clinician.

3. **Thought reversal:** The client begins to reduce and eliminate negative cognitions. Essential to this process is the technique of "thought stopping" when negative self-talk occurs. This requires the client to tell himself, initially out loud, to stop using the negative ways of thinking about himself and his speech; with practice this is done silently. The primary goal is for the client to begin disengaging from undesired thoughts and images. Near the end of this stage, the client begins taking steps to utilize positive and productive cognitions. These activities take place within the treatment setting.

4. **Vicarious observation:** Once the client is able to experience some success at disengaging negative (and often self-fulfilling) cognitions, the clinician begins to model positive cognitions. As the client observes the clinician successfully coping with challenges in her own life, the client's self-efficacy will be enhanced. Such modeling increases the client's hope that he too can perform as he desires, despite problems and setbacks.

5. **Speech modification:** In this initial stage of behavioral change, the client begins to improve his information-processing, decision-making, and problem-solving abilities. As Maxwell points out, clients typically are not accurate self-observers. However, even before the client is able to successfully modify specific stuttering events, the fact that he is able to accurately self-monitor his behavior tends to have a positive treatment effect in terms

of reduced avoidance and possibly even increased fluency (Cooper, Cady, & Robbins, 1970; Daly & Kimbarow, 1978; Wingate, 1959). Many aspects of the identification and termination steps as described by Maxwell are similar to the variation and modification stages of treatment as described by Van Riper (1973). Rather than thinking about his speech as something that "happens to him," the person eventually begins to understand the lawfulness of stuttering in different communication situations. An essential aspect of this modification stage of treatment involves the client describing what he does with his speech-production mechanism. With more accurate monitoring of his behavior, the speaker begins to see the cause-and-effect relationship of his choices and will be more likely to understand and predict his cognitions and behavior.

6. **Identification:** The client becomes proficient at identifying specific moments of stuttering, beginning with ten-minute segments using short words and progressing to reading and conversation.

7. **Termination:** The client terminates the old form of stuttering by following a moment of stuttering with a silent pause. The client then gradually replaces the fluency break with cognitive and behavioral responses (fluency- and stuttering-modification) that are more appropriate. Termination is accomplished first following (as in a cancellation), then during (as in a pullout), and finally before (as in a preparatory set) the stuttering moment. The client uses imagery to see, hear, and feel a new motor plan consisting of fluency-enhancing targets. The client is also asked to identify and modify avoidance or substitution behaviors.

8. **Cognitive restructuring:** As during the third stage of this treatment, the client is asked to "identify maladaptive speech-related emotions, and self-defeating cognitions on which these are based" (Maxwell, 1982, p. 415). This time, however, the client is asked to restructure his cognitions in more stressful extra-treatment speaking situations.

9. **Coping skills:** The client begins to use positive self-statements and imagery techniques to revise negative aspects of his covert verbal behavior. The client's ability to restructure his thinking about himself and his problem is often reflected in self-talk. As Egan (2007) suggests, clients often talk themselves out of things by verbalizing feelings such as "I can't do this. This technique won't work. I'm not good enough to do this yet." This self-talk is often disabling and tends to get the person into difficulty before he has given himself a chance to succeed. Egan indicates that clinicians can add value to the treatment experience by helping clients challenge negative self-talk that prevents them from taking action. With the clinician's modeling, the client reorganizes monologues in preparation for actual speaking tasks. Group sessions using role-playing activities are recommended.

Maxwell provides a clear example of how a client can alter his thought process about giving an oral report to an art history class. The first paragraph indicates the client's initial thoughts about this task.

> Oh, Lord, here I am in class with all of these people and soon I'm going to have to talk. What if my controls don't work? What if I fall on my face— make a fool of myself? Then, they'll think I'm stupid. Maybe I ought to quietly get up and walk out of here. Maybe there won't be time to get to my report. If I stutter, will they laugh or feel pity? (1982, p. 417)

Following analysis of the nonproductive content of that self-message, the clinician then models a revision of more positive internal monologue, as in this example:

> I am now in class with other students like me discussing the subject of art history. Soon I will be asked to speak on a topic that I know well. I have interesting information to share. When I speak, I plan to use to the best of my ability the controls that I've learned to use well in therapy. What I want to convey is the strong interest I have in my topic. I'll remember to smile, maintain eye contact with my listeners, and try to be open and friendly. (Maxwell, 1982, p. 417)

10. **Self-management:** During this final stage of treatment, the client takes ever-greater responsibility for setting his own goals and for self-management of the cognitive and behavioral features of his speech. From the outset there must be the recognition that the "majority of therapeutic work takes place between, rather than during, therapy sessions" (Maxwell, 1982, p. 418; see also Kanfer, 1975). The time for dismissal from formal treatment approaches as the client becomes able to self-manage without the assistance of the clinician. Related to the abovementioned activities are the recommendations of Daly (1992, pp. 135–136) for using positive affirmations for reinforcing and enhancing cognitive changes.

Applying Personal Construct Theory

In the previous chapter we briefly described the nature of personal construct theory (PCT) as it relates to principles of counseling. We will now present some of the findings of applied research with this theoretical perspective. The first to apply PCT to individuals who stutter, Fransella (1972) hypothesized that a person stutters "because it is in this way that he can anticipate the greatest number of events; it is by behaving in this way that life is most meaningful to him" (p.58). Although this may sound illogical and even offensive to some individuals who stutter, from a personal construct perspective it simply means that when the speaker stutters in a situation it is in line with what he would predict. A fluent interaction would not enable the speaker to prepare for and predict listener responses and the outcome of the situation with the same degree of experience and confidence. From a PCT perspective the speaker is likely to experience *fear* (an imminent *incidental* change in one's core structures), *anxiety* (the awareness that the events a person is experiencing are beyond the range of convenience of his construct system), or even *guilt* (the person is acting in a way that is contradictory to his or her core role structure). The speaker is "choosing" to stutter, not because he prefers it in the usual sense, but because it is what is familiar; it is how he understands the world (Dalton, 1983).

Fransella (1972) attempted to increase the meaningfulness of the fluent speaker role for individuals who stuttered using a technique called "controlled elaboration." That is, she used behavioral experiments (using repertory and implications grids) to assist each of the 16 participants in her study to examine the validity of their construct system and to focus on occasions where they had experienced fluency. The treatment focused on assisting the participants to develop a more meaningful construction of their experiences with fluent speech, and no attempt was made to directly alter the behavioral features of their speech. Fransella found that stuttering decreased as the meaningfulness of the fluent speaker role increased. Follow-up with nine of the 16 participants at both three months and one year indicated that one participant had regressed and eight had maintained or improved their level of fluent speech. Fransella (2003) suggests that the "crucial question" when using behavioral experiments to elaborate how the speaker is construing his fluency is "Did you predict you would be fluent?" As clients learn to be more aware of their fluent speech, predictions of fluency become more frequent, and they are able to attribute their fluency to themselves rather than to some "fluke" or external source; that is, their fluency becomes more *meaningful* to them.

Manning and DiLollo (2007) suggested that, along with questioning the speaker about their occurrences of fluent speech, there may be other ways to help the speaker to reconstrue the meaningfulness of their fluency. As Kelly (1955) described, controlled elaboration can also take nonverbal forms. For example, as speakers practice their fluency-enhancing abilities in hierarchies of increasing communicative difficulty, they can be asked to consider their thoughts and feelings and predict the outcome *before* going into the situation. After completing the "experiment" they can then consider the accuracy of their predictions, including their fluency, their feelings, and listener responses. As the speaker, along with the clinician, assesses the outcome of the experiment by contrasting predictions with the actual outcomes, a deconstruction of the speaker's stuttering role may begin. With continued progress in the achievement of fluency—and increasing predictions of fluency that are confirmed by further experiments—elaboration of the fluent speaker role is more likely to occur.

DiLollo, Manning, & Neimeyer (2003) conducted a systematic content analytic study that examined the cognitive anxiety (Viney & Westbrook, 1976) of 29 persons who stuttered and 29 fluent speakers with respect to "fluent" and "stutterer" speaker roles. Viney and Westbrook defined cognitive anxiety as the awareness that one's construct systems are inadequate to allow full and meaningful construing (and, therefore, prediction) of the events with which one is confronted. In this study, the two groups were interviewed and asked identical open-ended questions regarding what life was like as (a) a person who stutters and (b) a fluent speaker. Responses to the two questions were transcribed and analyzed using a modified version of Viney and Westbrook's Cognitive Anxiety Scale. The results indicated that both persons who stutter and fluent speakers demonstrated significantly higher levels of cognitive anxiety related to their "nondominant" speaker role compared to their "dominant" role, as they each dismissed experiences of the nondominant role as meaningless. The authors found that people who stutter tended to protect their "stutterer" self-image by ignoring or discounting episodes of fluent speech, referring to them as "lucky" or "a fluke," and always predicting a return to stuttering. In contrast, fluent speakers made little meaning out of their occasional disfluencies and reasserted their identities as fluent persons.

DiLollo, Manning, & Neimeyer (2005) again examined the meaningfulness of the fluent speaker role for the 29 persons who stuttered from the DiLollo et al. (2003) study, but re-analyzed the data applying a measure of *cognitive complexity* (Bieri, 1955; Crockett, 1965) to the transcripts. According to Crockett, the number of constructs participants use to describe a domain of interest will be a reflection of the complexity of their construct system with respect to that domain. In this study, the number of constructs used by persons who stuttered to describe the domains of their *fluent speaker role* and their *stutterer role* were taken to indicate the cognitive complexity—or meaningfulness—of each role. Again, results provided support for constructivist interpretations of stuttering, indicating that the participants in this study demonstrated significantly less complex construct systems related to the fluent speaker role compared to the stutterer role.

Plexico, Manning, and DiLollo (2005) took a constructivist perspective in attempting to understand the ability of adults who achieved the successful management of their stuttering. Seven participants described their experiences across three temporal stages (past, transitional, and current). Using a phenomenological approach, recurring themes were identified across participants in order to develop an essential structure of the phenomena at each stage. There were five recurring themes associated with past experiences when stuttering was being unsuccessfully managed: (1) gradual awareness, (2) negative reactions of listeners, (3) negative emotions, (4) restrictive lifestyle and avoidance, and (5) inadequate therapy. The ability to make the transition from unsuccessful to successful management of stuttering occurred gradually and was associated with six recurring themes: (1) support from others, (2) successful therapy, (3) self-therapy and behavioral change, (4) cognitive change, (5) utilization of personal experience, and (6) high levels of motivation and determination. The four recurring themes identified for the current situation where stuttering continued to be successfully managed were: (1) continued management, (2) self-acceptance and fear reduction, (3) unrestricted interactions and sense of freedom, and (4) optimism. This study provided information from a constructivist perspective in that it searched for evidence of meaning-making in the individual constructions of reality as part of the data collection process. The results of this study suggest that those who are able to successfully manage stuttering are able to reorganize a sense of the self and provide a cognitive and emotional context for the changes in their fluency.

Other personal construct theory-based methods have been used with persons who stutter. Botterill and Cook (1987), for example, discuss the use of a "problem solving" exercise based on Kelly's (1955) "circumspection, pre-emption, and control" (CPC) cycle, and a role-playing method based on Kelly's "fixed-role" therapy.

Applying a Constructivist-Narrative Approach

With the rationale for the constructivist-narrative approach provided in Chapter 7, we will now describe some suggested applications of a narrative therapy approach for assisting individuals who stutter. Along with traditional behavioral techniques, the narrative approach is offered as a way of facilitating fundamental changes in the ways in which individuals who stutter construe themselves as speakers and communicators (DiLollo, Neimeyer, and Manning, 2002; DiLollo, 2006; Manning & DiLollo, 2007). This is complementary to Fransella's (1972) application of personal construct methods such as controlled elaboration. The goal is to assist the speaker in elaborating his core constructs in order to accommodate spontaneous and treatment-induced episodes of fluency. As fluency increases, the speaker begins to consolidate a preferred story of an individual who is capable of fluency. As indicated above, this postmodern view also takes into account the social aspect of behavior, looking to secure social validation for the achievements made in treatment. In the following paragraphs we will provide some preliminary suggestions for using narrative therapy with adolescents and adults who stutter. Many of the following comments are derived from a presentation by DiLollo (2006) to the Fifth World Congress on Fluency Disorders in Dublin, Ireland.

Reconstructing the Narrative

Mapping the influence of the problem on the person. The clinician questions the client with curiosity, enthusiasm, and persistence in order for both of them to develop a better understanding of the problem-saturated story that has dominated the client's identity. As the speaker tells and reconsiders his story he begins to organize a coherent account and map the influence of "Stuttering" on his life to this point. Examples of questions could include, "What has *Stuttering* persuaded other people to think or say about you?" and "What decisions does *Stuttering* make for you?" The clinician is careful not to interrogate the speaker, and may, on occasion, ask permission to pose questions. Also implicit in the conversations is the acknowledgement that the person is not to blame for stuttering. Nonetheless, it should become clear that the speaker's position is one of responsibility in altering his relationship with stuttering. The clinician looks for experiences that may allow the speaker to loosen *Stuttering's* hold on his life and reconstruct the relationship, perhaps by identifying talents and abilities that have been hidden or veiled by the problem (Monk, 1997). Throughout the conversations the clinician provides encouragement for the speaker's ability to become the origin of action rather than a pawn in his relationship with stuttering.

Externalizing. The use of "externalizing" language encourages the speaker to move from interpreting their situation as a "problem person" (i.e., "I'm a stutterer") to a "person with a problem" (i.e., "I am a person who stutters").[10] Conceptualizing "Stuttering" as an external "entity" can help in recruiting the client's involvement as an active participant in the treatment process rather than feeling like a problem person that requires "fixing" by the clinician. The externalizing process serves to separate the person from the problem, placing the cognitive and behavioral factors of the problem "on the table or workbench" so that they can be considered and rearranged. It does not, however, attribute supremacy to the characterization of the problem. Some readers may be familiar with the admonitions of authors in the decades of the 1950s and 1960s warning about conceptualizing stuttering as an external force, which resulted in the speaker interpreting the stuttering experience as "something is happening to me" rather than "the things I am doing to make speaking difficult." In both cases, the point is the same in that the purpose is to empower the speaker to separate from and reinterpret the impact of stuttering. One example of an externalizing conversation with the clinician and client might sound something like:

Clinician: "How did you do at the party you were going to last night?"

PWS: "I knew I'd mess up at the party, so I didn't go."

Clinician: "What was Stuttering telling you as you prepared to go to the party?"

PWS: "That I'd mess up and look stupid."

Clinician: "So Stuttering was telling you that you'd mess up? That you shouldn't go because he'd make you look stupid."

---

[10]Although this suggestion may appear to be at odds with findings by St. Louis (1999) regarding the lack of an effect of "person-first" terminology, St. Louis's research was conducted to assess the effect of the terminology on the *listener,* not the *speaker* as is being suggested here.

PWS: "Yes, I guess so."

Clinician: "And you allowed stuttering to make that decision for you?"

Mapping the influence of the person on the problem. As the person begins to separate from and understand their relationship with Stuttering, the speaker can now begin to consider the influence he may have on the life of Stuttering (How am I able to influence the effect of stuttering?). Considering the speaker's relationship with Stuttering in this way permits a further deconstruction of the dominant narrative of Stuttering's influence and a construction of an alternative or preferred story that is less restrictive and more fulfilling to the speaker. The client can begin to author a new story with the assistance of the clinician in the role of co-author or editor. Similar to Kelly's (1955) controlled elaboration, the influence of the *speaker* on the life of "Stuttering" may be facilitated by the use of questions that help the individual identify "sparkling moments" (Winslade & Monk, 1999), or times when the individual has experienced unique outcomes that have been contradictory to the problem story (e.g., getting the client to elaborate on times when he or she was fluent). This process is facilitated by "unique outcome questions" (McKenzie & Monk, 1997) designed to facilitate the speaker's understanding of actions and intentions that run counter to the dominant story (e.g., "You have mentioned several occasions when you have been able to resist Stuttering's hold on you. How did you accomplish this and how did you feel when you achieved that? " or "There have been times when Stuttering began to grab the spotlight when you were making that presentation and you managed to nudge him aside. How did you accomplish that?").

Creating an alternative, preferred story. Questions and comments by the clinician are now intended to help the speaker further focus on the preferred experiences. The speaker is invited to make sense of the exceptions to their dominant narrative of stuttering and to retain them as part of an emerging narrative. Questions focus on facilitating the development of a preferred alternative story centered on previously identified unique outcomes (e.g., "How might you stand up to Stuttering in the future and refuse its requirements of you?" "What can you tell me about your history that would help others to understand the emergence of your ability to defeat Stuttering?"). Conversations include the ability of the client to redescribe themselves and to speculate about various personal and relational alternatives that can be derived from their emerging alternative narrative. Although this new narrative includes the speaker's role as a creator of fluent speech, it can also incorporate the speaker's ability to comfortably alter their old stuttering into minor disfluencies that are effortless and smooth.

Construing meaning for the fluent speaker role. As McKenzie & Monk (1997) suggest, even small changes in behavior and thinking are seen as victories and as sources of material to be worked with and expanded. However, the victories that are recognized by the clinician as an indication of a possible new plot to the story may be ignored or unappreciated by the client. Rather than the clinician highlighting the change, it may be more effective for the clinician to inquire about other changes that have occurred, creating opportunities for the client to uncover the meaning of his choices and behavior.

With the narrative approach there is an important distinction to be made between behavior change and cognitive change. Although the primary way of facilitating change is by experimenting with alternative constructions of events and testing these constructions via new behaviors, the behavior is less important than how the individual construes the outcome of the behavior (Monk, 1997). What is suggested is that, in many instances, *the behavioral changes seen during therapy are not as important as the act of experimenting with alternative constructions about the client's role as a speaker.* Questions from the clinician which serve to develop alternative meaning might include "What does your achievement reflect about the sort of person you are that is important for you and others to know?" or "What will the future be like without Stuttering's dominate, influence on your life? How will your future be different from the one that Stuttering would have planned for you?"

Anchoring the preferred story in a social and historical context. It is important to establish the speaker's new story that is now focused on the role of a more fluent speaker in a broader historical context. Rather than being buried or denied, the story of the speaker's journey is viewed as an important and valued part of the person's history. This perspective helps to facilitate the meaningfulness of the fluent speaker role for the client and establish predictions of fluency. As described in Chapter 12, this process of establishing the new story in daily experiences is important not only for the speaker but also for the significant others in his or her environment. As McKenzie and Monk (1997) explain, the process helps to develop the still fragile but emerging story, establish it as having a memorable history, and increase the likelihood of it being carried forward into the future. Examples of questions the clinician may consider for historicizing the new story include "Now that you have overcome Stuttering's influence in your life, who else should know about it?" "Of the people who knew you growing up, who would have been most likely to predict that you would break free from Stuttering's influence?" "Of the significant people in your life, who do you anticipate would have difficulty accepting the new life you have chosen?"

DiLollo and Neimeyer (2008) provide examples of questions used to help map the influence of stuttering on the life of the person and to investigate the influence of the person on his or her "Stuttering" (Table 8-1). The questions are

Table 8-1   Examples of questions that might be used in narrative therapy with a person who stutters.

Stage	Sample Questions
Mapping the influence of the *problem* in the life of the person:	What has *Stuttering* persuaded other people to think or say about you?
	How does it convince them of these things?
	What has it persuaded you to think about yourself?
	What decisions does *Stuttering* make for you?
	What are its intentions for your future?
Mapping the influence of the *person* on the life of the problem:	
a. Unique Outcome questions	Have there been times when you have been able to overcome *Stuttering's* hold over your speech?
b. Unique Account questions	How might you stand up to *Stuttering* in the future and refuse its requirements of you?
c. Unique Redescription questions	By freeing yourself from *Stuttering's* hold over you, do you think in any way that you are becoming less of "a stutterer"?
d. Unique Possibility questions	What will the future be like without *Stuttering's* influence dominating your life?
e. Unique Circulation questions	Of the significant people in your life, who do you anticipate would have difficulty accepting the new life you have chosen, free from *Stuttering's* influence?
f. Questions that Historicize Unique Outcomes	Of the people who knew you growing up, who would have been most likely to predict that you would break free from *Stuttering's* influence?
	What qualities would this person have seen in you that would have led him/her to believe that you would have been able to achieve what you have?

DiLollo, A., & Neimeyer, R. (2008). Talking back to stuttering: Constructivist contributions to stuttering treatment. Appeared in J. D. Raskin & S. K. Bridges (Eds). *Studies in Meaning 3: Constructivist Psychotherapy in the Real World* (pp. 165–182). NY: Pace University Press. Reprinted with permission of the author.

also designed to identify "unique outcomes" that contradict the problem-saturated story and give meaning to occasions when the person created exceptions to the dominance of stuttering in their life. As the person begins to deconstruct the influence of stuttering and integrate new alternatives for responding to the problem, a reconstruction of the story as well as the person becomes possible.

Guidelines for Clinicians

Perry and Doan (1994) provide guidelines for clinicians as they assist their clients to understand and revise their stories. Although there are 12 guidelines, we will present five that appear to have the most obvious utility for clinicians assisting individuals who stutter.

Be Curious. Be extremely curious but know little. Do not assume that you know all there is to know and that you fully understand your client's story. Perry and Doan suggest that if clinicians finds themselves becoming bored it is because they have put their curiosity on hold and have begun to assume that they know all they need to know about the person.

Have a Broad Focus. As we noted in Chapter 1 when discussing the effective clinician, Perry and Doan suggest that we should expand the focus of treatment by looking beyond the basic characteristics of the client's speech and pattern of communication. We need to understand the person we are assisting from a broad social and cultural perspective. This is particularly the case when we are having a difficult time understanding the client's story and the patterns of cognition and behavior we are observing. On occasion, there are powerful influences in the form of the client's gender, culture, religion, family, or ethnic heritage.

Use Resistance. Avoid an oppositional stance and allow yourself to "go with the resistance." That is, in spite of the natural tendency to do so, do not attempt to edit the client's story from the position of an expert. To the extent that we try to revise their story by telling them how to live it we escalate the person's resistance and possibly invite resentment and defensiveness. By going with clients' resistance we can provide them with the space to create their own story. As clients describe the ways they have selected to make their decisions and develop their story we might respond with "How is that working for you?"

Find unique outcomes. As the client describes their current situation listen closely for quality words that provide examples of client strengths. These examples can provide clues of successful authorship in the emergence of the new narrative. Look also for examples of the sparkling moments or unique outcomes that run counter to the dominance of stuttering in the speaker's life. Listen for examples where the speaker describes solution-focused rather than problem-saturated responses to their experiences. Often these counterthemes are found in other areas of their lives and can be used to inform the speaker about new responses to their stuttering (Plexico et al, 2006).

Share responsibility with the client. Although our instinct as members of a helping profession is to do all that he can for those who come to us for assistance, Perry and Doan caution that we should not work harder than our clients in helping them to revise their narratives. These authors suggest that the more the clinician (or parent) works the less the client (or child) is invited to participate. In other words, the more responsible the clinician the less responsible the client is likely to be. As Perry and Doan suggest, "'Working Harder than My Clients' is also an excellent title for a book whose final chapter will be titled 'Burned Out'" (p. 127).

The Special Case of Adolescents

Although it was probably recognized long before, in 1971 Van Riper commented that adolescents are often difficult cases. Daly, Simon, and Burnett-Stolnack (1995) suggest that this age group is particularly challenging because the teenage years are often characterized by emotional conflicts, fears, and frustrations. And, of course, these typical characteristics of adolescence may be compounded by the anxieties and negative consequences of stuttering. In acknowledging the special nature of this population, Blood (1995) noted that the extensive treatment some adolescents experience during elementary school tends to reduce their motivation to continue working on the problem. Blood also noted that often an adolescent's many social and school activities leave little time for treatment. A 1997 survey of 287 school-based clinicians by Brisk, Healey, and Hux found that the clinicians felt that they had fewer successes with adolescents who stutter than with any other age group. Others, including Manning (1991a) and more recently Zebrowski (2002), have pointed out the difficulties often encountered when attempting to convince an adolescent who stutters to enroll in treatment. Achieving success with this population requires understanding at least as much about adolescence as it does about stuttering.

Zebrowski's (2002) discussion of building relationships with teenagers who stutter should be required reading for clinicians working with these clients. Relying on her personal experience as well as an insightful book by Wolf (1991) whose title is worth mentioning—*Get Out of My Life, But First Could You Drive*

Clinical **Insight**

A long time ago in a galaxy far away . . . I was a high school student who stuttered at a moderate-to-severe level. At least that was the case when I was unable to avoid a classroom presentation. Eventually, I was referred to the speech therapist (the title at the time) who served the school. Although I was certainly embarrassed by stuttering in front of my peers, I was also embarrassed and somewhat angered by being singled out and asked to report to the speech therapist. I marched myself across the street to the office where I had been told to report and found not one, but two young men in their early twenties, both of whom were the therapists! With absolute fluency I told them that I was asked to report to the office, that I didn't have a problem, and that I wasn't at all interested in receiving any help. My fluency, as well as my agitated state, must have convinced them for they immediately responded by saying something like, "Well, I guess you're right. You don't seem to have a problem and don't need any help." And thus ended my first encounter with the field I would enter as a graduate student some seven years later.

During my two years as a speech clinician in the public schools (as well as on other occasions), I had adolescents provide me with their own versions of denial. My response was to engage them long enough to show them that I had some understanding of their situation. If I could interest them enough, I could take the opportunity to tell them about some of the many stories of success I have seen and inform them about organizations such as The Stuttering Home Page, The National Stuttering Association, Friends: The National Association of Young People Who Stutter, and The Stuttering Foundation. As they were running out the door I would tell them that good help is available when they were ready.

Me and Cheryl to the Mall?—Zebrowski provides some suggestions for understanding adolescents and for facilitating treatment for those who stutter. Of course it is not always the case, but teenagers tend to be intensely self-focused, appear to be immune to the many stresses facing them, strive to be cool and collected in social situations, value the relationships with their peers above all else, and tend to see adults as "jerks" who are irrelevant and clueless.

In many instances the handicapping effects of stuttering often increase as a young person reaches the early adolescent years. Peer pressure becomes a major factor in the social life of middle and high school students and teasing and bullying, if they have not already occurred, often peak at this time. In fact, it is not unusual for these inappropriate actions of others to be the catalyst that drives an adolescent or teenager to seek help. Not surprisingly, teenagers who stutter may respond to these pressures by expanding their tendencies of avoidance and denial, and coping strategies may become further refined and sophisticated.

Despite all of the problems presented by stuttering during the years of adolescence, there are many reasons why these individuals are likely to resist treatment:

- Priorities during the adolescent years make it difficult to convince those who stutter about the advantages of treatment. Although stuttering may be seen as a problem, it is not usually seen as the most pressing one. Other issues take higher priority, including social activities, sports, and work.

- Many teenagers harbor the hope that, with time and maturity, they will "outgrow" stuttering or that, at least for now, facing the problem can be postponed.

- In some instances, adolescents who are willing to give treatment a try soon find it difficult to take responsibility for practicing and committing to the tasks necessary for change. While they may be willing to come to the treatment sessions, they are unlikely to use behavioral techniques in daily speaking situations socially or at school.

- Many of the activities and techniques associated with treatment strategies tend to highlight the speaker and set him apart from his peers, a crucial issue for teenagers.

- Adolescents are especially sensitive to overstatements by adults who are attempting to make a point (Zebrowski, 2002) or to the possibility of being talked-down to (Haig, 1986). This may be exacerbated somewhat if clinicians are unable to communicate that they truly understand the experience of stuttering. Because adolescents are unlikely to credit adults with great insight and understanding about the things that are important to them, it is all too easy for clinicians to show them that stuttering is simply another thing that adults are clueless about. As Zebrowski (2002) explains, adolescents are not likely to tell you this. They are more likely to demonstrate their displeasure in a passive-aggressive manner by refusing to communicate, not showing up for appointments, or by failing to do the activities that have been agreed upon.

- Some teenagers are not particularly good at confronting emotions, often assigning responsibility or blame to others, including clinicians, parents, and teachers.

- Particularly aversive for some adolescents is the fact that successful therapy requires the involvement of their family. Many teenagers are characteristically striving on many levels to become independent of adults (often with limited success). However, the involvement of the parents is often critical because they often have wonderful insight about their children and know what they are capable of doing. Accordingly, parents are sometimes able to push their child harder than we can, come up with problem-solving

Clinical Insight

As we commented in Chapter 3, there are many reasons for stereotypes and there are always many exceptions to each of these conceptualizations. In many ways adolescents are more like adults than children, but it's frequently painfully clear that they have several more miles to go before reaching adulthood. The literature suggests that adolescents can be (select one or more from the following menu) noncompliant, difficult, complex, uncooperative, resistive, rebellious, sensitive, contentious, and argumentative. And this is only a short list. Another way of categorizing adolescence is an old psychiatric adage suggesting that "Adolescence is not a stage of life; it is a psychiatric diagnosis" (Chapman & Chapman-Santana, 1995, p. 154).

strategies, and help set up contingencies that will enable their child to modify their behavior and their attitudes. The fact that a child's parents are willing to take an active part in therapy demonstrates their sincerity and commitment. Of course, having other family members or friends involved in the therapy process can be important for understanding, support, disclosure, and activities related to transfer and maintenance.

- As a function of their desire for independence, teenagers are sometimes less likely to enter into a trusting clinical relationship with adults. Given the importance of the clinical alliance described in earlier chapters, this may impede therapeutic progress.

- Finally, there are also some interesting gender issues that may hinder the therapy process with adolescents. For example, adolescent males who stutter—and of course there are more males who do—may have some hesitancy about being seen by a female clinician. For a teenage boy to be forthright and honest about his stuttering behavior as well as his feelings of helplessness, loss of control, and shame with a female clinician is not something that necessarily happens naturally or spontaneously. Curiously, this has not been a topic of discussion in the literature on the treatment of stuttering.

Treatment is more likely to be successful for adolescents if they are able to locate a clinician who specializes in stuttering. The Special Interest Division 4 of the American Speech-Language-Hearing Association and groups such as the National Stuttering Association, Friends, and the Stuttering Foundation of America provide lists of such specialists. These groups also provide important sources of information and support including newsletters, informative pamphlets and videos. Furthermore, in the security and privacy of his or her own room, the adolescent can make contact with others around the country and the world via the Internet. Such contacts allow like minds to share information in a non-threatening way. The isolation of being a person who stutters can be dramatically lessened by contact with other people who are likely to have many shared experiences. Each of these options enables the adolescent to understand that he is not alone and is, in fact, far from being the only person with this problem. This information can help to inform, desensitize, and encourage the adolescent so that he or she may find effective help.

Adolescents are often ideal examples to demonstrate that, as clinicians, we "cannot push the river" (see Chapter 6) and that it is usually best to show that we are willing to follow their lead. Zebrowski (2002) stresses the importance of placing the teenage client in the role of the expert about their stuttering and emphasizing that the therapeutic alliance with the clinician is one of mutual dependence. This is especially important given that a teenage client is likely to be carefully scanning for efforts by the clinician to direct or monopolize the therapeutic narrative. By following the client's lead the clinician can elaborate the client's understanding of his or her problem. This strategy also facilitates the clinician's ability to explain the nature of therapy based on the speaker's interests and to demonstrate the knowledge and genuineness of the clinician. Several therapy suggestions provided by Zebrowski include the use of humor for strengthening the therapeutic relationship, writing activities by the client for developing responsibility and expanding insight and coping responses, developing positive self-talk, imagery, motor and mental focus (as used with athletes), and cognitive restructuring for altering core beliefs about themselves and their interactions with others. She also stresses the importance of developing the teenager's ability to effectively communicate with his or her parents about their experience with stuttering.

Given all the potentially thorny aspects of working with adolescents, it should also be said that spending time with them can be enjoyable. It is enjoyable to hear about the many activities adolescents are energetically participating in at this stage of their lives. They often display high levels of enthusiasm and they generally appreciate an occasional enlightened or even humorous perspective about the difficult speech situations (as well as other social predicaments) they find themselves in. Such moments may provide the opportunity for the clinician to reveal embarrassing or uncomfortable occurrences in his or her own life. Timely and spontaneous humor has been suggested as a way to prevent talking down to adolescents and to lessen the problem as we talk playfully and informally about their stuttering (Haig, 1986). Metaphors such as sports or related activities that promote a shared understanding of the experience of stuttering and the progress that is being made in and out of therapy also work well with adolescents (Manning, 1991a). A young person, for example, may appreciate how the persistence and hard work necessary for success on an athletic team (or other school or club activity) easily translates to their experiences with changing their stuttering.

Clinical **Insight**

As suggested in Chapter 1, humor can be justifiably conceived as an important variable in the process of cognitive change and healing. In his book *Social Intelligence*, Daniel Goleman (2006) describes the value of humor in the establishment and enhancement of the therapeutic alliance. Goleman explains that playfulness is a source of joy for all mammals, often beginning with tactile stimulations and visual–auditory interactions among parents and offspring. The strong neurological responses from the brain indicate that playfulness is a natural and often instantaneous response that fosters synchrony and resonance between two creatures.

As we have discussed in earlier chapters, the playfulness and spontaneity of humor are not apt to characterize the therapeutic alliance until the child or adult feels secure and understood in the treatment environment. However, understanding and sensitivity to the other person and their story often create experiences where humorous connections can be made. The opportunities for shared understanding provided by the humorous interpretation of events often forge a powerful connection. As Goleman suggests, "Laughter may be the shortest distance between two brains" (p. 45).

It should also be said that a realistic option for the adolescent is to decline therapy, and we may want to take the lead in presenting the possibility of doing just that. We can acknowledge that the decision for taking the therapeutic journey is largely theirs. It makes little sense to be dragging them along on a trip only their parents, their teachers, or their potential clinician want to take. Nevertheless, though we may be unsuccessful in convincing teenage clients to pursue treatment at this stage of their life, we can leave them with two take-home messages:

- It is possible to have a happy and productive life even though you stutter. Many things tend to improve with age, particularly as one develops a variety of skills and achieves different forms of success. With a broader understanding of relationships, social skills, and life in general, individuals often develop greater insight and confidence, even if they happen to stutter.

- There are qualified professionals who enjoy working with people who stutter who will be willing to help when you are ready.

A few years ago, a teenager demonstrated remarkable insight when he wrote an article describing the common themes he noted as he simultaneously learned to rock-climb and to work through treatment for his stuttering. His name is Brad Sara, and he was 14 years old when he wrote the following article that appeared in the National Stuttering Association Newsletter *Letting GO* in April, 1999 (see also the NSA web site).

Lessons I Learned While Rock Climbing

My name is Brad Sara, and I am a 14-year-old eighth-grade student who stutters. Last year I attended a monthly "speech group." I have also been learning to rock climb. In indoor rock climbing, there are two people; one who is climbing while the other is holding the rope that is connected to the ceiling. So if you fall, that person will catch you. The lessons I learned about rock climbing were many, but they also taught me about speech. Here's how they are similar.

You have to learn and then practice. In rock climbing, we had to practice over and over before we could even get on the wall. This is just like in speech, where you have to practice speech tools in order to get better at them.

You have to take on more responsibility. As we paired up for climbing, I remember thinking that I had not expected to be in charge of another person's safety. This meant that I had to be really responsible. This reminded me of how I used to feel about working on speech. I have learned that dealing with stuttering is my responsibility, and I have to accept more and more of it as I get older.

You have to trust the other person. While climbing, I needed to trust that my partner would not drop me. With stuttering, you have to trust listeners, teachers, friends, your speech therapist, and your parents that they will listen to you and say positive messages. You also have to trust yourself to follow through on your goals.

Effective communication is essential. When people are rock climbing, they have to talk to each other for safety. In speech, the most important thing is to get your point across, whether you stutter or not. The message is more important than how you say it.

You have to conquer your fear. When we started up the wall I think we were all afraid at first. But we faced it because we trusted the person hanging onto our rope. I also had trust in my training, and got less afraid by watching others being successful. So I went up and climbed, too. When I speak in front of a large group, I get afraid. Fear has a big deal to do with speech. If you don't face it, you will hold yourself back. If you conquer your fear, you will learn to be less afraid each time.

It's OK to make mistakes. One thing is very obvious to me. It's OK to make mistakes. Because if we felt we had to climb perfectly all the time, we were most likely to do worse. If you stutter, it's not the end of the world. If you say it's not OK, you're putting too much pressure on your speech to be perfect, and then if you do make a mistake, you will discourage yourself.

It's OK to get frustrated; eventually you will get it. There were many times while climbing that we got frustrated. Just like in speech, you keep on trying and you are going to "get it" someday. Have faith in yourself.

(continues)

It's OK if you fall. You catch yourself and start from there. Sometimes on the wall, I would slip and then catch myself. I just started again from where I was. If you stutter, it's OK and you can pick up your message from where you left off.

If you fall all the way down, start over again. When I fell a long way down while climbing, I started from the bottom, but knew I had learned the skills I needed to begin again. We have bad spells in our speech, sometimes. It's OK. We have learned what to do, and can start again.

Remain calm. I thought of this because one of our speech teachers is afraid of heights. When she got to the top, she was very scared to start down again, and we all talked to her to help her remain calm. In dealing with stuttering, I have had to learn how to deal with fear and to calm myself down when I am nervous so that I can manage my speech better.

When you're facing the edge, have faith in your support. When we got to the top of the wall, we had to stand on a ledge and then lean out to start going down again. We had to really have faith in the person who was supporting us. When I am real anxious and nervous about my speech, I have faith in the people who are behind me and who support me in whatever I do or say.

You just have to find the right rocks. When I was climbing, my partner and I were giving each other advice about which way to go and which rock might be the best one to go to next. In learning to manage my stuttering, I have found that I need to find the things that work for me. I need to use my own best words to express myself, find my best chances or opportunities to talk, and discover which tools work best for me. Other people can guide me, but I have to find my own "right rocks."

Source: "Lessons I Learned While Rock Climbing," National Stuttering Association Newsletter, *Letting Go*, April 1999. Reprinted with permission.

Group Treatment

One of the earliest applications of group treatment in the field of communication disorders was the work of Backus (1947), who advocated the use of speech in social situations beyond the usual speech-production drills popular at the time (Backus, 1957). The popularity of group treatment for adults increased as a result of World War II. The many men in need of treatment for psychological and medical problems, in combination with the relative shortage of therapists and counselors, resulted in group meetings replacing individual treatment. Conture (2001) suggests two trends that contributed to a decrease in the use of group therapy for individuals who stutter: the increased application in the 1970s of behavioral modification procedures necessitating prescribed individual therapy protocols, and a more recent emphasis on a "bottom line mentality" (p. 289) emphasizing the time and cost of treatment.

Luterman (1991) suggests that there are two basic types of groups: therapy groups and counseling groups. Group meetings for clients with fluency disorders typically serve both functions. The group setting provides opportunities for enhancing as well as maintaining change in both the surface and intrinsic aspects of the problem. Unless there happens to be a local support-group chapter, the group treatment meeting will be the only way for the client to understand that he is not alone. The group provides a social setting where the client can discuss his problem openly. As the client adjusts to the roles and expectations of the group setting, he is more likely to become desensitized to stuttering in general as well as his own stuttering in particular.

The Advantages of Group Therapy

Nearly anyone who has taken part in group therapy experiences as a clinician or participant knows that the opportunities provided by group interaction are a valuable part of a comprehensive treatment program. The activities that are possible in a group are a natural extension of the individual treatment session. The social environment permits a greater variety of treatment choices as well as a more comprehensive treatment approach than would be possible with individual treatment alone (Levy, 1983). The group provides an ideal setting for "divergent thinking," as members have the opportunity to observe how others have dealt with similar problems. Of course, as Egan (2007) points out, divergent thinking (e.g. "lateral thinking," "thinking outside the box") is uncomfortable for individuals who are bound to the idea that there is a single "correct way to approach issues or problems" (p. 228–231). Perhaps most important, the support in terms of understanding, motivation, and courage provided by the members of the group to each individual can hardly be underestimated, effects that are difficult to explain to someone who has never had the experience.

Depending on the therapeutic philosophy of the clinicians who have organized the group, there are many other potential benefits of the group therapy experience. The group meeting is likely to be the only place in the community where a person who stutters can feel safe; the only place they will not be penalized for stuttering. If they are able to stutter openly and easily, they can have the unique experience of being rewarded for stuttering well. The structure provided by a group setting provides the client with the opportunity to practice the techniques learned during individual treatment sessions. Conture (2001) points out that in some instances, group meetings can also provide social and speaking opportunities for people who might otherwise go for days or weeks without communicating with others. The group provides an audience for gaining confidence during many activities such as public speaking, making introductions, role-playing, discussion, and even debate.

Group interaction also provides the clinician with the opportunity to monitor the client's progress in a social context (Conture, 2001). When the treatment is taking place in an academic program, the group setting provides an opportunity for student clinicians to observe a broad range of behavior and to note the dynamics of progress in other clients. Group sessions also provide an ideal way for clients to gradually phase out of the more intensive individual treatment schedules. Following the conclusion of formal treatment, clients can readily return again to the group meetings if they desire support or experience signs of relapse (Levy, 1983) or simply feel the need for a booster session.

Luterman (1991) also indicated several characteristics of group treatment that are beneficial:

The instillation of hope: As other members of the group are able to make positive changes in their speech and ways of interpreting their situation, the client can increase his belief that he is also capable of such success. The client can often gain momentum from others in the group who are becoming more assertive and taking risks. Much like being a member of an athletic team, group participation often motivates a client to extend him- or herself beyond his or her original notions of what is possible.

The promotion of universality: By being a member of a group of individuals who share a common problem, the client comes to recognize that he is not alone. The group provides a means for coping with feelings of isolation and loneliness. The group setting also provides the client with the opportunity to practice recently learned modification techniques in a more realistic setting than alone with the clinician. For most speakers, publicly speaking in a group situation is a good initial step in generalizing newly acquired behavioral techniques to a social situation; successfully using the techniques in a group setting helps to reduce the client's dependence on his clinician.

The imparting of information: Information is provided not only by the group leader, as in individual treatment, but also by the other group members and, in some cases, other clinicians. All members of the group, whether or not they stutter, are able to provide examples and advice based on their own, unique problem-solving experiences. The inclusion of other clinicians, spouses, or friends provides the opportunity for individuals who stutter to understand, many for the first time, that nonstuttering speakers share many of the same fears about speaking in public or about risk-taking in general.

The provision of altruism: Each group member provides not only information to other members, but also support, reassurance, and insight. Furthermore, as the group members are helping others, they also tend to experience an increase in their own self-esteem.

The enhancement of group cohesiveness: As with most small groups, the treatment group develops its own history and evolves through the stages of "forming," "storming," "norming," and "performing" (Tuckman, 1965). That is, group members learn to adjust to the group protocol, discover how to identify roles and resolve conflicts, become committed to working with each other, and eventually focus on group objectives and goals. As this process occurs, the group becomes more self-directed, and individual members experience an increased desire to maintain their role in the group and look forward to group meetings. As group unity increases, group activities will be more likely to facilitate growth and change of individual members.

The possibility of catharsis: As the group provides a safe place for individual members to release and share feelings concerning their own problems, there is often a release from the control these feelings have had over the individual. This can be especially obvious as members become desensitized to their long history of fear associated with fluency failure and begin to achieve increased agency in daily communication situations. The group provides a safe place to ventilate feelings of embarrassment, shame, and social failure associated with previous stuttering experiences. Participants are often able to revise their interpretation of these past experiences. With greater distance and objectivity from these events, the possibility of humorous interpretation often occurs.

The development of existential issues: The group can provide the opportunity for individual clients and clinicians to deal with questions concerning anxiety associated with daily living, such as feelings of loneliness, dependency, and meaninglessness. The discussions can help reduce anxiety and allow the members to improve the quality of their decision making, including the many interpersonal aspects of their lives.

Determining Group Membership

The selection of those who will participate is an important part of assuring the success of the group. Each individual participant must be committed, motivated, and willing to contribute to the group process. It is also good to keep in mind that once an individual is included, it will be difficult to remove him. As Luterman suggests, individuals must have "a willingness to examine their lives and to share their insights with the group" (1979, p. 199). Furthermore, the group will be more likely to be dynamic and self-directed if the members are motivated and share a common interest for introspection and contributing to the success of others in attendance (Luterman, 1979). Individuals who tend to be argumentative, who consistently attempt to dominate group discussions, or who consistently withdraw from participation are generally not good candidates for group sessions.

Group treatment is not appealing to all clients, and it can be difficult to get adults who stutter to commit to a group setting. Silverman and Zimmer (1982) found, for example, that women who seek treatment for stuttering tend to prefer individual rather than group settings. On occasion, some individuals will express the fear that their problem will become more severe by being exposed to others who stutter (Conture, 2001). For some people with a long history of stuttering, even an informal group can be intimidating and carry with it the threat of social penalty. Some individuals may need to become desensitized somewhat before engaging in a group session. Thus, simply getting a client to attend his first group meeting can be a major success. Telling the reluctant individual that is alright for him to observe and not take part in the discussions for several sessions usually increases the possibility of participation. Most people are attracted by the interest, support, and energy provided by the other participants.

The Group Leader

As in individual treatment, the group leader is likely to be somewhat more directive during the initial meetings. At the outset, the effective clinician will need to establish credibility by demonstrating both knowledge of stuttering and people who stutter as well as a genuine interest in the members of the group. Just as the characteristics discussed in Chapter 1 describe the actions of an ideal clinician during individual treatment, these same features of empathy, warmth, and genuineness are necessary requirements of an effective group leader. Furthermore, the leader should be flexible and not only be able to sufficiently structure the group so that the participants have a sense of direction, but also willing to discard prearranged plans when necessary. One of the most difficult aspects of group therapy is striking a balance between the concerns of the individual members and group issues and goals. Another concern is finding a balance between a focus on the use of behavioral techniques that enhance fluency and issues of cognitive and affective change. As Conture (2001) points out in a commentary on the dynamic nature of group meetings, the meeting "is no place for those who have a low tolerance for ambiguity" (p. 292). Once the norms of the group become established and the goals and direction of the group have been defined, the group leader will be less instructive, creating increased opportunity for the members to be self-directive and interact with one another (Luterman, 1991). Of course, the group is more likely to become self-directed if group attendance remains consistent over several weeks. If the membership of the group is constantly changing, it will be more difficult for the group members to assume their own direction and develop their own norms.

Establishing Group Norms

Because a primary goal of group therapy is to create an environment where the individual members will interact with one another, it is usually *not* helpful for the group leader to assume to the role of asking and responding to questions from the group. In order for the group to become self-directive, the leader must promote the primary goal of members taking responsibility for the activities and topics. Another norm or characteristic of the group is one of self-disclosure. As the leader and other clinicians model disclosure of their experiences and attitudes the group members are likely to become more comfortable about revealing their own feelings, beliefs, and attitudes. However, group members should not feel pressure to self-disclose before they are ready. A good guideline is that no one has to talk unless they want to, and no question has to be answered. The trick is to encourage participation without eliciting judgmental statements by other members. A basic guideline used in many support groups is for the participants to describe their experiences but refrain from telling others what they should think or do. Finally, members must be reassured of the confidentiality of the group's discussions (Luterman, 1991).

Other Considerations with Group Activities

As might be expected, there are apt to be a variety of problems with attendance and schedules. In some settings it can be a major hurdle simply to find a time and a place to meet. It may be necessary for some participants to arrive somewhat after the starting time or leave prior to the end of the session in order to maintain consistent participation. It may be difficult to gather enough clients to form a critical and consistent mass. The number of people in groups varies widely. Most authors suggest a group size of around seven members, with a range of six to ten (e.g., Conture, 2001; Van Riper, 1973). Luterman (1991) suggests an upper limit of 8 to 15 members. A general rule might be that the group should be large enough for a variety of interactions but small enough that members have the opportunity to get to know and trust one another. If clinicians are included (something that is highly recommended for student clinicians), the group can easily become too large. One solution is to break up the larger group into smaller subsets so that all members have the opportunity to participate. At the conclusion of the session, all members can gather together for summary comments.

Achieving diversity among the members is desirable for promoting the divergent thinking described at the outset of this section. In most instances, clients will have been in treatment for varying lengths of time or will be at different stages of change. It has been our experience over the years that a wide range of diversity is usually achieved in terms of age, social, cultural, educational, and occupational background. Of course, group members will bring a variety of personalities and experiences to the meetings and, as Sheehan (1970b) suggested, a group is only as good as its membership. On occasion, some participants may impart inaccurate or unhealthy information or provide feedback to others that is less than constructive. In a few cases, members may fail to demonstrate any efforts at self-improvement, being content to use the group as their basic means of socializing (Levy, 1983).

Suggestions for Group Activities

Ideally, group meetings should be held in an adequately sized room with comfortable seating. A degree of privacy is preferred (Levy, 1983), and if relaxation and imagery activities are to be conducted, the area must be quiet. It is also useful if the room (or adjacent rooms) is large enough for public-speaking activities and can be divided into areas for small-group discussion or role-playing. Some availability of outside speaking situations is helpful so that group members (usually in pairs) can leave the building, conduct brief speaking assignments, and return to evaluate their experiences. Of course, arranging the participants in a circle is useful for enhancing conversation as well as for promoting eye contact and allowing the clinicians and clients to read each other's body language (Luterman, 1991). Once the group's structural and procedural norms have been established, the group culture will begin to evolve and specific activities can be considered.

Relaxation-Imagery Exercises. Many of the activities that are done in group meetings for fluency disorders are useful for all members, regardless of the quality of their speech. This is clearly the case with this category of techniques (Kirby, Delgadillo, Hillard, & Manning, 1992). It is not necessary or even desirable to be extremely relaxed in order to produce fluent speech. However, being able to relax in the midst of life's many anxiety-producing stimuli is a valuable skill for anyone. The process can be done anytime during the meeting, but often it works well to begin the meeting with these activities. Assuming the meeting is taking place in a reasonably quiet room with comfortable seating, the lights are dimmed. Playing quiet, relaxing music designed for such activities is helpful. Each group member closes his or her eyes and gradually focuses his or her thoughts on the instructions being delivered by a member of the group. The instructions direct each participant to progressively relax groups of his or her skeletal muscles, eventually focusing on the muscles of respiration, phonation, and articulation. The emphasis is on slowing and smoothing one's breathing, as well as visualizing an open vocal tract with cool air smoothly flowing through and out of the oral cavity. Participants are asked to imagine themselves in a serene and natural setting. Once relaxed, they are led through images of success, which include speaking activities. They are asked to remember the positive feelings associated with each success.

The process usually lasts approximately 10 minutes. Often, a relaxed state is created that carries over into the remainder of the group session. Initially, the responsibility of leading this portion of the session can be directed by a clinician. However, the instructions, which are delivered slowly and smoothly, provide an ideal speaking situation for speakers who have limited experience in speaking in front of a group.

Relaxation has been advocated as a way of promoting fluency for many years. In and of itself, relaxation is not a comprehensive solution to the problem of stuttering. Such techniques can, however, contribute to the learning that takes place during treatment. The goal is not to promote fluency per se but to teach the client better ways of responding to stress-producing situations, whether giving a presentation to a large audience, flying in turbulent weather, or undergoing dental work. Some members of the group will respond more readily to this experience than others, and some will be better able than others to make use of the relaxation and imagery skills in everyday situations. Of course, it takes consistent practice for these skills to be available when needed.

Role-Playing. The acting out of real-life situations is facilitated by group treatment sessions. The exercises can be useful in helping the speaker reconsider especially negative experiences associated with past fluency failure and experiment with various coping responses for future anxiety-provoking situations. Such situations may include ordering food at a restaurant or drive-through window, taking an oral exam for certification, giving an oral presentation, exchanging marriage vows, or dealing with threatening or confrontational situations at home, work, or school.[11] Role-playing activities by the group lend themselves to creativity and sometimes humorous responses to the situation. Participants are free to experiment with role-reversals, alternately taking on the personality of different characters in the exchanges. Observers can analyze the interpersonal aspects of the situation and offer constructive feedback and alternative ways of responding to the situation.

Public Speaking. Public speaking has been consistently shown to be a highly threatening situation for nearly everyone. For many individuals who stutter, the therapy group is likely to be the only opportunity they have ever had to assume such a role before an audience. Group members have the opportunity to experience the preparation of different types of presentations (informative, demonstration, storytelling, extemporaneous) and to practice responding to questions from the audience. Group members can practice upcoming presentations at school or work. Although the speakers have the opportunity to practice their fluency-enhancing techniques, it is important to also stress basic communication skills (e.g., eye contact with all members of the group, clarity, organization and sequencing of ideas, appropriate rate and timing of speech). Public speaking can be done in the same room where the group session normally takes place or (eventually) in a more formal setting such as a classroom or auditorium, sometimes making use of a microphone and amplification system. During the final stages of preparing for a speech at work or school, the individual or the entire

---

[11] Role-playing in response to bullying and teasing will be described in the following chapter.

group can meet at the site where the actual presentation will take place. When it comes time for the actual presentation, the group members can share in the success of the event by being there or by viewing the presentation on videotape. A particularly interesting possibility for achieving success in a variety of progressively more challenging communication situations is the use of virtual reality environments (Brundage, Graap, Gibbons, Ferrer, & Brooks, 2006). Used in the clinical setting, the procedure enables the clinician to evaluate the ability of the client to generalize their new capabilities to beyond-treatment speaking situations in a controlled and repeatable manner (see also Chapter 11).

Demonstration of Client Skills and Progress. During the group meeting, each participant has the opportunity to demonstrate techniques being worked on during the individual treatment sessions. For example, each group member can explain, demonstrate, and respond to questions about the use of specific techniques. Voluntary stuttering is a good example of such an activity. Other activities involve demonstrating examples of decreased avoidance behavior, providing examples of risk-taking activities, and describing humorous situations that occurred as a result of potential or real stuttering.

Clinical **Insight**

In order to complete their assignment of posing as a moderately severe stutterer, two graduate students walked through a local mall and engaged in conversations with people at several stores. As they entered a bookstore, one of the students realistically stuttered as she asked for a book on the topic of physical therapy. The clerk checked her computer and indicated that no books on that topic were available. The student, still obviously stuttering, asked for something on the topic of occupational therapy. The clerk's search was unsuccessful yet again. After a brief pause, the clerk turned to the student and cautiously asked, "Would you be interested in something on speech therapy?"

In many instances, the group therapy experience is considered as an adjunct to individual therapy. However, if attendance in a group is possible, it often provides critical impetus for successful change. As discussed in more detail in Chapter 12, the group experience may also set the stage for participation in support groups that are often essential for long-term success.

Conclusion

For the clinician who understands the surface behaviors as well as the underlying cognitive and affective components of stuttering as they are manifested in a particular individual, the fundamental treatment decisions become reasonably obvious. The creative challenges for the clinician center on how we can assist the speaker to achieve the goals of enhanced fluency, improved communication abilities, and especially a more agentic lifestyle. In contrast to the young person who stutters, the adolescent or adult client typically enters treatment with well-developed and sometimes subtle coping responses; responses that have helped the speaker to negotiate within a generally fluent culture. Because the person has learned to survive with their problem and because the coping responses are ingrained and tightly bound together with anxiety and fear, treatment for older speakers is typically more complex and requires more effort and time. The many subtle adjustments for coping behaviors, some of which the speaker may be unaware of, may take even the most experienced clinician time to detect. Working together, the client and the clinician can begin the process of identifying and varying the behavioral and cognitive patterns that have for so long informed the person's choices about communicating with others.

The experienced clinician recognizes that, in many ways, it is the client who will lead the way throughout the process of therapeutic change. What is possible during treatment is often determined by treatment variables such as the availability, setting, and cost of services. At the outset of treatment, the clinician, although being realistic about the level of fluency that the speaker may eventually achieve, should include spontaneous and natural fluency as a real possibility. For some adult speakers, however, controlled or acceptable fluency is the more likely outcome. Nevertheless, regardless of the eventual level of the person's overt fluency, it is possible to greatly reduce the limiting effects of the problem and enable the speaker to improve his or her quality of life.

Treatment for adults typically includes many features of both stuttering- and fluency-modification strategies. Fluency-modification techniques can help adult clients learn how to use their speech production mechanism more effectively and produce stable fluency in progressively more challenging speaking situations. However, most adult speakers who are able to achieve controlled or acceptable fluency also need to be able to confidently use stuttering-modification techniques that will enable them to repair the fluency breaks that do occur. Following the client's lead, the clinician can determine how to sequence and blend the variety of strategies and techniques for altering the behavioral features of the person's speech. Both stuttering- and fluency-modification protocols can result in the achievement of spontaneous fluency for some speakers. Regardless of the treatment protocol, the support and understanding provided within the therapeutic alliance facilitate all-important cognitive changes that provide the scaffolding for the behavioral changes. Group meetings often serve as an essential part of treatment, providing information, support, and insight that are otherwise unavailable. The activities of the group provide the members with an opportunity to practice skills learned during individual meetings, try out new speaking roles, and test new perceptions with others who share the same problem. The group experience reinforces the basic ideas that the speaker is not alone and that they do have choices about communicating and how they want to live their lives.

Topics for Discussion

1. What are several indicators to the clinician that the client is not yet desensitized enough to move to the variation or modification stages of stuttering modification?

2. During the next week take part in three activities (ideally communication situations) that you typically avoid. Journal a description and your reaction to each experience.

3. Use Brad Sara's description of rock climbing to create a similar set of guidelines in preparing for a challenging activity of your own.

4. Given the potential problems in getting an adolescent to give therapy a try, describe the basic take-home messages you would choose to impart during a 30-minute meeting.

5. Describe your response to an adult who has been stuttering for many years when he asks you, "What are my chances of success?"

6. What are the some common misconceptions that clinicians typically have about stuttering-modification techniques?

7. Write a short paragraph describing your use of negative self-talk about an upcoming event. Indicate whether or not you were able to change your negative self-talk to neutral or more positive self-talk.

8. Describe the possible benefits of group treatment meetings to a potential participant.

9. Describe the most important characteristics of an effective group therapy leader.

10. Given the discussions in Chapters 6, 7, and 8, prepare a short paper describing your philosophy about the therapeutic process that you would be willing to give to a potential client.

Recommended Readings

DiLollo, A., & Neimeyer, R. (2008). Talking back to stuttering: Constructivist contributions to stuttering treatment. In J. D. Raskin & S. K. Bridges (Eds.). *Studies in Meaning 3: Constructivist Psychotherapy in the Real World* (pp. 165–182). NY: Pace University Press.

Drewery, W., Winslade, J., Monk, G., (2000). Resisting the dominating story: Toward a deeper understanding of narrative therapy. In R. Neimeyer & J. D. Raskin (Eds.). *Constructions of Disorder* (pp. 253–263). Washington, D.C.: American Psychological Association.

Fransella, F. (2003). From theory to research to change. In F. Fransella (Ed.). *International Handbook of Personal Construct Psychology* (pp. 211–222). West Sussex, England: John Wiley & Sons.

Ramig, P. R., Ellis, J. B., & Pollard, R., (2010). Application of the SpeechEasy to Stuttering Treatment: Introduction, background, and preliminary observations. In B. Guitar & R. McCauley (Eds.). *Treatment of Stuttering: Traditional and Emerging Approaches* (in press). Baltimore: Lippincott, Williams & Wilkins.

CHAPTER 9

Facilitating Fluency for Preschool and School-Age Children

A lot of times, after I'd been outside playing and had gotten real thirsty, I'd run into the kitchen and ask her to give me a glass of water. I was still stuttering badly, of course, so it took some time. And early on, she would stop washing dishes or whatever she was doing and just reach down, pat me on the back, and encourage me: "C'mon Robert Earl, spit it out now, son." After a while though, whenever I ran in there and started tripping over my words, she'd say the same thing, but instead of patting me on the back she'd take the dishrag and pop me upside my head with it. It didn't help me "spit it out" any quicker, but I learned to stop asking and get that water for myself, real quick.

Bob Love (2000). The Bob Love Story.
Chicago, IL: Contemporary Books.

Chapter Objectives

The purpose of this chapter is to describe therapeutic approaches for assisting preschool and young school-age children who have been confirmed to be stuttering. The primary objectives of this chapter are to provide the clinician with examples of both indirect and direct forms of intervention that have been demonstrated to be effective with young speakers who stutter. Strategies to help the young speaker to enhance the amount and quality of fluent speech as well as alter stuttering in the direction of effortless and smooth disfluencies are described. Beyond describing the essential role of the parents in the process of therapeutic change, counseling strategies focus on desensitizing the child to the experience of stuttering and procedures for mitigating the impact of the all-too-frequent problem of bullying by peers. We discuss the possible effects of a variety of coexisting problems—particularly speech and language problems—that are likely to impact the therapeutic process. Finally, we provide recommendations for ways the classroom teacher may best respond when he or she discovers a child who stutters in the classroom.

The Age of the Stuttering and the Likelihood of Success

The largest number of individuals who stutter are found among children in their preschool and early school years; there are far more children who stutter than adolescents or adults. Consequently, several authors have suggested that clinicians will have the greatest impact by providing service to this group of speakers. As described in Chapter 2, the literature strongly suggests that by the early teenage years, there is a notable decrease in the number of individuals who stutter. As Bloodstein and Bernstein Ratner's (2008) review of many prevalence studies indicates, stuttering remains consistent through the elementary grades and begins to gradually decline during the high school years. Although a child's chronological age is a factor influencing the behavioral features and severity of stuttering, age is not as meaningful as the length of time stuttering has been taking place. As Conture (2001) puts it, the age of the stuttering is usually more meaningful than the age of the child. Children as young as two or three years old can present with strikingly complex stuttering behaviors and with high levels of tension, struggle, and fear. As described in earlier chapters, the longer a child has been stuttering, the more likely it is that the problem will become chronic.

In contrast to the sometimes more demanding challenge of facilitating successful treatment for adolescents and adults who stutter, the literature indicates that assisting preschool and early school-age children is often successful (Adams, 1984; Bloodstein & Bernstein Ratner, 2008; Conture, 1996; Conture & Guitar, 1993; Conture & Wolk, 1990; Fosnot, 1993; Franken, Van der Schalk, & Boelens, 2005; Gottwald & Starkweather, 1995; Lincoln, Onslow, & Reed, 1997; Onslow, Packman, & Harrison, 2003; Starkweather, 1987; Starkweather, Gottwald & Halfond, 1990). Interventions for young speakers typically make use of techniques that help the child to make slower and easier movements for voicing and articulation, decrease sensitivity to the stuttering event, increase self-confidence and problem solving as it relates to speech and communication, and promote an enjoyment of speaking. The reports of successful treatment for preschool children are undoubtedly aided (and confounded) by the fact that many children would have recovered on their own during the first months following onset. As a result, there has been some debate about the cost-effectiveness and ethical considerations about early intervention (Curlee & Yairi, 1997).

The literature indicates that treatment for somewhat older school-age children also is effective (Conture, 1997; Runyan and Runyan, 1993). However, as children experience the socialization process and the penalties associated with less than acceptable fluency during the early years of school, treatment tends to become more complex. Depending on the child and the coping behaviors that can rapidly evolve, clinicians may also make use of stuttering-modification procedures such as voluntary stuttering, cancellations, and pullout techniques. In other words, clinicians tend to employ a multifactorial approach whereby the clinician, often with the assistance of one or more parents, helps the child to improve skills or capacities in a number of areas that facilitate a smooth flow of language and speech.

Clinicians have also observed a history of increasingly direct forms of intervention with younger speakers during the last decades of the 20th century. According to Gottwald and Starkweather (1995), this increase is partially a result of the implementation of federal legislation in 1975 of Public Law 94-142, calling for the education of all handicapped children, and in 1986 of Public Law 99-457, requiring early intervention for children three to five years old. Perhaps even more influential were the results of research findings with young children by Yairi and his associates described in Chapter 2 that documented the characteristics of very early childhood stuttering, indicating that 75% of the risk for stuttering onset occurs before the age of three years, five months (Yairi & Ambrose, 1992a, 1992b). The increased understanding of early childhood stuttering, in combination with successful intervention for children who are seen as soon as possible following stuttering onset, began to make it clear that such treatment offers the best chance for altering the development of the problem. As we will see in the following pages, early intervention with young speakers has been found to be both effective and long-lasting.

Basic Considerations When Treating Young Children

There are, of course, many salient distinctions between intervention with children and with older speakers. In earlier chapters, the natural variability of fluency was noted and this is especially true for younger speakers. Variability in the frequency and form of early developmental stuttering makes both assessment and therapeutic change somewhat more difficult to determine for this age group. There is always the question of how much behavioral change is due to treatment and how much is due to the natural variability of the stuttering. In contrast to older speakers, there are several other important factors that are likely to influence how we assist young children who stutter:

1. Children are functioning with conceptual, linguistic, affective, and neuro-physiological systems that are far from adult-like and are still in the process of maturation.

2. The clinician is more likely to place emphasis on the evaluation and possible treatment of other communication, learning, and behavioral problems.

3. Teasing and bullying at school and in other social situations may occur.

4. Depending on the child's level of awareness and reaction to the stuttering experience, the clinician may select treatment techniques that are less direct than those used with adults.

5. Parents and a variety of other professionals, including the child's classroom teacher, play essential roles in the treatment process.

6. There tends to be somewhat less effort needed for helping the child to transfer and maintain treatment gains into extra-treatment environments.

7. The likelihood of achieving natural and spontaneous fluency is much greater for young children than for adults.

8. Relapse following treatment is not as likely as with adults.

Another thing that is unique about children who stutter is the setting where they are likely to be receiving therapy. Most children are seen in a public school setting under conditions that sometimes limit the effectiveness of therapy. It is not unusual for clinicians to be responsible for double or triple the maximum caseload of 25 to 40 children recommended by the ASHA direct service itinerant model (*ASHA*, 1984; Kelly, et al., 1997; Mallard & Westbrook, 1988). The lack of time available for individual treatment often results in children who stutter being seen along with children who have a variety of other communication problems. In most cases, children attend treatment, at most, twice a week for 20 to 30 minutes each (Kelly, et al., 1997; Healey, 1995). Finally, because children who stutter typically make up only 3% to 4% of a clinician's caseload (Blood & Seider, 1981; Kelly, et al., 1997; Slater, 1992), it is usually difficult to organize group therapy for these children with distinctive problems and treatment goals. All these issues combine to create what are often obviously inadequate services for children who stutter. It is not unusual to hear public school clinicians express their frustrations concerning these and other conditions that hamper the delivery of quality services for children who stutter. The frustration and anger expressed by persons attending local and national self-help meetings also reflect the less-than-adequate service delivery experienced by individuals who have attended school-based treatment programs. Clearly, this is not always the case, and there are examples of school systems that provide outstanding service to these children and their families, often made possible by clinicians specializing in fluency problems and the creation of after-school and summer programs.

An issue that is not unique to children has to do with how we, as clinicians, assign value to and describe both fluent and stuttered speech. That is, when we are speaking to younger as well as older individuals who stutter, how do we express ourselves about stuttering and the importance of fluency? Do we, by our verbal and nonverbal behavior, imply that fluency is "good" and stuttering is "bad" (or at least not as good as fluency)? If so, we could easily be engendering feelings of shame in the young speaker, who may already feel as though stuttering is his or her fault. Regardless of the overall treatment strategy, the effectiveness of many treatment techniques requires that the child be free to experiment with a variety of fluent and nonfluent speech behaviors. An overemphasis on fluent speech as the only valued goal of treatment can easily lead to the child trying too hard not to stutter, something he or she is already likely to be doing. Although it is true that listeners react negatively to most forms of stuttered speech, one of the clinician's basic goals is to break up the simplistic, conceptual dichotomy that all fluent speech is good and that stuttered speech must always mean that the speaker is out of control and helpless. As described in the previous chapter, an important aspect of treatment is to break the link between stuttering and being out of control. The speaker can, in fact, learn to tolerate "being in" the stuttering and choose from several responses that lead to a smooth and effortless form of stuttering. The speaker can understand that surface fluency, at the cost of many forms of avoidance and word substitution, is not control at all. All these aspects that are unique to the nature of stuttering in younger speakers combine to produce a number of clinical choices that the clinician must consider. One of these is the directness of the intervention process.

Indirect and Direct Treatment Strategies

In order to fully appreciate the current thinking regarding treatment for young children who stutter, it is useful to provide some historical context. Except for the latter years of the last century in the United States, the treatment for young children who stuttered was indirect. That is, the children themselves were not the recipients of the intervention activities and few specific instructions were given to the child about modifying their fluency. Rather, the adults in the child's environment—the parents, family members, grandparents, and teachers—received advice concerning procedures for altering the child's environment. The choice of this general approach was due to the many cautions from authorities who, over the years, recommended that the clinician avoid making the child aware of the problems he was having with his speech. Clinicians were extorted not to bring the child's disrupted speech to his or her attention or to respond in ways that might associate negative emotion with speaking. This view was especially popular during the decades of the 1940s through the 1960s and coincided with the prominence of the diagnosogenic theory of stuttering onset and development described in Chapter 3. The following series of quotes from a popular textbook of the time by Eisenson and Ogilvie (1963) reflects the then-current thinking about intervention for young children who were considered to be experiencing *primary* stuttering. Described by Bluemel in 1932, primary stuttering is seen as a transient phenomenon during which the child does not yet show awareness of his or her problem or demonstrate struggle behavior while speaking:

> The emphasis of treatment for the primary stutterer was to prevent the child from becoming aware that his speech was in any way different from others and a cause for concern. (p. 318)

> Essentially, therefore, the primary stutterer is to be treated through his parents if he is not of school age. If he is of school age, teachers as well as parents become the recipients of direct treatment. (p. 318)

Parents were instructed to respond in the following ways:

> If the child is a primary stutterer or is showing any of the speech characteristics associated with stuttering, it is essential that signs of parental anxiety be kept from him. Do not permit the child to hear the word stuttering used about his speech. Do not . . . do anything that makes it necessary for him to think about speaking or to conclude that he is not speaking well. (Bluemel, 1932, p. 323)

Another good example of this indirect approach is seen in Wendell Johnson's 1962 "Open Letter to the Mother of a Stuttering Child," which contained this statement:

> Do nothing at any time, by word or deed or posture or facial expression, that would serve to call Fred's attention to the interruptions in his speech. Above all, do nothing that would make him regard them as abnormal or unacceptable. (p. 3)

Finally, Van Riper (1939), in the first edition of his popular text, *Speech Correction: Principles and Methods*, wrote, "The way to treat a young stutterer in the primary stage is to let him alone and treat his parents and teachers."

With such cautions, few clinicians and parents were likely to intervene directly to assist a young child with his or her communication problems. The thinking was that direct intervention could make the stuttering more severe, a fear that permeated the decision-making process for clinicians at the time. Although these views are not likely to be held today by authors, instructors, and clinicians, there are undoubtedly many clinicians who are overly cautious about assisting young stuttering children and associate the natural variability and sometimes increased stuttering with greater severity.

Although there is considerable overlap between indirect and direct methods of treatment for children (Conture, 2001), an indirect approach may be appropriate for a child whose stuttering is characterized by relatively easy fluency breaks with little tension or struggle and who is generally unaware of any speaking difficulty. In such cases, the clinician is likely to model and encourage easier and perhaps slower ways (e.g., "turtle speech") of speaking but make little or no effort to directly modify specific features of the child's stuttered speech. The child's parents are provided with information concerning the developmental nature of language and fluency and encouraged to adjust the various environmental factors that tend to both disrupt and promote fluency. For example, by decreasing demand speech; promoting turn-taking; desensitizing the child to fluency-disrupting stimuli; and rewarding open, easy, and forward-moving speech, the child is guided toward increased fluency.

Treatment is more likely to be direct if the child has been stuttering for several months and is experiencing tension and struggle behavior or fragmenting monosyllabic words. In addition, the child may be exhibiting the nonverbal characteristics of more developed stuttering such as breaking eye contact with the listener (Conture, 1990). If the child shows these reactions on measures of awareness and negative reactions to communicating described in Chapter 5, the clinician will be more likely to initiate activities directly with the child that are designed to enhance fluency and, in some cases, modify moments of stuttering. Fluency modification techniques are most likely to be used for such children (Gregory, 1995; Healey & Scott, 1995; Guitar, 2006). However, depending on the success of these techniques, stuttering modification techniques may also be employed. That is, rather than focusing solely on enhancing fluent speech the child can follow the clinician's model in producing and contrasting both fluent and stuttered speech with the eventual goal of enabling the child to choose the easier and smoother form of speaking. Of course, the clinician can select the most appropriate activities along a continuum of directness according to the needs of the child and his or her response to treatment.

Regardless of how directly the clinician works to enhance the child's fluency, treatment for a young child who stutters should be characterized by a high degree of understanding, reassurance, and encouragement by the clinician. A major focus of both indirect and more direct approaches is to make speech enjoyable for the child. A highly supportive treatment environment enables the child to approach and explore the speaking experience and to enhance the ability to make choices about how speech is produced. Primary messages to the child via verbal and nonverbal modeling of both the parents and the clinician include such concepts as (1) stuttering is not the child's or the parents' fault, (2) speaking can be easy and enjoyable, and (3) the child is capable of selecting and producing forms of fluent speech.

The Importance of Parent Participation in Treatment

There is a wealth of information supporting the idea that parents play an influential role in the successful management of communication problems and this is certainly the case with stuttering. Since stuttering is typically a developmental problem beginning during childhood and parents are the most important models for their children, successful intervention requires the participation of the parents. Conture (2001) wisely points out that parents need to be rewarded for their insight and courage when they ask for help for their nonfluent child. The last thing parents need is for the clinician to lecture or reprimand them for their previous patterns of parent-child interactions. Parents should be informed at the outset that they have not caused this problem to occur nor do they bear the responsibility for eliminating it. However, parents can be shown how to assist in providing vital understanding and support. In some cases, parents will play a major role in administering and monitoring therapy techniques.

As influential as their participation in treatment for their child may be, on some occasions parents are unconcerned or uninterested in taking part in their child's treatment. Conture (2001, p. 154) provides a sensitive and insightful description of parents who for a variety of reasons, are unable or unwilling to become involved. They may be unable to take part due to work, travel time, or financial concerns. They may feel that the child will outgrow the problem. In such cases simply observing the child or initiating individual treatment is likely to be counterproductive. However, if the child's pattern of stuttering as well as his emotional and social maturity warrant, Conture suggests intervention in the form of parent/child fluency groups or a period of trial therapy (p. 167). Ramig (1993c) also points out that parents have many priorities, including work schedules and financial survival, which are likely to be regarded as more important than the current status of their child's speech fluency. Additionally, in rural or poor urban areas, there may be no way to contact the parents by telephone or internet, the parents may not be able to read or write, or English may be a second language. There may be only one parent in the home, making transportation of the child to treatment difficult or impossible.

Nevertheless, as we have indicated, it is the consensus of many experienced clinicians who have achieved therapeutic success with young children who stutter that parental involvement in treatment is crucial (Bluemel, 1957; Bottrill, W., Kelman, E., & Rustin, L., 1991; Conture, 1990; Conture & Schwartz, 1984; Ham, 1986; Johnson, et al., 1967; Peters & Guitar, 1991; Riley & Riley, 1983; Rustin, 1987; Starkweather, Gottwald, & Halfond, 1990; Wyatt, 1969). Rustin indicates that, if there is going to be any realistic chance for therapeutic success, the parents must play a major role. She states that "without the involvement of parents, clinicians become powerless to help the child beyond the confines of the clinic room" (Rustin, 1995, p. 125). Likewise, Ramig (1993c) and Bronfenbrenner (1976) state that without the parents' developing ability to help their child, the effects of treatment will likely deteriorate. Our experiences in running summer programs for children who stutter consistently show that those children whose parents attend sessions make considerably more progress than children whose parents, for one reason or another, do not attend.

Parental involvement not only assists the child in making behavioral and cognitive changes but also permits a form of mental hygiene to occur for the parents. Through counseling and parent group contact, the parents can accumulate the necessary information to become stronger and more confident about helping their child (Rustin & Cook, 1995). Although it may not be necessary for the clinician to spend a great amount of time desensitizing the young child to his fluency breaks, other people in the child's environment—including grandparents and teachers—often receive great benefit from these activities (Silverman, 1992). It is also worth considering that increasing numbers of children from nontraditional families are being seen in clinical facilities. In such cases, the major caregiver may not be the child's parent. Whoever takes on this role will play a central role during the stages of assessment, therapeutic change, and maintenance.

Ratner (1993) provides a helpful metaphor that clinicians can use to explain the nature of stuttering to parents. She points out the similarities of stuttering to allergies or juvenile diabetes. "Parental behaviors are not presumed to play a role in the onset of either allergies or juvenile diabetes. However, it is clear that the response of parents to these disorders can either mitigate or aggravate their consequences" (p. 238). To the degree that parents are able to adjust the child's environment in regard to such problems (e.g., exposure to allergens or adjustments in diet), the symptoms will become less severe. In the case of stuttering, parents can come to understand that although the etiology or the problem is unlikely to change, the maintenance of the symptoms can be significantly altered by the actions and support of the child's parents.

In order to assist the parents in understanding the problem and making good decisions on their own, the clinician can provide behavioral models as well as information. Still, the clinician needs to be cautioned to provide information in reasonable amounts. When counseling parents it is easy to provide too many recommendations too quickly (Conture, 1990; Luterman, 2001). As a result, parents can become overwhelmed and discouraged. Rather than lecturing the parents, it is more effective to follow their lead by listening to their questions and responding to—and expanding on—the issues they want to know about. Parents can select from a wide variety of helpful sources and obtain informative pamphlets, watch instructional videotapes, search the Internet, and observe treatment being conducted with their child. By taking such action they will be much more likely to provide the clinician with insightful ideas and suggestions.

One way to consider the levels of parental involvement throughout fluency therapy for their children is suggested by Ramig (1993c), who describes three stages of parent involvement of (1) facilitating communicative interaction, (2) educational counseling, and (3) involving parents as observers and participants.

During the initial stage of *educational counseling*, a primary role of the clinician is to help demystify stuttering and increase the parents' understanding of their child's situation. The clinician explains the difference between normal breaks and stuttering-like-disfluencies (SLDs), discussed in Chapter 2. Parents are informed that, although the etiology of stuttering is not completely understood, a great deal is known about the dynamics of stuttering and much can be done to decrease the problem, especially in young speakers. With increased understanding, parents will become less anxious and inhibited about stuttering and see how their involvement in treatment will support rather than somehow hurt their child. As parents become more knowledgeable and desensitized they will be better able to make intuitive and helpful responses to their child.

As Ramig (1993c) suggests, parents are likely to bring along many myths about stuttering including that as parents, by omission or commission, they have somehow caused the problem (Conture, 1990, 2001; Peters & Guitar, 1991; Rustin, 1987; Van Riper, 1982). As Ramig (1993c) suggests, the reduction of possible feelings of guilt by the parents should be viewed as a major achievement by clinicians. Group meetings of parents provide an invaluable forum for dealing with these frustrations as parents begin to realize that they are not alone. Used in a variety of settings, including public schools and support groups, the meetings provide an opportunity for the more seasoned parents to provide the support and insight that are especially helpful to other parents who are new to the experience (Berkowitz, Cook, & Haughey, 1994; Ramig, 1993c). Detailed descriptions of parent/child fluency group dynamics may be found in Conture (2001, pp. 167–177).

It is also helpful for parents to understand that, *as a group*, parents of stuttering children behave no differently than those of normally speaking children. As Ratner (1993) points out, there is no evidence for the view that the parental interaction style is related to the severity of a fluency disorder. Furthermore, no correlations were noted between stuttering severity at initial assessment and parental conversational behaviors of speech rate, frequency of questions, and interruptions. In addition, Weiss and Zebrowski (Weiss, 1993; Weiss & Zebrowski, 1992) found that parents of children who stutter do not produce significantly more requests for verbal responses than parents of nonstutterers. Furthermore, the parents of children who stutter show no psychological differences when compared to the parents of fluent children (Adams, 1993).

According to Ramig (1993c), a second stage of parent involvement involves the *facilitation of communicative interaction* with the child. The goal of the clinician is to model for the parents the interpersonal styles that facilitate fluency during parent-child interactions. The overall communication and interpersonal characteristics of the child, as well as the child-parent interaction style, should be continuously evaluated. These characteristics include linguistic as well as paralinguistic variables, many of which have been studied in recent years in an attempt to determine their effect on children's fluency (see Kelly, 1994 for a summary). Such studies have investigated the rate of the speech (Conture & Caruso, 1987; Kelly, 1994; Meyers & Freeman, 1985); parent verbal and nonverbal responses to the child's fluency breaks (LaSalle & Conture, 1991); the amount and type of interruptions of the child's speech by the parents (Meyers & Freeman, 1985); turn-taking behaviors and response-time latency (Kelly, 1994); the complexity of the questions posed to the child (Stocker & Usprich, 1976); and the tendency for the parent to provide verbal and nonverbal corrections to the child as he or she is speaking (Gregory & Hill, 1980). As these features are identified, the parent can be shown how to alter some aspects of their interactive style. For example, the mother can be shown how to slow her speech, provide more time for turn-taking, interrupt the child's speech less, and positively reinforce the child for using fluency-enhancing techniques.

Conture and Caruso (1987) and Ramig (1993c) advocate the use of "Mr. Rogers" speech (referring to the soft-spoken television figure) as a prototype for slower, smoother speech and longer turn-taking pause times. Silverman (1996) suggests having the parents view videotapes of themselves and their child while the clinician points out both the less and more desirable ways they are responding to their child's fluency breaks. For example, the parents may be speaking rapidly and frequently interrupting or indicating by their body language (e.g., breaking eye contact) that they are not interested in what their child is saying. Recall, for example, the study by Winslow and Guitar (1994) mentioned in Chapter 3 who found that the fluency of a 5-year-old child increased when conversational demands were lessened by the implementation of turn-taking rules, while stuttering increased when these rules were withdrawn. During an obvious or severe stuttering moment, parents may unconsciously freeze or show anxiety or concern. They may have a pattern of asking their child difficult or abstract questions that require complex responses. On the other hand, of course, the parents may also be doing many appropriate things, including modeling slow, easy speech and responding with an unafraid attitude to stuttering behavior. Videotapes of clinician–child interactions also can be used to demonstrate desirable parent behavior.

A third and final stage of parental involvement places the parents in the role of *observers and participants* in the process of therapeutic change. The participation of both parents is often the ideal situation, although there is minimal research on the role of the father in this process. Ramig (1993c) indicates that even if only one parent is able to take part, the result is still likely to be beneficial for the child. Initially the parent's role is to observe the interaction of the child and clinician as the clinician models changes in the previously described interactive style. The clinician also demonstrates strategies for expanding the child's fluency and modifying moments of stuttering, using techniques described in the previous chapter as well as in later sections of this chapter. Parents gradually join in this process with the clinician and the child and eventually interact with the child on their own.

The Lidcombe Program

A treatment strategy that places the parents in a central role is illustrated by the Lidcombe Program (Harrison, Onslow, & Rousseau, 2007; Onslow, Costa, & Rue, 1990; Onslow, Packman, & Harrison, 2003). Responding to the need to treat children who stutter at a community health center in a suburb of Sydney, Australia, the developers of the program were influenced by the success shown in a series of direct, response-contingent treatments for young stuttering children conducted in the United States in the 1970s (e.g., Martin, Haroldson, & Kuhl, 1972a; Martin, Kuhl, & Haroldson, 1972; Siegel, 1970).

At the outset of the Lidcombe Program (Stage I) parents attend weekly 45- to 60-minute sessions in the clinic and observe the clinician's use of verbal contingencies in response to the child's fluent and stuttered utterances. Following the clinician's model, parents learn to administer verbal response-contingent stimulation. Fluent responses are acknowledged with what is termed a neutral response (e.g., "That was good talking. Those words were smooth.") or praised (e.g., "Wow, good smooth talking!"). Unambiguous stuttering is highlighted by the clinician with responses such as "That was bumpy speech." or "That was a bump there." The clinician is continually supportive, responding to the child's examples of stuttering intermittently in order not to overwhelm the child. The clinician (and eventually the parent) responds to fluent and stuttered events on a five-to-one ratio. Two "non-essential" child responses include self-evaluation of stutter-free speech (e.g., "Was that smooth?" or "Where there any bumps there?") and self-correction of stuttering (e.g., "Can you say 'orange' again smoothly?"). Self-corrections are praised (e.g., "Great talking, you smoothed out that bumpy word by yourself!"). As the parents learn to administer the verbal contingencies during structured activities they begin to assume the role of the clinician, conducting the program at home during short (10–15 minutes) structured sessions, often using games. As the parent and the child adapt to the nature of the activities the parents begin providing verbal contingencies during unstructured, everyday activities.

The primary goal during Stage 1 is stutter-free speech or near-zero stuttering. Treatment sessions in the clinic occur once a week, resulting in a median number of 11 visits. Harrison, Onslow, and Rousseau (2007) describe three fluency measures that are obtained to document therapeutic change. Parents are taught to obtain a reliable (within one scale value) perceptual measure of the severity ratings (SRs) of their child's stuttering and a count of the child's stuttering frequency, or stutters per minute of speaking time (SMST). The SRs are rated on a 10-point scale (1 defined as "no stuttering," 2 as "extremely mild stuttering," with 10 representing "extremely severe stuttering"). Parents may obtain SRs for an entire day or for a 10-minute period one or more times each day. The SMST measure is optional and is used to supplement the parental SRs. The SMST is obtained by the parent listening to the child's conversational speech for an amount of time and then dividing the number of stutters by the duration of the speech. A third measure is obtained by clinicians during clinic visits and takes the form of a percentage of syllables stuttered (%SS) during conversational samples (300 syllables or 10 min).

During Stage I of the program, children demonstrate a decrease in both the variability and frequency of their SRs as they produce more frequent and longer stutter-free utterances in nonstructured, everyday situations. At this point the clinician (and the parent) may choose to use self-evaluation contingencies following a series of stutter-free utterances. Once the child is able to achieve and maintain Stage I criteria for three consecutive weeks, Stage II begins. Stage II criteria are (1) weekly average SRs of less than 2.0 with no more than three scores greater than 2 in a week, (2) less than 1.0 %SS in the clinic, and (3) less than 1.5 SMST outside the clinic (assuming that SMST scores are used).

The primary goal of Stage II is to maintain the gains the child has achieved during Stage I. Clinic visits are gradually decreased to once every two, then four, then eight weeks and so on. In cases where the child is unable to maintain Stage II criteria (which occurs about half the time, often during the outset of Stage II), clinicians and parents confer and make adjustments.

Because of the methodical, manualized nature of the approach and the focus on the child's frequency of stuttering, the program facilitates the ability of researchers to conduct controlled research. As a result, the Lidcombe program has received extensive documentation in the literature. The investigators have demonstrated consistent and impressive efforts to demonstrate the efficacy of the approach. However, although many of the initial investigations showed high levels of treatment efficacy with well-trained clinicians, there was little control for natural recovery. Fortunately, more recent investigations controlled for natural recovery and continued to show impressive results. Phase III randomized controlled trial data controlling for natural recovery demonstrated large effect sizes for children who received the Lidcombe Program versus preschoolers who received no treatment for a 9-month period (Jones, Onslow, Packman, Williams, Ormond, Schwartz, et al., 2005).

In much the same way that Ingham (1993) indicated that the reasons for the reduction of stuttering with operant programs are unknown, the explanation for the success of the Lidcombe Program with children is unknown. Yairi and Ambrose (2005) point out six features of the Lidcombe

Program that may account for reduced stuttering, although it is not clearly understood which of these features (or combination of features) specifically account for the change: ". . . treatment in the clinic, treatment by parents at home, reinforcement of fluency, disapproval of stuttering, direct modification of stuttering, and self-evaluation" (p. 455). In contrast to many other treatment programs for young children, parents are not asked to change the characteristics of their language, rate of speech, and interactions (Bonelli, Dixon, & Bernstein Ratner, 2000; Harrison, Onslow, & Rousseau, 2007; Onslow, Costa, & Rue, 1990; Onslow, Packman, & Harrison, 2003). However, the parents are directed to respond in important ways to their child's fluency (acknowledgement and praise) and stuttering (highlighting, modeling, and encouragement of self-corrections).

Bonelli, Dixon, and Bernstein Ratner, (2000) attempted to identify the possible variables accounting for changes in the fluency of the young children treated in the Lidcombe Program. These authors found no changes in child or parent speech rate, interspeaker turn-taking latencies, or pragmatic function that accounted for the treatment effects. In all but one case, the mothers showed an increase in their articulation rate during conversation with their children following treatment. The speech rate of the children showed no consistent rate change accounting for treatment effects. A variety of language measures for the children fell within normal limits for their age, both pre- and post-treatment. On the other hand, many of the children had pretreatment language scores that greatly exceeded the mean expectation for their ages. As others have done (Camarata, 1988; Ratner, 1997; Tetnowski, 1998), Bonelli et al. (2000) suggest the possibility of a trading relationship among the various components of the language-speech production system in children. That is, because many of the children who were receiving treatment produced advanced pretreatment language, the reductions in expressive language demand to more age-appropriate levels may have facilitated the production of stutter-free speech. Bonelli et al. also point out that the contingent responses prescribed by the Lidcombe Program selectively reinforces fluent utterances of the children and, as a result, is likely to disproportionately reward the production of short utterances. Because short utterances are more likely to be fluent they are also more likely to be praised, and it may be for that reason children will choose shorter utterances, thereby producing less stuttering (Muma, 1969).

There are several additional characteristics that may inform clinicians about the success of the Lidcombe program that are also worth considering. Ratner and Guitar (2006) provide a list of factors extending beyond operant explanations that are likely to facilitate successful therapeutic change across a variety of treatment protocols, including the Lidcombe Program: (1) development of an active role for the parents in the therapeutic process, providing the parents with a sense of control over a difficult parenting problem; (2) achievement of high levels of parental understanding, learning, and commitment; (3) reduction of parental anxiety as a result of understanding and participation in their child's treatment program; (4) acknowledgement and normalization of stuttering by the parents, making it an acceptable topic for discussion; (5) administration of parental praise by a sincere and involved praise-giver; (6) facilitation of a bonding process via the interaction of the parents and the child; (7) conduction of the majority of the treatment sessions in the child's home environment; and (8) reduction in the child's expressive language complexity to more age-appropriate levels. In addition, based on the increased attention given to "stutter-free" speech by the child's parents, Dilollo and Manning (2007) suggest the possibility that yet another mechanism of change may result from the *construction of a meaningful fluent speaker role* for the child.

It may be that, to the extent that one or more of these factors (especially those related to parent participation) are also common to other treatment programs, increased fluency is likely to occur for young children who stutter. Support for this possibility (and the common factors model described in Chapter 6) was provided by the results of a preliminary investigation by Franken, Van der Schalk, and Boelens (2005). A comparison of the Lidcombe Program and the demands and capacities protocol (Starkweather, Gottwald, & Halfond, 1990) by Franken et al. found that both programs demonstrated a significant decrease

Clinical Insight

Some of the most poignant comments by adults who stutter, including those who have successfully managed their stuttering, describe the silence that surrounded the topic of stuttering when they were children. They describe the frustration and shame that was heightened by the unwillingness of their parents to address a problem that was so obvious. Most parents are willing to address and try to help their child with other problems they may have. But stuttering is too often viewed as an embarrassing and taboo topic, and the silence is easily interpreted by the child to mean that stuttering is something that is plainly too shameful to mention. Dr. Alan Rabinowitz, in his 2005 keynote address to the Stuttering Foundation (Speech Foundation CD # 8500), recalled that "My parents never knew what to do with me. . . . I loved my parents but their greatest mistake was their denial of my stuttering and their belief that to talk about the problem with me or in front of me would only hurt me more." Clinicians play a valuable role in helping parents to bring stuttering out of the closet and making it an acceptable topic of conversation. Clinicians can model an enlightened approach to an issue that is fascinating, help to alter the myths about stuttering, and mitigate the pain and humiliation so often and so unnecessarily experienced by young children and adolescents who stutter.

in both stuttering frequencies and severity ratings. Interestingly, both programs emphasize high levels of parent involvement in the treatment process, with a large portion of the therapy occurring in the child's home environment.

Another program for children that places the parents in a key role is the *parent-child interaction therapy (PCIT)* developed by Rustin, Botterill, and Kelman (1996). The program combines both indirect and direct procedures with the overall objective of empowering parents to manage their children's stuttering and to develop confidence in their own skills. The first of the two major components of PCIT are *management strategies* that enable the parents to reduce their anxiety about stuttering, cope with the sensitivities of the child, set boundaries, develop consistent routines, and understand the positive effects of providing helpful forms of praise. The second component takes the form of *interaction strategies* that are unique for each family. Accordingly, rather than the clinician demonstrating targets or acting as a role model, the parents select their own targets based on videotaped observation of interactions with their child. Possible targets include the parents reducing the rate of their speech to match their child's, increasing response time latency, and reducing the linguistic complexity of their language to a level appropriate for the child. A basic rule during interactive play is to "follow the child's lead."

Using a longitudinal, multiple single-subject design, Millard, Nicholas, and Cook (2008) investigated the effectiveness of the PCIT program with six children aged from 3 years, 3 months to 4 years, 10 months who had been stuttering more than 12 months following onset (three of the six children had been stuttering for up to two years). Treatment consisted of indirect therapy during six sessions of clinic-based therapy and six weeks of home consolidation activities. During the consolidation period the children took part in a 5-minute "special time" (playtime) with each parent three to five times each week in order to implement the management strategies. This daily period consisted of engaging the child in a one-to-one communicative setting where parents practice their interaction target goals. Speech samples were videorecorded during these play periods, and the parents provided a written record of the interactions. Stuttering frequency and variability in %SS were analyzed during a pretreatment baseline phase, during therapy, and up to 12 months following therapy.

Analysis procedures that uniquely took into account the typical variability of stuttering found a pattern of systematic, nonrandom decrease in the children's stuttering. The patterns of change for the children indicated that the decreases in stuttering were attributable to the treatment rather than natural recovery. As expected, the response to the treatment was distinctive for each child. Four of the six children significantly reduced the frequency of their stuttering with both parents by the end of the therapy phase. One of the two children who did not show a significant decrease with either parent during the 12-week period of indirect intervention required further direct intervention and significantly reduced her stuttering with both parents during a follow-up phase. The second child reduced his stuttering with the father but not the mother during therapy. In this case, a direct program was initiated and continued with further decreases with the father but not with the mother. It seems apparent from these as well as other recent investigations (Jones et al., 2000; Yaruss et al., 2006) that parent participation in the therapeutic process is a key factor in the success of relatively short treatment programs for young children who stutter.

Goals of Treatment for Younger Speakers

A realistic goal of treatment, particularly with preschool age children, is a high level of spontaneous or normal fluency (Conture, 2001; Healey & Scott, 1995; Guitar, 2006). The future for fluency is bright for such children who receive good, early intervention. Of course, it is possible that some children may recover on their own without intervention. Depending on the weight the clinician places on the factors related to chronicity of stuttering described in Chapters 2 and 5, clinicians and parents may or may not opt for some formal assistance in facilitating fluency for these young speakers. The child's familial history of stuttering, as well as indications of the child's awareness and negative reactions toward his or her fluency breaks, will need to be considered. For preschool age speakers it is reasonable to consider the frequency and quality of the child's disfluent speech as a primary indicator of successful change.

For the child who is somewhat older and undergoing the early stages of school and the socialization process, issues beyond basic measures of fluency are more likely to come into play. A short quote from Healey and Scott (1995) provides a broader view of the situation for these children.

> We are reluctant to base treatment effectiveness exclusively on pre- and post-treatment fluency data. This seems to be a rather narrow definition of "success." Some children in our program have demonstrated increased levels of fluency but were unable to achieve a positive attitude about themselves as fluent speakers. (p. 153)

As with adolescents and adults, focusing on the child's fluency may provide the clinician with both a restricted view of the problem and a narrow definition of progress. However, there is little question that, even for young children, both affective and cognitive changes take place during effective therapy. It's not uncommon to encounter children who have stuttered for only a few weeks or months who demonstrate reactions of frustration, anger, and avoidance in response to their inability to easily produce speech. In any case, the monitoring of changes in these intrinsic features will provide the clinician with a broader view of progress and long-term success.

Other experienced researcher-clinicians (Conture, 2001; Guitar, 2006) also express the same comprehensive therapeutic view when assisting young children who are at the outset of stuttering. That is, along with a focus in reducing the frequency and form of stuttering, intervention also includes the goals of reducing negative feelings and thoughts about stuttering, decreasing avoidance, involving the parents in altering the child's environment, and enhancing the child's abilities and enjoyment associated with communicating.

Conture (2001) suggests that most children will take approximately 20 weeks (with a range of 10 to 30) of weekly therapy before they are ready for dismissal. He also advises, however, that the clinician should be careful not to force treatment into a parent's busy schedule. The clinician should be prepared to give both the parents and the child an intermission from weekly treatment sessions and be available for consultation with the parents during such intervals. These children may be more likely to have a family history of fluency disorders or one or more other problems that make communicating or learning more complicated. In such cases, treatment may take somewhat longer.

A Consideration of Treatment Strategies

Although most current authors writing about treatment for young children recommend reasonably direct treatment, there is some question as to whether many practicing clinicians feel the same way. Based on several recent surveys of professional clinicians (see Chapter 1), some clinicians continue to be hesitant—or at least highly cautious—about working directly with young children who stutter. Whether the clinician chooses to work more or less directly with the younger child, the essence of treatment consists of some combination of both facilitating the child's capacities to produce effortless fluent speech and reducing the demands placed on the child that result in fluency disruption. As Starkweather (1999) suggests, "We can prevent the complexity of stuttering from developing, or if it has developed, we can undo it, untie the knots of frustration and struggle. And the younger the child is, the easier the knots are to untie" (p. 233). Certainly there will also be several associated goals, including desensitizing the child to the experience of stuttering, and increasing the child's resistance to fluency-disrupting stimuli.

It is also worth noting that many of the strategies and techniques used with adolescents and adults can be applied, in many cases with only minor alterations, to older school-age children. Of the two major strategies, various versions of fluency-enhancement approaches are most often used with younger speakers. Many stuttering modification techniques may also be appropriate depending on the level of struggle and emotional reactivity indicated by the child. Particularly with younger clients, the techniques associated with fluency enhancement and stuttering modification strategies become quite similar. Both strategies emphasize easy, often slowed, and smooth articulatory movements; light articulatory contacts; and attention to monitoring and producing consistent airflow and voicing. Perhaps most importantly, underlying these behavioral techniques is the cognitive set that the child is able to make choices and be in charge of his or her speaking mechanism.

Assisting the Child in Responding to Stuttering

For many children, particularly if they have been stuttering for a short time and have yet to incorporate high levels of avoidance behavior, modeling and instruction of fluency-enhancing techniques may be all that is needed to promote fluency. In other instances, the clinician may decide to also provide the child with strategies for helping him or her respond to stuttering in more positive ways. In order for the child to learn ways of changing the form of his or her stuttering, it is essential to identify both the desirable and the less undesirable characteristics of the fluency breaks. Some clinicians are undoubtedly concerned about using the "S" word (stuttering), and it is not uncommon for parents to avoid using the word *stuttering* in front of their children. Most clinicians and authors believe that referring to what the child is doing as stuttering is not a major issue with young children. Assigning unnecessary power to the word *stuttering* and making great effort to avoid its use is unnecessary (see Conture, 2001, p. 141). As Murphy (1999) suggests in his discussion of shame as it relates to stuttering, it is good for everyone to talk openly and forthrightly about stuttering. It is true that if we assign positive or negative value to any word, the word tends to become more powerful. However, using the word stuttering in a normal conversational manner is not, in and of itself, likely to make the situation worse. Whether the word stuttering is used or avoided, contrasting descriptors such as easy–difficult, slow–fast, gentle–hard, and smooth–bumpy are likely to be much more meaningful to a young child. These are also words that others (teachers, relatives, friends) are less likely to interpret in a negative fashion.

One of the most efficient ways to identify and discriminate between different forms of fluency–disfluency is for the clinician to produce examples for the child. The style of the clinician when demonstrating these examples is important, and doing it in a matter-of-fact manner, with enthusiasm, curiosity, and a sense of fun is apt to be the best approach. Underlying these activities is the child's appreciation that he or she has the power to produce speech in a variety of forms. The contrasts between bumpy and fast versus easy and slow speech can be illustrated with body movements and toys. The clinician and the child can, for example, alternately tighten and relax various parts of their bodies (including the speech mechanisms), helping the child to differentiate between tightness and relaxation and giving the child a sense of control when using his or her "speech helpers." Both the clinician and the child can introduce intentional brief and easy stutters into their speech, experimenting and playing with alternative ways of easing or smoothing through them. It is not necessary to demonstrate extreme forms of stuttering—only a degree of mild tension and fragmentation is necessary to make the point. It is often especially instructive for the child to take the role of the "teacher" and direct the clinician (or the parents) as the adult speaker makes the suggested adjustments.

Of course, the primary goal of these activities is not fluency *per se* (although that is often the result) but the child's ability to vary and purposely control and vary his or her speech production (Williams, 1971). The child learns that he or she is not helpless and, in fact, has many choices about how to produce sounds and words. Once children are able to consistently alter their stuttering moments into easy, effortless productions, they will become able to revise real moments of stuttering in a similar fashion. The point is to assist the child in making the experience of speaking enjoyable while giving the child a sense of power over his or her speech, concepts that are emphasized by virtually all writers on the topic of treatment for young children.

Of course, it is important that parents understand the importance of highlighting their child's moments of difficult speech in a sensitive way and reward smooth and easy speech as it occurs. Parents can note such speech and respond with verbal praise, "Ah, that was easy (or smooth)!" or nonverbally, with a smile or eye contact, when they notice the child turning a bumpy form of speech into a smoother and easier version. However, Conture (2001) cautions that not all parents will be able to do this without some observation and practice. He notes that some parents tend to reprimand, correct, nag, or badger the child regarding his or her speech; they must be taught instead to assist in a gentle and appropriate manner. Without practice, some parents are likely to be inhibited about mentioning their child's stuttering or afraid of doing something wrong. Until they become desensitized, some parents will resist intentionally producing anything that resembles even easy and smooth stuttering in their own speech. The success of these experiences depends on the sensitivity of the clinician in guiding the parents toward a less reticent response when experimenting and "playing" with different forms of fluency.

Analogies that are appropriate for children can assist them in producing speech with an open and flowing vocal tract, often facilitating fluency and helping to alter the form of stuttering. As Conture explains, the creation of airflow in

Clinical **Insight**

Although the clinician will be able to detect the many successes that the child is achieving as he or she is able to change his or her habitual forms of stuttering into less effortful and smoother forms, less sophisticated listeners are unlikely to take note of such success. Parents and teachers (and perhaps other family members and friends) can be taught that, although the child may continue to stutter for a time following the initiation of treatment, there are other important indicators that provide evidence of important victories in the development of improved fluency: a slight slowing in the rate of repetitions, a continuation of airflow and voicing, an easy articulatory contact, and smooth transitioning through the sounds and syllables. To the extent that these important people in the child's life are able to respond to the child's increasing ability to make these changes during daily speaking situations, further success is enhanced.

garden hose and balloon analogies (alternately constricting and releasing the flow of water or air) and lily pad analogy (lightly touching each sound or word while "talking across" the lily pads) enable the child to visualize the necessary flow of air and voicing as well as smooth and effortless speech production. For somewhat older children, it can be useful to use finger tapping (lightly touching the thumb and fingers while producing the sounds or syllables of a word) and gradually changing a tightly closed fist to an open hand corresponding to changing a voluntary (or real) moment of stuttering to effortless and forward-moving speech. A particularly appealing example of the closed fist to open hand example is demonstrated by Barry Guitar in the Stuttering Foundation video (#47), *The School-Age Child Who Stutters*. Williams' (1971) technique of instructing the child to momentarily "freeze" the stuttering for a moment followed by "moving on" into the following sequence of sounds, and Conture's (2001) recommendations to the child to "change and move forward," are both useful adaptations of stuttering-modification procedures suggested by Van Riper (1973) for older speakers. The many suggestions found in textbooks, pamphlets and videos focus on suggesting and modeling for the young speaker ways to achieve air flow; voicing; and gentle, effortless movement of the articulators.

Also noteworthy is the concept of negative practice, whereby the child is asked to produce the very behavior we wish to alter. That is, rather than constantly urging the child to produce fluent speech, we are also requesting (and rewarding) examples of voluntary disruptions of fluency, and, importantly, showing the child that he or she is able to change and alter the situation. The child, by using such suggestions, can become adept at releasing the struggled speech behavior and make the necessary transitional gestures that enable movement to subsequent sounds and syllables. As the clinician comes to know a child, terminology and analogies appropriate for the child's maturity can be selected to most effectively convey these principles.

Guitar (2006) suggests that young speakers who have been coping with stuttering for many years are likely to have incorporated responses that are characterized by avoidance and motivated by shame and embarrassment. Because of this possibility and depending on a variety of other factors including the age and maturity of the child, the severity of the stuttering, and the child's reaction to the experience of stuttering, therapeutic activities that address desensitization and cognitive restructuring about stuttering are likely to be important features of intervention. The case study of a 9-year-old boy by Murphy, Yaruss, and Quesal (2007a) provides a good example of ways to incorporate these features.

Noah, age 9, had a history of intermittent therapy, his score of 28 on the SSI-3 (Riley, 1994) was *severe*, his frequency of stuttering was 11 SLDs/100 words, and his CAT-R (DeNil & Brutten, 1991) score (negative responses on 21 of 32 items) indicated strongly negative attitudes about communicating. Noah was coping with his stuttering by using many avoidance behaviors and was distraught as a result of being bullied by others at his school (a topic addressed later in this chapter). Murphy et al. describe activities designed to assist Noah in becoming desensitized to stuttering and to cognitively restructure his response to his stuttering in order to use stuttering and fluency-modification techniques. Because Noah had been unwilling to use these behavioral techniques in the past, goals were designed to help Noah in becoming less sensitive to stuttering and to consider alternative responses to his experience with stuttering. The techniques were guided by the principle of approaching the problem and involved (1) learning key facts about stuttering in order to reduce Noah's uncertainty and increase his understanding, (2) learning about other people who stutter, (3) exploring and learning to tolerate his moments of stuttering (e.g., freezing and experimenting with variations of effort and movement as modeled by the clinician, including pseudostuttering with examples that were sillier and more extreme than those produced by the clinician), (4) changing negative to positive self-talk, and (5) self-acknowledgement to friends, his teacher, and classmates. Noah brought several classmates to therapy to help them learn about stuttering and what he was doing to improve his speech. As a result of these activities Noah was able to employ his speech management techniques in daily speaking situations beyond the treatment setting. Following these experiences his scores on the SSI-3 were within the mild range, his frequency of stuttering decreased to 2% syllables stuttered, and his communication attitudes (a score of 10) approached those of normally fluent children of his age on the CAT-R. Noah's satisfaction with his speech was self-evaluated as an 8 on a 1–10 scale (in contrast to ratings of 1 and 3 prior to the initiation of therapy). Finally, his teacher

Clinical **Insight**

In earlier chapters we discussed the value of "using silence" and "leading from behind" in order to promote creativity and problem solving on the part of the speaker. There is real value in using similar strategies with younger speakers. For example, clinicians can ask the child to instruct them about how to do various techniques, often feigning misunderstanding ("You want me to do what?" or "Why do you want me to say it like that?") in order to encourage the child to demonstrate and expand his or her understanding of a technique. The clinician may pause, not responding immediately to a client's statement, encouraging the child to take action by reinterpreting or elaborating his or her question. Or, the clinician might ask the parent or the child a question such as "What do you think we should do next?" Such actions by the clinician, even early in the treatment process, set the tone for the transference of problem solving by the parents and the child to beyond the treatment setting and facilitate the eventual maintenance of behavioral and cognitive changes following formal treatment.

reported that Noah was talking more in class (even if he did not choose to use his management techniques) and no longer using avoidance behaviors.

Ramig and Bennett (1995) provide a list of suggestions for the clinician, parents, and teachers when using a stuttering modification approach with younger children. They indicate that the clinician can:

1. Explain the nature of the speech production system to the child and the parents, providing the child with understanding and the means of manipulating fluency.

2. Illustrate the physical behaviors associated with his smooth and bumpy fluency, using terms that the child can understand.

3. Show the child how to vary his or her speaking behaviors by adjusting his or her levels of effort. Making use of modeling (including bumpy fluency), the clinician and the child can explore ways of altering the features affiliated with effortful and disrupted fluency, gradually working in the direction of easier, forward-moving fluency breaks. The child's speech does not have to become completely fluent, but simply easier and smoother. Gregory (1989), for example, suggests that after a child experiences a difficult and tense moment of stuttering, the clinician should direct him to produce the word again, this time reducing the tension by half. The incorporation of fluency-initiating gestures at this point is a good example of how the two general strategies can be intertwined during treatment with young children.

4. Discuss, with the child leading the way, strategies for responding to people and situations that arise in the child's world. Together, the clinician and the child (as well as parents and teachers) can role-play responses to teasing, participation in social and class activities, relaxation in preparation for stressful situations, changing negative into positive self-talk, using visualizations and positive affirmations, and responding to time pressures.

5. Help the child and his or her parents to prepare for the possibility of relapse by considering responses to possible increases in fear, avoidance behavior, struggle behavior, and fluency breaks. The clinician, the child, and his or her parents can discuss self-assessment procedures as well as prescribe possible responses.

6. Develop a schedule for the maintenance and use of both stuttering-modification and fluency-maintaining skills in real-world contexts.

Assisting the Child in Producing Fluent Speech

Techniques for creating and promoting fluency go by several names. These techniques have been called fluency-initiating gestures (FIGs), fluency-enhancing techniques, fluency-facilitating movements, and easy speech. Regardless of the names for these techniques, they consist of procedures described in the previous chapter concerning older speakers that also assist the child in more efficiently managing fluent speech production (e.g., efficiently using the breath stream and vocal folds, creating lighter articulatory contact and movement, smoothing the transitions from one sound or syllable to another). Conture (2001, pp. 193–210) provides a variety of useful suggestions for explaining the nature of constricted versus open and smooth production in ways that children will understand, including the use of cursive writing as an analogy for slow and easy speech production. The child is shown how to smoothly make writing movements transitioning between letters at the same time that he or she is saying the sounds or syllables of the word. Not only is the clinician able to demonstrate the value of easy and flowing (versus hard and erratic) movement during serial motor tasks, the activity also provides an opportunity to show the child that speech is something he or she is producing rather than something that is happening to him or her. Of course, in order to make the activities enjoyable for the child, the clinician can incorporate puppets, games, or cartoon pictures with these activities. The clinician can choose from a wide variety of therapy techniques designed for children found in many sources, including Guitar (2006), Ramig and Dodge (2005), and Reitzes (2006).

One way to provide the child with a sense of his or her ability to create the necessary ingredients for fluency may be a sequence of solo, tangential, and interactive forms of play combined with sound production. For example, as the clinician and the child play separately with their own sets of toys (solo play) the clinician begins to model nonspeech sounds associated with the toys (sounds of animals, trains, and airplanes). Gradually, the clinician moves to producing one-word utterances to describe the movements. Little or no emphasis is placed on the child communicating; the focus is on the child's enjoyment when producing sounds and one- and two-syllable utterances. The clinician next begins to create minimal interactions with the child, briefly commenting on the child's activities with the toys. As the child becomes increasingly interactive, the activities become more cooperative, allowing for playing of games. Still, the emphasis is on having fun and enjoying the experience of producing speech. This sequence of activities was originally presented by Van Riper (1973), and various interpretations are also presented by Conture (1990) and Shapiro (1999). As Conture suggests, games provide the opportunity to move into cooperative play and experience turn-taking during verbalization. The clinician can then begin to direct the level of communicative demand and model a variety of other interactive activities. Guitar (2006) suggests that this form of gradually increased interaction can be particularly helpful for children who are reluctant to separate from the parents or who refuse to talk with the clinician.

It is interesting to note that although children usually respond with greater fluency to slower and less complex speech produced by the parent or the clinician, the reasons for this effect are not well understood. Although there are a few investigations (each with relatively few participants) suggesting that modeling of slower speech by a parent is likely to result in greater fluency by children, Bernstein Ratner (2004) notes that such advice is universal and often suggested in the major training texts. To say to a parent, "Slowing down may help your child to be somewhat more fluent" is correct, but it is not understood why this is often the case (Bernstein Ratner, 1993, p. 244). She suggests that it may be that a request to slow speech production assists in the motor planning and motor sequencing of sounds and syllables as well as decreasing self-imposed time pressure to complete the utterance.

It also may be that the pragmatic aspects of communication come into play more than the actual complexity of language. For example, Weiss and Zebrowski (1992) found that responsive utterances were significantly more likely to be produced fluently than assertive utterances. Although it is commonly suggested to parents that they model less complex speech and language for their nonfluent child, this has received little empirical support. Bernstein Ratner (2004) suggests that because the sophistication of linguistic input by the parents is a strong predictor of the child's subsequent language profiles, such modeling should not be recommended. More general approaches for both increasing the child's tolerance for and modifying communicative disruptors (interruptions, aggressive over-talking by others, lack of patient interest in the child when he or she is talking, over stimulation—particularly when the child is tired) may be more helpful components of successful intervention with young children who stutter.

Finally, Bloodstein & Bernstein Ratner (2008) emphasize that the clinician should make it clear to the parents that recommendations for altering their communication style do not suggest that they are the source of the child's fluency problem. However, as with many other physical, academic, or social issues their child will encounter, the parents' thoughtful and supportive response to stuttering will improve the situation.

Another way to conceptualize treatment for a young speaker in the early stages of stuttering is to consider the demands and capacities (Starkweather & Gottwald, 1990) or the component model (Riley & Riley, 1979; 2000) framework described earlier. That is, the clinician can determine what capacities are likely to increase the child's ability to produce fluent speech and facilitate the child's ability to achieve a sense of mastery over a speech-production system that is still in the process of maturation. In some cases, an initial response may involve adjusting communicative and environmental patterns in the home. Many of these behaviors (slow rate, more leisurely turn-taking, shorter utterances, and more frequent use of paraphrase) are already characteristic of parental or child-directed speech (Ratner, 1993). Gottwald and Starkweather (1995) provide a succinct description of this combined approach, including the goals of fluency enhancement, reduction of demands, and desensitization of the child to normal fluency breaks:

> Depending on the child's specific needs, the clinician may use a reduced speech rate, many silent periods and pause times, and the language stimulation techniques of self-talk and parallel talk, but at a slow rate. Also, the clinician may reduce the number of language demands made on the child, including limiting questions requiring complex answers and reducing implied expectations for ongoing oral communication. Finally, the clinician will use normal disfluencies, such as whole word and phrase repetitions. (p. 122)

A similar strategy would be employed for clinicians who are using a diagnostic-treatment model such as Riley's component approach. The clinician would quite naturally facilitate and help the child to improve those components that have been associated with fluency failure for a particular child. Children with attending problems would be treated in a similar fashion as nonstuttering children in need of such help. Likewise, assisting children in the improvement of their speech motor control may be a basic part of treatment for some children who stutter. Combining procedures that have much in common, Daly,

Riley, and Riley (2000) employ a series of exercises that combine speech-motor training and fluency-shaping techniques. If a child appears to be unusually sensitive, with high self-expectations (for fluency as well as other activities), the Rileys suggest helping the child to cognitively reframe those expectations that are unrealistic and are contributing to anxiety and tension. They suggest creating absurd situations in which the child could not possibly perform perfectly and responding with laughter that recognizes the impossibility of performing the task "just right." As the child is given the opportunity to choose among completely unrealistic and more realistic possibilities, he begins to develop the freedom of choice, the ability to laugh at him- or herself, and the ability to let go of unrealistic expectations. The Rileys suggest that many children who are especially sensitive feel powerless—a reaction that may be triggered by the feeling that they are not being listened to. The clinician can assist children in verbalizing their feelings and analyze, with the parents and the child, stimuli that appear to trigger these reactions.

Fluency-enhancing procedures provide the child with techniques for creating and expanding fluency. Ideally, the speech that is to be expanded and rewarded should have high-quality fluency that is characterized by smooth and effortless production rather than unstable movements. As with adults, it is good to keep in mind that the achievement of fluency should be enjoyable and empowering. The videos produced by the Stuttering Foundation provide concrete examples of how to implement many useful fluency-enhancing techniques. Underlying the documented success of therapy for younger speakers are the same principles that inform successful therapy for adolescents and adults. A successful therapeutic experience for younger speakers is enhanced to an extent that the clinician who:

1. understands the nature of stuttering and is willing to help the young speaker to experiment with and vary forms of nonfluent speech;

2. provides a supportive therapeutic experience that allows the child to become desensitized to and explore the characteristics of his or her stuttering;

3. enables the child to understand the basic features of speech production and promotes the child's ability to control these features, resulting in effortless and forward flowing speech; and

4. elicits the understanding and support of parents and other important individuals in the child's daily environment.

Guitar (2006) describes the concept of *superfluency*, an idea that seems particularly useful with older children who have been stuttering continuously into early adolescence. This idea involves four basic skills that parallel the fluency-shaping targets for older speakers described in Chapter 8. The skills are first modeled by the clinician, who then refines the child's responses. Guitar suggests that these skills can be introduced in any sequence, although, depending on the child, they are usually introduced according to those that are easiest for the child. *Flexible rate* involves showing the child how to slow the production of the initial syllables of a word or syllable on which the child expects to stutter (rather than slowing down all words in the utterance). All of the sounds in the word or syllable are slowed and lengthened, as is the transition to the subsequent sounds. *Easy onsets* emphasize the gradual onset of voicing (and the necessary air flow) rather than a sudden glottal attack. Physical movements with toys or bodily movements are often helpful to convey the concept. *Light contacts* for modeling easy articulatory postures (rather than pushing through an effortful stuck position) can be practiced on all types of sounds, many of which require a slightly distorted (but desired) production to create and maintain the light contact (particularly for plosives). *Proprioception* and heightened feedback for the locations and degree of contact and associated articulatory movements are used for both nonspeech and speech sounds. The sensory feedback can be heightened with exaggerated or slowed movements, closing the eyes, or using masking noise. The components of superfluency are gradually expanded, initially using three-word sentences with considerable modeling by the clinician and then with longer sentences and progressively less modeling by the clinician. Although the purpose is to use superfluency as stuttered words are anticipated, the child may also want to use these techniques on words where stuttering is not anticipated. The final goal is to increase the child's confidence in his or her ability to replace reflexive patterns of stuttering with these superfluent responses in progressively more difficult speaking situations beyond the therapy setting.

By using fluency-facilitating activities the clinician assists the child in reaching a basal level of fluency in the treatment setting. Fluency-disrupting activities are then gradually introduced (e.g., listener loss, time pressure, and greater linguistic demands). As the child's fluency becomes unstable—but prior to the point at which a child will produce fluency breaks—the clinician minimizes the disrupting activities. As a result of these procedures, the child will gradually become able to increase his or her tolerance and will become "toughened" to various forms of demands, including communicative stress (Van Riper, 1973).

Beyond the specific techniques used, Ramig and Bennett (1995) provide a list of suggestions for the clinician, parents, and teachers when using a fluency-modification approach with younger school-age children. The clinician, parents, and teachers who are assisting the child can:

1. Use basic and understandable terms when explaining and demonstrating what they want the child to do. Whatever terms are selected by the clinician (or better yet, the child) for describing the quality of the child's fluency (e.g., "easy" or "turtle speech," or "bumpy" or "rabbit speech"), they should be used consistently when identifying and rewarding target behaviors.

Regardless of the methods used, children need to have terms and concepts that enable them to conceptualize their ability to produce speech and language (Cooper & Cooper, 1991a).

2. Model (rather than instruct) the child about how to perform target behaviors.

3. Model slow and easy speech when interacting with the child in a variety of treatment and extra-treatment settings.

4. Model slow and easy body movements when interacting with the child, again in a variety of treatment and extra-treatment settings. These movements can be coordinated with easy, slow, and smooth speech movements. Such activities are especially good to use at the outset and end of treatment sessions.

5. Reinforce the child's accomplishments and feelings of self-worth in the context of as many experiences as possible.

Counseling Recommendations for Parents and Children

Parents of children who stutter receive great benefit from counseling that emphasizes an understanding and a corresponding reduction of their anxiety concerning stuttering. During treatment sessions the clinician can provide the parents with valuable models, not only for facilitating behavioral change but also for creating an open, uninhibited style of addressing the cognitive and affective experiences of stuttering with their child. One primary goal is to help the parents make stuttering a topic that can be tolerated and discussed. Small group meetings of parents of children who are attending treatment provide a forum for developing an uninhibited attitude about discussing their child's stuttering and for providing supportive reassurance for the parents' active participation in therapy. In a related matter, it is important to appreciate that a child is apt to feel pressure to speak fluently when talking to his or her parents. Older children, in particular, are apt to recognize that parents are anticipating a successful result from the effort and cost of therapy. While spontaneous and effortless fluency is a realistic outcome, parents can also learn to recognize and appreciate easy and smoother forms of stuttering. Such understanding and attitudes about stuttering as modeled by the clinician and adopted by the parents are infinitely better than the "conspiracy of silence" recommended in the past.

For children who have been stuttering for a year or two, and especially those children who have experienced the socialization process associated with attending school, counseling is likely to be helpful and possibly essential. The relatively few sources that exist that specifically describe counseling with young children who stutter (rather than their parents) may be due to the view that children are too young to benefit from counseling or the acknowledged discomfort that many speech-language pathologists have with regard to conducting counseling activities with children who stutter (DiLollo and Manning, 2006; Luterman, 2001; Shames, 2000). While the child may be aware of the breaks in his or her fluency and, in fact, associate negative feelings with that difficulty (Brutten and Hernandez, 2005), these emotions are not likely to be well developed or firmly established. This may help to explain the natural recovery for many young speakers as well as the success of treatment approaches intended to modify the speaking patterns of preschool children.

To one degree or another, most older children and adolescents are in the process of attaching negative feelings of shame and fear to their attempts to communicate. They are apt to be adjusting to their predicament by elaborating ever more sophisticated coping behaviors manifested by an overall pattern of avoidance and a restricted lifestyle. This is not to say that all children who stutter experience unhappy or unaccomplished lives. But their daily activities, particularly as they relate to verbally connecting with others and establishing themselves as autonomous individuals, are apt to be considerably more difficult than they would otherwise be.

Logan and Yaruss (1999) provide a comprehensive approach for helping clinicians and parents respond to the cognitive and affective features of stuttering in young children. They describe modeling and listening activities that help parents respond to their child's stuttering that not only facilitate fluency but also an improved response to the emotional and attitudinal features of the stuttering experience. With the clinician leading the way, parents can become truly desensitized to stuttering behavior in general and their child's pattern of stuttering in particular. Following the principal of approaching rather than avoiding the occurrences of stuttering as described in Chapter 8, parents can become comfortable enough to begin showing interest and curiosity about their child's stuttering behaviors. Examples of modeling behaviors by the parents include practice (by role-playing with the clinician) of a calm, objective, and interested response to their child's stuttering. As parents become aware of their feelings about stuttering, they are better able to stay in the moment and openly discuss possible responses to their child's speech, such as experimenting with purposely producing a variety of hard or easy fluency breaks as described earlier by Murphy, Yaruss, and Quesal (2007a).

With experience, parents can evaluate and monitor their nonverbal responses to stuttering. The parents' mind-set about what stuttering is and what it is not will begin to change for the better. They will be able to model easy, open, and relaxed fluency breaks in their own speech. They will be able to show their child that it is possible to discuss stuttering and speaking in general in an open and matter-of-fact manner rather than taking an all-or-none view about fluency and stuttering. Daily ratings of their child's fluency enable the parents to play an active role in documenting changes in the frequency and quality of their child's speech. Parents can become better listeners and learn to affirm their child regardless of whether or not stuttering is occurring; they can reassure and encourage their child regardless of their child's level of fluency. Parent support groups (either via meetings or a telephone network) are extremely useful in helping parents to understand that they are not alone and that their feelings about their child's stuttering are both natural and acceptable. Although there are many options for parents who want to help their child, often only a few of these will be necessary.

Another important feature of programs designed for children who stutter is the development of problem-solving skills (Gregory, 1986; Riley & Riley, 2000). With the clinician as a model, children are shown how to evaluate their usual ways of thinking about themselves and their problems, including, of course, their stuttering. As a result of the therapy experience, children should be able to provide more objective descriptions of their speech behavior and, depending on the age of the child, listener reactions. Beyond the achievement of increased fluency, are there indications that the child is experiencing a sense of command or

Clinical **Decision-Making**

How is the clinician to know whether or not to ask children about their concerns regarding their speech? As described in Chapter 3, children are not as likely as adults to describe their frustrations and fear related to the experience of stuttering but rather to show it in other ways (pitch rise; cessation of air flow or voicing; substitution of the schwa vowel; or avoidance of sound, words, and speaking situations). A few years ago, a friend of mine, who is an accomplished clinician, told me of a telephone call she received from another speech-language pathologist who worked with children who stutter. The caller explained that she had worked for several months with a young child who stuttered and had been able to teach him several techniques for achieving fluency. However, despite the child's ability to understand and use the fluency-enhancing techniques, he continued to be anxious about speaking and stuttered on many occasions both in and out of the clinical setting. Her question to my friend was whether or not it might be a good idea to "do emotions" with this child. Chances are that to some degree at least, all children who stutter are bothered by the experience. If the child is not highly reactive to the stuttering experience, the clinician may not need to spend much time "doing emotions." In most cases, however, spending time on the affective and cognitive aspects of the stuttering experience is an essential part of the treatment process from the outset and will be well worth the effort.

power as he or she plays and experiments with different forms of fluency? Can the clinician find indicators that the child is beginning to change the interpretation of him- or herself and his or her overall problem-solving abilities? Such indicators may take the form of comments to the clinician, parents, or teachers. The child may demonstrate increased participation in class and social activities. Subtle changes may appear in drawings or comments recorded in a journal. The clinician or the parents may be able to identify in the child an increase in positive rather than negative self-talk related to many activities, as well as a more agentic view about his or her behavior and choices. As Logan and Yaruss (1999) report, as a result of therapeutic change, children also show more sophisticated coping reactions to other forms of adversity and stress, a response we have also noted with adults.

Descriptions of many current treatment programs designed for children are found in Bloodstein & Bernstein Ratner (2008, pp. 353–379) and throughout Guitar (2006). It is worth noting the comments about the development of expertise in Chapter 1, as well as Ham's (1999) advice that the accomplished clinician needs to be aware of many approaches. Children as well as adults will respond in unique ways to different therapeutic approaches. Furthermore, as we discussed in earlier chapters, the influence of any approach will always be somewhat different because of the characteristics of the clinician who is delivering the treatment as well as the child receiving it. As Starkweather states:

> The technique that works so dramatically for one child does not necessarily work dramatically, or at all, for other children. Stuttering is so variable and so highly individualized that, few would disagree, no one method works for all children. (1999, p. 235)

As illustrated by the earlier discussion of the Lidcombe Program, clinicians who employ fluency-shaping strategies are likely to tabulate the resulting decrease in %SS or corresponding increase in fluent utterances. For some approaches, these tabulations are often the major (or only) criteria for moving a child from one step of the program to another. The emphasis in most fluency-shaping strategies is to reward periods of fluency and (less frequently) comment on or highlight instances of stuttering. As we have seen, however, analysis of these programs indicates that there are critical elements of support and reassurance taking place by the clinician and the parent. In a straightforward and uninhibited manner, the adult helps the child to objectively identify the features of both stuttered and fluent speech. The child begins to understand that he or she has a choice about ways of speaking.

Some clinicians emphasize a stuttering-modification approach, which is characterized by a less structured interaction between the clinician and the child. This approach tends to place somewhat less emphasis on tabulating percentages of stuttering and greater emphasis on the child's cognitive and affective response to speaking. Depending on the age, maturity, and temperament of the child; the nature of the stuttering; the extent of parental participation; and the child's response to treatment, many clinicians use a combination of both fluency-enhancing and stuttering-modification strategies often employed with older speakers. The therapeutic approach selected for a particular child is also apt to be influenced by the clinicians' academic and clinical background as well as their clinical experience and interactive style. Certainly, it is appropriate for clinicians to have allegiance to a particular protocol but, in fact, experienced clinicians are likely to adapt protocols, sometimes providing a direct instruction for rewarding fluency and highlighting moments of stuttering while at other times providing indirect modeling and suggestions for promoting fluency and cognitive and affective change. Undoubtedly, the enthusiasm and optimism of the clinician also plays a critical role when implementing any empirically informed (or validated) treatment.

Treatment approaches for the preschool children who stutter contain several common factors that the clinician can draw from in planning treatment strategies for individual children. While there are exceptions, clinicians using virtually all programs include activities designed to achieve the following goals:

- Enhancing the child's enjoyment of speaking.
- Improving the child's self-confidence as a communicator.
- Facilitating an active role for the parents.
- Making certain that the child enjoys the therapy activities.
- Providing the child with verbal praise or tangible rewards for success (easier forms of stuttering or fluency).
- Modeling easier forms of speech with good air flow, an open vocal tract, and light articulatory contacts.
- Moving from less to more complex utterances (both motorically and linguistically).
- Altering fluency-disrupting factors in the child's environment (time pressure, overtalking by others, self-imposed demands for fluency).
- Desensitizing the child to fluency disrupting factors (including teasing and bullying).

A Constructivist-Narrative Approach for Children

DiLollo and Manning (2006) provide a constructivist-narrative framework for counseling preschool and school-aged children. Following a working definition of counseling as "an *interactive, communicative* process that involves a *relationship between clinician and client,* and is focusing on *facilitating effective change*" (p. 116), the authors suggest a counseling process for children that focuses on improving attitudes toward self; deconstructing the concept of "self-as-a-stutterer"; activating and building personal strengths and resources; and guiding the child's "relationship" with stuttering so that it is the child, not "stuttering," who is in control.

Drawing from constructivist theory (Kelly, 1955; Fransella, 2003), DiLollo and Manning (2006) point out two factors that influence the child's development of constructs: (a) Events are repeated; the more repetitions of an event, the greater the chance for the child to extract consistent themes; and (b) Events have characteristics that clearly stand out to the child, such as a consequence or an outcome, so that they may be abstracted across repetitions of that event. For the child who stutters, some of the characteristics of stuttered events are abstracted across reoccurrences of the event to produce constructs about the child's role as a speaker and predictions about how such events will unfold. The experiences with stuttering and its social consequences can have a powerful effect on the development of "core" constructs about the self that the child finds meaningful and predictive. Early awareness of stuttering by young children is likely to impede the development of a meaningful speaker role. In addition, individuals typically protect "core" constructs about the self through processes of denying, ignoring, or trivializing invalidating experiences. Fortunately, for young children who stutter, constructs relating to their role as a speaker tend to be permeable and relatively easily influenced.

Reconstructing the Self: Moving from Behavior to Meaning

An obvious implication for therapy and counseling with young speakers is that a focus of attention (therapeutic and parental/social) is placed on the child's production of *fluent* speech rather than his or her disfluent productions. Moreover, beyond the behavior of producing fluent speech it is important to provide the young speaker with opportunities to make his or her generation of fluent speech meaningful on cognitive and emotional levels that will have an impact on the child's self-concept as a speaker. For example, fluent speech can be made "meaningful" by bringing the child's attention to comments by parents and other caregivers in the child's environment. Young speakers may produce highly fluent utterances but ignore or trivialize the act in order to protect their existing constructs (e.g., "It wasn't me, it was just the techniques"). Alternatively, prior to experimenting with a speaking event, the child can be asked to *predict* the likely outcome of the activity and to write down his or her predictions. Following completion of the experiment, the clinician and child can discuss the experiment—describing their own emotion reactions as well as response of others—and compare what happened to what the child predicted. This has the effect of (a) elaborating or increasing the child's ability to construe the experience of "being a fluent speaker," as he or she will typically report *more* observations from the experiment than were initially predicted; and (b) contrasting the child's current constructs (i.e., the predictions) with actual outcomes, in essence *forcing* meaningful consideration of an event that might have previously been ignored or trivialized (DiLollo & Manning, 2006).

This constructivist-narrative approach to counseling provides a theoretical framework for assisting children in altering their stuttering-dominated self-narratives and to mitigate issues such as fear, anxiety, guilt, and helplessness. DiLollo and Manning (2006) suggest a variety of therapy activities designed to alter these issues.[1]

Telling the "Problem-Saturated Story"

The counseling process can be initiated by the clinician simply asking to hear the child's story. The clinician will need to be patient and allow children to tell their stories on their own terms. The clinician may choose to model the story-telling mode of communication, even throwing in some easy disfluencies in the narrative production, suggesting to the child that fluent speech is not the goal of the interaction. The clinician takes the role of interested listener, asking clarifying questions and inviting as detailed a description of the problem as the child can provide. The clinician accepts the child's story and takes it seriously, all the while understanding that it is not likely to be "the whole story" (Payne, 2000). In the retelling of a problem-saturated story over one or more meetings, the child will almost always provide the clinician with "clues" to an ignored or overlooked alternative storyline—one that is resistant to the problem and its effects on the child (Payne). It is from these brief, mentioned-in-passing clues that an alternative story might emerge.

Using Externalizing Language

Following the child's telling of his or her narrative, the clinician may encourage the child to give their problem a name (White & Epston, 1990). This is likely to be the first opportunity for children to reposition themselves and consider stuttering as external to themselves rather than an enduring, internal trait (Payne, 2000; White & Epston, 1990). Such repositioning can facilitate the

---

[1]For an in-depth discussion of these activities see DiLollo, A. & Manning, W. H. (2006). Counseling children who stutter and their parents, In E. Conture & R. Curlee, *Stuttering and Related Disorders of Fluency* (3rd Edition, 115–130). New York: Thieme Medical Publishers, Inc.

child's role as an *active* participant in *resisting* the problem rather than a passive *recipient* of treatment.

Naming of the problem also provides the opportunity for the clinician and the child to engage in "externalizing language" (White & Epston, 1990) whereby the problem is portrayed as a separate entity, with its own feelings, motivations, strengths, and weaknesses. Following an example of stuttering by the child, for example, the clinician might ask the child, "I wonder why 'Stuttering' decided to come to visit you just then?" Similarly, the child and the clinician might talk about the things "Stuttering" is telling the child when he or she chooses not to answer a question in class, or how powerful "Stuttering" felt when it convinced the child not to order what he or she really wanted at a restaurant. This form of conversation not only helps children to separate themselves from their problem but also promotes a "lighter," more "playful" atmosphere during therapy (Freeman, Epston, & Lobovits, 1997). In addition, the process of externalizing discussions will identify instances during which the child has been able to resist or neutralize the influence of stuttering on his or her speech as well as his or her daily decisions.

Clinical Insight

Some readers may take issue with the above techniques designed to externalize stuttering from the speaker. As an example, Williams (1957) provided a contrasting view in his classic paper, "A point of view about stuttering." Williams identified the difficulties that can occur when a person who stutters thinks of stuttering as a "part of him" in a similar way that White and Epston (1990) talked about the "problem person." Williams also suggested, however, that "animistic" thinking—thinking of stuttering as a "thing that lies inside him"—may be a significant part of the stuttering problem and should be discouraged.

On closer consideration, however, Williams's discussion of animistic thinking is actually supportive of the use of externalizing language with persons who stutter. Williams's argument against "animistic" thinking is that it prevents the person from recognizing his or her alternative ways of behaving by handing over control of behavior to the "thing." However, the purpose of using externalizing language in narrative therapy is to make any animistic thinking that already exists overt and more real to clients so that they can then deal with its influence in their thinking—effectively neutralizing it. The key issue in both perspectives (and in both stuttering- and fluency-modification protocols) is to provide speakers with a choice about speaking and about how they interpret both themselves and their problem.

Identifying Unique Outcomes and Redescriptions

As examples of the child's ability to resist the influence of stuttering are discovered, these "clues" to an alternative story can be elaborated. By using externalizing language, the clinician can help the child to expand these clues into a "unique outcome" (White & Epston, 1990) that describes the basis for a preferred, alternative narrative to the problem-saturated one. The clinician again takes the stance of a curious listener, sometimes feigning misunderstanding, encouraging the child to restate and expand his or her description of the alternative story (Freeman, Epston, & Lobovits, 1997).

With the development of an alternative story, children can be invited to explore how this new story will affect their relationships with themselves, others, and the problem (White & Epston, 1990). Clinicians might consider "unique redescription questions" (Epston & White, 1999) that can be used to aid clients in this process—although such questions would need to be adapted for use with children who stutter.[2] For example, the clinician might ask a child to think of him- or herself as a "superhero" and to describe his or her "superpowers" that enabled him or her to battle "Stuttering." The goal is to facilitate the ability of the children who stutter to resist stuttering's influence, thus undermining it and altering the relationship between the child and the problem so that "Stuttering" is no longer "in control."

Elaborating Alternative Stories Through Creative Play

When children (and adults, for that matter) engage in a creative process, they can often express emotions, thoughts, and insights that may not have been available to them at a more conscious level (Neimeyer, 2000). In addition, children are likely to find it easier to express some events and experiences in a creative or dramatic form rather than talking about them with the clinician (Barrager-Dunne, 1997). Through the spontaneity and security of creative play the child can experiment with new behaviors and reveal "clues" to unique outcomes and an alternative story.

Cattanach (1992, 1994) describes three kinds of play that could be useful in expanding a child's experiences:

1. *Embodiment play* provides the child with the opportunity to explore the world through the senses and utilizes such items as play-dough, slime, clay, and other tactile materials that can be manipulated. Particularly for young children who stutter, embodiment play may provide a safe, playful environment in which further exploration of their fluent speaker role is made possible.

---

[2]See DiLollo, A., Neimeyer, R., & Manning, W. (2002). A personal construct psychology view of relapse: indications for a narrative therapy component to stuttering treatment. *Journal of Fluency Disorders, 27*(1) 19–42.

2. *Progressive play* enables children to discover and explore the world outside of themselves through the use of toys, dolls, and other objects. Like embodiment play, progressive play may facilitate understanding about the concept of "externalization" and provide the opportunity to explore alternative stories. For example, a child and clinician might agree that a certain doll or toy will represent "Stuttering." By using externalizing language the child can talk to the doll or toy, providing it with its own voice to describe its motivations and feelings. Puppets can be used to act out alternatives to an experience that did not go well for the child or an experiment that the child is going to eventually try out.

3. *Role-play* permits the child to play him- or herself in a familiar situation and then switch to take on the role of someone else. This type of play may also aid in the externalization process by allowing the child to take on the role of "Stuttering" and to talk about how and why it likes to push the child around.

For children who are especially creative, various forms of artistic expression such as drawing, painting, sculpture, collage, mask making, poetry, and other forms of creative writing can help to verify the emerging alternative story. For example, a child can create a mask for "Stuttering," making use of various images, colors, patterns, and/or icons that reflect the child's feelings about, and understanding of, this lifelong "companion." As therapy progresses, such creations (masks, drawings, and paintings) can help to document successful changes in the child's cognitive and emotional responses to stuttering.

Supporting the Alternative Story

In order to promote *meaningful* change for the child's emerging alternative story, DiLollo and Manning (2006) refer to suggestions of narrative therapists who recommend the use of *therapeutic documents* (Payne, 2000; White & Epston, 1990; Winslade & Monk, 1999). Such documents are simply tangible and durable descriptions of the child's alternative story. These may take the form of letters, e-mails, certificates, pictures, or videos that give the child specific feedback regarding his or her alternative story. The documents may coincide with a favorite theme or topic of the child and, with appropriate materials (a gold star, trophy, or medal), can be used with preliterate children. Such documents also help to engage significant others in the process of supporting the child's emerging alternative role.

Responding to Teasing and Bullying

For some younger speakers, and certainly for older individuals, *shame* is one of the major affective features of the stuttering experience that influence their overall self-interpretation (Bloodstein & Bernstein Ratner, 2008; Corcoran & Stewart, 1998;

Murphy, 1999; Plexico, et al., 2005). As Murphy (1999) points out, teasing is one of the ways that the emotion of shame becomes attached to stuttering. A major aspect of shame is our interpretation of how we are viewed by others. A feeling of shame can pervade the individual's self-concept and typically results in a high degree of social inhibition and the desire to avoid or hide from others. In contrast, the feeling of *guilt* is generally associated with a particular behavior or act and is less apt to influence a person's self-concept (Murphy, 1999). Shame typically originates in the reactions of others in a child's environment, including parents, classmates, and teachers.

As noted in Chapter 5, one of the components of Riley and Riley's revised component model (2000) for diagnosing and treating children who stutter is Teasing and Bullying. The Rileys found that 31% of children reported that they had experienced such treatment by their peers. Using a questionnaire developed to determine the nature of teasing and bullying experienced by children, Langevin, Bortnick, Hammer, and Wiebe (1998) found that approximately 60% of children who stutter (age 7 to 15 years) experienced this negative treatment by peers. The effect of these experiences continues into adulthood. For example, Riley and Riley (2000) reported that adults often associate their first remembrance of stuttering with the experience of being laughed at or teased. Hugh-John and Smith (1999) found that as many as 75% of adults who stutter recalled that bullying during their school years had negatively influenced their academic performance.

Murphy, Yaruss, and Quesal, (2007b) suggest the utility of making a distinction between teasing and bullying. Citing Tattum (1989) and Coloroso (2003), Murphy et al. define bullying as the conscious effort of someone to hurt or control another person. Teasing, on the other hand, is described as "an enjoyable, often good-natured exchange between friends, without the intention of being hurtful" (p. 140). Murphy et al. (2007b) also describe the many negative emotional effects of bullying that may include emotional (lowered self-esteem, depression, loneliness, anxiousness, and insecurities), academic (negative feelings about school, school dropout, social failure), and physical problems. Of course, children are likely to be bullied about a variety of physical or personal characteristics. Nonetheless, for the child who stutters the behaviors associated with the struggle to speak provide an obvious and sensitive target. The child who stutters may also be a relatively safe target, since disfluent children may be unable to provide a verbal retort to the bully. In fact, taunting often results in increased stuttering (Blood & Blood, 2004).

Murphy et al.'s (2007b) case study of a young boy, Noah, described earlier in this chapter indicates that the primary impetus for his return to treatment was his experience of being bullied by his peers at school and on the school bus. The authors describe an intervention strategy designed to assist Noah in developing effective responses to those who bullied him while at the same time educating others about stuttering and the consequences of bullying. With the clinician's help, Noah first learned to distinguish between statements that were clearly intended to be hurtful ("Hey, stutterhead!") and normal inquisitive comments ("Why do you talk that way?"). As the clinician validated Noah's concerns and at the same time indicated empathy for his experiences, Noah learned to assess what the children were actually saying and to differentiate statements that were intended as hurtful from those that indicated a natural curiosity. Noah was instructed about the nature of bullying and the nature of those who tend to do it; while some may be well-liked, many children who bully others have low-self esteem, insecurity, and low self-confidence. As Murphy et al. point out, it is not unusual for bullies to come from hostile environments or homes where they are neglected (Olweus, 1993).

Because role-playing activities can be especially useful for approaching and becoming desensitized to particularly aversive situations, this was a major part of the program described by Murphy et al. (2007b). Noah and the clinician alternately took both sides of a bullying situation, and a wide range of possible responses were brainstormed and practiced. Primary goals were to create coping responses that Noah could rely on and to assist him in achieving a sense of control over the situation. While all possible responses were considered, several that have been shown to be less effective for bullies were discouraged. For example, crying or ignoring the situation may escalate the bully's attempts to get a reaction. Although it is an instinctive response for some children, for many reasons physically fighting back is not likely to be helpful in the long run. For some children, clever or humorous retorts may be effective but for the child who experiences considerable disfluency when being ridiculed this too is unlikely to be helpful.

Role-playing activities also provide the child with the opportunity to ventilate his or her frustration and anger. For example, the clinician and the child can take turns giving and receiving specific taunts. The child is usually then able to become desensitized to the expected comments and to discuss alternative responses. The child also may be able to defuse or redirect the sting of the comments by overt acceptance of his or her stuttering (Guitar, 2006; Van Riper, 1973) and acknowledging the obvious, thereby defusing the situation. Guitar suggests that a forthright statement such as "I know I stutter, but I'm working on it" (p. 367) may disarm the bully. Murphy et al. cite the work of Cooper (2000), who provides a variety of possible responses to hurtful comments such as the "Shrug" response (the child with an accompanying shrug says "I don't care" or "So what?"), a "broken record" response (consistent repetitions of "Because I want to."), or the "Mighty-might" response (consistent responses of "You might be right."). Murphy (1999), citing Crosby (1997), suggests that for a child who is likely to be disfluent in such a situation, a consistent response of "So?" may be particularly fitting. If a child is mature enough and reasonably fluent, he or she

Clinical **Decision-Making**

A few years ago, a 13-year-old girl whose speech was characterized by both stuttering and cluttering sought my help. Like Noah, the primary reason she asked her parents to seek a clinician was her profoundly negative reaction to the bullying of others (primarily two boys at her school). For the most part, she was unwilling to discuss her experiences of being bullied and on those occasions when she did, she would begin to cry. Following some minimally successful attempts to role-play her experiences, I suggested that she try to write about one or more of her experiences and her reactions to what had occurred. I stipulated, however, that whatever she wrote was "for your eyes only"; there was no suggestion that she show her thoughts to her parents or to me. I was hoping that the experience of journaling would help to organize her thoughts about her experience. I was especially hopeful that the act of putting her thoughts on paper would help her to externalize, objectify, and achieve some distance from her experience. Not only was she able to create a written description of and begin to reinterpret the events but also, within a few weeks, took some pride in showing her parents and me what she had written. We still had some work to do on her fluency, but a major barrier to progress had been diminished.

may respond to imitations of his stuttering by saying something such as "Look, if you're going to stutter you ought to learn how to do it correctly. Prolong the first sound like this and add a little more tension. If you get really good at it and you're brave enough, see if you can do it with me at school tomorrow."

The second major goal of the strategy designed by Murphy et al. (2007b) was to assist Noah in educating his classmates and others about stuttering and the effects of bullying. The major focus was on the development of a classroom presentation to Noah's classmates. The activity has many advantages, including putting the child in the position of an expert (Blood & Blood, 2004; Murphy, 1989, 1999), and accomplishing self-acknowledgement of stuttering and desensitization (Dell, 1993; Ramig & Dodge, 2005; Reardon & Yaruss, 2004). Murphy et al. suggest that the response of most individuals to those who stutter will improve as the nature of stuttering becomes less mysterious and better understood.

The rationale and advantages of a class presentation will need to be explained to the child's parents and teachers, who will, of course, be closely involved in the stages leading up to the presentation. Although for some children the challenge may be daunting, the process is broken into steps that are incorporated in the treatment sessions (e.g., presentations to the clinician, the child's parents, the teacher, groups of selected students). As described in detail by Murphy et al. (2007b), the clinician and child can make a series of videos of experimenting with different versions of the presentation. Murphy et al. provide an extensive sequence of topics that can be included in the presentation. Describing the heroic life stories of famous people who stutter who have achieved great success [see the Stuttering Home Page for links (http://www.mnsu.edu/comdis/kuster/stutter.html)] is a good place to begin. Other topics include the nature of stuttering, examples of therapy techniques, ways to respond to stuttering, the experience of being bullied, and how to handle bullying.

Obviously, the classroom teacher should ensure that bullying in the classroom is off-limits. However, there will be situations where the teacher will be unable to prevent this behavior by other children. Certainly, the teacher or parent may discuss the injustice of such behavior with those involved. Of course, this is not always helpful and, in some instances, may increase the problem. Another possibility is to ask an adult who has undergone successful treatment to speak to the class. Volunteers for interesting and informative explanations about stuttering can be found through nearby clinics or local chapters of self-help groups. Such speaking opportunities are often welcomed by these individuals, who are often more than pleased to practice their public-speaking skills. There is a wealth of good information and suggestions contained in several publications that have been designed specifically for assisting with problems created by children who stutter being bullied (Cooper, 2000; Dell, 1993; Langevin, 2000; Langevin, Kully, Ross-Harold 2007; Reardon & Yaruss, 2004; Yaruss, Murphy, Quesal, & Reardon, 2004).

Children with Coexisting Problems

Although it has often been noted that children with fluency disorders tend to have other communication problems, both Nippold (1990) and Bernstein Rater (1997) suggest that it is best to think of children who have co-occurring problems (particularly language and phonological/articulatory problems) as subgroups of children who stutter. Blood and Seider (1981) reported that 68% of 1,060 children being treated for stuttering in elementary schools had other speech, language, hearing, or learning problems. Most often noted is the frequent co-occurrence of articulation and phonological problems (Blood & Seider, 1981; Bloodstein & Bernstein Ratner, 2008; Conture, 2001; Daly, 1981; Louko, Edwards, & Conture, 1990; Paden, Yairi, & Ambrose, 1999; Schwartz & Conture, 1988; St. Louis & Hinzman, 1986; Riley & Riley, 1979; Thompson, 1983; Yairi et al., 1996; Williams & Silverman, 1968). As we described in Chapter 5, Riley and Riley (2000) found that 50% of the 50 children they assessed had moderate to severe articulation or phonological disorders. Daly (1981) also found that more than half of children being seen for fluency intervention also have articulation disorders. Just how these other communication problems relate to the onset or maintenance of stuttering is unclear. It is clear that the experience of communicating with others is apt to be a challenge for these children. Depending on the reactivity of a child faced with this situation it is not surprising that the stuttering may be more severe and that remediation may be somewhat more complex for these speakers.

The co-occurrence of fluency disorders and language impairment is less well-documented but also has been noted (Blood & Seider, 1981; Louko, Edwards, & Conture, 1990; St. Louis & Hinzman, 1986; St. Louis, Murray, & Ashworth, 1991). More recent studies (Silverman & Bernstein Ratner, 2002; Anderson & Conture, 2000, 2004) have either indicated subtle or nonclinical differences (Bloodstein & Bernstein Ratner, 2008) or that young children who stutter are no more likely to also have depressed language abilities than their fluent peers (Watkins, Yairi, & Ambrose, 1999; Bonelli, Dixon, Bernstein Ratner, & Onslow, 2000). Furthermore, the presence of coexisting disorders may not always be apparent at the outset of treatment. For example, a child's language impairment may only become evident after fluency has improved (Merits-Patterson & Reed, 1981).

Two Effects of Coexisting Problems

There are two basic issues the clinician will want to consider with coexisting communication problems. First, it has been observed by some clinical researchers that, on occasion, children who are being treated for language disorders become more disfluent as a consequence of treatment (Conture, 1990; Merits-Patterson & Reed, 1981; Meyers, Ghatak, & Woodford, 1990). Conture (1990) suggests that if a child is receiving treatment for severe articulation problems or unusual phonological problems, the possibility of stuttering onset may be increased. Treatment for articulation or language impairments also may precipitate fluency breaks if children are placed in treatment too early. That is, premature treatment may require the child to improve his or her articulation before he or she is capable of producing sounds correctly with relative ease and without excessive scanning or effort. As a result, treatment demands may exceed the child's still-limited capacities for producing speech fluently, something Conture (1990) suggests is more likely to occur for children who are approximately five to six years old.

> We are inclined to speculate that increases in the length and complexity of verbally expressed languages increases the opportunities for instances of disfluency to emerge and is probably a natural byproduct of improved but still unstable expressive language skills. (p. 105)

A related therapeutic issue for children who are being treated for fluency and other impairments is the "trading" relationships among the fluency, language, and phonological capabilities of the child. Such reciprocal interactions have been suggested between fluency disorders and both language and phonological capacities (Crystal, 1987; Masterson, & Kamhi, 1992; Ratner, 1995, 1997; Ratner & Sih, 1987; Stocker & Gerstman, 1983; Stocker & Usprich, 1976; Watkins et al., 1999). This relationship has been particularly well-documented for expressive syntax and fluency (Gaines, Runyan, & Meyers, 1991; Gordon, 1991; Gordon, Luper, & Peterson, 1986; Ratner & Sih, 1987; Stocker, 1980). The affiliation of a child's expressive and receptive capabilities is a major influence on clinical decision making for young children who stutter. That is, the clinician should introduce fluency skills at carefully graded levels of linguistic demand (Ratner, 1995; Stocker, 1980). According to Bernstein Ratner,

> Imitation and modeling tasks designed to address syntactic or morphological deficits, shown to be most efficient clinically in inducing changes in expressive language performance[,] . . . may evoke fluency failure. Similarly, fluency practice, if structured in such a way that it does not address the demand it poses on a child's expressive language capacity, may not produce desired changes in fluency. (1995, p. 183)

As discussed in Chapter 3, such trading relationships and their resulting effect on a child's ability to produce fluent speech provide clinical support for a capacities and demands model (Adams, 1990; Starkweather & Gottwald, 1990). That is, at least for some young stuttering children, any task that requires a child to formulate complex ideas with greater levels of language demand may result in decreased fluency. In fact, that is what Weiss and Zebrowski (1992) found with eight child–parent pairs. When these young stuttering children (average age 6 years, 11 months) were asked to respond to questions requiring greater linguistic sophistication, there was a greater occurrence of fluency breaks. That is, higher levels of language demand (Stocker & Usprich, 1976) resulted in significantly more disfluencies than lower-level parent requests. In addition, disfluent utterances were significantly longer and more complex than those produced fluently.

Although clinical decisions are made more complex with the presence of multiple problems, the answer to the question of whether to initiate treatment of a child who is disfluent and has other concomitant communication problems or disorders is usually "yes." Articulation and language problems require long-term treatment, and the clinician is unlikely to be able to wait until these problems are resolved before initiating treatment for fluency problems. Given the success that is likely for early intervention of fluency disorders, waiting may only aggravate the problem. Many clinical researchers support the view of focusing on the combination of communication problems the child may have (Conture, Louko, & Edwards, 1993; Gregory & Hill, 1980; Guitar, 1998; Runyan and Runyan, 1993; Wall & Myers, 1995). Guitar (2006) has not found that treating other speech or language problems exacerbates the child's stuttering. Guitar provides some particularly good examples of how the clinician may adapt clinical activities to a child with multiple problems. For example, if the clinician is using the Lidcombe Program in order to facilitate fluency, Guitar indicates that other communication problems may be addressed prior to, or (more typically) following Stage I of treatment.

Depending on the nature and extent of other associated problems, the clinician will have to decide whether the problems should be addressed sequentially or concurrently. Conture, Louko, and Edwards (1993) advocate a concurrent approach for children with both fluency and phonological problems, making use of a fluency-shaping protocol along with indirect phonological intervention. These authors, however, advise the clinician to avoid any overt correction of the child's speech. It is agreed by most authors that children should not receive any direct feedback concerning the accuracy of their articulation, to prevent possible communicative or emotional stress from impacting the child's capacities. Obviously, the response of each child to feedback will be different, with their unique capacities and responses to communication demands. For example, Conture (2001) recommends that the clinician assist the child to develop a "more physically easy, less hurried, less hesitant or rushed means of initiating and manipulating speech rather than an over careful, cautious, physically precise, and overarticulated productions of sounds" (p. 161). Ratner (1993) indicates that subtle forms of feedback in the form of imitation, recasts, and selective emphasis on language structures that children are finding difficult may facilitate overall communication development. The clinician should feel free to model fluency-enhancing gestures in his or her own speech. Certainly, the child's distinctive response to linguistic as well as emotional demands must be carefully considered, both within and beyond the treatment environment.

Ratner (1995) suggests that the blending of treatments (e.g., phonology and fluency) during a treatment session may work well for those children whose fluency system does not appear to be stressed by the requirements of feedback monitoring. However, if the clinician determines that working on one aspect of speech or language production places stress on the child's ability to produce fluent speech, it may be better to sequence treatment, achieving a stable level in one area before tackling the other. Whether or not to sequence treatment is a good example of the kind of clinical decision the experienced clinician must be entrusted to make. If, for a particular child, fluency problems appear to be related to expressive language formulation, the clinician may choose to emphasize language intervention skills prior to fluency treatment. Obviously, as Ratner (1995) points out, an inappropriate justification for targeting language prior to—or in place of—fluency is the lack of confidence a clinician may have for conducting fluency therapy. Given the evidence concerning clinician attitudes about people who stutter and about treatment with this population of clients (see Chapter 1), this is a valid concern.

Finally, Ratner (1995) suggests some principles that clinicians can use for making clinical decisions for children with fluency and other concomitant problems:

1. The clinician should recognize that demands for phonological and grammatical processing compete with resources that permit fluent speech production.

2. The clinician should organize treatment hierarchically, proceeding from language and articulation activities that the child has established and stabilized to tasks that involve greater demands.

3. Even though it may slow progress in articulatory and linguistic growth, the clinician should structure interventions for children who stutter with minimum overt feedback.

4. The clinician, based on the child's individual capacities and responses to communicative demands, should determine whether a child's multiple impairments should be treated concurrently, sequentially, or cyclically. Furthermore, this strategy should be subject to change in the event that progress in one domain comes at the expense of regression in another.

Intervention for all clients is likely to be most efficient when a careful analysis of the speaker's capacities and responses to demands are factored into the treatment strategy. Clients can—and should—be pushed to the upper ranges of their ability in order to help them to change the many features of their fluency disorder. The clinician working with young children who stutter should be able to help them to learn to easily produce difficult sounds or new grammatical structures without introducing the idea that they need be concerned or frightened or should struggle with their speech. It is possible to model a smooth and flowing manner of speech production while also giving the child a real sense of command over him- or herself.

Problems That Reduce or Impact Fluency

Not only do co-occurring speech and language problems influence the clinician's decisions for providing treatment for children who stutter but there are also a variety of neurological and behavioral conditions that result in various forms of disrupted fluency. Interesting commonalities exist among many of these conditions, not the least of which is the executive function or regulatory activities associated with the basal ganglia. However, as Conture (2001) points out, this association does not necessarily imply that stuttering is the result of problems with this portion of the central nervous system.

Tourette's syndrome (TS) is a neurological disorder with childhood onset (Donaher, 2006; Donaher, Healey, Sisskin, Daly, & Graham, 2005) and is thought to be secondary to abnormal metabolism of the neurotransmitter dopamine. By age seven, children with this syndrome may exhibit motor, phonic, and mental tics that are repetitive and involve rapid, involuntary movements or vocalizations (e.g., facial grimaces, eye-blinking, shrugging, head-jerking, face-rubbing, lip-licking). Phonic tics may include throat-clearing, snorting, grunting, sniffing, repeating words, barking, and impulsive remarks. These characteristics tend to be episodic and situational in nature and are more likely to occur under stress. Children with TS are also found to have other, often more debilitating, problems, including obsessive-compulsive disorder (OCD), attention deficit hyperactivity disorder (ADHD), learning disabilities (LD), and anxiety disorders or phobias. Associated communication problems may include a wide variety of language, pragmatic, and intelligibility (particularly due to rapid speech) problems.

For our purposes, an important characteristic of children with TS is that most of the disfluencies are not the SLDs typical of developmental stuttering but rather are fillers, phrase repetitions, and sentence revisions. Facial tics that are unrelated to stuttering may occur, for example, during silence or when speech planning is not taking place (Conture, 2001). Because, as Van Borsel and Vanryckeghem (2000) have noted, so many speech characteristics of these children are similar to cluttering, Donaher (2006) recommends intervention strategies that focus on teaching the child to monitor his or her speech during structured interactions and increasing the ability to read social cues. Speech rate is addressed by emphasizing clear articulation with natural speech prosody. Other goals may include enhancing the child's ability to comprehend abstract or figurative language, accurately process verbal information, and formulate ideas. General communication goals include improving eye contact, listening skills, and developing appropriate volume.

Autism spectrum disorders (ASD), including *Asperger's syndrome,* are an assortment of developmental problems including impairments in social interaction, communication, play and imagination, and restricted interests and activities (Sisskin, 2006; Sisskin and Scott, 2007). Disfluencies, including SLDs, are common. A review of two speakers with both autism and stuttering by Sisskin and Scott (2007) illustrates the range of possible communicative characteristics. An 8-year-old male with autism had average nonverbal cognitive functioning but severe delays in the personal/social, adaptive, motor, and communication and cognitive domains. He also had poor nonverbal communication skills. A sudden onset of SLDs occurred at the age of eight. Iterations occurred as many as 15–20 times on the same sound, syllable, or word and were accompanied by a lowering of the head, phonating on residual air, and jerking of the torso as he completed the disfluency. Otherwise, the child indicated few reactions to his stuttering. Because the child had no family history of stuttering and was seen shortly after onset of stuttering, it was decided not to immediately initiate fluency treatment.

The second speaker, a 20-year-old man with both autism and intellectual disability, spoke with one- and two-word utterances and displayed a variety of stereotypical behaviors, including rocking and hand movements as well as a variety of ritualistic behaviors (touching windows, rotating his body prior to sitting). Onset of stuttering was sudden at age 18. Disfluencies occurred on half of his spoken words, with 50% whole-word repetitions and 50% sound/syllable repetitions. Most of his disfluencies occurred when making requests rather than when answering questions or during social interaction. There were no associated physical concomitant behaviors and no awareness of his disfluencies. Although the form of his disfluencies was similar to developmental stuttering, the quality was not. That is, the disfluencies were more like palilalia, with the units of repetition being longer and the iterations more numerous than those of developmental stuttering (Van Borsel, Bontinck, Coryn, Paemeleire, & Vandemaele, 2007). Sisskin and Scott noted that the number of iterations appeared to be related to the time it took for a conversational partner to grant verbal requests, with the repetitions ceasing once the function of the communication was complete. The authors speculated that this man's repetitions may have served as a communicative function, as a form of self-talk, and as a self-regulatory function as suggested by Prizant & Rydell (1984). As a result, his disfluencies were not addressed during treatment and the establishment of functional verbal and non-verbal communication was seen as a higher priority.

Asperger's syndrome is regarded as a milder form of autism and is characterized by no delay in general language ability or cognitive development. These children may, in fact, score in the superior range on standardized intelligence tests (Sisskin, 2005; 2006). Although semantic and syntactic language ability appear to be age-appropriate, these children experience problems with pragmatic skills, illustrated by egocentric or one-sided monologues. They are likely to have obsessive interests, a tendency to monopolize conversations, poor markers for topic change, an inability to suppress internal thoughts, and an over-intellectualized conversational manner. In addition, speech and voice quality are atypical with unusual prosody, rapid rate, restricted intonation patterns, and poor volume modulation. Fluency for children with Asperger's syndrome is "jerky" (Klin, McPartland, & Volkmar, 2005), with many filled pauses and content mazes (excessive repetitions, revisions, and/or filled pauses as described by Loban, 1976) and fillers which may mask their disfluencies (Klin, Volkmar & Sparow, 2000).

Sisskin (2006) provides a disfluency analysis for two speakers with Asperger's syndrome. The pattern of disfluencies for the 7-year-old was atypical of developmental stuttering. Word-final disfluencies ("ones-uns, train-ain, stores-ores") made up approximately one-fourth of the part-word disfluencies and mid-syllable insertions (characterized by a short exhalation in the middle of the syllable) made up one-third of the within-word breaks. This young speaker showed little or no awareness of his disfluencies and provided no indication that he felt speaking was difficult. The pattern of fluency breaks of the 17-year-old was similar in that 90% of his disfluencies were also atypical of developmental stuttering. In this instance, word-final repetitions made up about half of disfluencies, and mid-syllable insertions made up one-third. This speaker indicated no awareness of his disfluencies and did not display any avoidance, word substitution, or fear of speaking. With yet another speaker, a 10-year-old female, Scott and Sisskin (2007) noted prolongations and blocks accompanied by both tension and audible inhalation. No other secondary behaviors were noted. Although this child indicated some awareness of her disfluencies, she was unable to identify them as they occurred.

Although disfluencies are evident for these speakers, Scott and Sisskin (2007) and Sisskin (2006) indicate that pragmatic issues are likely to detract the most from the person's ability to communicate. Therapeutic goals therefore may emphasize ways to enhance effective communication by focusing on improved nonverbal communication and the development of pitch, stress, and intonation patterns that match intent or meaning. In order to develop executive function skills, self-monitoring activities and practice in verbal problem solving (e.g., role reversal, perspective taking, generate solutions to problems) are recommended. For some children, pausing and formulation strategies in conversational contexts are helpful for minimizing typical fluency breaks. If the child's fluency breaks are SLDs and he or she is aware of and reacting to them, the use of fluency strategies (easy onset, pullouts, continuous phonation) is suggested.

Attention deficit hyperactivity disorder (ADHD). ADHD occurs in 3–5% of school-age children (American Psychiatric Association, 2000). However, Healey and Arndt point out that there is good evidence that ADHD is commonly misdiagnosed, with error rates as high as 30% to 50%. The hallmark of these children is "consistent inconsistency" in two or more environments such as school, home, and other social settings (Healey & Reid, 2003) and is characterized by inattention, hyperactivity, and impulsivity. Based on a variety of symptoms, children are classified into three patterns: (1) primarily hyperactive-impulsive (without inattention), (2) predominately inattentive type (without significant hyperactivity), or (3) a combination of the first two types (American Psychiatric Association, 2000). Child psychiatrists, child psychologists, neurologists, or developmental pediatricians are suggested for providing a diagnosis of ADHD (Graham, 2006; NIMH, 2003). In order for a child to be diagnosed as ADHD, some of the symptoms must occur prior to age seven but often appear around age three (Healey & Reid, 2003). The many characteristics of these children, including restless and overactive behavior, lack of attention to detail, inability to complete tasks, distractibility, excessive talking, and lack of turn-taking, are likely to negatively impact learning in general as well as the effectiveness of treatment.

Conture (2001) and Arndt and Healey (2001) point out that most children who stutter do not have ADHD. However, preliminary studies indicate that the co-occurrence of ADHD and stuttering has been estimated at 4% (Arndt & Healey, 2001) to as high as 26% (Riley & Riley, 2000). Conture (2002) suggests that when this is the case, therapy for stuttering is likely to take longer or result in little improvement. Healey and Arndt (2001) and Graham (2006) describe research supporting the use of a treatment protocol that combines behavioral, environmental, and pharmacological (often a stimulant medication such as Ritalin®, or Methylin®, or Dexedrine®). These authors also stress the importance of advocating a combination of approaches to the parents of children who stutter.

Because the positive effects of medication vary according to how long it has been since the child ingested it, Graham (2006) recommends that, to the extent possible, the clinician schedule therapy activities that require the greatest amount of concentration at a time when the child's medication is at its peak effectiveness. Healey and Reid (2001, p. 84) provide guidelines for the maximum effectiveness for various medications and the duration of their effects (short, intermediate, or long-acting). They also indicate that for the most commonly used stimulates, such as Ritalin® (short-acting) and Adderall® (intermediate-acting), it takes approximately 30 minutes for the medication to become effective, with effects lasting from 2 to 6 hours.

In some instances, stimulate medications have been found to result in the onset of disfluencies (Burd & Kebeshian, 1991; Lavid, Franklin, & Maguire, 1999; Riley & Riley, 2000), although this is less likely if the right prescription and level of medication is achieved. Because of this possibility, Graham (2006) advocates that clinicians consider the temporal relationship of the administration of a stimulant medication and the subsequent onset of stuttering. Understanding ADHD and its manifestations for a particular child who stutters is critical, as well as promoting an interactive intervention that involves parents, teachers, and physicians. Healey and Arndt (2001) provide several principles of intervention for children with ADHD (pp. 87–90) that should be useful to clinicians assisting children who also stutter.

Down syndrome. Bloodstein and Bernstein Ratner (2008) provide a summary of what is known about the occurrence of stuttering in individuals with intellectual disabilities as well as those speakers with Down syndrome (pp. 232–234). The results of several investigations beginning in the early to mid-1900s have consistently shown that stuttering is more likely to occur in individuals of lower intelligence than in the typical population. Van Borsel, Jozefien, Charlotte, Rijke, Evy Van, and Tineke (2006) found that children in a "special needs" classroom in Belgium had a prevalence of stuttering four times greater than in the general school enrollment (2.28% vs. 0.56%). A significant and somewhat greater than typical male to female ratio of 4.6:1 was found. It is worth noting, however, that no definition of stuttering was provided and that children were largely identified by their classroom teachers (54.7%) or speech-language pathologists (22.2%), which may have influenced the outcome. In contrast to children attending regular schools, Van Borsel et al. (2006) found that younger children (ages 6–10 years) attending special schools had a lower prevalence of stuttering than older children (ages 11–15). Van Borsel et al. suggested that this unusual trend may be the result of the typically delayed onset of speech of such children or the presence of other communication problems that masked the presence of a fluency problem. Bernstein Ratner and Bloodstein note that while these individuals are generally aware of their disrupted fluency, few secondary behaviors are noted and the speakers, for the most part, are not concerned about their speech.

In the specific instance of the most common cause of intellectual disability, Down syndrome, the occurrence of stuttering occurs with greater frequency. Bloodstein and Bernstein Ratner (2008) provide prevalence estimates in the 25–35% range, with several as high as 42–48%. Along with the possible reasons for the relatively late onset of stuttering for speakers with intellectual disability suggested by Van Borsel et al. (2006), Bloodstein and Bernstein Ratner proposed that, like more typical children, these children are also more likely to develop normal disfluencies when they reach a language level at which they are combining 2–3 words, usually at a chronological age of 8 to 10 years. The disfluencies are often easy repetitions of part and whole words and phrases. Younger children with Down syndrome are unaware of their disfluencies and do not attempt to avoid or hide their stuttering. As the children become older, however, avoidance and shame may develop, along with secondary behaviors. As with many of the speakers described in this section, there is a lack of self-monitoring abilities, which will influence the nature of treatment. Preus (1972) provides a description of the disfluency characteristics of Down syndrome children, citing high frequencies of whole-word repetitions, part-word repetitions, and prolongations. Using a threshold of 5 disfluencies/100 words, including only part-word repetitions and prolongations, 34% of the children were determined to be stuttering.

Conture (2006), citing the work of Preus (1981), points out that individuals with Down syndrome also have many characteristics of cluttering (see Chapter 10), including variable and often fast speech rate, decreased intelligibility, and the lack of self-monitoring. For these speakers, Conture (2001) recommends direct therapy with "clear, unambiguous reinforcement for changes in disfluency that are repeatedly and clearly modeled for the child" (p. 166). He suggests treatment goals that emphasize the improvement of overall communication abilities, including practice in language formulation and word-finding skills. Short periods of oral-motor activities combined with practice on pausing, slowing rate, and speech phrasing may be helpful in decreasing disfluencies.

If avoidance has evolved as a coping behavior for the child, it is important to provide support and encouragement for increased participation (Conture, 2001). The Stuttering Foundation brochure #66, *Down's Syndrome and Stuttering* provides information that clinicians and parents will find helpful.

Transfer and Termination Issues

Throughout treatment and certainly prior to the child's dismissal from formal treatment, the clinician will want to determine how well the child has been able to transfer new capabilities and techniques to the world beyond the treatment setting. Of course, the understanding and motivation of the parents will be the major factor in facilitating transference. Fortunately, as Conture (2001) points out, for many children the skills learned in the treatment setting transfer quite easily. Guitar (2006) notes that progress with younger children can be determined by such accomplishments as the improving use of techniques, decreased reliance on cueing by the clinician, increased control of fluency, decreased avoidance of speaking and speaking situations, and greater risk-taking in speaking situations.

Criteria that the clinician may consider for the termination of formal treatment are provided by Gottwald and Starkweather (1995). Parents and teachers should feel confident about their ability to manage the child's improving fluency. These adults can assess the child's progress and make independent decisions concerning how to alter fluency-disrupting stimuli

Clinical **Decision-Making**

The participation of the clinician in providing modeling and support for the child when practicing beyond the treatment environment cannot be overemphasized. As described in the first chapter of this text, the willingness to do yourself what you ask the speaker to do is critical. Guitar (2006) provides vivid examples of "scaffolding" the child's ability to use the techniques associated with the fluency-enhancing skills described earlier in this chapter. When making telephone calls and seeking out face-to-face speaking situations of gradually increasing difficulty, the clinician takes the first turn when speaking with others. During telephone calls the child and clinician can signal each other or the clinician coaches the child in freezing the stuttering and then gently moving through or sliding out of a moment of stuttering. As the child indicates the onset of fear, the loss of control, or a moment of stuttering, the clinician may touch the arm of the child to cue the use of the skills. Continued desensitization and assertiveness are often necessary for expanding the child's confidence and success in daily speaking situations.

such as time pressure and linguistic demands across a variety of social and educational settings. Parents can create an environment that corresponds to the child's capacity to maintain fluency. In addition, the young child should be normally fluent for his age; some mild fluency breaks, particularly whole-word and phrase repetitions produced without effort, are unexceptional for three- to four-year-old children. Even fluency breaks produced with mild levels of tension may be acceptable if the clinician anticipates that the child will make continued improvement. Of course, termination is also facilitated by a gradual phase-out of treatment that provides the clinician with the opportunity to monitor the child's progress. Ideally, such monitoring should take place through age seven or eight, when basic skills underlying fluency are thought to be internalized. Finally, parents and teachers should be informed about the characteristics of relapse, made aware of the signs of incipient stuttering, and be encouraged to contact the clinician if such indicators occur.

The Possibility of Relapse with Children

In contrast to the situation for older speakers, the maintenance of the gains made during formal intervention is far more common with children (Bloodstein & Bernstein Ratner, 2008). Several investigators indicate that once formal treatment has been successfully completed, the chance of regression is much less likely with children than it is with adolescents and adults who have been stuttering for many years (Hancock, Craig, McCready, McCaul, Costello, Campbell, & Gilmore, 1998; Gottwald & Starkweather, 1995; Starkweather, 1999; Starkweather, Gottwald, & Halfond, 1990). However, a comprehensive treatment program will include periodic checks for as long as two years following the conclusion of formal treatment. As with older speakers, follow-up or refresher sessions of fluency-facilitating skills may be necessary for some children if fear, avoidance, or increased stuttering reoccur.

Starkweather (1995) estimates that the relapse rate following successful treatment for young children is approximately 2%. In a summary of the families seen from 1981 through 1990 at the Temple University Stuttering Prevention Center in Philadelphia, Gottwald and Starkweather (1995) indicate the following:

> Forty-eight of these families received individualized intervention services, ranging from parent counseling only to family counseling and direct therapy for the child. At the time these results were reported, three children and their families were still in therapy, and seven families had withdrawn from the program for a variety of reasons. The remaining 45 youngsters and their families completed the program. All 45 children were speaking normally at the time of discharge. Follow-up telephone calls to each of the

families 2 years following program completion revealed that fluency had been maintained according to parent report. (p. 124)

Partial or even complete relapse can occur, of course, and one procedure that may prevent such regression is the use of a "buddy system." This may be especially helpful for the child who is having difficulty with motivation, carryover, or maintenance. When entering into new and difficult speaking situations outside the treatment setting, the presence of someone who understands the dynamics of the situation can have a powerful supporting effect. If the clinician or parent is not there, the presence of a speech buddy may be extremely beneficial. This strategy may be particularly useful with preadolescent or adolescent clients, who tend to spend the vast majority of their time with their peers rather than their parents or clinicians.

Hancock et al. (1998) conducted a two-to-six year follow-up of 62 children who had received one of three stuttering treatments (intensive smooth speech, parent-home smooth speech, and intensive electromyography feedback). These children, age 11–18 years, were older than those followed by Gottwald and Starkweather (1995). Children were assessed overtly during a clinic conversation with the clinician, while speaking on the clinic telephone talking to a family member or friend, and talking at home. The authors found that most of the children had maintained the gains they had achieved one year post-treatment. About half of the children had less than 1% syllables stuttered across the three speaking contexts, and nearly 70% of the children achieved less than 2% syllables stuttered two to six years following treatment. From a parent's perspective, eight of the parents (13%) believed that their child had relapsed to pretreatment levels and 33 parents (53%) felt that their child's speech had deteriorated but not to pretreatment levels.

Suggestions for the Classroom Teacher

For school-age children, classroom teachers can play a major role in facilitating therapeutic change. In some instances, the child's classroom teacher will have as much influence on a successful therapeutic outcome as the child's parents. However, in order for teachers to have a positive influence they must have some understanding of the nature of stuttering and the objectives and rationale of treatment. Many authors provide a variety of suggestions for the classroom teacher who finds a child who stutters in his or her class (Conture, 2001; Cooper, 1979a; Dell, 1970; Guitar, 2006; Van Riper, 1973, pp. 446–450). Of course, the character of the clinician–teacher relationship will depend on the model used for service delivery in the school. One possibility is a consultative model, where the clinician works through the teacher and parents to help the child. A collaborative-consultative model has the clinician working with the child on an individual basis but also collaborating with the teacher and parents in planning appropriate activities in the child's daily world. According to Gregory (1995), a pullout model, where the children are taken out of the classroom and seen individually or in small groups by the clinician, is probably the strategy that is least apt to create meaningful professional interaction or long-term change for the child.

An efficient first step for involving classroom teachers is for the clinician to present a workshop for teachers and related school personnel. For many reasons, it is preferable for the clinician to be proactive in explaining the nature of stuttering to classroom teachers rather than waiting for them to one day discover such a child in one of their classes. Perhaps the most important reason is that many children who stutter can go undetected or be misunderstood. Some children who stutter will refuse to answer, intentionally saying "I don't know" despite knowing the correct answer to the teacher's question, or give the wrong answer due to the fear of stuttering on the correct answer. The story of the former football player (see Chapter 5) and the following examples are particularly effective stories to relate to classroom teachers.

Highly effective presentations can result from discussing the informative videotapes and pamphlets available through such groups as the Stuttering Foundation or the National Stuttering Association. Nearly everyone is interested in stuttering, and it is usually easy to draw an appreciative audience for such presentations. One good possibility is to show the 20-minute DVD (#0126) and accompanying handbook (#0125) available from The Stuttering Foundation titled *Stuttering: Straight Talk for Teachers*. The materials, presented by both young students who stutter and experienced clinicians, provide the audience with essential information about stuttering. Topics include information about responding to the child who stutters in the classroom, the basic principles of treatment, recommendations for teasing and bullying, and suggestions for assisting the child

Clinical Insight

Over the years, students have provided many examples of attempts to hide their stuttering from their teachers and classmates. More than one individual has reported piercing him- or herself with a pencil in order to be excused from speaking and be allowed to go the nurse's office with a bloody hand. Many have pretended to be sick on the day of a presentation or have feigned illness when faced with an unexpected assignment to speak in class. Others describe suffering the consequences of getting caught scribbling on or tearing out a page of a book in order to avoid taking their turn at reading in front of the class. One of the more poignant descriptions was that of a young boy who found himself frequently getting in trouble for talking during class; a boy the teacher viewed as an undisciplined student. The boy explained, however, that because he typically stuttered severely when called on by the teacher to speak before the entire class, he would fluently talk out of turn to a classmate in order to show his peers "that I really could talk."

who stutters with oral presentations. Reardon (2000) provides a helpful checklist for helping classroom teachers in identifying students who stutter and for following their progress as they receive treatment (Figure 9-1). The reader is also referred to a Stuttering Foundation workbook designed for speech-language pathologists working in a school, titled *Practical ideas for working with feelings and beliefs about stuttering* (Publication No. 5) by Chemla and Reardon (2000).

Teacher Checklist—Fluency

Student: _____ Birthdate: _____ C.A.: _____ Grade: _____

School: _____ Teacher: _____ Section: ____ Date: _____

Speech/Language Pathologist: _____

The child above has been referred for or is receiving services regarding fluency skills. Please help me gain a better overall view of this student's speech skills by completing the following information.

Informational Checklists:

1. This student: (check all that apply)

    ___ doesn't mind talking in class.

    ___ seems to avoid speaking in class. (Does not volunteer, if called upon, may frequently not reply.)

    ___ speaks with little or no outward signs of frustration.

    ___ is difficult to understand in class.

    ___ demonstrates frustration when speaking (please describe): _____

    ___ performs average or above average academically.

2. This student is disfluent or stutters when he/she: (Check all that apply)

    ___ begins the first word of a sentence.

    ___ speaks to the class.

    ___ speaks an entire sentence.

    ___ gets upset.

(continues)

Figure 9-1   A checklist to assist classroom teachers in identifying students who stutter and for following their progress as they receive treatment. Source: Reardon, N.A. Working with teachers. Presentation to the Stuttering Foundation of America Conference, Stuttering therapy: Practical ideas for the school clinician. Charleston, SC, June, 10, 2000. Reprinted with permission.

___ uses little words.

___ shares ideas or tells a story.

___ uses main words.

___ answers questions.

___ talks with peers.

___ carries on a conversation.

___ gives messages.

___ reads aloud.

___ talks to adults.

___ other _____

3. Check any of the following behaviors you have noticed in this child's speech:

___ revisions (starting and stopping and starting over again)

___ frequent interjections (um, like, you know)

___ word repetitions (we-we-we)

___ phrase repetitions (and then, and then)

___ part-word repetitions (ta-ta-take)

___ sound repetitions (t-t-t-take)

___ prolongations (n--------obody)

___ block (noticeable tension/no sound comes out)

___ unusual face or body movements (visible tension, head nods, eye movements)

___ Other _____

In the Classroom:

1. I do/do not have concerns about this child's speech because . . .

2. I observe the most disfluency when . . .

3. When this child has difficulty speaking he/she reacts by . . .

4. When this child has difficulty speaking, I respond by . . .

Figure 9-1   Continued.

Your Perceptions:

1. I have/have not had prior experience with a child who stutters.

2. I feel stuttering is caused by . . .

3. Some questions I have about stuttering are . . .

4. Some questions I have about helping this child be successful in the classroom would be:

5. The amount of knowledge I currently have regarding the disorder of stuttering is . . .

    Nothing _____ A Lot

    　　　　1　　2　　3　　4　　5　　6　　7

6. My confidence level regarding dealing with stuttering in the classroom would be . . .

    No confidence _____ Very Confident

    　　　　1　　2　　3　　4　　5　　6　　7

7. My comfort level when communicating with this child is . . .

    Uncomfortable _____ Very Comfortable

    　　　　1　　2　　3　　4　　5　　6　　7

Your Observations:

This child with PEERS . . .

1. Please describe this child's relationships with others of the same age.

2. Has this student been teased or mimicked because of his/her speech?

3. When this child has difficulty speaking, the other children react by . . .

4. Following a reaction by a peer, this child . . .

Figure 9-1 Continued.

<u>This child in GENERAL . . .</u>

1. Have other students or this student's parent(s) ever mentioned his/her fluency problems? If yes, what was discussed?

2. Has this student ever talked to you about his/her speech problem. If yes, what was discussed?

3. What other information might be pertinent regarding this child's speech and language skills?

4. Do you have any other concerns regarding this child's <u>speech and language</u>, <u>academic</u>, or <u>social</u> skills?

Thank you for taking time to share this helpful information.

Please return this form to _____ by _____

Speech-Language Pathologist   Date

> Note: Because follow-up is so important, I would like to observe this child in at least three different speaking situations. Please list some times that this student:
>
> Goes to lunch _____
>
> Has the most opportunity to share in the classroom _____
>
> Attends gym class _____

Figure 9-1   Continued.

As the goals and techniques of treatment are explained to the child's teacher, he or she is more likely to become involved in treatment. As with parents, it is often better to show, rather than tell, colleagues what takes place during the treatment sessions with the child. Live or taped demonstrations are especially important if the child is taken from the classroom for intervention. As the classroom teacher recognizes that a child is choosing to participate in class in spite of some stuttering, the teacher will be able to reward that response (either during or following the event, and either verbally or nonverbally). When a child successfully uses a fluency- or stuttering-modification technique in the classroom, the teacher will be more likely to recognize what the child has done and know how to respond. When a child successfully alters his or her usual tense and fragmented speech into a more open and forward-moving pattern, the teacher has an opportunity to reward the accomplishment. Until the teacher is able to interpret these seemingly small events as victories, they will go unrecognized and unrewarded. As the teacher gains this brief experience with the child, the choice of how to respond in the classroom, playground, or the school lunchroom becomes apparent. With this understanding, the teacher will be much more likely to discuss the problem with the child and be another important source of support and encouragement in the child's daily school environment. The clinician may also want to consider communicating with the child's teachers via informal newsletters or e-mail messages in order to document the nature of the progress the child is making.

The clinician should also alert classroom teachers that possible outcomes of successful treatment are increased participation, increased speaking, and possibly an increase in the occurrence of fluency breaks. As the child achieves success in diminishing his avoidance behaviors and increasing speech assertiveness, one possible result may be greater participation in the classroom. A child who may have chosen to sit quietly prior to treatment may begin to communicate more, begin to talk to his friends and, on occasion, stutter more as a result of his or her increased involvement in classroom activities.

Perhaps one of the most important concepts the clinician can impart to the classroom teacher is that unless he or she is a totally insensitive and uncaring person, he or she is not likely to harm the child who stutters. Yes, certainly it would be possible for an insensitive teacher to make things worse for the child. Clearly such people do exist, as reflected by reports in the newsletters of support groups. More often than not, however, classroom teachers are well-intentioned and need to be given permission to respond naturally without fear of somehow damaging "this fragile child who stutters." As with parents, when the teacher understands the basic characteristics of stuttering behavior and avoidance responses, it becomes obvious that it is possible to discuss the topic of stuttering openly without hurting the child.

Many suggestions provided to parents can be applied, with slight modification, to the classroom teacher as well. For example, although there may be some exceptions, children who stutter should generally not be permitted to escape from school assignments and responsibilities. Just as the other children are required to take their turn, the child who happens to stutter must also take his or her turn in reciting, reading, and answering questions. To allow a child to escape these responsibilities may foster more harassment from his peers than the fact that he or she occasionally stutters. If they could, some children who are fluent would also choose not to face the threat of class participation and public speaking. These decisions, of course, vary with the child and the circumstances, and it would be inappropriate to say that a child must always be required to take part in every speaking situation. However, the exceptions should be rare. Even children who stutter severely are able to take part in class presentations or plays. When the teacher understands that children who stutter are unlikely to stutter when playing a role—speaking with a dialect, singing, or speaking in unison with other children—the teacher is more likely to have the child participate. At the very least, the child could have a nonspeaking part or play a character that makes mechanical or animal sounds.

As the teacher begins to appreciate the effect of time pressure on fluency, he or she may decide, on occasion, to call on the child unexpectedly or early in the class, when he or she is less likely to stutter. The child can then relax a bit and attend to the rest of the class. By understanding the dynamics of fluency-enhancing or disrupting stimuli for a particular child, the teacher may choose to call on him or her when the anticipated response is a short, perhaps one-word, answer. Of course, the teacher can reward the child for not avoiding and taking the opportunity to participate. With the assistance of the clinician, the teacher can talk privately with the child before or after class so there can be a mutual understanding about an anticipated or past speaking experience. Stuttering can be a serious topic, but, with the assistance of the clinician, the teacher can become desensitized to it and show the child that it is possible to openly and easily discuss the problem.

Like parents, teachers can be shown the powerful effects of listener loss on the child's fluency. The ability of the teacher to remain calm, even during a moment of severe stuttering, communicates understanding and support to the child. Nonverbal indicators of anxiety and avoidance, such as becoming tense or rigid, turning away, or breaking eye contact, can be monitored and changed with some practice. Voluntary stuttering during role-playing activities with the clinician or other teachers and desensitization activities using videotapes also can be especially helpful. Generally, but again with some few exceptions, the teacher should not help the child say a word when he or she is experiencing an extended long block. There may be some occasions when there is no other choice but to help the child, but this should be infrequent.

Certainly the teacher should not let other children interrupt a child while he is stuttering. Similarly, it is never beneficial for the teacher to suggest to the child that he or she stop and think about what he or she is going to say. Such comments simply indicate the naïvety of the listener about the true nature of stuttering. A better response is for the teacher to restate to the class what the child has said. That is, even though the child may have struggled through his or her comments, the teacher can increase the value of the child's comments by paraphrasing his or her words. Such a restating of the child's words gives him or her increased importance and allows the other children in the class to appreciate the content of the child's response. It may take some practice to do this gracefully, but providing such a response is clearly much better than reacting with silence and pretending that no stuttering has occurred or unintentionally conveying the impression that what the child has said is unimportant. An open and forthright response by the teacher also carries a strong statement of unconditional acceptance of the child despite his manner of speaking.

Perhaps most importantly, the classroom teacher can become an advocate for the child. By showing understanding, being available to the child, and rewarding what he or she recognizes as progress in the direction of behavioral and attitude change, the child's teacher, like the parent, can be a powerful force for decreasing the handicapping impact of stuttering and for preventing the maintenance and further development of the problem.

On those occasions when the clinician is working with a child privately or in a clinical setting outside of the child's school, making contact with the school is an important part in helping the child to transfer his or her ability to modify his or her stuttering in this important setting. The following letter can serve as a model for informing the teachers about how to respond to a child currently undergoing treatment.

A sample letter for informing classroom teachers about how to respond to a child who stutters.

To the Teachers of Fred Smith at   Date _____
South Park Elementary School

Dear _____,

Fred has been attending the Speech and Hearing Center for the past few months in order to learn how to modify his stuttering and enhance his fluency. He has been doing well as he learns how to monitor and modify specific features of his speech, both in the clinic setting and at home with his family and friends. As he begins a new school year it is important that his teachers have an understanding of the techniques he is using so that his efforts to smooth his speech and take part in speaking activities are rewarded. Here are some suggestions for helping Fred.

- Encourage Fred's participation in all speaking activities. Avoidance of speaking situations and specific words or sounds are a significant part of the daily impact created by stuttering.

- Of course, progress is indicated by decreased moments of stuttering. However, success is also indicated by Fred's ability to change his more typical stuttering moments into easier and smoother forms of stuttering; ask him to show you what this looks and sounds like.

- As Fred approaches an anticipated moment of stuttering he will begin to slow his speech slightly and stretch out the initial sounds and syllables of the word he is going to say. Although his speech at this point may not always sound perfectly normal, his best response at this time is to move through the word with this "easy form of stuttering." Your recognition and positive response to his ability to do this is extremely helpful.

- You can find additional information about the nature of childhood stuttering and how to respond to a child who stutters in your classes by contacting any of the following groups via the Internet: The Stuttering Foundation, The National

Stuttering Association, Friends, The National Association of Young People who Stutter. There is also a very informative website called the Stuttering Home Page that has a lot of good information for children and adults who stutter (as well as parents and teachers) and links to additional sites.

I would be happy to come to your school to speak with you and other teachers concerning these and other suggestions for Fred as well as other children in your school who stutter. Thank you for your help assisting Fred to increase his participation and his fluency. Please feel free to contact me if you have any questions concerning any of the recommendations I have suggested.

Clinical Decision-Making

Throughout this text there are many examples of the countless decisions that clinicians need to make. Some children require more direct intervention than others. Some parents are willing participants in the process of therapeutic change and others are not. Some children are especially sensitive or have experienced the added sense of shame brought about by bullying. Some classroom teachers are more adept than others in providing support and recognizing success. In many cases, the clinician will not know what might be the best decision until a choice is made and the outcome considered. With this in mind, consider the following circumstances and describe one or more possible choices or responses that could be made.

- A third-grade boy who has just begun treatment comes to a therapy session and states, "I feel really great. I haven't stuttered at all today!"

- A child tells you that the fluency-enhancing technique he learned and used perfectly in therapy last week "doesn't work at school."

- A child's teacher informs you that a child you are seeing for therapy refuses to take his turn presenting a report to the class.

- The parents of an 8-year-old child who stutters want their child to receive treatment, but the child refuses to attend individual or group treatment sessions.

- An elementary school student tells you that his preferred method of coping with his stuttering is to avoid words.

- A child tells you that his parents do not want to talk with him about what he is learning in treatment.

- The parents of a young client inform you that their child is being bullied by a child in the neighborhood because of his stuttering.

- The parents of an 8-year-old child are resistant to do easy voluntarily stuttering during a treatment session.

- The parents of a child who is about to begin therapy ask you "How long will it take for my child to stop stuttering?"

Conclusion

In comparison to older speakers, treatment for young children who stutter is of much shorter duration and often more successful. Some of this success is undoubtedly the result of a natural process of recovery from stuttering during the preschool and early school-age years. In most cases, the length of the time that the child has been stuttering is liable to be more informative to the clinician than the chronological age of the child. Nevertheless, even for children who have been stuttering for as long as 6 to 12 months, the behavioral and cognitive patterns associated with stuttering are rarely embedded to the extent they are for older speakers. Nonetheless, many of the principles and techniques of change that allow older speakers to expand their fluency and modify their stuttering can be applied to children, keeping in mind, of course, that the young speaker's conceptual, linguistic, affective, and neurophysiological systems are still in the process of maturation. Regardless of the specific techniques that may be used, children can learn how to more efficiently manage their breath stream, create a gentle onset of voicing, slow their articulatory rate, make easy transitions from one sound or word to another, and use light articulatory contacts. They can also become skilled at varying and changing the effort associated with the struggle responses they may have developed.

During recent decades, treatment for children has become increasingly direct. Clinicians are now more likely to model behavioral techniques that directly assist the young speaker in changing fluency rather than primarily focusing on altering the child's environment. Depending on the child, indirect techniques that help to alter the family's communicative style may also be useful for enhancing fluency. No matter the therapy approach, the involvement of the parents and other family members is crucial for promoting and maintaining successful therapeutic change. The documented success of the Lidcombe Program provides support for such direct approaches and points to the importance of parental understanding and commitment for transferring and maintaining the fluency of young speakers in their daily environment. Recent research also indicates that the therapeutic success may be accounted for by important common factors that are found in several treatment protocols. Such factors as the active participation of the parents in the child's everyday environment, the reduction of parental anxiety, the acknowledgement of stuttering in an open and forthright manner, praise-giving by the parents conveying that the child has a choice about how he or she speaks, and the construction of a meaningful speaker role appear to play important roles in therapeutic success. Perhaps most essential, regardless of the particular treatment protocol and associated techniques, is the ability of the clinician and the parents to convey to the child that he or she is not helpless and has a choice about how to produce words and sounds.

As research increasingly points to both the awareness and reactive nature of some children to the experience of stuttering, counseling for children and their families has become even more vital. Consequently, the clinician, beyond modeling behavioral change, should also promote cognitive and affective change for the child as well as the parents. In cases where the child is particularly sensitive or experiencing the effects of bullying, understanding and support from the clinician becomes especially important. Activities that promote desensitization will allow the child to approach and explore his or her experience with stuttering, lessening shame and guilt. Related activities allow the child to ventilate his or her frustration and anger and become desensitized and knowledgeable about stuttering. Some children will become secure enough to acknowledge their stuttering to others, perhaps educating listeners concerning interesting facts about the topic. Parents are especially likely to benefit from counseling that emphasizes an understanding and a corresponding reduction of their own anxiety concerning stuttering. The clinician can play a key role in modeling an open, uninhibited style of addressing many stutter-related issues, showing the parents that it is possible for stuttering to be an acceptable topic of discussion. A clinician's coordination of informal group meetings of parents can be particularly helpful for becoming desensitized and exchanging helpful information about stuttering.

In contrast to older speakers, clinicians are more likely to evaluate and determine the impact of co-occurring communication, learning, and behavioral problems on children. Although there are many children for whom stuttering is their only communication difficulty, there are most certainly subgroups of children who also have various degrees of phonological, language, and learning problems that impact fluency. The "trading" relationships across the various prerequisite abilities necessary for producing fluent, age-appropriate speech and language will need to be considered when selecting the sequence of intervention activities for such speakers. Although even less common, there are some conditions that can result in the reduced ability to produce fluent speech, including Tourette's syndrome (TS); autism spectrum disorders (ASD), including Asperger's syndrome; attention deficit hyperactivity disorder (ADHD); and Down syndrome. To the extent that it is appropriate, most experienced clinicians will assist the child who stutters while also helping the child to deal with other coexisting problems.

While exchanging information with the classroom teacher of a child who is receiving fluency therapy is essential, most teachers will appreciate knowing something about stuttering prior to discovering such a child in their classroom. The informed teacher can play an important role during transfer and maintenance of therapeutic successes. The presentation of a brief workshop with accompanying video and written materials is a highly efficient method of imparting key information. As classroom teachers achieve enhanced understanding about the basic characteristics of stuttering and the realization that a caring teacher is unlikely to harm the child, they are more likely to recognize and praise positive changes in the child's attitude and behavior. Working with clinicians, the classroom teacher can find many ways to include the child who stutters in class activities and can become an important advocate for the child.

The future for fluency is bright for young children who receive good, early intervention. Issues of transfer and maintenance are generally less difficult for younger speakers, particularly if the clinician, from the outset of treatment, works with the child's parents and teachers to promote these activities beyond the immediate treatment environment. Several investigators have demonstrated that regression and relapse to pretreatment levels following treatment is much less apt to occur with children than it is with adults. As described in Chapter 1, the clinician who models a confident, curious, and enthusiastic style can make the process of therapeutic change successful and enjoyable for the young child who stutters.

Topics for Discussion

1. What characteristics of younger children who stutter are likely to influence both your diagnostic and treatment decisions?

2. What were the views about direct intervention for young children who stuttered in the middle of the 20th century? How do these ideas contrast with current ideas?

3. How would you describe the primary goals and overall direction of therapy to the parents of a preschool child who is beginning treatment?

4. What are the basic principles and goals when providing counseling to the parents of a young child who stutters?

5. Describe the primary objectives and associated activities that are likely to be helpful for a school-age child who is experiencing bullying by peers?

6. Describe to a friend the techniques you would consider using to help a child who stutters to deal with his fear and shame associated with stuttering.

7. What are the fluency-enhancing techniques you would consider using with a young child who stutters?

8. With a friend, model techniques that will assist a young child who stutters in varying and modifying her stuttering behavior.

9. What decisions will you need to make when deciding to treat a child who stutters and also exhibits one or more additional communication problems?

10. Prepare an outline of an in-service training for a group of 30 classroom teachers. What are the main points you want to make about the nature

of stuttering, the nature of therapy, how they may help to identify a child who stutters in their class, and how they can assist in the treatment process? What pamphlets, videos, and Internet addresses would you make available to your audience?

Recommended Readings

Chmela, K. A., & Reardon, N. A. (2000). *The school-age child who stutters: Practical ideas for working with feelings and beliefs about stuttering.* Publication No. 5. Stuttering Foundation of America.

DiLollo, A. & Manning, W. H. (2006). Counseling children who stutter and their parents, In E. Conture & R. Curlee (Eds.), *Stuttering and Related Disorders of Fluency* (3rd Edition, 115–130). New York: Thieme Medical Publishers, Inc.

Langevin, M. Kully, D, Ross-Harold, B. (2007). Treatment of School-Age Children who Stutter: A Comprehensive Approach with Strategies for Managing Teasing and Bullying. In E. Conture & R. Curlee (Eds.), *Stuttering and Related Disorders of Fluency* (3rd Edition, pp. 131–150). Philadelphia, PA: Thieme Medical Publishers Inc.

Millard, S. K., Nicholas, A., & Cook, F. M. (2008). Is parent-child interaction therapy effective in reducing stuttering? *Journal of Speech, Language, and Hearing Research, 51,* 636–650.

Murphy, W. P., Yaruss, J. S., & Quesal, R. W. (2007). Enhancing Treatment for school-age children who stutter I: Reducing negative reactions through desensitization and cognitive restructuring. *Journal of Fluency Disorders, 32,* 121–138.

Murphy, W. P., Yaruss, J. S., & Quesal, R. W. (2007). Enhancing Treatment for school-age children who stutter II: Reducing bullying through role-playing and self-disclosure. *Journal of Fluency Disorders, 32,* 139–162.

Ramig, P. R., & Dodge, D. M. (2005). *The child and adolescent stuttering treatment and activity resource guide.* Clifton Park, NY: Thomson Delmar Learning.

CHAPTER 10

Assessment and Management for Atypical Fluency Disorders

Make everything as simple as possible, but not simpler.

Albert Einstein[1]

Chapter Objectives

As the title of this text suggests, humans can experience fluency disorders other than the more common form of developmental stuttering that we have focused on up to this point. Although less common than developmental stuttering, it is not unusual for clinicians who specialize in fluency disorders to encounter individuals with fluency problems associated with cluttering, neurogenic stuttering, and psychogenic stuttering. The first of the two primary objectives of this chapter is to describe assessment procedures that enable the clinician to differentiate between these less common forms of fluency problems. As we will see, the disfluencies of these individuals are not only distinguishable from typically fluent speakers but, in many ways, including the nature of their disfluencies, are uniquely different to speakers with developmental stuttering. The second objective is to provide treatment protocols and procedures that have been found to be useful for promoting fluency and improving the ability of these speakers to communicate.

We begin this chapter by discussing the assessment and treatment of cluttering, the most common of these fluency problems. Another rationale for discussing cluttering at the outset is that it is not unusual for speakers with developmental stuttering to also possess some characteristics of cluttering. Most individuals who clutter also stutter, a combination that occurs most often in

---

[1]Robins, G. www.cs.virginia.edu/~robins/quotes.html

children (Bloodstein, 1987; Daly, 1986; St. Louis & Hinzman, 1986). Indeed, Weiss (1964) suggested that stuttering often is the result of the child's attempts to cope with cluttering. Although the onset of cluttering usually occurs only slightly later than developmental stuttering, fluency problems of neurogenic and psychogenic origin tend to occur later in life, often in the middle years of adulthood and typically in individuals with a history of fluent speech.

The Characteristics of Cluttering

Cluttered speech appears to be just that, cluttered and chaotic. The most prominent feature of speech is a rapid rate and often uneven rate. An already rapid rate of speaking often accelerates as the speaker produces longer sentences (Daly, 1986). The speaker seems to be in a hurry, even driven, sometimes displaying a compulsive and tense demeanor. Sounds and syllables are omitted and there are few, if any, gaps between words or sentences. The speaker pauses only long enough to take a breath before continuing. Words are often poorly articulated and produced at a rate that, in extreme cases, is unintelligible. Both during speaking and writing, the person seems to lack the ability to attend to the details of the task. The speaker appears to take a gestalt view of communication and only with concentrated effort is he or she able to attend to the individual words or the punctuation on a page of text. Oral reading sounds as though the person is demonstrating speed-reading aloud, as though he or she is attempting to produce the entire page of text in a single utterance. The speech is frequently unorganized and the speaker may have difficulty describing the specific features of an activity or event. There are many false starts, irrelevant words, and superfluous or meaningless words. Although disfluencies occur, they appear to be the result of the speaker's attempts to rapidly formulate and produce the utterance. Complicating the problem is the speaker's lack of awareness concerning his or her ineffective communication.

Cluttering is unlikely to be detected until a young child begins to produce longer and more complex utterances (St. Louis, Myers, Bakker, & Raphael, 2007). Thus, onset is not usually recognized until about age 7 years, later than the 33-month average for stuttering as indicated in Chapter 2. A review of the literature by St. Louis, Myers, Bakker, and Raphael (2007) indicates that little is known about the possibility of recovery or therapeutic outcome.

Although cluttering has been described in the European literature for many decades (e.g., Weiss, 1964), until the 1980s few authors in the United States showed much interest in the problem. Because we tend to find what we are looking for, and because few clinicians were looking for speakers who cluttered, few were identified. This began to change with the work of authors such as (Daly, 1992, 1993; Myers, 1992, 1996; St. Louis, 1986, 1992; St. Louis & Myers, 1995). Recent investigations by these and other authors have resulted in an increasing understanding of the occurrence of cluttering both in its "classic" or "pure" form and as cluttering co-occurs with stuttering. St. Louis, et al. (2007) indicate that cluttering may occur in conjunction with stuttering approximately 22–32% of the time. Daly (1992; 1996) estimated the occurrence of this combination of problems at 40% based on the clients he had seen over 20 years. Both St. Louis et al. (2007) and Daly (1996) estimate that approximately 5% of these speakers demonstrate a pure form of cluttering. St. Louis et al. (2007) indicate that these figures may be underestimates, because few individuals who clutter recognize their problem and ask for assistance. These authors also suggest that an absence of a working definition of the problem, as well as a lack of knowledge about cluttering by many clinicians, has also contributed to underestimates of the problem.

The various definitions emphasize the complexity of cluttering and highlight the many etiological and behavioral aspects of the problem. Most authors agree that cluttering involves aspects of perception, learning, and expression (both verbal and written). Extensive lists of the features associated with cluttering are provided by many authors, with St. Louis and Hinzman (1986) developing a list of 65 different characteristics. Weiss (1964, 1967) considered cluttering to be the consequence of a central language imbalance that affected all language modalities. Luchsinger and Arnold (1965) described cluttering as an inability to formulate language, with associated organic, familial, and aphasic-like symptoms. St. Louis and Rustin (1992) describe the problem as a speech-language disorder, characterized by abnormal fluency that is not stuttering and a speech rate that is rapid, irregular, or both. The American Psychiatric Association's *Diagnostic and Statistical Manual of Mental Disorders, Fourth Edition-Revised* (DSM-IV-TR) (2000) classifies cluttering as an Expressive Language Disorder (DSM 315.31) and provides a single sentence indicating that the diagnostic features include ". . . a disturbance in fluency and language formulation involving an abnormally rapid rate and erratic rhythm of speech and disturbances in language structure (p. 59)."

Daly (1992; 1996) provides a behavioral description that includes what he felt to be the primary features of the problem:

> Cluttering is a disorder of speech and language processing resulting in rapid, dysrhythmic, sporadic, unorganized, and frequently unintelligible speech. Accelerated speech is not always present, but an impairment in formulating language almost always is. (Daly, 1992, p. 107)

Distinguishing Cluttering from Stuttering

For the relatively few individuals (approximately 5–7%) who produce purely cluttered speech, the nature of the problem is usually obvious. But since the majority of individuals with cluttering characteristics also stutter, distinguishing the two patterns of fluency problems is useful. For example, the lack of self-awareness of speakers who clutter makes both assessment and especially treatment difficult. While individuals who stutter typically have more fluency breaks when asked to monitor their speech, people who clutter often show an immediate improvement in both rate and naturalness. To the extent that they are able to continue monitoring their speech, people who clutter are able to speak at a consistent rate and without fluency breaks, even when under communicative pressure. However, their ability to monitor their production is short-lived. Although treatment includes increasing self-awareness and monitoring skills, for the person who stutters that is only a part of the battle. Individuals who stutter must also become adept at modifying behavior.

Another subtle difference between individuals who clutter and those who stutter has to do with formulating and organizing language. For those who clutter, the disorganized flow of information, false starts, interjections, and phrase repetitions suggest that the speaker is having difficulty finding the word they want to use. In addition, Daly and Burnett (1999) provide examples of transpositions by speakers who clutter such as "at this plant in time/at this point in time" and "taking/talking." Much the same thing may seem to be occurring for the person who stutters when they approach but hesitate to attempt a word for fear of stuttering. However, the person who stutters usually knows the word they want to say but uses avoidance, substitution, or circumlocution to conceal the stuttering. As St. Louis et al. (2007) explain, "Stutterers know what they want to say but are interfered in their attempt to produce various words, whereas clutterers do not necessarily know all of what they want to say—or how—but say it anyway" (p. 304).

The Assessment of Cluttering

Cluttering as a Rate-Regulatory Problem

St. Louis et al. (2007) constructed a working definition that includes cluttering within the realm of fluency disorders. Although these authors view cluttering as a fluency problem, it is *not* considered to be stuttering. In fact, as the authors explain, some speakers who clutter do not produce excessive disfluencies. The definition, somewhat different to that of Daly's presented earlier, emphasizes the central issue of rate: a speaking rate that is too rapid and too irregular and that hinders the speaker's ability to produce clear and intelligible speech. St. Louis et al. include in the definition only those features that they believe are essential features of cluttering, not those that often co-occurred (e.g., disfluencies, language component, lack of awareness). Accordingly, their definition indicates that

> Cluttering is a fluency disorder characterized by a rate that is perceived to be abnormally rapid, irregular, or both for the speaker (although measured syllable rates may not exceed normal limits). These rate abnormalities further

are manifest in one or more of the following symptoms: (a) an excessive number of disfluencies, the majority of which are not typical of people who stutter; (b) the frequent placement of pauses and use of prosodic patterns that do not conform to syntactic and semantic constraints; and (c) inappropriate (usually excessive) degrees of coarticulation among sounds, especially in multisyllabic words. (St. Louis, et al., 2007, p. 299)

The authors explain an important distinction in that the term *manifest* in the second sentence of the definition indicates that the rate alterations *cause* many of the other co-existing symptoms often found with cluttering. The best example of this cause-and-effect relationship is seen in the deletion and neutralization of sounds and syllables, particularly during the production of multisyllabic words. Acoustic analysis of cluttered speech by Martin, Kroll, O'Keefe, and Painter (1983) indicated a lack of distinct vowel formant structure, release of energy for stop bursts, and aperiodic fricative energy. Substitutions and distortions of phonemes such as /s/, /r/ or /l/ have also been noted by Daly & Burnett (1999).

An investigation employing spectrographic analysis of cluttered speech by Baker, Raphael, Myers, and St. Louis (2000) indicated that although listeners perceived the rate of cluttered speech as extremely fast, spectrographic analysis indicated that the number of syllables per second fell within the normal range. The perception of a rapid rate of speech was the result of the speaker's omission of many sounds and syllables. When the authors considered the number of omitted or "intended" syllables that could have been tabulated (and that listeners were undoubtedly processing) the "perceived rate" was indeed much higher than normal. Recent research (Raphael, 2004, 2005) comparing speakers who clutter with matched normal-speaking controls indicated that clutterers self-selected comfortable diadochokinetic (DDK) and analogous real words (e.g., "pattycake") at speaking rates that were somewhat slower than the matched controls. Raphael and colleagues suggest that a possible interpretation of this result is that clutterers produce conversational speech at a rate faster than their systems can handle. For such nonconversational DDK tasks in which clutterers can concentrate on articulation but do not have to formulate speech to convey a message, they are more likely to select a rate they can handle.

As also described in the definition by St. Louis et al. (2007), the fluency breaks are not those typically produced by individuals who stutter (part-word repetitions, monosyllabic word repetition, and dysrhythmic phonations) but, rather, take the form of interjections, unfinished words, revisions, and repetitions—especially one syllable words and phrases. Also unlike the person who stutters, the clutterer is not likely to associate fear or avoidance with specific sounds or words. Accordingly, clutterers rarely show the accessory or secondary coping behaviors often seen with speakers who stutter. The clutterer may, however, indicate concern about certain speaking situations. The intrinsic features of the person who stutters—loss of control, helplessness, and fear—do not appear to be operating here. In fact, in some speakers, especially with those considered to be pure clutterers, there may be no awareness that there is any problem at all with their speech.

Finally, there are several other features, that although they are commonly found with people who clutter, are viewed as nonobligatory characteristics. Although this differs from the views of Weiss (1964; 1967) and Daly (1992; 1996) who view problems with language processing as a core aspect of cluttering, St. Louis et al. (2007) view language problems as co-existing rather than central or essential features of their definition. Likewise, maze activity (Loban, 1976) consisting of false starts, disfluent speech, and words irrelevant to the message are common. As a result of this activity, individuals who clutter are often unable to communicate in a coherent manner, resulting in pragmatic issues and an inability to consider the listener's perspective. Clutterers are also often reported to possess attention deficit/hyperactivity disorders (ADHD) resulting in distractibility, an inability to attend to details, and a lack of follow-through with activities. Specific learning disabilities (LD) are also common as well as poor handwriting and musical ability. Apraxia is another common characteristic of individuals who clutter, with the effects being more pronounced during the production of longer and more complex words. Speakers often will make several attempts before producing the word correctly.

Efforts to explain the etiology of cluttering reflect the many, widely varying characteristics of the problem and are well summarized by St. Louis et al. (2007). Models include cognitive and linguistic processing problems (e.g., Daly, 1986, 1992; Daly & Burnett, 1999; Molt, 1996; Myers, 1992; St. Louis & Hinzman, 1986; Tiger, Irvine, & Reiss, 1980; Weiss, 1964), genetic models suggesting a predisposition for disfluent speech (Arnold, 1960; Daly and Burnett, 1999; St. Louis & Myers, 1995; Weiss, 1964), and models suggesting that the central nervous system may contain lesions in the region of the basal ganglia that impede the "executive functions" of the brain (Myers, St. Louis, Bakker, Raphael, Wiig, E., et al., 2002a; 2002b). Such individuals tend to experience problems with behavioral regulation, initiation of action, organization and planning, monitoring, responding to feedback, and self-motoring. Myers et al. point out that there are several other disorders that manifest such characteristics, including Tourette's syndrome, autism, Asperger's syndrome, pervasive developmental delay, obsessive-compulsive disorders (OCD), learning disabilities, and ADHD.

The many core and accompanying characteristics that are often associated with individuals who clutter require that the assessment process be multidimensional—even more so than is often the case for speakers who stutter. An example of such a multifaceted approach is illustrated by the work of St. Louis, Myers, Faragasso, Townsend, and Gallaher (2004). Two groups of 48 listeners (a group from New York and a group West Virginia) rated two young male speakers who cluttered across five attributes: naturalness, articulation, language, disfluency, and rate. Listeners used 9-point equal-appearing interval scales similar to the naturalness scale of Martin, Haroldson, and Triden (1984). Scores of 1 represented "highly natural" or "excellent" and scores of 9 represented "highly unnatural" or "very poor," depending on the attribute being considered. Listeners found the attributes of *rate* and *naturalness* to be least acceptable, followed by the speaker's *articulation*. The results supported the concept that an essential characteristic of cluttered speech is the rapid and irregular rate of speech. The attributes of *disfluency* and *language* were rated most acceptable. In fact, disfluencies were not seen to be a prominent characteristic of cluttered speech, even when the rate of speech was moderately high. The authors felt that the global measure attribute of *naturalness* best captured the most important aspects of all five attributes.

St. Louis et al. (2007) suggest the use of an experimental *Cluttering Assessment Program* (Bakker, 2005).[2] Designed to provide a molar/perceptual rather than a molecular/behavioral approach, this computer-based tool consists of two tracks for indicating severity. The first track provides a computation of the percentage of talking time from individual or cumulative samples that is cluttered or noncluttered. The second track provides a visual-analog scaling procedure for the listener to rate the perceptual effects of nine features associated with cluttered speech: speaking rate, rate regularity, disfluency, syllable-production integrity, overall articulation accuracy, naturalness, pragmatic language appropriateness, language coherence, and thought organization.

Because of the lack of self-awareness for many people who clutter, St. Louis et al. (2007) recommend using a variety of assessment measures typically used for individuals who stutter (see Chapter 4) in order to determine the level of the speaker's self-awareness associated with speech and communication. In addition, they suggest using the *Self-Awareness of Speech Index* (SASI) (St. Louis & Atkins, 2005), a 14-item measure that provides a criterion-referenced indication of a speaker's lack of awareness of their own speech characteristics (Table 10-1). In addition, St. Louis et al. (2007) also recommend the use of several diagnostic measures that provide information about a wide variety of difficulties, including oral motor problems and general coordination, handwriting, central auditory problems, reading comprehension, spelling, and mathematical skills (Table 10-2). Testing for LD and ADHD may also be warranted based on school reports and related therapeutic history.

Cluttering as a Cognitive-Linguistic Problem

Another group of clinicians who have considerable experience with speakers who clutter is Daly and his associates. Although there is considerable overlap in the characteristics of cluttering as described by St. Louis et al. and Daly et al., Daly takes more of a cognitive-linguistic perspective and deemphasizes the

---

[2]The *Cluttering Assessment Program* is available as freeware at the Stutteringhomepage.com

Table 10-1   Self-Awareness of Speech Index.

Name   Date

Instructions: Please check (✓) the appropriate box for each question. Work rapidly and do not look back or change your answers.

		Never	*Rarely*	*Usually*	*Always*
1	I notice differences in the way I say words as compared with the way other people say words.	❏	❏	❏	❏
2	I notice when other people use fillers when they talk, such as "uh," "ya know," and "um."	❏	❏	❏	❏
3	I try to copy the way other people say certain words.	❏	❏	❏	❏
4	I listen to whether someone else's voice is high-pitched or low-pitched.	❏	❏	❏	❏
5	I am aware of other people's accents as they talk.	❏	❏	❏	❏
6	I know when I repeat a sound, word, or phrase.	❏	❏	❏	❏
7	I notice pitch changes in my own voice.	❏	❏	❏	❏
8	I pay attention to how fast other people talk.	❏	❏	❏	❏
9	I notice repetitions of sounds, words, or phrases when other people talk.	❏	❏	❏	❏
10	I am aware of how other people say words.	❏	❏	❏	❏
11	I pay attention to how fast I talk.	❏	❏	❏	❏
12	I notice when I stumble over words.	❏	❏	❏	❏
13	I notice my own accent.	❏	❏	❏	❏
14	I am aware when I use fillers when I talk, such as "uh," "ya know," and "um."	❏	❏	❏	❏

Reprinted with permission of St. Louis and Atkins (2005).

(continues)

Summary Form

Instructions: Count the number of checks in each of the 4 columns of the completed *SASI* form. Write the totals in the boxes in the 1ˢᵗ row. Multiply these numbers by the weights provided in the 2ⁿᵈ row and write Weighted Totals in the boxes in the 3ʳᵈ row. Write the sum of these four numbers in the Grand Total box in the 4ᵗʰ row. On the line below, divide the Grand Total by 14 to determine the Average *SASI* Score. Round the Average *SASI* Score to the nearest tenth, e.g., 2.4.

	Never	*Rarely*	*Usually*	*Always*
Total Checks in Each Category	❏	❏	❏	❏
Weights (Multipliers)	×1	×2	×3	×4
Weighted Totals	❏	❏	❏	❏
Grand Total		❏		

Average *SASI* Score: _____ /14= _____
                              Grand Total

Table 10-1   Continued.

Table 10-2   Clinical Signs of Diagnostic Significance.

	Key
FD—Fluency Disorder RD—Rate Deviation Cl—Cluttering St—Stuttering ArtD—Articulation Disorder LangD—Language Disorder ADHD—Attention Deficit/Hyperactivity 　　Disorder LD—Learning Disability	X̲—Important sign that is important for 　　inclusion in the category (sometimes in 　　combination with other X̲s) x—Sign frequently present but is not 　　necessary for inclusion in the category ?—Sign that may or may not be present and is 　　not necessary for inclusion in the category

Sign	*FD*	*RD*	*St*	*Cl*	*ArtD*	*LangD*	*ADHD*	*LD*
Excessive typical disfluencies	X̲		?	X̲		x		x
Excessive atypical disfluencies	X̲		X̲	?				
Excessively rapid rate	X̲	X̲		X̲				

(continues)

Table 10-2 Continued.

Sign	FD	RD	St	Cl	ArtD	LangD	ADHD	LD
Excessively slow rate		X	x					
Excessively irregular rate	X	X	x	X		?	?	?
Atypical pauses	X	x	x	X		x	?	?
Pragmatic errors				?	x	X	x	x
Semantic errors						X		x
Syntactic/morphological errors			?	x	x	X		x
Lexical (word finding) errors	x			x		X		x
Mazes	?	x	?	x		x	?	?
Phonological errors				?	X	x		
Consistent developmental misarticulations			x	x	X	x		
Excessive neutralization of vowels		x		X	?			
Excessively "over-coarticulated" (collapsed) syllables		x		X	?			
Atypical coarticulation patterns	X	x		X	?			
Distractible				x			X	x
Hyperactive				x			X	x
Reading difficulties				x		x	x	X
Writing difficulties				x		x	x	X
Mathematical difficulties						x	?	X

importance of a rapid speech rate. Daly and Burnett (1999) stated that they have yet to evaluate a person who clutters who did not exhibit at least one disturbance in each of the following five dimensions:

1. Cognitive—People who clutter demonstrate a near-total lack of awareness of their inability to communicate. They characteristically have poor self-monitoring abilities, inadequate thought organization, poor attention span, verbal and nonverbal impulsivity, and show signs of perceptual deficits (auditory or visual processing or poor auditory memory).

2. Language—These individuals show some form of language difficulties that are expressive, receptive, or both. This may be related to their poor auditory memory, attention deficits, and inability to concentrate. They are often poor readers and show little interest in music and literature. Daly and Burnett (1999) also report the occurrence of transpositions such as "The Lord is a shoving leopard."

3. Pragmatics—Clutterers are notoriously poor at turn-taking as well as the introduction, maintenance, and termination of topics. They fail to recognize subtle nonverbal signs indicating turn-taking, and show a lack of interest or attention in the conversation.

4. Speech—The fluency breaks of people who clutter are characterized by irregular rate, accelerations, sporadic bursts of speech, variable intensity, and overall poor rhythm. Some fluency breaks are typical of stuttering.

5. Motor—People who clutter tend to be clumsy and uncoordinated and demonstrate impulsive motor movements. The client may appear to be physically immature. Lack of coordination also may be reflected in the poor legibility of handwriting, which tends to disintegrate during the writing of a paragraph. There is often a lack of ability to imitate a simple rhythm or to sing.

These characteristics are presented as the major components of a "linguistic disfluency model" provided in Figure 10-1. Linguistic disfluency is characterized by Daly and Burnett (1999) as "frequent verbal revisions and interjections, excessive repetitions of words or phrases, poorly organized thoughts, lack of cohesion in discourse, and prosodic irregularities" (p. 226).

Given the perspective by Daly and colleagues that cluttering involves the inability to formulate language, it is not surprising that the writing of people who clutter also tends to be disorganized and often illegible. Daly (1986, 1992) recommends procedures for obtaining writing samples. In many ways, handwriting vividly illustrates many of the features of cluttering. Williams and Wener (1996) describe the handwriting of a young man in his twenties who was diagnosed with both stuttering and cluttering behaviors. His writing was composed of simple declarative sentences with short, simple words. Of 148 words, 54 were stricken due to grammatical errors or misspellings. Legibility was poor, and there were many punctuation errors, particularly misused commas. Figure 10-2 is an example of handwriting by a 16-year-old male who possessed virtually all of the classic characteristics of cluttering.

Daly (2006) provides an updated version of a series of checklists originally created by Daly and Burnett (1996, 1999). Based on the responses of 60 clinicians and researchers experienced in fluency problems who rated the factors they felt to be most important for identifying cluttering, Daly (2006) developed a 33-item *Predictive Cluttering Inventory* (PCI) (Figure 10-3).

Cluttering

Cognition	Language	Pragmatics	Speech	Motor
Awareness - listener perspective - self-monitoring Attention span Thought organization - sequencing - categorization Memory Impulsivity	Receptive - listening/directions - reading disorder Expressive – Verbal - thought organization - poor sequence of ideas - poor story telling - language formulation - revisions and repetitions - improper linguistic structure - syllabic or verbal transpositions - improper pronoun use - dysnomia/word finding - filler words, empty words Expressive—Written - run-on sentences - omissions and transpositions of letters, syllables, and words - sentence fragments	Inappropriate topic introduction, maintenance, termination Inappropriate turn-taking Poor listening skills; impulsive responses Lack of consideration of listener perspective Inadequate processing of non-verbal signals Verbose or tangential Poor eye contact	Speech disfluency - excessive repetition of words/phrases Syllabic or verbal transpositions Prosody of speech - rate (rapid or irregular) - poor rhythm - loud, trail off - lacks pauses between words - vocal monotony Slurred articulation - omit sound(s) - omit syllable(s) - /r/ and /l/ Dysrhythmic breathing Silent gaps/hesitations	Poor motor control Slurred articulation Dysrhythmic breathing Speech disfluencies, - excessive repetitions of sounds or words Silent gaps, hesitations Prosody problems - rate (rapid or irregular) - poor rhythm Clumsy, uncoordinated Poor penmanship Impulsivity

Figure 10-1   The Linguistic disfluency model for individuals who clutter, indicating possible impairments across five broad communicative dimensions. [From Daly, D. A. & Burnett, M. L. (1997). Cluttering: Traditional views and new perspectives. In R. Curlee (Ed.), *Stuttering and Related Disorders of Fluency* (2nd Edition, pp. 222–254). New York: Thieme Medical Publishers, Inc.] Reprinted with permission.

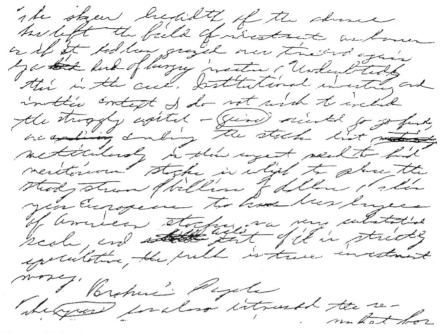

Figure 10-2   An example of cluttered writing.

The inventory includes four categories or speaker characteristics (Pragmatics, 10 statements; Speech-Motor, 10 items; Language-Cognition, 8 items; and Motor Coordination-Writing Problems, 5 items). Listeners indicate the frequency of occurrence of the characteristics using a 7-point scale from "always" (6 points) to "never" (0 points). The two items that clinicians ranked as the most frequent characteristics of cluttering were "omits, transposes sounds and syllables" (Item 8) and "lack of effective, sufficient self-monitoring skills" (Item 27). A total score of 120 or greater is indicative of a "pure clutterer," which, according to Daly, rarely occurs. Scores ranging from 80–120 are more typical and indicate the more common classification of "Clutterer-Stutterer".

Treatment Options for Individuals who Clutter

There are a variety of factors, such as the speaker's lack of awareness of speech rate and the inability to effectively communicate with others, that make treatment for cluttering difficult. To the degree that a person who clutters becomes aware of these problems, he or she may accordingly deny that they occur. This response, along with other personality characteristics such as compulsivity, poor concentration, and a host of pragmatic issues, can make these individuals particularly difficult to interact with. Individuals who clutter tend to be intolerant of interruptions (Van Riper, 1992b) and are particularly resistant to suggestions

PREDICTIVE CLUTTERING INVENTORY (PCI)
David A. Daly (2006)

INSTRUCTIONS: Please respond to each description section below. Circle the number you believe is most descriptive of this person's cluttering.

Descriptive Statement	Always	Almost Always	Frequently	Sometimes	Infrequently	Almost Never	Never
PRAGMATICS							
1. Lack of effective self-monitoring skills	6	5	4	3	2	1	0
2. Lack of awareness of own communication errors or problems	6	5	4	3	2	1	0
3. Compulsive talker; verbose; tangential; word-finding problems	6	5	4	3	2	1	0
4. Poor planning skills; mis-judges effective use of time	6	5	4	3	2	1	0
5. Poor social communication skills; inappropriate turn-taking; interruptions	6	5	4	3	2	1	0
6. Does not recognize or respond to listener's visual or verbal feedback	6	5	4	3	2	1	0
7. Does not repair or correct communication breakdowns	6	5	4	3	2	1	0
8. Little or no excessive effort observed during disfluencies	6	5	4	3	2	1	0
9. Little or no anxiety regarding speaking; unconcerned	6	5	4	3	2	1	0
10. Speech better under pressure (improves short-term with concentration)	6	5	4	3	2	1	0

Figure 10-3 Predictive Cluttering Inventory (PCI), Daly, David (2006). Copyright © David Daly. Reprinted with permission.

(continues)

	SPEECH-MOTOR							
11.	Articulation errors	6	5	4	3	2	1	0
12.	Irregular speech rate; speaks in spurts or bursts	6	5	4	3	2	1	0
13.	Telescopes or condenses words	6	5	4	3	2	1	0
14.	Rapid rate (tachylalia)	6	5	4	3	2	1	0
15.	Speech rate progressively increases (festinating)	6	5	4	3	2	1	0
16.	Variable prosody; irregular melody or stress pattern	6	5	4	3	2	1	0
17.	Initial loud voice trailing off to unintelligible murmur	6	5	4	3	2	1	0
18.	Lack of pauses between words and phrases	6	5	4	3	2	1	0
19.	Repetition of multi-syllablic words and phrases	6	5	4	3	2	1	0
20.	Co-existence of excessive disfluencies and stuttering	6	5	4	3	2	1	0
	LANGUAGE-COGNITION							
21.	Language is disorganized; confused wording; word-finding problems	6	5	4	3	2	1	0
22.	Poor language formulation; poor story-telling; sequencing problems	6	5	4	3	2	1	0
23.	Disorganized language increases as topic becomes more complex	6	5	4	3	2	1	0
24.	Many revisions; interjections; filler words	6	5	4	3	2	1	0
25.	Seems to verbalize before adequate thought formulation	6	5	4	3	2	1	0

Figure 10-3 Continued.

26.	Inappropriate topic introduction, maintenance, or termination	6	5	4	3	2	1	0
27.	Improper linguistic structure; poor grammar; syntax errors	6	5	4	3	2	1	0
28.	Distractible; poor concentration; attention span problems	6	5	4	3	2	1	0
	MOTOR COORDINATION-WRITING PROBLEMS							
29.	Poor motor control for writing (messy)	6	5	4	3	2	1	0
30.	Writing includes omission or transposition of letters, syllables, or words	6	5	4	3	2	1	0
31.	Oral diadochokinetic coordination below expected normed levels	6	5	4	3	2	1	0
32.	Respiratory dysrhythmia; jerky breathing pattern	6	5	4	3	2	1	0
33.	Clumsy and uncoordinated; motor activities accelerated or impulsive	6	5	4	3	2	1	0

TOTAL SCORE: _____

COMMENTS:

Figure 10-3 Continued.

to monitor the details of their speech production. The prognosis for success is not particularly good, but, as always, the prognosis for a successful treatment outcome is better for children than adults (Daly, 1986, 1993; Luchsinger & Arnold, 1965; Myers & St. Louis, 1992; Silverman, 1995; Weiss, 1964).

In more extreme cases, individuals who clutter may display immature responses, a short temper, and a history of emotional problems. On occasion, such individuals can appear defensive and even antagonistic, characteristics that make it difficult to develop a successful therapeutic alliance. Daly has often pointed out that individuals who clutter can provide a challenge to our ability and especially our patience. In addition, the person often finds it difficult to tolerate speaking at what seems to him an exceedingly slow rate. The "driven" quality of these clients becomes obvious after even a brief period of attempting to speak at a slower rate. On the other hand, because these speakers are usually oblivious to their communication problem, as they develop the ability to monitor their speech, intelligibility and fluency can often be dramatically improved. As the person becomes aware of his irregular and rapid speech, appropriate alterations in production are likely to occur, even without specific instruction.

As with the assessment of cluttering, the multidimensional characteristics of these speakers also require a wide-ranging approach to treatment. It is likely that the clinician will want to consult with a variety of other professionals (psychologists, mental health specialists, neurologists, and specialists in LD or ADHD). In fact, during the initial contact with the speech-language pathologist, it is not unusual for adults to report that they have seen or are currently seeing one or more of these professionals. The focus of treatment will vary somewhat depending on whether the speaker manifests the relatively infrequent pure form of cluttering or the more commonly occurring combination of stuttering-cluttering. Following the primary assumption of St. Louis et al.'s (2007) definition of cluttering, that individuals who clutter are attempting to speak at a rate that they are unable to manage, these authors recommend a synergistic therapy approach (Meyers, 1992; Louis & Myers, 1995). That is, the underlying goal of treatment is to help the speaker to enhance the synchrony of language formulation and the rate of speech production. Primary emphasis is on enhancing the coordination of the linguistic and articulatory levels in order to prevent "derailment" of the speech sequence at either of these levels. Another key element is increased awareness by the speaker of the excessive rate, or "haste," during both linguistic organization and motoric/articulatory production. With these principles as a guide, the clinician can experiment with the variety of techniques that clinicians have found to have clinical utility for individuals who clutter. A detailed compendium of techniques from which the client and the clinician can select is found in both St. Louis and Myers (1995) and St. Louis, et al. (2007). These authors suggest that a focus on these principles often results in improvement in articulation and intelligibility as well as fluency. These principles are nearly identical to those suggested by Daly and Burnett (1999), who suggest three basic principles of intervention:

(1) Because the speaker is usually unaware of their communication behavior as well as listener reactions, the frequent repetition of therapy goals and rationale will be necessary.

(2) Because of the speaker's lack of awareness, the clinician should provide immediate and direct feedback.

(3) Parents and significant others should play a major part in providing feedback, correction, and reinforcement. Regardless of the techniques that are selected, all authors stress the importance of daily practice as well as the understanding and encouragement of family, friends, and support groups.

Even for those individuals with a pure form of cluttering, several stuttering-modification and particularly fluency-shaping techniques used with individuals who stutter may also be used to heighten awareness and facilitate changes in rate and fluency. Readers will find it especially useful to consult the list of techniques designed for individuals who clutter provided by such authors as Daly (1996, 1999, 2006), St. Louis and Myers (1995, 1997), St. Louis, et al. (2007), and Van Riper (1992b). The following are examples of such techniques that can be employed by the clinician or by the client (in some cases with the assistance of family or friends), organized according to categories suggested by St. Louis, et al. (2007). Of course, many of these activities, particularly when done in written or verbal form, can serve a variety of functions across several categories.

Awareness and Self-Monitoring Skills

- Play back audio and video recordings to identify and monitor speech.
- Vary the rate of nonspeech (e.g., hand) movements prior to speech movements.
- Heighten awareness of listener indicators of unintelligible speech.
- Increase proprioceptive and kinesthetic feedback associated with the articulatory movements (possibly using altered feedback devices).
- Purposely vary the rate of speech from extremely slow through very fast.

Rate, Articulation, and Intelligibility

- Read in unison, beginning with a fast rate, and systematically change speed while the client shadows the clinician's rate changes.
- Imitate and vary rhythmic patterns by tapping a finger or other object; perform verbally with numbers or word sequences.

- Use a window-card so that one or a few words are visible to the client.
- Read a passage backwards one word at a time in order to increase tolerance for a slower rate.
- Repeat phrases using different tempos, altering the stress placed on different words or syllables.
- Say words as they are written or produced on a keyboard.
- Slow speech rate during reading by using the natural pauses afforded by punctuation and clause boundaries.
- Heighten the awareness of final sounds and syllables.
- Shadow the speech of the clinician (and others).

Linguistic and Narrative Skills

- Write down the words of a sentence prior to speaking.
- Heighten turn-taking ability during conversation to decrease overtalking.
- Describe sequencing of steps for a moderately complex task.
- Practicing selecting one of several thoughts or words that occur at once.
- Organize the sequence of a story in writing, then verbally.
- Practice telling jokes requiring precise sequencing and timing.

Fluency

- Analyze recorded speech samples for repetitions, misarticulations, revisions, and interjections.
- Use rate-altering techniques and fluency-shaping targets of respiration, phonation, and articulation (Chapter 8) to enhance fluency.

Ability To Understand and Describe the Characteristics of Cluttered Speech

- Contrast the proprioceptive feedback associated with slow, fast, and irregular speech rates.
- Contrast the nature of the emotions (e.g., anxiety, sense of urgency) and behaviors (avoidance, anticipation, types of fluency breaks) associated with stuttering and cluttering.
- Contrast the influence on communication of helpful and poor pragmatic skills.
- Role-play nonverbal and verbal cues of listener confusion.

Phonatory, Respiratory, and Motor Skills

- Practice fluency-shaping targets of respiration, phonation, and articulation; begin with shorter, and then longer, breath groups.
- Prolong vowels during progressively longer utterances.
- Engage in oral-motor skills training.
- Practice writing or printing skills using graph paper.

Family, Friend, and Employer Support

- Request feedback of clear and poor communication from family and friends; role-play in clinic environment.
- Interact with others who have similar communication problems (e.g., local chapters of the National Stuttering Association, cluttering@yahoo.com).
- Consider involvement in group-speaking activities socially or at school or work.

A comprehensive treatment approach is also provided by Daly (2006), who describes a strategy for treatment called the Cluttering Treatment Profile Analysis (Figure 10-4). Information obtained on the Predictive Cluttering Inventory is converted to this profile. Rather than focusing on rate alone, treatment can focus on other commonly occurring characteristics, such as #17 (Initial loud voice trailing off to unintelligible murmur) and # 2 (Lack of awareness of own communication errors or problems). The profile analysis is intended to facilitate individualized treatment according to the areas where the speaker is in particular need of assistance.

Acquired Stuttering

The next two fluency problems have been referred to as "acquired stuttering" because they tend to occur for the first time in adults, long after the onset of developmental stuttering in childhood and after many years of fluent speech. With adult onset of stuttering it is possible that we may be observing the result of a relapse following previously successful therapy or the occurrence of overt stuttering characteristics for speakers who have been able to manage their stuttering in a covert or "interiorized" manner (Van Riper, 1971; Deal, 1982). Although developmental stuttering may have a rapid onset, this is more likely to be the case for older speakers with neurogenic and psychogenic stuttering. Although far less common than both developmental stuttering and cluttering, more recent reports suggest that acquired neurogenic and psychogenic stuttering occur more often than previous literature suggests. Like cluttering,

CLUTTERING TREATMENT PROFILE ANALYSIS
David A. Daly (2006)

NAME _____

INSTRUCTIONS: Transfer the scores from the PCI, and then connect the scores. Higher scores indicate more severe deficit areas. For best results, clinicians should focus on at least two deficit areas, in additon to "rapid rate."

CLUTTERING CHARACTERISTICS	Very Severe	Severe	Moderate	Mild	Very Mild	Inconsistent	Not a Problem
PRAGMATICS							
1. Lack of effective self-monitoring skills	6	5	4	3	2	1	0
2. Lack of awareness of own communication errors or problems	6	5	4	3	2	1	0
3. Compulsive talker; verbose; tangential	6	5	4	3	2	1	0
4. Poor planning skills; misjudges effective use of time	6	5	4	3	2	1	0
5. Poor social communication skills; inappropriate turn-turn-taking; interruptions	6	5	4	3	2	1	0
6. Does not recognize or respond to listener's visual or verbal feedback	6	5	4	3	2	1	0
7. Does not repair or correct communication breakdowns	6	5	4	3	2	1	0
8. Little or no excessive effort observed during disfluencies	6	5	4	3	2	1	0
9. Little or no anxiety regarding speaking; unconcerned	6	5	4	3	2	1	0
10. Speech better under pressure (improves short-term with concentration	6	5	4	3	2	1	0

Figure 10-4   Profile analysis for planning treatment with cluttering clients. Copyright © David Daly. Reprinted with permission.

(continues)

	SPEECH-MOTOR							
11.	Articulation errors	6	5	4	3	2	1	0
12.	Irregular speech rate; speaks in spurts or bursts	6	5	4	3	2	1	0
13.	Telescopes or condenses words	6	5	4	3	2	1	0
14.	Rapid rate (tachylalia)	6	5	4	3	2	1	0
15.	Speech rate progressively increases (festinating)	6	5	4	3	2	1	0
16.	Variable prosody; irregular melody or stress pattern	6	5	4	3	2	1	0
17.	Initial loud voice trailing off to unintelligible murmur	6	5	4	3	2	1	0
18.	Lack of pauses between words and phrases	6	5	4	3	2	1	0
19.	Repetition of multi-syllabic words and phrases	6	5	4	3	2	1	0
20.	Co-existence of excessive disfluencies and stuttering	6	5	4	3	2	1	0
	LANGUAGE-COGNITION							
21.	Language is disorganized; confused wording; word-finding problems	6	5	4	3	2	1	0
22.	Poor language formulation; poor story-telling; sequencing problems	6	5	4	3	2	1	0
23.	Disorganized language increases as topic becomes more complex	6	5	4	3	2	1	0
24.	Many revisions; interjections; filler words	6	5	4	3	2	1	0
25.	Seems to verbalize before adequate thought formulation	6	5	4	3	2	1	0
26.	Inappropriate topic introduction, maintenance, or termination	6	5	4	3	2	1	0
27.	Improper linguistic structure; poor grammar; syntax errors	6	5	4	3	2	1	0
28.	Distractible; poor concentration; attention span problems	6	5	4	3	2	1	0

Figure 10-4   Continued.

	MOTOR COORDINATION-WRITING PROBLEMS							
29.	Poor motor control for writing (messy)	6	5	4	3	2	1	0
30.	Writing includes omission or transposition of letters, syllables or words	6	5	4	3	2	1	0
31.	Oral diadochokinetic coordination below expected normed levels	6	5	4	3	2	1	0
32.	Respiratory dysrhythmia; jerky breathing pattern	6	5	4	3	2	1	0
33.	Clumsy and uncoordinated; motor activities accelerated or impulsive	6	5	4	3	2	1	0
	Totals							

Grand Total _____   Diagnosis _____

Figure 10-4   Continued.

there have been relatively few reports and nearly all in the form of case studies. De Nil, Jokel, and Rochon (2007) stress the need for continuing systemic literature reviews, meta-analysis, and prospective investigations in order to develop a better understanding of these speakers.

The differential diagnosis of these forms of acquired stuttering can be difficult, not only because these speakers are seen relatively infrequently in most clinical locations (with the exception of large medical centers), but also because they can occur together—particularly with neuropathologies related to closed head injuries and medications. In the following paragraphs we will discuss the characteristics of these forms of acquired stuttering, as well as the speaker characteristics that assist the clinician in distinguishing between the two. Because speech and language characteristics can reflect the overall health of a person, speech-language pathologists are often able to play a vital role in the diagnostic process. Based on the speaker's characteristics and the results of trial therapy, the clinician may be able to detect the presence of neuropathology, including possible sites of lesion (Baumgartner, 1999).

Characteristics of Neurogenic Stuttering

Neurogenic stuttering is likely to occur post-puberty, characteristically occurring in the decade of the forties (Jokel & De Nil, 2003; Market et al., 1990; Mazzucchi, Moretti, Carpeggiani, Parma, & Paini, 1981; Stewart & Rowley, 1996). As with most fluency problems, the majority of individuals presenting with neurogenic stuttering are males (De Nil, et al., 2007; Market, et al., 1990; Stewart & Rowley, 1996). Clinicians who specialize in fluency disorders will eventually encounter these speakers, particularly if they work in a large clinic or medical environment. Estimates of occurrence are complicated by a number of factors, including the multiple linguistic, cognitive, and motor problems that often accompany and sometimes mask the speaker's disfluency as well as the sometimes transient nature of the problem (Helm, Butler, & Canter, 1980; Helm-Estabrooks, 1993; Rosenbek, Messert, Collins, & Wertz, 1978).

As others have done, we have chosen to use the term *neurogenic stuttering* (Helm, Butler, & Canter, 1980; Silverman, 1992). However, many other terms have been used to describe this form of acquired disfluency, including *late* or *adult onset stuttering, cortical stuttering* (Rosenbek, Messers, Collins, & Wertz, 1978), *organic stuttering* (Van Riper, 1982), and *stuttering associated with acquired neurological disorders* (SAAND) (Helm-Estabrooks, 1999). The variety of terms is a result of the many etiologies and resulting subgroups of individuals who experience forms of acquired fluency problems. These include onset as a result of stroke, head trauma, extrapymadial disease, tumor, dementia, and drug usage (Helm-Estabrooks, Yeo, Geschwind, & Freedman, 1986). Accordingly, neurogenic stuttering does not appear to be associated with a particular site of lesion. One or both hemispheres may be involved, although Rosenbek, Messert, Collins, and Wertz (1978) indicate that the left hemisphere is more likely to be implicated. More recently, De Nil, et al. (2007) describe the onset of neurogenic stuttering associated with many sites for head injury patients, including the internal and external capsule, low frontal white matter tracts, and the caudate and lentiform nuclei; and for stroke patients the thalamus and brain stem, basal ganglia, and cerebellum. The work of Alm (2004) indicates that the basal ganglia circuits are often involved. Certainly the wide variety of sites of anomalous brain function noted by many researchers and authors provides support for a multifocal view of stuttering etiology in which one, and perhaps several, regions of the brain associated with (at the minimum) linguistic and motor planning are involved. It is not surprising that authors have suggested that a more thorough understanding of neurogenic stuttering is likely to inform our understanding about the onset of developmental stuttering (De Nil et al., 2007; Watson & Freeman, 1997).

In some instances, the onset of neurogenic stuttering may be suddenly and unambiguously associated with head trauma, stroke, cryosurgery, drug usage, or anoxia. In other cases, when the speaker's fluency is slowly degraded, as with degenerative disorders, vascular disease, dementia, viral meningitis, or dialysis dementia, the association between neurological damage and fluency is less obvious (Helm, Butler, & Canter, 1980; Helm-Estabrooks, 1986). In other cases, a speaker's fluency may deteriorate as the result of a reoccurring medical condition (Helm-Estabrooks, 1999; De Nil. et al., 2007). In some cases, fluency problems are observed prior to what turns out to be a gradually evolving and yet-to-be-discovered medical condition. Complicating the diagnostic situation still further are other problems, including dysarthria, apraxia, and aphasia, that tend to accompany neurogenic stuttering.

Assessment Procedures

Certainly individuals with neurogenic stuttering tend to have some unique speech and fluency characteristics. However, Van Borsal (1997) cautions that the speaker's clinical symptoms alone do not provide adequate information for distinguishing neurogenic from developmental stuttering. Likewise, De Nil et al. (2007) also comment that generalized criteria do not provide the necessary specificity for individual speakers who have acquired fluency problems as a result particular insults or disease processes. Furthermore, De Nil and colleagues also point out exceptions to some of the fluency characteristics that have been used in the past to identify neurogenic fluency problems.

For example, Canter (1971) and later Helm-Estabrooks (1993) provide a list of six criteria that have traditionally been associated with neurogenic stuttering: (1) fluency breaks are produced on grammatical as well as substantive words. Compared to developmental stutterers, who are more likely to have fluency breaks on content words, neurogenic stutterers are equally likely to stutter on function and content words; (2) the speaker may appear annoyed but does not appear anxious about the stuttering; (3) repetitions, prolongations, and blocks are not restricted to the initial syllables. Unlike developmental stuttering, fluency breaks occur not only on initial sounds and syllables, but also in medial and final positions of words; for example, "gre-e-en" and "sto-o-o-ore;" (4) secondary symptoms such as facial grimacing, eye blinking, and fist clenching are rarely associated with the fluency breaks; (5) fluency does not improve with repeated readings of a passage (the adaptation effect); and (6) the speaker stutters regardless of the nature of the speech task.

De Nil, Jokel and Rochon (2007) suggest that an appreciation of the wide variety of problems that accompany neurogenic stuttering calls for a modification of the traditional diagnositic characteristics recommended by Canter (1971) and Helm-Estabrooks (1993). For example, in spite of the tendency for disfluencies to occur on medial and final positions of words, in their work with six stroke patients, Jokel and De Nil (2003) and Jokel, De Nil, and Sharpe (2007) found that 93–95% of disfluencies occurred in the initial position. The lack of an adaptation effect (a reduction in disfluency with repeated readings of the same passage) has often been offered as diagnostic criteria for neurogenic stuttering. Again, exceptions to this have been noted by Jokel and De Nil (2003) and Jokel et al. (2007) who found as much as a 30% reduction in disfluencies with successive readings for some stroke patients (adaptation was less likely to occur with head injury patients). Clinicians have also been advised that neurogenic stuttering tends to be consistent regardless of such factors as the speaking situation, time pressure, and grammatical complexity (Rao, 1991). Exceptions to this trend have been noted by Abe, Yokoyama, and Yorifuji (1993), who found a greater number of repetitions occurring during spontaneous speech than during reading and, by Jokel et al. (2007), who noted more disfluencies during monologue than in conversation as well as less stuttering with more complex reading material.

Two additional related characteristics have often been attributed to speakers with neurogenic stuttering: a lack of both secondary behaviors and anxiety or emotion associated with the disfluencies. As De Nil et al. (2007) point out, because of the variety and the difficulty in identifying and describing secondary behaviors, relatively little is known about them. Jokel and De Nil (2003) and Jokel et al. (2007) noted the occurrence of eye blinking, facial grimacing, head bending, foot tapping, and limb or head movements associated with occurrences of stuttering. De Nil et al. (2007) point out that Rosenbek et al. (1978) also reported accessory features in half of the patients (n = 7) they studied, particularly in the most severe patients. De Nil et al. (2007) suggest that the more time that elapses between the lesion or disease and the onset of disfluencies and the formal assessment, the more likely speakers are to develop accessory or coping responses. Likewise, it has been suggested that speakers experiencing neurogenic stuttering are likely to indicate annoyance rather than a high level of anxiety about their lack of fluency. It may be, of course, that such individuals have many emotions associated with their fluency problems but lack the ability to fully express themselves about their condition. Furthermore, although speakers may simply be annoyed about their ability to communicate at the outset, their emotions are more likely to become more elaborate after suffering the prolonged effects of disfluency. Jokel and De Nil (2003) and Jokel et al. (2007) found that six speakers with stroke-induced neurogenic stuttering scored an average of 18.3 on the S-24 Communication Attitudes Inventory, a score comparable to the average of 19.22 reported for individuals with developmental stuttering and significantly greater than the S-24 average for fluent speakers (9.42) (Andrews & Cutler, 1974). De Nil reports observing patterns of speaker withdrawal from social and professional situations associated with speech disfluencies. In addition, it has been suggested (Grant, Blousse, Cook, & Newman, 1999) that behavioral and emotional reactions to acquired, neurogenic stuttering are especially likely to occur in cases where a neurological problem triggers preexisting stuttering.

Two characteristics that appear to be uniquely associated with neurogenic stuttering are (1) the relative ineffectiveness of fluency-enhancing techniques that tend to immediately eliminate stuttering for most individuals with developmental stuttering (e.g., choral speaking, rhythmic speech, singing, prolonged speech, whispering, and silent speech) (Andrews et al., 1983; Bloodstein, 1949) (for example, Perkins (1973) noted that of over 100 people who stuttered, the only person who did not show a reduction in stuttering under such conditions was a woman who was later diagnosed as suffering from a neurological disorder); and (2) people with neurogenic stuttering are more likely than those with developmental stuttering to produce disfluencies during the production of automatic speech tasks such as counting, naming days of week, etc. (Helm-Estabrooks, 1993; Helm-Estabrooks, et al., 1986).

Given the multiple etiologies and resulting varieties of neurogenic stuttering, it is clear that the assessment process needs to be both thorough and individualized. De Nil et al. (2007) suggest a battery of assessment procedures (Assessment Battery for Acquired Stuttering in Adults [ABASA], Table 10-3) for obtaining case history, general communication functions (language, speech, and cognition), speech fluency assessments, and speaker self-assessment of attitudes (S-24, LCB).

The guidelines provided by Canter (1971) and Helm-Estabrooks (1993) appear to be useful in identifying the occurrence of neurogenic stuttering. But as we have seen, particularly depending on the nature of the insult to the speaker's neurological system and the duration of the disrupted fluency, there are exceptions to these characteristics. The continuing research with these individuals suggests that there is likely to be individual variability associated with what may be too readily thought of as stereotypical behavioral characteristics for this population. It may be best to consider the following list as characteristics that *may* accompany the various forms of neurogenic stuttering and which can help the clinician to distinguish these individuals from those with developmental stuttering.

Clinical **Decision-Making**

Characteristics that *may* occur for speakers with neurogenic stuttering:

1. No reported history of previous fluency problems.
2. Evidence of sudden or progressive degrading of the speaker's central nervous system (CNS).
3. Fluency-enhancing techniques do not result in significantly improved fluency.
4. Fluency does not improve during automatic speech tasks.
5. There is a tendency for stuttering to occur on medial and final syllables of words.

   Compared to individuals with developmental stuttering, there is less of a tendency for speakers to demonstrate:

6. Improved fluency with repeated readings of a passage (adaptation effect).
7. Variability in fluency across speech tasks or speaking situations.
8. Struggle behavior and secondary behaviors, particularly at the onset of the problem.
9. Emotional reactions associated with their disrupted fluency, particularly at the outset of the problem.

Table 10-3 Assessment Battery for Acquired Stuttering in Adults (ABASA).

A. Case History

    a. Medical history, including neuroimaging data (structural and functional)

    b. Social and occupational history

    c. Personal/family speech and language history and current status

    d. Detailed history and current status of disfluencies (onset and development)

    e. Self-reported awareness of stuttering severity and secondary behaviors

B. Testing of General Functions

    a. Language (BDAE, BNT, PALPA, GORT, TROG, PPVT, PPTT)

    b. Speech: ABA, Motor speech examination

    c. Cognition: MMSE

C. Speech Fluency Assessment

    a. Reading: single words, short sentences, paragraph

    b. Spontaneous speech: monologue, conversation (minimum 200 syllables)

    c. More automatized speech (counting, days, months, singing)

    d. Fluency-enhancing techniques (slowed speech, delayed auditory feedback)

    e. Speech situation checklist

    f. Stuttering severity (SSI)

D. Self-Assessment of Attitudes (S-24, LCB)

BDAE, Boston Diagnostic Aphasia Examination (Goodglass, Kaplan, & Barresi, 2001); *BNT,* Boston Naming Test (Goodglass, et al., 2001); *GORT,* Gray Oral Reading Test (Wiederholt & Bryant, 1992); *LCB,* Locus of Control for Behavior (Craig, Franklin, & Andrews, 1984); *MMSE,* Mini-Mental State Examination (Folstein, Folstein, & McHugh, 1975); *PALPA,* Psycholinguistic Assessments of Language Processing in Aphasia (Kay, Lesser, & Coltheart, 1992); *PPTT,* Pyramids and Palm Trees Test (Howard & Patterson, 1992); *PPVT-III,* Peabody Picture Vocabulary Test (Dunn & Dunn, 1997); S-24 (Andrews & Cutler, 1974); *SSI,* Stuttering Severity Instrument (Riley, 1994); *TROG,* Test for Reception of Grammar (Bishop, 1989).

Source: Conture & Curlee, *Stuttering and Related Disorders of Fluency,* 3rd ed., p. 337, Thieme Medical Publishers, Inc., 2007. Reprinted with permission.

Treatment Procedures

An interesting aspect of treatment for individuals with the various forms of neurogenic stuttering is that not all speakers will require therapy. In some cases, the neurological problem will be transient and as the person recovers over a period of weeks or months, the fluency problem subsides. This is most likely to be the case for stroke patients (Helm-Estabrooks, 1999). For patients with closed head injuries associated with seizure activity, resolution of the seizures may result in improved fluency. Particularly interesting are the reports of clinicians who describe an improvement of fluency in clients with neurogenic stuttering who have suffered further damage to their central nervous system (Helm, Yeo, Geschwind, Froedman, & Wenstein, 1986; Jones, 1966; Manders & Bastijns, 1988; Van Riper, 1982). The additional trauma apparently resulted in further neurological change that facilitated speech fluency.

Because acquired neurological stuttering is far from a unitary disorder, no single therapeutic approach is preferred, and it is not possible to predict a particular speaker's response to intervention. For example, Helm-Estabrooks (1993) has found that Parkinson's patients tend to respond well to a variety of therapeutic approaches, while stroke patients tend to be less responsive. The treatment strategies and associated techniques described in Chapter 8 for speakers with developmental stuttering are routinely used for those with neurogenic stuttering. Clinicians experienced with this population indicate that the behavioral changes and cognitive restructuring promoted in stuttering-modification techniques and fluency-shaping techniques that facilitate easy, slowed, and relaxed, speech production can be successfully employed with these speakers (Helm-Estabrooks, 1999; De Nil, et al., 2007; Market, Montague, Buffalo, & Drummond, 1990; Meyers, Hall, & Aram, 1990; Rousey, Arjunan, & Rousey, 1986). In addition, since word finding is a common problem in neurogenic fluency disorders and may contribute to fluency breaks (Brown & Cullinan, 1981; Meyers, Hall, & Aram, 1990), a slow rate of speech production may also assist the speaker by providing more time for retrieval. Helm-Estabrooks (1986) suggests that for all forms of fluency disorders encountered, pharmacological treatment may be the most beneficial, although she also noted that undesirable side effects are possible (see Chapter 8).

Characteristics of Psychogenic Stuttering

In terms of personality and psychological characteristics, the vast majority of people with fluency problems do not differ from a matched group of normally fluent speakers (Goodstein, 1958; Sheehan, 1958). However, in any randomly selected group of people there will be some individuals with emotional problems. Van Riper (1979) indicates that only a handful of people who come to us with the complaint of stuttering are emotionally ill. To be sure, many of the people we will see are deeply troubled by what they correctly perceive as an extremely frustrating and sometimes devastating problem. For some people, the coping responses are far from normal and may take on the characteristics of extreme anxiety as well as neurotic and compulsive behavior. However, as Van Riper (1982) suggests, these behaviors are best interpreted as a result rather than a cause of stuttering. The behaviors are rarely the symptoms of some deep-seated conflict. Rather, they are learned and in some cases, maladaptive coping responses to the fear and helplessness of stuttering.

On occasion, however, clinicians may encounter people with more pronounced emotional problems resulting in stuttering. Acquired psychogenic stuttering occurs with roughly equal frequency in men and women (Baumgartner & Duffy, 1997). In some instances, the client will have a history of emotional problems and may be currently receiving professional help for his or her condition. Even in the absence of a serious or long-standing emotional problem, some people react strongly to the common stresses of life, and disrupted fluency is a result.

Baumgartner (1999) suggests, for example, that psychopathology is not always present in psychogenic stuttering; the symptoms may be a natural response to either the anticipation or the experience of life events. As one with considerable experience with acquired psychogenic stuttering, Baumgartner disagrees with the ASHA Special Interest Division technical paper (1999), which suggests that the term "psychogenic stuttering" should apply only to individuals who have been diagnosed with a psychopathology. He provides a convincing argument that, at least in many cases, such a diagnosis is not necessary for the speech-language pathologist to determine that a fluency problem is psychogenic in nature. Furthermore, Baumgartner suggests that waiting to begin therapeutic intervention until a formal psychiatric diagnosis is forthcoming negates the valuable information that may be gained through trial therapy.

As with neurogenic stuttering, the onset of disfluent behavior is likely to be relatively sudden, and the person may come to us without any previous history of fluency problems. There may be, however, a history of psychological problems, neurological problems, or both (Baumgartner, 1999). As Aronson (1992) suggests, speech and voice disorders may be caused by distress or "psychologic disequilibrium." Baumgartner and Duffy (1997) found that when a diagnosis of psychopathology does take place, the most common classifications are conversion reaction (Mahr & Leith, 1992), anxiety, and depression. Other possible diagnostic categories are reactive depression, personality disorder, drug dependence, and posttraumatic neurosis, with some individuals being placed into more than one category. For some individuals, there may be an interaction of psychogenic and neurological problems as a result of psychological reactions to a medical condition. As several authors indicate, a person's awareness of a serious neurological disease may quite naturally precipitate a psychological reaction resulting in psychogenic stuttering (Baumgartner & Duffy, 1997; De Nil et al., 2007; Helm-Estabrooks & Hotz, 1998; Van Borsal, 1997).

Assessment Procedures

One of the more striking aspects of this form of disfluency is the stereotypical nature of the fluency breaks. Some people with psychogenic stuttering may give the impression of "holding onto" their stuttering, in the sense that both the frequency and the form show little change. The listener may get the sense that it is as though the speaker has chosen a particular "brand" of stuttering and for a time, at least, that is the way he or she is choosing to speak. In some cases, speakers will stutter on nearly every word, show little adaptation during multiple readings, continue to stutter during fluency-enhancing activities, and produce stuttering-like movements during miming—mouthing words without voicing (Deal, 1982). Another characteristic of both neurogenic and psychogenic stuttering is the lack of an adaptation effect. In fact, if stuttering becomes more severe with successive readings of a passage, it is a strong indicator of psychogenic stuttering (Baumgartner & Duffy, 1997).

Distinguishing between Neurogenic Stuttering and Psychogenic

Distinguishing among possible neurological and psychological etiological factors presents one of the most difficult aspects of assessment for these speakers. In a retrospective study of 69 patients diagnosed at the Mayo Clinic for psychogenic stuttering, 20 patients were found to have confirmed neurologic disease. Baumgartner and Duffy (1997) note the considerable overlap between the characteristics of both etiologies, and the two forms of acquired stuttering cannot be distinguished solely on the nature of the disfluencies (Helm-Estabrooks, 1999; Baumgartner, 1999). One potentially helpful fact is that many more cases of neurogenic stuttering are reported in the literature than psychogenic stuttering (Helm-Estabrooks & Hotz, 1998).

Information obtained in the speaker's case history is particularly important in the assessment of acquired stuttering. Baumgartner (1999) recommends a careful and systematic "psychologic interview" process in order to determine events that may indicate a temporal relationship between the patient's speech problems, evidence of CNS impairment, and possible sources of emotional stress in the person's life. Baumgartner suggests that the clinician look for patterns of unexplained problems and communication difficulties in the near or distant past. In order to achieve this goal, it is critical that the clinician approach this interview by creating a setting that allows the client to describe these events, as well as his or her reaction to them. As Baumgartner describes:

> The skilled interviewer creates an atmosphere that encourages and supports discussions of feelings, fears, and information not previously disclosed (very possibly to anyone). It is not enough to find out what has happened in an individual's life. The truly successful interview explores how people feel about these things, how they have dealt with them, and whether they would "really like" to do something else about them. (p. 272)

If the clinician is able to facilitate such an exchange of information and the speaker is, in fact, experiencing acquired psychogenic stuttering, speech fluency is likely to show an immediate change, either by becoming more or less severe. In some cases, stuttering may disappear (Baumgartner, 1999). This can be taken as a clear diagnostic sign: "Symptom resolution, a marked disclosure of emotionally sensitive information, is powerful evidence in support of psychogenicity and argues strongly against organicity" (Baumgartner, 1999, p. 272). Clearly such an approach lays the groundwork for subsequent treatment and counseling activities.

Baumgartner (1999) also suggests a series of tasks to further define the nature of the problem with these speakers and to rule out the possibility of coexisting neurogenic communication disorders. The quantity and form of the stuttering may have little etiological value, since these may closely parallel those in speakers with developmental stuttering. Although disfluencies are more variable than those of neurogenic speakers, a pattern of worsening of symptoms during the performance of less difficult speaking tasks is a clear sign of psychogenicity. In addition, bizarre movements (e.g., of the head and eyes) that are unrelated to speech production and unusual speech patterns are a sign of psychogenicity.

Considering the suggestions of Baumgartner and Duffy (1997) and Mahr and Leith (1992) for identifying psychogenic stuttering, as well as the research presented in the previous paragraphs, the following is a list of 10 characteristics that may assist the clinician in identifying speakers experiencing this acquired fluency problem. Because of the similarities of psychogenic and neurogenic stuttering, a good first step is to rule out evidence of CNS impairment. As mentioned, it is also useful to consider that there are many more reported instances of neurogenic than psychogenic stuttering.

Treatment Procedures

Because of the relatively small number of speakers with acquired psychogenic stuttering, there are few empirical studies documenting treatment strategies and the nature of recovery for this population, especially over the long term. Roth, Aronson, and Davis (1989) recommend "traditional fluency treatment" in combination with counseling from a psychologist or psychiatrist. According to Roth et al., these patients are receptive to both stuttering- and fluency-modification procedures. These authors stress the importance of encouragement and optimism concerning a successful outcome on the part of the clinician. Psychiatric referral is not typically the treatment of choice (Baumgartner, 1999). However, in cases where the patient continues to be affected by environmental stress or if there is little change in the patient's fluency following several sessions, such referrals are in order.

Clinical **Decision-Making**

Characteristics that may occur for speakers with psychogenic stuttering:

1. Case history information indicates a history of emotional problems such as personality disorder, posttraumatic stress, drug dependence, acute anxiety, or depression. (A diagnosis of psychopathology is not necessary.)

2. The speaker gives the impression of "holding onto" stuttering, and continues to stutter during fluency-enhancing activities, including miming.

3. A rapid improvement in fluency occurs following the disclosure of emotionally sensitive information.

4. The speaker shows a rapid and favorable response to a brief period of trial therapy.

5. The speaker shows a pattern of worsening symptoms during the performance of less difficult speaking tasks.

6. Stuttering becomes more severe with successive readings of a passage.

7. The speaker demonstrates bizarre struggle behaviors and signs of anxiety that are not associated with breaks in fluency.

8. The speaker produces unusual grammatical constructions, e.g. "Me get sick."

9. The speaker shows unusual forms of fluency disruptions such as multiple repetitions of nearly all phonemes with simultaneous head bobbing, facial grimaces, and tremor-like movements.

10. There are intermittent or situation-specific episodes of stuttering.

Baumgartner (1999) indicates that because behaviors vary so much across patients and because even the initial assessment procedures may be highly therapeutic, treatment goals should be open ended. The initial goals of treatment, which can occur during the first (diagnostic) session, are to provide the client with an explanation of the evaluation and the development of an atmosphere whereby "the patient becomes receptive to the idea that these findings are good news and indicate that a total resolution of symptoms is possible" (p. 279). Because many patients with acquired psychogenic stuttering believe that the problem is organic in nature, it is important for the patient to have a positive reaction to the news that no organicity is present and that this an unsurprising result of the evaluation. As Baumgartner explains:

A "cognitive set" must be achieved so that the lack of organicity is perceived in a positive light by the patient, as is the clinician's belief that this is a reasonable, not unexpected finding. If this is not achieved, a patient may have received indirectly the message that the clinician is surprised or that the findings are somehow mysterious. Worse yet would be the message that a lack of organicity indicates that there is not a real problem. In my opinion, a prerequisite for patients achieving such a cognitive set is the clinician's belief that psychogenicity is a valid concept and that findings pointing to such a diagnosis are reasonable and not uncommon. (1999, p. 279)

Treatment should proceed with the same confidence on the part of the clinician about the possibility of achieving normally fluent speech. According to Baumgartner (1999), it is not unusual to achieve much improved fluency during the first treatment session. If improvement occurs the patient should be informed that this is a positive sign. On those occasions when this is not the case, the clinician can focus on helping the speaker to reduce struggle behavior associated with abnormal movements that are unrelated to speech production (e.g., movements of the limbs or torso or bizarre movements of the eyes) and to alter such aberrant behaviors as speaking only when lying down or when grasping an object. Baumgartner (1999) recommends that it is often helpful to focus treatment activities on the area of the body that is associated with excessive effort or tension. He has found that touching or manipulating of these areas by the clinician is particularly effective in reducing musculoskeletal tension (see Baumgartner [1999, 284–285] for a description of this technique).

Baumgartner stresses that it is important not to "rush" the speaker with these therapeutic activities, but rather to emphasize the fact that the speaker's improving fluency represents a good prognosis. He argues that it is more essential to change the patient's "belief system" than to elicit fluent speech or practice speech-related movements. As these measures are successful, the clinician can then show the speaker how to expand his or her fluency. In contrast to the prognosis for persons with acquired neurogenic stuttering, individuals with acquired psychogenic stuttering are more likely to demonstrate a rapid achievement of fluency. For example, Baumgartner and Duffy (1997) reported that more than 50% of their patients improved to normal or near normal fluency following one or two sessions of symptomatic treatment.

The Possibility of Malingering

There exists another—perhaps the least likely—possibility for explaining the sudden onset of stuttering in adults. It may be that the speaker is malingering in an effort to gain some advantage by posing as a person who stutters. Based on diagnostic criteria described by Morrison (1995), Seery (2005) describes two levels of malingering. Pure malingering involves intentional faking all of the symptoms of a physical or mental disorder. Partial malingering is the exaggeration of existing symptoms. Both forms of malingering are motivated by the intention of achieving some form of gain or advantage (e.g., money or avoidance of responsibility). Seery notes cases of malingered stuttering found in the literature (Bloodstein, 1988; Culatta & Goldberg, 1995; Shapiro, 1999) that involved partial malingering, the exaggeration of true stuttering.

The few documented instances of this behavior are forensic cases whereby individuals are attempting to demonstrate their innocence (Bloodstein, 1988; Seery, 2005; Shirkey, 1987). Seery provides an especially interesting example of a man accused of armed robbery. Part of his attorney's defense was that his client's severe stuttering would have prevented his complete fluency when uttering a statement made during the robbery. When asked to consult on the case Seery adapted procedures by Resnick (1993) for detecting malingering for psychosis. Her assessment protocol included elements of speech sampling under multiple speaking conditions, a thorough examination of case history information, and indirect tests of malingering. Although some indicators suggested developmental, psychogenic, and neurological stuttering, Seery (2005) found the strongest evidence supporting partial malingering. Specifically, she found little variability from a consistently high frequency of stuttering across speaking tasks, little or no decrease in stuttering frequency with multiple readings, a lack of consistency of stuttering on specific words during multiple readings, direct and relaxed eye contact with the examiner during even the most severe stuttering events, a lack of secondary or struggle behavior during stuttering events, stuttering on the last rather than the first words of a statement, and reports of "islands of fluency" by witnesses in spite of the speaker's report of consistent stuttering during all communication situations. Perhaps most revealing was the speaker's maintenance of consistently severe stuttering during conditions that often elicit enhanced fluency (automatic speech tasks, finger tapping while talking, prolonged speech, as well as both lipped and unison speech. It was apparent that this speaker was able to make use of his history of developmental stuttering in order to call attention to and magnify his stuttering.

Clinical Insight

Several years ago we had the opportunity to interview a woman in her early thirties who complained of a sudden onset of severe stuttering. Approximately three weeks prior to our assessment, she had been raped. One week following the attack, she lost her ability to speak, and when she began speaking again, approximately three days later, she demonstrated well-developed stuttering. She reported no personal or family history of stuttering. At the time of the assessment interview, she was stuttering on nearly every word and showed a high level of anxiety. The frequency of her fluency breaks was uniform throughout the interview and consisted almost entirely of tense prolongations of whole words. We were unable to elicit any periods of fluent speech through using a variety of fluency-enhancing activities.

(continues)

We also had the opportunity to interview a 41-year-old man who complained of a sudden onset of stuttering. As was the case with the woman described earlier, this man also had no previous history of fluency disorders. In this instance, however, there appeared to be no single traumatic event preceding the onset of his disrupted fluency. During the evaluation and for many years following this interview I had conceived of this speaker as an example of psychogenic stuttering, but now believe there was a good chance that he was malingering. He had been receiving ongoing inpatient treatment at a local Veterans Administration hospital for an emotional disorder for several years. We were also unable to get this man to produce fluent speech using a variety of fluency-enhancing activities. The frequency of his stuttering was consistent throughout the entire two-hour assessment interview. His fluency breaks consisted of relatively easy one- and two-unit repetitions produced at the same rate as the rest of his speech, rather than at a relatively more rapid pace characteristic of stuttering. Although he explained that he was very concerned about his fluency problem, he showed no struggle or tension during his fluency breaks, nor did he report any avoidances or fear associated with this problem. Perhaps the most interesting aspect of his stuttering was the way he watched listeners as he stuttered. He constantly maintained eye contact, and while we cannot say for sure that he "enjoyed" watching his listeners for their reactions, he clearly did not appear embarrassed or upset by his disfluencies. He appeared to remain detached from his stuttering, sometimes smiling as he both stuttered and closely watched the interviewer. As with the woman, it was apparent to us that stuttering was not his most important problem—a characteristic response that the clinician is likely to have when interviewing such clients. However, while the woman's speech seemed to indicate a profound emotional reaction to a specific and documented trauma, this man's speech appeared to be contrived and manipulative.

Conclusion

The increasing interest in the less common forms of disrupted fluency has resulted in an appreciation of the complexities as well as the possible etiological and epidemiological characteristics of these problems. Of these less typical fluency problems, cluttering is by far the most prevalent either in a pure form or, more frequently, co-occurring with stuttering. The combination of stuttering and cluttering will dramatically influence the plan of treatment, possibly making treatment more complex, in large part because of speakers' difficulty in self-monitoring the rate and quality of their speech. While individuals who stutter occasionally have problems formulating language and coordinating speech production, these are especially important issues for those who clutter. Fortunately, many of the fluency- and stuttering-modification techniques employed with individuals who stutter are helpful for enhancing the fluent speech of those who clutter. However, a multifaceted approach is necessary that also includes activities that assist the individual to develop self-monitoring, linguistic, rate-control, and motor skills.

Even less common are those persons who, often in the middle years of adulthood, experience the onset of an acquired fluency problem in the form of neurogenic or psychogenic stuttering. It can be difficult to distinguish these two forms of acquired stuttering from one another, for while there are many important behavioral and cognitive-affective differences there is also considerable overlap, including the possibility of coexisting neurological damage. Both assessment and treatment for acquired fluency disorders will depend on the nature and extent of the insult to the person's neurological system. It is not possible to distinguish forms of neurogenic stuttering based solely on the speaker's clinical symptoms. The greater occurrence of neurogenic stuttering than psychogenic stuttering is of some help in differentiating between the two forms of acquired stuttering.

Although a diagnosis of a psychopathology may not be necessary for individuals with psychogenic stuttering, case history information is likely to provide important information for an accurate diagnosis. The unique speech and behavioral characteristics of individuals presenting with what may be psychogenic stuttering during assessment procedures, as well as the often positive response to intervention, provide key indicators for making an appropriate diagnosis. In some cases the initial assessment and trial therapy procedures may be therapeutic. Recommended therapeutic strategies emphasize enhancing the speaker's belief that improved fluency is highly likely rather than improving the individual's fluency. In rare instances of adult onset of stuttering—sometimes having to do with forensic matters—it may also be necessary to consider the possibility of malingering.

Each of these problems that humans may confront as they attempt to communicate fluently present clinicians with unique challenges. They may even provide the exciting opportunity to operate for a time "on the edge of our incompetence."

Topics for Discussion

1. In what ways would your diagnostic and treatment choices differ for speakers who present with characteristics of stuttering versus speakers with both stuttering and cluttering?

2. What are the core and accessory characteristics of cluttering as described by St. Louis, et al. (2007)? How does this view of cluttering differ from that of Daly and colleagues?

3. What differences may be noted in the disfluencies of speakers with developmental stuttering, speakers who clutter, and speakers with acquired neurogenic stuttering?

4. According to St. Louis and colleagues, what are the primary goals of treatment for cluttering?

5. What are the speech, fluency, linguistic, and emotional characteristics of individuals presenting with neurogenic stuttering?

6. Why is it appropriate to consider a variety of treatment options for speakers with neurogenic stuttering?

7. What activities would you ask a speaker to carry out in order to propose a diagnoses of psychogenic stuttering?

8. What are the speech, fluency, linguistic, and emotional characteristics of psychogenic stuttering?

9. What would you say are the primary considerations when developing a therapeutic strategy for a speaker with psychogenic stuttering?

10. Differentiate between pure and partial malingering. What activities would you consider in order to identify the possibility of malingering?

Recommended Readings

Baumgartner, J. M. (1999). Acquired Psychogenic Stuttering. In R. Curlee (Ed.), *Stuttering and Related Disorders of Fluency* (2nd Edition, pp. 269–288). New York: Thieme Medical Publishers, Inc.

Daly, D. A. (1996). *The Source for Stuttering and Cluttering*, East Moline, IL: LinguiSystems, Inc.

De Nil., L. F., Jokel, R., & Rochon, E. (2007) Etiology symptomatology, and treatment of neurogenic stuttering. In E. Conture & R. Curlee (Eds.), *Stuttering and Related Disorders of Fluency*, (3rd Edition pp. 326–343). New York: Thieme Medical Publishers, Inc.

Seery, C. H., (2005). Differential diagnosis of stuttering for forensic purposes. *American Journal of Speech-Language Pathology, 14,* 284–297.

St. Louis, K. O., Myers, F. L., Bakker, K., & Raphael, L. J. (2007). Understanding and treating cluttering, In E. Conture & R. Curlee (Eds.), *Stuttering and Related Disorders of Fluency.* (3rd Edition, pp. 297–325). New York: Thieme Medical Publishers, Inc.

CHAPTER 11

Indicators of Successful Change During Treatment

We cannot reject plausible forces because we do not see them directly. Most of science relies on ingenious and rigorous inference, not passive observations alone (p. 167).

Steven J. Gould (1995). Dinosaur in a Haystack.
New York: Crown Trade Paperbacks.

There are, of course, observable aspects of this disorder, but do we want to say that efficacious therapies are those that deal only with the observable aspects? If anything, it should be the other way around. . . . The unobservable events seem more important than the observable ones.

C. Woodruff Starkweather (1999). The effectiveness of
stuttering therapy: An issue for science?
Chapter 16 (231–244) in N. B. Ratner and E. C. Healey (Eds.),
Stuttering research and practice: Bridging the gap.
Mahwah, NJ: Lawrence Erlbaum.

Chapter Objectives

Traditionally successful therapeutic change has most often been informed by the clinician's observation and interpretation of data which appear to indicate the speaker's progress. More recently there is growing appreciation of the importance of locating these data in the context of the unique lived experience of the speaker, giving value to the specific knowledge of the individual experiencing the phenomenon. From the outset of therapy, there will be many opportunities for speakers to inform the clinician about the goals that are important to them in their journey from being dominated by stuttering to the achievement of successful management. This philosophical position is consistent with recommendations by clinicians to focus on individual, rather than group, data as a means for assessing treatment efficacy. For example, Starkweather (1999) and Quesal (1989) suggested that a primary reason for our lack of success in understanding and combating relapse following initially successful therapy is a result of a tendency to study the commonalities of group studies rather than considering patterns of individual change. Furthermore, it is apparent that many clinicians and clients understand the nature of successful therapy in very different ways (Bothe, 2004; Finn, 2003; Krauss-Lehrman & Reeves, 1988; Yaruss & Quesal, 2002; Reeves, 2006; St. Louis, 2006; Yaruss, Quesal, & Murphy, 2002). For example Krauss-Lehrman and Reeves (1988) found that 75% of National Stuttering Association members surveyed felt that their therapy had been mildly or very successful even though many continued to display varying degrees of stuttering. It is unlikely that some individuals who describe a successful therapy experience or self-report recovery from stuttering would meet the threshold of fluency that some professional clinicians or researchers would judge as acceptable (see Reeves, 2006). Nonetheless, many of these former clients indicate a clear sense of accomplishment and genuinely feel that their lives are unrestricted by the occasional occurrence (or even the possibility) of stuttering. It seems clear that clinicians and researchers need to be asking individuals who have undergone treatment what they consider to be a successful therapeutic outcome. It is also clear that their answers should influence our views of evidenced-based treatment.

Therapeutic progress goes far beyond the changes that take place during the time the client is immersed in formal treatment. Formal treatment may be thought of as that time when the client is receiving and paying for the services of a professional clinician. It is important, however, to view the speaker's long-term progress as a continuum of both formal and informal treatment. As discussed in the next chapter, informal treatment may be regarded as the much longer time following formal treatment during which the client is fully independent of the clinician. In many important ways this latter stage of treatment is the most critical part of the process and provides the true measure of treatment efficacy. To the extent that the speaker is able to make consistent use of the strategies and techniques acquired during formal treatment, that treatment can be regarded as a success. Will the person take the time to expand his or her ability to monitor and modify his or her fluency in an increasing variety of challenging communication situations? Will the person be able to gather the energy necessary to cultivate the cognitive and affective changes necessary to reduce the influence of stuttering? Or will relapse—to a greater or lesser degree—dictate additional periods of formal intervention?

The Multidimensional Nature of Therapeutic Change

Van Riper (1973, pp. 178–199) provides a comprehensive overview of ways to consider progress during treatment. His fundamental point is that any view of progress should be comprehensive and consider multiple factors. That is, several overt or surface characteristics, as well as many of the more subtle, intrinsic features of the problem, must be taken into account. Otherwise, success will be either overstated or unrecognized. As Sheehan (1980) points out, the more trivial the criteria for improvement, the greater the likelihood of success.

The changes in the surface behavior of the client often occur relatively early in the treatment process. On the other hand, cognitive changes are reflected in the quality of the client's self-management and patterns of decision making, aspects of change that generally take longer (Emerick, 1988; Manning, 1991). Some authors have provided reports suggesting what seems intuitively correct—that desired changes in the surface behaviors will be more likely to be permanent if changes in the cognitive features also occur (Emerick, 1988; Guitar, 1976; Guitar & Bass, 1978; Maxwell, 1982).

In some cases, the speaker actively begins to make important changes prior to the initiation of formal treatment (Andrews & Harvey, 1981; Bordeau & Jeffrey, 1973; Gregory, 1972; Ingham, Andrews, & Winkler, 1972; Ost, Gotestam, & Melin, 1976; Peins, McGough & Lee, 1972; Webster, 1979). For example, Andrews and Harvey (1981) obtained data on 132 adults who were placed on a list awaiting treatment. A variety of measures were taken approximately eight months prior to treatment and again immediately before treatment. The speakers showed significant decreases in the percentage of syllables stuttered (18.2% to 14.4%) and a significant increase in the rate of speech in syllables per minute (91.5 to 129.8), changes that became evident after the first three months on the waiting list. No significant changes, as measured by the S-24 scale (Andrews & Cutler, 1974), were found in the speakers' attitude about speech communication. Furthermore, no significant change was found in two of the three measures (perceived avoidance and severity of stuttering) indicated by the Stutterers Self Rating of Reactions to Speaking Situations (Johnson, Darley, & Spriesterbach, 1963). If, as suggested in Chapter 4, adults are apt to seek treatment when their problem is the greatest, this regression toward the mean is not surprising. Furthermore, the process of seeking professional help and asking for assistance indicates that an individual is in the preparation stage of change (see Chapter 6). Even though formal intervention has not yet taken place, the speaker has demonstrated some degree of assertiveness, and being included on a waiting list provides a measure of support.

Certainly, clinicians will interpret progress differently, depending on the overall treatment strategy and the associated techniques. An indicator of progress for a speaker taking part in a treatment program emphasizing fluency enhancement will not necessarily be thought of as progress for another client who is taking part in a program where stuttering modification is the major goal. Conture and Guitar (1993) suggested that treatment can be considered successful if a child begins to communicate easily whenever and to whomever he or she chooses. This also seems to be a reasonable approach to take with adults.

The Variability of Change

Just as speech fluency itself can be highly variable, change as a result of treatment is far from linear. As our comments in earlier chapters on the nature of the counseling and the therapeutic processes suggest, although successful change is apt to be the result of good and timely treatment, we cannot force the process and "fix" the problem in every instance. The pace and direction of change is often dictated by the speaker. In addition, at different times and for different people, fluctuations in some features of stuttering are better indicators of change than others. For example, while treatment may focus on decreasing stuttering and avoidance behavior, it is often the case (particularly early in treatment) that decreased avoidance results in greater stuttering. Depending on the context, increased stuttering may be desirable as the speaker becomes more assertive about communicating and entering into more challenging speaking situations. The nature and rate of change are influenced not only by the primary focus of a particular treatment strategy but also by many other factors, including the treatment schedule, the quality of the therapeutic alliance, the agentic nature of the speaker, and the support available to the speaker from family and friends.

On occasion, clients as well as clinicians are confused by information on the internet and even in professional journals describing impressive levels of success for individuals undergoing treatment or using unique treatment techniques or devices. Often, closer examination of these reports indicates a variety of factors accounting for "success," such as a highly restrictive selection process for those enrolled in treatment (e.g., the only individuals who took part in treatment were highly motivated, could afford the time and expense of treatment, were responsive to the diagnostic tasks, and had few or no concomitant learning or communication problems). In addition, it is not unusual for individuals who decline or drop out of a treatment protocol to be excluded from the experimental cohort, resulting in an inflated sense of treatment effectiveness. It may also be that the criteria for success include only an overt measure of the percentage of syllables stuttered within the clinic environment.

As we have described in earlier chapters, children, especially those of preschool age, typically enjoy good success rates as a result of treatment (again, partly because some of them would have recovered anyway). For adolescent and adult speakers, however, regardless of the particular treatment strategy, clinicians who have studied these populations seem to accept what could be called the "one-third rule." That is, regardless of the overall treatment strategy, and everything else being equal in terms of client motivation and intelligence, clinician experience, and the timing of intervention, approximately one-third of clients will make good progress; one-third, moderate progress; and one-third (often because they prematurely drop out of treatment) little or no progress.

Of those speakers who make good progress, there are some that do extremely well and conclude formal treatment exhibiting little or no stuttering behavior. Some also begin to demonstrate cognitive changes suggesting a reinterpretation of their situation that result in a greatly improved quality of life. Should these speakers experience a break in their fluency, they are unlikely to panic. They are able to analyze what it is they are doing and employ fluency or stuttering modification techniques. They are gradually more assertive and able to assess the circumstances and adjust to the situation in an ever-widening array of communication situations. Other clients, while not showing such marked change, make good progress. As they move away from the security and support provided by the clinic environment, the quantity and quality of their fluency may regress to a degree. Still, they are able to maintain many of their new coping responses and stutter with considerably less frequency and struggle. The fact that they are a person who stutters incrementally plays a smaller role in their lives. They learn to avoid less and are progressively less likely to be at the mercy of a possible stuttering event.

Of course, there is the perplexing final third of all clients, those who make little progress or fail to maintain the gains they achieve within the supportive therapy environment. Every clinician has seen these people. They range from people who stutter in extremely overt to extremely covert ways—although the latter are unlikely to seek our help to begin with. Our chance to interact with these people may be fleeting, and we are able to have contact with them only during an initial diagnostic meeting or perhaps one or two treatment sessions. As we help them approach and begin to unpack their situation, they begin to realize the full nature of their stuttering and the importance of their role in the change process. Their motivation quickly fades, attendance becomes inconsistent, and eventually ceases. When we suspect that we are with people who will respond in this manner it would seem that we should attempt to do what we can for them while we have the chance. It may well be our only opportunity to provide them with encouragement and hope by showing them a few techniques that will provide them with immediate, if temporary, fluency. We can provide them with sources of information about support groups and useful websites so that they might acquire greater understanding and some new insights, as well as the knowledge that they are not alone, there are helpful support groups out there, and that when they are ready good help is available. In some cases, we are able to stay in contact with these people for a few sessions, long enough to facilitate some positive changes. Nevertheless, often for reasons unknown to us, they eventually fail to show up for their sessions. It may be that they found our information and suggestions helpful and they feel that they have made enough progress for now. They may feel that the cost of additional change, at least at this point, is not worth the time and effort. Or maybe the timing and the quality of the therapeutic alliance were not satisfactory.

Several clinical investigations support the notion of the one-third rule. In a review of 13 clinicians and their associates, Martin (1981) determined that one-third of the clients achieved and maintained satisfactory fluency, one-third achieved fluency during therapy but regressed over time, and one-third either failed to complete treatment programs or were unavailable for follow-up assessment. Martin stressed that a major problem preventing a complete interpretation of the data was the fact that many clients left treatment prior to completion of the therapy program. Prins (1970) found comparable results, noting that 67% of 94 male clients taking part in an intensive residential program completed questionnaires indicating "much or complete" improvement. Interestingly, 65% of the subjects indicated that little or no post-treatment regression had occurred in terms of morale. In addition, Prins noted that once they occurred, interpersonal changes were more durable than the level of fluency or decreased avoidance of words. Even speakers who are fortunate enough to take part in an intensive, comprehensive and elaborately constructed treatment program with repeatedly documented success, such as the ISTAR Comprehensive Stuttering Program[1] (Boberg & Kully, 1985), are not always able to maintain behavioral and cognitive changes following treatment. Langevin et al. (2006) found that as many as 28% of such individuals are unable to maintain clinically meaningful speech gains, results that were comparable to earlier investigations of the ISTAR program (Boberg & Kully, 1994; Franken et al., 1997).

Chronic Stuttering

There is one other distinct category of clients that can be included in a discussion of therapeutic progress. These people would most likely fall into the second or third of the three groups discussed in the previous section. Cooper (1986a, 1987) argues that there is a significant group of individuals for whom fluent speech is an unrealistic goal. Any clinician who has worked for several years in the area of fluency disorders will recognize their patterns of behavior. Cooper describes this group as manifesting *chronic perseverative stuttering* (CPS). These speakers are adolescents or adults who have stuttered for several (at least 10) years.

---

[1]For a detailed description of the ISTAR Comprehensive Stuttering Program see Kully et al. (2007).

Cooper indicates that these clients typically respond to treatment with increased fluency, only to experience profound levels of relapse shortly after completing formal treatment. Their predominant self-perception and core constructs (see Chapter 6) are those of a person who stutters. They demonstrate some degree of obsessive striving for completely fluent speech as well as a deep fear of fluency loss, even though such loss may occur infrequently.

Cooper suggests that if clinicians are unwilling to recognize that fluent speech is not a realistic possibility for these people, they are likely to create and perpetuate unwarranted feelings of guilt on behalf of their clients. He has found that an acknowledgement of this pattern of stuttering by clinicians results in a profound relief for clients who see themselves as chronic stutterers. Whether this view would predispose a client to failure is debatable. It may be that accepting the fact that some people who stutter will always have a chronic problem is simply being realistic. Still, it is important to point out that although these speakers may always have a degree of obvious stuttering present in their speech, they may be able to alter their stuttering to the degree that they can communicate more effectively and improve the quality of their life. These speakers may also be ideal candidates for fluency-enhancing devices to supplement more traditional treatment.

Speaker and Clinician Judgments of Change

Determining progress during and following treatment is most often accomplished by client observation in a variety of settings and by administering paper-and-pencil measures of change. In most cases these are the same measures used during the diagnostic session or at the outset of treatment (see Chapter 4). Comparison of current results with baseline measures obtained prior to or at the outset of treatment can, of course, be used to indicate progress. The clinician can determine what measures are most appropriate according to such factors as the speaker's age and his or her social, educational, and career goals.

As the period of formal treatment comes to a conclusion, it becomes increasingly important to determine the client's performance and response in speaking situations beyond the treatment environment. Some assessment measures, although useful for obtaining initial diagnostic information, are specifically devised to determine progress during and following treatment. That is, they are designed to assess the speaker's behavioral and cognitive characteristics in daily situations. As with diagnostic procedures, there are a wide variety of protocols for determining progress and selecting criteria for termination from formal treatment. In Chapter 4, we presented several diagnostic measures that have been used to determine change as a function of treatment. The following section provides some examples of such research.

The LCB

Craig, Franklin, and Andrews (1984) administered the LCB scale to a group of 45 adults who stuttered and who received treatment in the fluency-modification program at the Prince Henry Hospital in Australia. Stuttering subjects averaged scores of 32.0, while a nonstuttering control group averaged 27.0, a difference that was statistically significant. (Recall from Chapter 4 that higher scores indicate greater externality and lower scores indicate greater internality.) Following treatment, 32 of the subjects maintained fluency levels 10 months post-treatment, and 13 subjects showed relapse (more than 2% syllables stuttered). Twenty-eight of the 32 subjects who maintained fluency also showed increased internality on the LCB scale during treatment. Of the 13 subjects who relapsed, 11 either had no change in LCB scores or increased their scores (greater externality) during the three-week program. These results were replicated by Craig and Andrews (1985). Madison, Budd, and Itzkowitz (1986) used the locus of control (LOC) with children 7 to 16 years old and found that those subjects who had a more internal locus of control prior to treatment tended to achieve more fluent speech during treatment. They did not, however, find a significant relationship between pre-treatment LOC values and fluency levels at two follow-up measures taken two and six months post-treatment.

De Nil and Kroll (1995) found less encouraging results for the ability of the LCB to predict long-term change. These authors studied 21 adult subjects who had been enrolled in a three-week Precision Fluency Shaping Program (PFSP) designed by Webster (1975). While two-year follow-up measures with 13 participants indicated that the fluency gains achieved during treatment were maintained by most clients, no predictive relationship was found between LCB scores and the client's percentage of words stuttered. There was a significant decrease in LCB scores from pre- to post-treatment, indicating increased internality. The results did not support previously reported findings that the amount of change in locus of control toward more internality during treatment predicted success two years after treatment.

De Nil and Kroll's (1995) results supported the findings of Andrews and Craig (1988), that total LCB scores alone were of limited help in predicting treatment outcome. Moreover, as pointed out by De Nil and Kroll as well as Ladouceur, Caron, and Caron (1989), the predictive value of locus of control is likely to be significantly affected by the focus of the treatment program. If the program includes techniques designed to alter the speaker's longstanding and powerless response to stuttering (e.g., desensitization, acceptance, decreased avoidance/increased risk taking), LCB scores are more likely to change in the direction of internality. In fact, such changes can occur regardless of the individual's fluency level. In addition, intensive but relatively brief (two- or three-week) treatment programs may not allow adequate time (particularly for some speakers) for cognitive changes to occur and are therefore are not reflected in LCB scores.

The SESAS

Blood (1995) noted a clear improvement in SESAS scores during and following a successful cognitive-behavioral treatment program for three high school clients. Treatment consisted of 25 hours of intensive work on changing speech (a modified version of the Shames and Florance [1980] fluency-shaping program), 50 hours of relapse prevention, and two follow-up phases (6-months and 12-months post-treatment). All three clients showed gradual improvements in overall (Approach plus Performance) scores, which averaged 56.3% Performance (baseline), 77.6% (post-treatment change), 87.3% (post-relapse management), 89.7% (6-month follow-up), and 86.7% (12-month follow-up).

Hillis (1993) pointed out that the pragmatic nature of the SESAS Approach scale may be interpreted as an indication of the scale's content validity. In addition, the construct validity of the SESAS Approach scale is supported by a 28-point difference (effect size of 3.50 nonstuttering standard deviations; $p < .05$) found on the 100-point SESAS Approach between 20 subjects who stuttered and the 20 who did not. The construct validity of the SESAS Performance scale is supported by a 42-point difference between means on the 100-point scale between the 20 subjects who stuttered and the 20 who did not (effect size of 11 nonstuttering standard deviations, $p < .05$).

In order to decrease the uncontrolled variance resulting from the different levels of fluency selected by clients, Hillis (1993) modified the instructions for the Performance section of the SESAS. Rather than using the original (Ornstein & Manning, 1985) instructions that had the client determine a "level of fluency" based on his or her stage of treatment when scoring this section, Hillis asked the client to define fluent speech as "speech [that] would be so fluent in a given situation that, in the client's opinion, a listener would not recognize that the client had a history of stuttering" (1993, p. 28).

Hillis (1993) also provided data on a variety of measures, including the SESAS for an adult male stuttering client (see Figure 11-1). Despite two relapses during which the client's pauses per minute and stuttered syllables per minute increased (to less than pretreatment levels), there was continued progress in that the client was judged by himself, the clinician, and an independent observer to be speaking in a natural and fluent manner. Because this was not the case in speaking situations outside the clinic, this fluency was termed "clinical fluency." At the end of treatment the client was maintaining a high level of fluency, both in the treatment environment and in selected beyond-treatment situations. Nevertheless, Hillis points out that the SESAS Approach score remained less than 70 and SESAS Performance score less than 80 at the end of treatment—less than the scores of typically fluent speakers of 94 and 96, respectively. Hillis notes that even successfully treated clients rarely score much above 80 on the modified SESAS Performance scale. This is still within the range of normal speakers reported by Ornstein and Manning (1985) of 74–100,

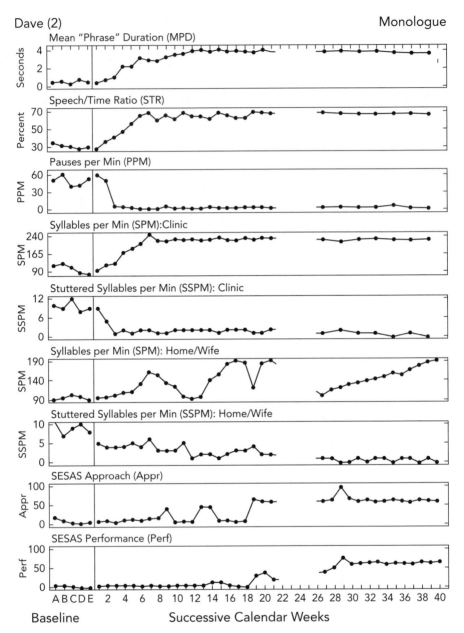

Figure 11-1 Baseline and treatment effects for an adult man on nine measurement parameters across a baseline period and 45 calendar weeks of treatment. (PPM—Pauses per Minute, MPD—Mean Phrase Duration in Seconds, STR—Speech-Time Ratio, SPM—Syllables per Minute, SSPM—Stuttered Syllables per Minute, APPR-SESAS Approach, PERF-SESAS Performance). From Hillis, J.W. (1993). Ongoing assessment in the management of stuttering: A clinical perspective. *American Journal of Speech-Language Pathology, 2 (1)*, 24–37. Reprinted with permission.

but well less than one standard deviation (8.0) of 86.2. Thus it is likely that clients can demonstrate high levels of fluent behavior but nevertheless be lagging behind in terms of cognitive change (SESAS Approach) and speech performance in extra-treatment performance (SESAS Performance).

The following figures (11-2, 11-3, and 11-4) indicate the changes for an adult female (SSI score of very severe) over a period of six years for the 17-item Locus of Control of Behavior Scale (Figure 11-2), and Approach (Figure 11-3) and Performance (Figure 11-4) portions of the Self-Efficacy Scale for Adult Stutterers (SESAS). This person was seen once a week for both individual and group therapy. Figure 11-2 indicates extremely high LCB scores at the outset of treatment (the highest we have ever recorded) with scores progressively decreasing (indicating the desired greater internality). With absences from treatment, scores would often increase in the direction of greater externality. After some two years of treatment, scores began to reach the range expected for fluent speakers.

Figure 11-3 indicates gradually increasing SESAS-Approach scores, and Figure 11-4 shows SESAS-Performance scores lagging behind, as noted by Hillis (1993). It took some five years for this speaker with very severe stuttering to begin to achieve a level of fluency where she believed listeners would not be aware that she had a history of stuttering. Near the end of the fifth year of treatment, periods of spontaneous and natural fluency began to be observed.

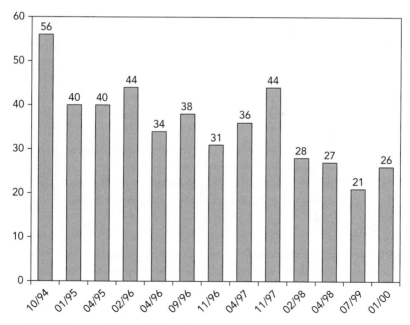

Figure 11-2   Locus of Control of Behavior (LCB) scores for an adult female with severe stuttering over six years of treatment.

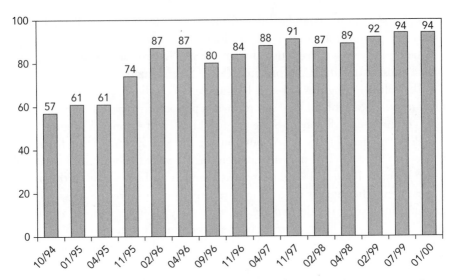

Figure 11-3   Approach scores for the Self-Efficacy Scale for Adult Stutterers for an adult female with severe stuttering over six years of treatment.

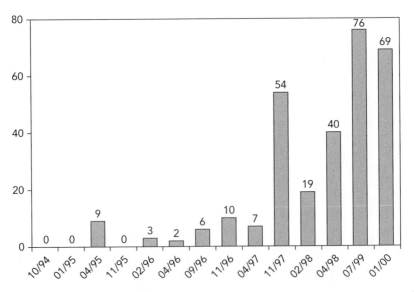

Figure 11-4   Performance scores for the Self-Efficacy Scale for Adult Stutterers for an adult female with severe stuttering over six years of treatment.

The S-24

Guitar and Bass (1978) studied 20 adults who underwent a three-week intensive fluency-shaping program. The study has been frequently cited for two reasons: (1) it provided support for the idea that the failure to change communication attitudes (as measured by the S-24) may be predictive of relapse within 12 to 18 months, and (2) it questioned the desirability of an entirely operant view of therapy (a popular approach at the time). Young (1981) used a combination of regression analysis and causal modeling to reconsider the results of the Guitar and Bass study. He found that pretreatment S-24 scores were unrelated to either pre-or post-treatment %SS or to post-treatment S-24 scores. Although the causal modeling technique did indicate that post-treatment S-24 scores were moderately predictive of post-treatment %SS, Young questioned how much communication attitudes might change during a three-week treatment program that was not intended to focus on attitude change. He concluded that to the degree that the S-24 is capable of measuring such attitudes, the results of Guitar and Bass did support the notion that treatment programs (including behavior modification) should consider such aspects of change. Finally, the results of a study by Andrews and Craig (1988) also found a relationship between attitude change as indicated by the S-24 and long-term success.

A long-term evaluation of the ISTAR Stuttering Program conducted by Langevin et al. (2006) demonstrated a successful outcome for client groups both from the Netherlands (N = 25) and Canada (N = 16). Follow-up two years after formal treatment indicated that participants maintained significant reductions in their frequency of stuttering as well as improvement in their cognitive adjustments. Cognitive and attitude changes were determined by the S-24, the SESAS Approach Scale, and the PSI (see Chapter 4). Comparisons of pre-therapy and two-year follow-up scores for these measures were statistically significant for both client groups. Participants were divided into groups of "maintainers" and "non-maintainers" based on pre- and post-treatment percent syllables stuttered (%SS). In order to be classified as maintainers, individuals had to achieve *follow-up* fluency levels that were at least 50% higher than pre-treatment levels *and* maintain a %SS that was equal to or less than their post-treatment %SS plus 3% (speakers were allowed up to 3% regression during follow-up relative to post-treatment). The authors suggest this as a more clinically meaningful approach than using a standard threshold of 2–4 %SS, and it also takes into account low pretreatment levels of stuttering as well as the assumption that treatment is unlikely to eliminate all stuttering. Those participants who were classified as maintainers improved 36.44% and 28.1% on the S-24 and SESAS, while participants classified as non-maintainers showed improvements of 23.81% and 17.93% for the S-24 and SESAS, respectively. Effect sizes (Cohen's kappa) for each of these measures were much larger than is typically found in the behavioral sciences.

Paper-and-pencil measures provide helpful information for the clinician's decision making during treatment, but these measures are not without their problems. Some can be tedious to complete, and there tend to be sequencing effects associated with multiple administrations of the measures. Clients may tire of completing the forms; may fail to take the task seriously; and may become "test wise" about the intent of the measure, filling it out the way they believe they "should" respond rather than indicating what they truly think or feel.

Listening to the Client

When considering the nature of therapeutic change, experienced clinicians rely on a variety of data obtained during treatment as well as current findings gleaned from both descriptive and experimental research. Sometimes the patterns in the data are clear and sometimes they are not. It is helpful to keep in mind that even the best and most comprehensive of assessment measures are the creation of the researcher and clinician. That is, although these measures usually provide ways of estimating change and progress, there is also the possibility of getting information directly from the source, that is, the person we are assisting. Listening closely to speakers when they respond to a question as simple as "How are you doing?" can yield a wealth of information.

Clinical **Insight**

One of the events that motivated the writing of the first edition of this text was a presentation I attended at the annual meeting of the American Speech-Language-Hearing Association. The six presenters were experienced researchers, and in some cases clinicians, in the area of fluency disorders. The panel members were charged with discussing criteria for determining successful treatment. After listening for most of the one and one-half hour session, I found myself becoming progressively frustrated. I suspected that, with the possible exception of one presenter, the speakers had managed to alienate a large portion of the approximately 100 clinicians in attendance about the experience of assisting those with fluency disorders. The speakers managed to impart their frustration with the inconsistency of the data concerning the efficacy of different treatment strategies. The emphasis was group data: the lack of data, inaccurate data, and conflicting data. There was no recognition of the many indicators of success that take place during treatment. The presenters failed to recognize the ability of clinicians themselves to identify progress in their clients and indicated little appreciation for the integrity of clinicians' decision-making abilities. There was no enthusiasm concerning the exciting process of therapeutic change. It was a fine example of being unable to see the people for the data.

(continues)

Near the end of the session there was a glimmer of hope. One panel member who was also clearly frustrated with the discussion made the suggestion that perhaps the most useful data is sitting right in front of us during treatment. "If you want data," he suggested, "try asking the client. That person might have some good information for you about what is helpful and what is not. He might be able to inform you about whether the therapy is successful or not."

Just as the frequency of stuttering is the dependent variable, often the only one, in the majority of the research concerning treatment, many clinicians look to the frequency of stuttering as a primary measure of change or progress—and to some degree this makes sense. For example, for young children who stutter and older clients who clutter or exhibit a combination of stuttering and cluttering characteristics, the frequency of the fluency breaks may provide a reasonably straightforward indication of progress. In most instances these are speakers who are less adept or interested in concealing their stuttering. Younger children, especially those who are in the early stages of developmental stuttering, usually have not yet developed sophisticated methods of hiding or avoiding their stuttering. The percentage of stuttered moments may also provide a relatively unencumbered picture of the situation for speakers with a psychogenic or neurogenic etiology. Moreover, there is also some indication that the surface behavior in the form of stuttering frequency may more clearly reflect progress for the developmentally delayed individual who stutters. Despite the fact that developmentally delayed individuals who stutter typically demonstrate high levels of stuttering frequency (Cooper, 1986b), these speakers often appear generally unconcerned about their fluency (Bonfanti & Culatta, 1977; Cabanas, 1954). These speakers also tend to use fewer avoidance and postponement behaviors and indicate less anxiety associated with stuttering. However, for the more common case of developmental stuttering, the frequency of stuttering is only one of many features of the problem, and by itself typically fails to provide an accurate picture of the speaker's status.

A decrease in the frequency of stuttering obviously indicates change, and such change may indicate progress. Many others, however, argue that the intrinsic aspects of the problem, the attitude and cognitive features, are at least as important (and possibly more so) for determining long-term progress (e.g., Cooper & Cooper, 1985b; Rubin, 1986; Sheehan, 1970; Starkweather, 1999; Van Riper, 1973). In addition, studies on the quality of fluent speech (also referred to as speech naturalness) following both stuttering-modification as well as fluency-modification strategies, indicate that the absence of stuttering, in and of itself, is not necessarily an indicator of successful treatment (Onslow & Ingham, 1987). As described on more than one occasion earlier in this text, progress may be indicated by an *increase* in stuttering if this is the result of the speaker's decreasing use of avoidance as a coping response and the resulting increase in opportunities to communicate. Fortunately, the trend of considering the frequency of stuttering as the sole indicator of success has decreased in recent years, in part because of increased appreciation of the importance of the cognitive features of the stuttering experience and the development of procedures for obtaining this information.

Many of the speaker's characteristics associated with the stuttering will begin to change as a function of treatment. The rate of these changes will depend on variables such as the treatment strategy, specific treatment techniques, the nature of the fluency disorder, the age of the speaker, the severity of the problem, the needs of the client, and the intensity and duration of treatment. As several authors have noted, when a fluency problem is further complicated by other difficulties such as excessive anxiety, psychological or social issues, or articulation or language disabilities, individually tailored therapy techniques become mandatory (Gregory, 1984; Riley & Riley, 1983, 1984, 2000; St. Louis, 1986b; Van Riper, 1973).

Variables Influencing Progress

It would be comforting to think that our understanding of the cause-and-effect relationships we attend to during treatment can be explained by our theoretical understanding about the nature of stuttering and the empirical and experiential evidence we accumulate. Whatever the level of understanding, it appears that clinicians most often choose strategies and techniques because they believe they work (Apel, 1999; Kamhi, 1999; Fey and Johnson, 1998). But just as individuals have widely varied reactions to identical levels of medications (not to mention the effects of drug interactions), people respond to behavioral intervention in diverse and unpredictable ways. The variables that influence such diverse responses are probably too numerable to mention, but we will suggest some of the more obvious ones that are likely to influence therapeutic success for individuals who stutter.

Age of the Speaker

The major focus for much of this chapter has been on adolescents and young adults who stutter. Of course, there are similar indicators of progress among all people who stutter. However, there are at least three age groups that are distinct enough in their response to treatment that they should be considered further: young (particularly preschool) children, adolescents, and older speakers.

Young children often have good success during both direct and indirect intervention for fluency disorders. They are relatively easy to work with, and the behavioral, attitudinal, and cognitive aspects of the stuttering tend to be responsive to intervention. Therapeutic progress with these speakers can be measured in the frequency of stuttering, increased rate of speech, lessening of speaking effort, and increased spontaneity and enjoyment of communication.

As described in Chapter 8, adolescents present an entirely different set of circumstances. Van Riper (1982) stated that adolescents are some of the clinician's most difficult cases. Motivation for change is relatively rare in adolescents. Daly, Simon, and Burnett-Stolnack (1995) explain that it is often extremely difficult to get adolescents to even take part in treatment. "Many adolescents drop out of therapy, miss sessions, or attend begrudgingly. [They may] downplay the effects of their stuttering on their communication and social interactions. . . . Student rationalizations for poor attendance or for not practicing are common" (1995, p. 163).

As Daly describes, adolescents are apt to be highly sensitive and easily give up during the treatment. Many teenage clients find great difficulty confronting their problem and strongly resist being singled out for anything that carries the potential of social stigma. The importance of peer affiliation is a much more powerful force than the problems originating from their disorder. To complicate matters even further, adolescents often challenge the clinician's qualifications, clinical experience, and overall expertise (Daly, Simon, & Burnett-Stolnack, 1995). Consequently, for adolescents, progress may be measured by the consistency of attendance at treatment sessions, the level of interaction with the clinician, interest shown in the topics and techniques, and even a minimal decrease in avoidance behavior. If the clinician is unable to achieve great change in the way of modification, he or she can begin to demystify the problem, explain some of the cause-and-effect relationships of the stuttering, and let the client and his or her parents know that—when the adolescent is ready—help is available from professionals who specialize in the area of fluency disorders. It may be possible to sow some grains of knowledge and understanding that another clinician can someday harvest.

The third group of speakers consists of older stutterers who have been coping with their lack of fluency for decades. Clients over the age of 50 are rarely seen in treatment or included in research reports (Manning, Dailey, & Wallace, 1984; Manning & Monte, 1981; Manning & Shirkey, 1981; Yaruss et al. 2002). This is unfortunate, because to fully understand a fluency disorder, it would appear to be essential to follow the development of the stuttering throughout the life cycle. Models of stuttering cannot be completed until the developmental changes that take place during the middle and late adult years are understood. A review of the literature, however, indicates that this subgroup of stuttering adults has received almost no investigation. Assuming a prevalence of at least 0.7% and population data from the 2005 census (U.S. Census Bureau), there should be nearly 800,000 people in the United States alone over the age of 45 who stutter.

Anecdotal reports have indicated that stuttering is less of a problem for older individuals. The few data available indicate some support for this argument. Manning, Dailey, and Wallace (1984) obtained attitude and personality information from 29 adults ages 52 to 82 years old who were members of two national self-help groups, the National Stuttering Project and the National Council of Stutterers. Scores on six paper-and-pencil self-assessment stuttering severity measures indicated that the scores of older stuttering individuals were minimally higher than the typical scores for young adults who were about to enter treatment. Scores on the Perceptions of Stuttering Inventory (PSI) (Woolf, 1967) averaged 20.3 (standard deviation of 12.0) for the older subjects, in contrast to pretreatment scores for young adults who stutter of 21.1 (Manning & Cooper, 1969) and 27.2 (Ornstein & Manning, 1985). Responses to the S-24 Scale (Andrews & Cutler, 1974; Erickson, 1969) for the older speakers averaged 16.0, in contrast to mean pretreatment scores for younger speakers of 19.4 (Howie, 1981), 20.0 (Guitar & Bass, 1978), and 15.6 (Ornstein & Manning, 1985). Scores on the Self-Efficacy Scale for Adult Stutterers (SESAS) (Ornstein & Manning, 1985) averaged 70.5% for approach items and 60.5% on the Performance items, in contrast to 66.2% and 55.8% for young adults who stutter (Ornstein & Manning, 1985). In addition, the older participants ranked the Approach tasks significantly higher than the Performance tasks, just as the younger subjects had done ($p < .05$) (Ornstein & Manning, 1985). Finally, responses to a 25-item bipolar-adjective scale (Woods & Williams, 1976) designed to describe the personality characteristics of individuals who stutter indicated no significant differences between the 29 individuals who stuttered and matched group of 13 nonstuttering individuals.

When asked to indicate whether the handicap associated with stuttering had lessened over the years, the large majority of the subjects agreed that this had been the case. Using a seven-point, equal-appearing interval scale to rank their perceived severity as young adults and at the present time, subjects scored their current severity as significantly less ($p < .005$). Furthermore, in response to open-ended queries concerning past and current perceived severity, subjects responded with statements such as "Stuttering is less of a problem now [since] there is not so much competition"; "I accept myself more now than when I was younger"; "I've become more insightful about personal problems as I grow older"; and "Stuttering has less of an all-consuming hold on me than when I was younger." Because of the way the subjects were selected, this group of older stutterers best represents those older individuals who are actively involved in self-help groups. Nevertheless, the results suggest that although the severity of stuttering in older speakers is similar to or slightly less than their younger counterparts, they consider themselves significantly less handicapped by the problem.

Treatment Strategy and Intensity

If a fluency-enhancement approach (e.g., Onslow, Packman, & Harrison, 2003; O'Brian, Onslow, Cream, & Packman, 2003; Ryan & Van Kirk Ryan, 1995; Webster, 1975) is the primary therapeutic strategy, a reduction in the frequency of stuttering is, of course, considered the basic indicator of progress. However, if stuttering modification is the primary focus of treatment, a decrease in stuttered moments (particularly early on in treatment) is not necessarily desirable and will, in fact, prevent speakers from having the opportunity to identify, become desensitized to, and modify their stuttering. Furthermore, if a decrease in avoidance behavior is also a primary goal of treatment (which it often is), increases in the frequency of stuttering are likely to occur as a result of increased speaker assertiveness and participation in speaking opportunities.

Intensive treatment is often desirable for many behavioral problems. For many people, becoming totally immersed in the treatment process increases the possibility of changes in the behaviors and attitudes that have persisted for many years (Gregory, 1983; Ingham, 1984; Shames & Florance, 1980; Webster, 1975, 1986). Azrin, Nunn, and Frantz (1979) and Webster (1975) have advocated short-term, intensive approaches on the grounds that it takes a big push for speakers to alter their habitual responses of coping with stuttering and begin moving in a new direction. The support, energy, and challenge provided by intensive programs can provide such a push. The commitment of time, effort, and money required for such programs suggests a readiness for change that may not be the case for individuals taking part in a therapeutic experience one or two hours a week.

However, as described in Chapter 8, many people are unable to attend intensive programs. Intensive treatment often presents logistical problems. Some people are unable to leave their work for weeks at a time or cannot commute to and from the treatment site. Potential clients cannot always afford the cost of intensive treatment. Moreover, while intensive programs can result in rapid behavioral change, treatment is sometimes followed by dramatic relapses (Kuhr & Rustin, 1985; Prins, 1970). An intensive program, especially if it requires the person to live apart from his or her typical environment, may yield rapid behavioral and cognitive changes. However, the transition back to their daily world can be traumatic, especially if it is not well thought out and approached in a systematic manner. The old discriminative stimuli and expectations, on the part of the speaker as well as the listener, are powerful and usually still operating. Therefore, relapse is sometimes the case, even for those who practice diligently and attend follow-up or "booster" sessions. Perhaps the suggestion by Cooper (1979a) provides the ideal situation. He suggests a period of intensive treatment to modify the surface behaviors followed by less intensive maintenance sessions in the person's typical environment to allow for changes in the cognitive and affective features of the stuttering to occur.

Related Problems

As we discussed in Chapters 4 and 5, clients come to us with a wide range of communication skills, sometimes involving language, learning, phonological, and cluttering problems. Some have difficulties with school performance, social interaction, general physical and emotional health, and in some instances, alcohol and various drugs. Virtually anything that makes learning, formulating, and producing language and speech difficult is likely to make therapeutic change more challenging for individuals who stutter. On the other hand, children and adults who have a history of good school performance, self-esteem, and support from parents and family members are more likely to experience therapeutic success. Still, regardless of where the speaker begins, his or her resilience and motivation, combined with the assistance and support of the clinician, can help to create change.

Patterns of Avoidance

There are, of course extreme examples of avoidance and denial regarding stuttering. On the rare occasion when we are able to see these individuals in the clinic, they may well refuse to consider that the problem they are facing is stuttering. Denial has served as a primary coping response and any suggestion that it may be better to approach and discuss stuttering is likely to be met with resistance. The speaker may refer to what clearly seems to the clinician to be stuttering as a "communication problem," "stammering," or as in the case of the young woman described at the beginning of Chapter 8, a "social anxiety disorder." These people may need our help as much or more than any others we have the opportunity to see. But their primary response is to run from the problem, and getting such individuals to attend even a few sessions requires an artful interaction on our part as well as support from others.

Most of the people who seek our help have begun to move beyond such extreme levels of denial and are able to tolerate some degree of discussion of the stuttering experience. At the outset of treatment almost every speaker will benefit from some amount of desensitization. Often we need to metaphorically take the person by the shoulders and slowly turn them around to face the problem, initially with more of a side glance and eventually facing full on. In some cases, we have to be extremely sensitive to the fear and stigma the person is attaching to the problem. However, as the individual is able to stay in the moment and experience some success at approaching and possibly even modifying some aspect of his or her stuttering, the likelihood of additional change is increased. With modeling, support, and some initial victories, the person may begin to believe that it is possible for him or her to achieve at least a tiny grasp on the wall that seems to be blocking their progress. These can be cathartic moments, moments we have all experienced as we accomplish, for the first time, something we have never done before and did not believe was possible. Working through hierarchies of increasingly difficult communication situations results in success for most speakers, but the extent of the effort made can vary greatly for different people.

Available Support

The appraisal by speakers of their situation involves self-assessment of their competence and available resources for problem solving (Plexico, 2008a, b). The availability of resources such as money, individual skills, physical health, energy, and a general sense of optimism are likely to be important components of a successful problem-solving approach. Social resources include the availability of social networks for providing informational and emotional support (Compas, Malcarne, & Banez, 1992), and, regardless of the speaker's age, the consistent involvement of family and friends can provide invaluable support for promoting and providing an historical context for successful change.

In some instances, the clinician may be unable to alter these and other factors that influence the chance of success for an individual speaker. However, if the time is right and the client is ready, significant progress can take place. Moreover, when important changes occur, it is critical for the clinician to recognize the presence and nature of the breakthroughs. He or she must recognize the victories when they occur, even though they may be small ones. If the clinician is unable to identify success—the sometimes small victories that nevertheless signal progress in the desired direction—it will go unrecognized and unrewarded. The following section describes the nature of such victories by describing several indicators of progress.

Indicators of Progress

Clues from the Speaker

Speakers provide both verbal and nonverbal clues as they describe themselves and their circumstances, clues that reflect their condition and whether or not progress is taking place. Clinicians may find it useful to consider the client's self-talk, journal entries, and e-mail communications for indicators of change. The language people use to describe their situation provides important clues about who they are and where they are going. The way a person depicts his or her situation or problem often indicates important signs of progress during treatment. Moreover, as described in our earlier discussions of cognitive restructuring approaches to counseling and treatment, by changing the way we describe a problem, we can often change the problem itself (Curlee, 1984; Fransella, 1972; Hayhow & Levy, 1989; Johnson, 1946; Kuhr & Rustin, 1985; Williams, 1979; Williams, 1995).

Early on in treatment the client typically feels helpless and his or her language may reflect his or her level of "stuckness." He may well believe that he is unable to do much to change his speech or himself. There is often a high degree of mystery associated with stuttering. He or she may say such things as "When it happens I feel helpless," "When I'm in a block I feel lost and I don't know what to do," or "That is a word that I can't say." As treatment progresses, the speaker slowly begins to develop the "language of fluency" (Blodgett & Cooper, 1988; Cooper & Cooper, 1985), as well as use more appropriate self-talk (Daly, 1986; Emerick, 1988; Maxwell, 1982). As speakers begin to successfully change their previously uncontrollable behavior, they will begin to change the way they interpret themselves and their ability to produce fluent speech. Moreover, they will begin to describe their behavior and actions in more objective, specific, and realistic ways. They will begin to interpret stuttering as something that they are doing rather than something that is happening to them. They will begin to say such things as "When I stutter, sometimes I stop the airflow at the vocal folds," "I was able to change the way I repeated that syllable into a smoother and easier way of stuttering," and "Even though that was a difficult telephone call, I was able to make it and successfully achieve most of my fluency targets."

On occasion, the clinician can take an active role and point out to clients how they are describing themselves and their problem. It may be possible for them to begin talking about their problem in a different way and, in turn, facilitate new and better ways of thinking about themselves and their speech (Daly, 1986; Emerick, 1988; Maxwell, 1982). As a result of a successful therapy experience, speakers' language will begin to reflect some degree of liberation from their problem. One adult female client related how she gathered the courage to enter a feared daily speaking situation she had always avoided. As she later related to her clinician, "You know, I believe that I stuttered as much as I always have in that situation. But this time when I walked away I didn't feel ashamed."

Clinical **Insight**

Even in the absence of formal therapy, change can be noted in the transcripts of conversations or written documents by the speaker. Making use of the Origin and Pawn Scales described in Chapter 4, we analyzed correspondence from a young man over a five-year period. Mickey first wrote to me in the fall of 2002. At the time, he was a 21-year-old college student living in Sarajevo, the capital of Bosnia-Herzegovina. He had come across something on the Stuttering Home Page that I had written a few years earlier for one of the International Stuttering Awareness Day (ISAD) conferences. My comments resonated with him and he contacted me with some general questions about stuttering.

Mickey's Internet searches had identified several sources of information, some good, some not so useful. Although I commented on some of the sites

(continues)

and the information he had discovered, my primary role in our subsequent correspondence was that of providing understanding, support, and feedback. I also offered encouragement and acknowledgement of his many successes. We spent some time discussing possibilities for problem-solving issues that were unique to his situation. We certainly were not conducting treatment in any formal sense in this long-distance relationship. Mickey viewed our exchanges that took place every two to three months as self-therapy.

As Mickey and I continued our correspondence it became clear that he was making important, often dramatic, changes in how he viewed himself and his ability to communicate. We began analyzing his e-mail letters using the Origin and Pawn Scales. Although the majority of Mickey's communications had to do with Mickey's experience with stuttering, the entire contents of the letters were included in the scoring process. For that reason, our analysis of his narratives also included topics such as politics, travel, weather, and family and social interactions. We analyzed a total of 22 letters from Mickey, which he sent from the fall of 2002 through the spring of 2007. Two judges independently identified Origin and Pawn statements and then compared their decisions. Item-for-item judgments matched an average of 85% of the time.

Examples from Mickey's letters during the first four years provide a sense of his progress, and this analysis helped to document the nature and extent of these changes. Two brief passages provide vivid examples of how Mickey was reinterpreting himself and his situation.

Examples of Pawn Statements (P), October 2003 . . . but sometimes it looks like progress is coming too slow and that demoralize me totally from time to time. (P) I am 22 years old now, and I don't know how much time I have left for overcoming stuttering in order to achieve normal life. (P) I feel like I'm spending best years of my life in the "mud", (P) not using all the available opportunities out there. (P) Despite the fact that I understand stuttering better now, some emerging fears are making progress difficult: (P) If I don't succeed in time I don't know how my life is gonna turn out. (P)"

Examples of Origin Statements (O), December 2004. But I am trying to enter them (stuttering blocks) without avoiding and using tricks. (O) But I am gaining more and more self-confidence, (O) and I think it is the most important thing in all this. Also I feel much more freedom (O) as I am accepting my stuttering (O) and decreasing emotional attachment and sensibility to it. I am now in position to feel and to see the full potential of the struggle free life (O) that I can achieve (O) if I put enough effort in this process of change. (O) Generally speaking I am now focusing more on reducing fear and emotional tension, (O) on improving the quality of my life, (O) than on techniques for improving fluency. I think it will be much

(continued)

easier to use those techniques (O) when I substantially improve my self-confidence and psychological health or life quality in general. I already achieved that in some extent (O) through facing feared situations, voluntary stuttering and changing negative attitudes, (O) but there is still a lot to be done in the coming weeks, months and years. (O) Also I am trying to increase physical activities (O) and to engage in some sport, (O) because I noticed such activities are contributing significantly to increasing my self-confidence. (O)

The results of the Origin and Pawns analysis (Figure 11-5) during the first four years (2002–2005) of our correspondence indicate a clear reduction in pawn statements and a corresponding increase in origin statements. There was a significant interaction of the sets of scores, with pawn scores showing a significant decrease in 2003 and origin scores significantly increasing through 2005. However, during the last 18 months, in 2006 and 2007, although not returning to the clear dominance of pawn over origin scores found in 2002, there was no significant difference between the two sets of scores. The pawn and origin scores during the final two years suggest a degree of relapse or possibly regression to the mean. According to Mickey, these values may also reflect his general dissatisfaction and frustration with other personal, social, and economic aspects of his circumstances at the time.

In any case, it is clear from this investigation that Origin and Pawn Scales can provide us with valuable information in many forms about the nature of their therapeutic progress.

The Speaker's Ability to Self-Monitor

Another primary indicator of progress is the speaker's ability to accurately monitor what he or she is doing when he or she stutters. Even if the speaker is not yet able to modify the way he or she is producing speech, he or she may be able to analyze what he or she is doing to make it so difficult to move through the desired sequence of sounds and words. Accurate self-monitoring of any behavior or thought process is a requisite step in taking responsibility and transforming the event. Martin and Haroldson (1982) demonstrated the value of self-monitoring in generalizing the reduction of stuttering, and Ingham (1982) found self-evaluation training to be associated with substantially reduced stuttering for up to six months post-treatment.

One place to begin monitoring is to identify listener reactions. The process of identifying and distancing from the stress and fear of listener responses can have an empowering effect on the speaker and begin to facilitate a conceptual

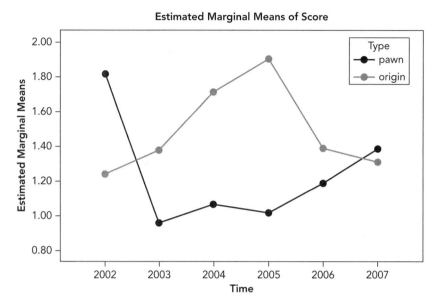

Figure 11-5   Pawns and Origins scores for Mickey over a six-year period.

shift concerning the communication process. What are the subtle and more obvious responses of individual listeners as they observe stuttering? By scrutinizing individuals before approaching them it is sometimes possible to predict (or even create) particular responses from them in terms of body language and verbal reactions. Role-playing can be particularly helpful as both client and clinician take turns portraying typical listener responses observed in daily speaking situations.

Early on in treatment, speakers tend to find it easier to confront and analyze stuttering behaviors in others. Using videos, the clinician can provide realistic examples of stuttering behaviors for the client to identify. Both the clinician and the client can replicate as closely as possible the unique and often interesting features of stuttering. Progress is seen in the ability of speakers to identify progressively more subtle moments of stuttering both in others and themselves. Speakers can learn to separate the features of their own stuttering into component parts that may be strongly linked together. That is, speakers may find that they repeat the initial syllable of the word and also constrict the vocal tract at the level of the glottis, consistently shift their eyes to the side, and insert the starter sound "ah" in order to postpone an upcoming feared word. It may not be necessary to identify all possible features, but a thorough appreciation of the speaker's typical and highly reflexive coping responses is often necessary for systematic and substantial change.

Eventually the client will be able to monitor his or her own speech production via both auditory and, more importantly, proprioceptive feedback. Auditory feedback provides some indication of the nature and quality of fluent speech, but proprioceptive feedback provides a more timely and direct indication of the status of the vocal tract and both the accuracy and ease of articulatory movement. Self-monitoring of the auditory output alone allows little or no opportunity to alter the motoric aspects of speech production. Proprioceptive feedback provides an instantaneous way to monitor the quality of fluency and the extent that speech is being produced in an open, flowing, and effortless manner. It is a major step in treatment for speakers to be able to monitor their own speech in this fashion.

Self-monitoring will continue to be a critical element of long-term success. Van Riper reported that his stuttering increased in frequency (although not, he felt, in severity) after an initial heart attack at age 65. He described "little sluggish prolongations" (1978) that mostly disappeared after his recovery. Following his retirement, he again noticed an increase in the frequency and, occasionally, the severity of his stuttering. He found that he was experiencing more frequent and longer tremors as well as some laryngeal blocks. Because these fluency breaks were surprising, he thought that these changes were probably due to his lack of monitoring of his speech. He speculated that the hard work of closely monitoring his speech and "stuttering fluently" was no longer worth the effort.

Increasing Approach Behavior

As we have discussed in this and in earlier chapters, patterns of denial and avoidance are natural coping responses to situations with high levels of stress and which the individual feels powerless to change. Speakers come to us with various levels of this coping pattern and virtually all adolescent and adult speakers manifest some of these responses to stuttering. Patterns of avoidance and escape are deeply embedded and involve more than the simple act of substituting one word for another or avoiding particular speaking situations. Accordingly, altering what have become reflexive avoidance responses and slowly developing and expanding forms of approach behavior takes considerable effort and persistence. This is often a major component of therapeutic change and the mentorship and support of the clinician (and perhaps other clients) as well as the speaker's family and friends often play a critical role.

Open and Effortless Speech

As the speaker develops the ability to enter into previously avoided communication situations, victories can be observed at every speaking opportunity as the speaker's stuttering pattern eventually begins to signal an open and relaxed vocal tract. At the outset of treatment the speaker's fluency breaks are typically characterized by noticeable vocal tract constriction and effort. As the speaker begins to understand the structure and function of the various parts of his or her speech production system, progress can be observed in greater airflow, easier articulatory positioning, and smoother transitions between sounds and words. With an increased ability to monitor his or her speech production, the speaker is able to contrast the difference between the tension and constriction of his or her old, habitual way of speaking and the new flowing and less effortful pattern. With less effort, the stuttering event becomes not only easier but shorter. As Conture (1990) suggests, a shortening in the duration of stuttering (even though the frequency may not change) is a good sign of progress. The speaker as well as the listener can hear (and see) the increased openness and ease of movement. The changes are obvious and satisfying, even with the occurrence of some stuttering. To the extent that the speaker is able to effectively employ modification techniques, the stuttering that does occur is likely to be smooth and relatively effortless.

Developing Agentic Behavior

Coinciding with the speaker's ability to approach rather than avoid the stuttering experience is the increasing ability to make choices about communicating that are based on information beyond the possibility of stuttering. As explained in Chapter 8, a person living an agentic lifestyle is able to act and speak on his or her own behalf (Monk et al., 1997), and the ability to live an autonomous and healthy life has more to do with the person's capacity for agency than the absence of the problem (Drewery, Winslade, & Monk, 2000). Successful treatment assists the speaker in opening his or her focus beyond the dominant influence of stuttering; he or she becomes able to consider other, more expansive possibilities and options. With this wider focus comes the recognition of new responsibilities and challenges. Speakers now have the obligation—if they are to be true to themselves—to act on this new information. If the initial hard-won progress of the therapeutic experience is to be maintained, the speaker must continue making new choices that result in new challenges. There will be many opportunities for open decision making during daily work and social activities. Years of avoidance and less-than-complete interpersonal involvement can gradually change. The clinician as well as the client will recognize that beyond the many behavioral changes related to speech and fluency, the person is also changing ways of approaching many of the challenges presented by life. It is not unusual to hear speakers describe how their increased confidence in their ability to successfully manage stuttering transfers to many other aspects of life, including competing for employment opportunities, taking part in public speaking opportunities, taking on organizational and leadership roles, and participating in a wide range of social interactions.

With increasing agency, it is not surprising that the speaker will also be likely to alter other related interpersonal characteristics. Greater levels of speech assertiveness are likely to translate into increased assertiveness in general. For example, it is a distinct indicator of progress when the speaker begins to decrease reflexive self-censorship and starts to consider entering into speaking situations once seen as daunting or even unimaginable. This is not to say that the person will now take part in these situations with ease or idyllic fluency. But the choice to take part, in and of itself, is a significant measure of progress. Closely associated with the development of assertiveness is an increase in risk-taking. Just as athletes, in order to improve their skills, reach to the edge of their ability (or sometimes, for a moment, just beyond), the speaker extends the envelope of his or her experience and performance. Each time speakers extend themselves into communication situations that involve factors such as competition, time pressure, and responsibility, they are expanding their world. It is worth considering that many of these experiences are not only challenging but also exciting. There is always the risk of failure, and sometimes degrees of disappointment will occur. Taking on the challenges of new adventures is more indicative of progress for some speakers than others. However, for many people, the ability to expand the sphere of risk-taking activities provides evidence of the cognitive changes that are part of long-term change.

Self-Concept and Self-Esteem

As the behavioral and cognitive changes evolve as a function of the support and encouragement provided by the therapy experience, the speaker is likely to undergo changes to his or her core structure as described in Chapter 7. Self-concept and self-esteem have been referred to many times in the literature on fluency disorders. According to Peck (1978), self-esteem is the cornerstone of psychological change. Although persons who stutter have not been found to have a unique self-concept or to be lacking in self-esteem, this concept has frequently been mentioned as an aspect of treatment programs (Van Riper, 1973, pp. 364–367).

Self-esteem is not something that can be given to you. Nonetheless, the stage can be set by supportive parents and friends as well as the clinician. The clinician is capable of providing a secure and stable therapeutic environment where growth and change will be likely to occur. As the speaker experiences the successful management of the behavioral and cognitive features of stuttering, self-esteem and self-concept are likely to begin shifting in a more favorable direction. This is certainly the case with preschool and early school-age children and a major reason why intervention for stuttering is much more likely to result in long-term success with these young speakers than with older individuals (Bothe, Davidow, Bramlett, & Ingham, 2006). The drawings by Brad, age 10, provide a clear description of how he interprets his stuttering (Figure 11-6) and the treatment process (Figure 11-7). Carol, age 6, is able to indicate her feelings about herself before and after three months of successful therapy, including how to deal with teasing (Figure 11-8). Adults are also able to redefine themselves and create an altered paradigm of their lives. Such changes can be quantified by self-reports during individual and group treatment sessions as well as by measures such as the locus of control (Kuhr & Rustin, 1985). The information described in Chapter 3 concerning the plasticity of the human brain provides direct support for the many cognitive and behavioral changes observed by clinicians.

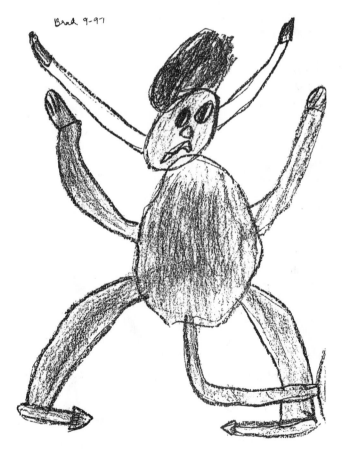

Figure 11-6   Brad's picture of the "stuttering monster."

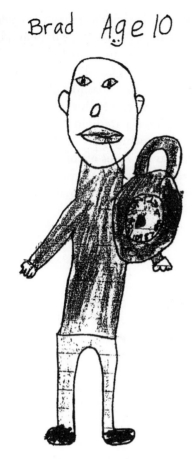

Brad   Age 10

my lips are locked up. I'm stuttering. The lock has a combination to open it. And the combination is to use tools and practice.

Figure 11-7   Brad's picture of treatment for stuttering.

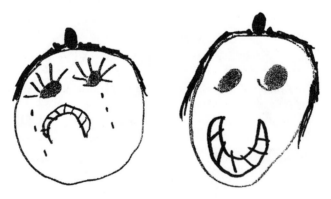

Figure 11-8   Carol's self-drawing before and after three months of treatment.

Clinical Insight

In his book *Social Intelligence* Daniel Goleman (2006) describes how the brain is capable of reorganizing itself in response to new experiences. Although stem cells produce new neurons at a much higher rate for children, the process continues, even in older adults. Given the number of connections in a limited space, those that are unused or unneeded are pruned while new ones are formed and integrated through constant use ("cells that fire together wire together"). Therapeutic procedures have long made use of what neuroscientists are now beginning to understand: that memory retrieval allows for the reconstruction of past events through a process of "reconsolidation" at the cellular level. The retrieved memory will be "slightly altered chemically by a new protein synthesis that will help store it anew after being updated" (p. 78). This allows, for example, a reduction of the fear associated with a recalled event according to how it is reprogrammed in the neurons and associated neural connections.

The Relationship of Formulative and Motoric Fluency Breaks

Nearly all clinicians would agree that progress during treatment is reflected by decreases in the occurrence of motoric fluency breaks. However, as Goldman-Eisler (1961) and Starkweather (1987) have indicated, fluency breaks are an important aspect of normal speech formulation. Preliminary findings by Manning and Monte (1991) suggest that adults who stutter, while they obviously produce more motoric fluency breaks than nonstutterers, also demonstrate significantly fewer formulative fluency breaks. If speech is to be normalized for people who stutter, one important aspect of that process, aside from a decrease in motoric breaks, may well be an increase to near-normal levels of formulative fluency breaks (Manning & Monte, 1981).

As the speaker produces fewer motoric fluency breaks as a result of treatment, there are fewer opportunities to formulate the content of the message. As with typically fluent individuals, the speaker may choose to include some fluency breaks (typically pauses or interjections) in order to consider alternate ways of formulating a message. Some speakers who stutter will be unwilling to voluntarily stop and use a formulative fluency break for fear of being unable to initiate speech again. Accordingly, with successful treatment the speaker may be less concerned about the ability to continue once the formulative break has provided the opportunity to organize his or her thoughts. Yairi (1993) found that children who recovered from stuttering continued to produce (or even increased their production of) other types of fluency breaks (revisions, interjections, phrase repetitions, and other between-word or formulative fluency breaks).

During the later stages of treatment it may be helpful for some speakers to engage in spontaneous monologues in order to practice sequencing and branching their thoughts. The process provides an opportunity for the person to speak "without putting on the brakes" and to free-associate out loud. Progress is seen as individuals are able to gradually free themselves from the practice of scanning ahead for feared words and "pretasting" feared sounds. Following a lifetime of speaking in a careful, cautious, or inhibited manner, some individuals are able to achieve remarkable levels of fluency and communicative competence.

Speech Naturalness

The impetus for studying the speech naturalness of individuals treated for stuttering came from observations that many people who had undergone successful treatment continued to sound unnatural (Onslow & Ingham, 1987; Runyan, Hames, & Proseck, 1982; Sacco, Metz, & Schiavetti, 1992). Their speech was perceived as effortful, uncomfortable to listen to, and contained auditory or visual features that prevented the listener from fully attending to the content of the message. Despite an otherwise successful treatment experience, many speakers found that they were still unsatisfied with their speech and were still regarded by others as having a problem (Schiavetti & Metz, 1997). Tasko, McClean, and Runyan (2007) found, for example, that of 35 adults who reduced their stuttering severity during an intensive fluency shaping program (mean *SSI-3* score reductions of 26 to 9.3), the speakers who showed the greatest success in decreasing the severity of their stuttering were also determined to be the most unnatural-sounding. Tasko et al. suggested that decreased naturalness ratings may have resulted from the effort the successful participants had to put forth in order to execute the behavioral therapeutic targets (e.g., increased abdominal breathing, continuity of airflow, pre-voiced exhalation, easy articulatory and phonatory onset, and continuous phonation). Although the strongest speech-motor correlate of the reduced speech naturalness was a reduced syllable rate ($r = -.40$) the authors also acknowledge that the increased inspiration and monitoring of speech movements required of the speakers may have also contributed to decreased speech naturalness.

In 1984, Martin, Haroldson, and Triden began the development of a reliable scale for rating speech naturalness. The scale consisted of a 9-point Likert scale, with 1 equivalent to highly natural-sounding speech and 9 equivalent to highly unnatural-sounding speech. This scale was subsequently used in many investigations of speech naturalness. Martin et al. found that mean naturalness ratings for the speakers who stuttered was 6.52, while normally fluent adult speakers averaged 2.12.

The naturalness of speech is recognized as an important consideration in determining the success of treatment. The scale developed by Martin, Haroldson, and Triden appears to be reliable for either oral reading or spontaneous speech. Some (but not all) clients improve their speech naturalness as a result of treatment, and listeners tend to judge treated clients' speech as being significantly less natural than that of normally fluent speakers (Runyan, Bell, & Proseck, 1990; Franken, Boves, Peters, & Webster, 1992; Kalinowski, Nobel, Armson,

& Stuart, 1994). Runyan et al. found post-treatment naturalness ratings of 4.26 for speakers judged to be mild, 3.82 for speakers judged to be moderate, and 3.68 for speakers judged to be severe. These findings coincide with Starkweather's (1992) observation that even with increased fluency, some therapy procedures often tend to diminish the quality of a person's speech. Speakers who differ on naturalness ratings at the outset of treatment may be rated much the same after treatment, although pre- and post-treatment severity ratings influence judgments of naturalness. Moreover, feedback appears to enhance the speaker's ability to improve naturalness (Ingham & Onslow, 1985; Ingham, Martin, Haroldson, Onslow, & Leney, 1985). It also appears that listeners and speakers may have different criteria for determining naturalness. Listeners tend to evaluate an audio recording of a speaker as being more natural than when both audio and visual signals are presented (Martin & Haroldson, 1992). Lastly, voice-onset time and sentence duration have been suggested as important acoustic features of speech naturalness (Metz, Schiavetti, & Sacco, 1990).[2]

The research on speech naturalness indicates that the goal of treatment is considerably more complex than assisting clients to decrease the frequency of their stuttering. Some moments of stuttering are not likely to detract from a speaker's naturalness and spontaneity, particularly if these breaks are brief and relatively effortless. Clinicians who understand the importance of these effortless and smooth fluency breaks are most likely to appreciate this change. However, the research suggests that even naïve listeners may prefer speech with fluency breaks to unnatural-sounding and highly controlled speech devoid of all fluency disruptions.

There is a wide range of speaking performance that is possible, but fluency without ease of production as well as listening represents something short of an ideal therapeutic success. If the client's nonstuttered speech is less than fluent—if it sounds unnatural and the fluency is tenuous—it may foreshadow the possibility of relapse. If clients' fluent but unnatural speech elicits a negative response from listeners, it may be that they will soon grow tired of the practice necessary to maintain their new and unnatural speech and will return to their original and familiar form of stuttering. Adams and Runyan (1981) state that the client who is ready for dismissal should have speech that is objectively and perceptively indistinguishable from that of normal speakers. The client's speech should not only be free of stuttering but should be produced at an acceptable rate, sound natural, and be free of perceptible signs of tenuous fluency. Some speakers, after several years of experience, may be able to achieve spontaneous fluency. However, as suggested earlier in this chapter, although this may be possible for younger speakers, these are lofty and perhaps unrealistic goals for many adults who stutter. Nonetheless, such changes in speech naturalness should certainly be viewed as important signs of progress.

---

[2]The author is unaware of any naturalness studies involving preschool and school-age children who stutter.

Success also can be observed through the reports of others in the speaker's environment, such as teachers, parents, a spouse, or friends, who indicate to the client or the clinician the desirable changes both in fluency and daily participation in activities. For example, Conture (1990) indicates that early signs of improvement often take the form of others reporting that they are noticing an improvement in speech or related behavior. These reports may appear spontaneously or may be elicited from those in the client's environment who are able to provide candid feedback. Such feedback should be taken seriously and regarded as an important indicator of success.

The Self-Discipline of Practice

The achievement of any moderately complex behavior requires repetition and persistence in order to obtain some degree of mastery. This is especially the case when stressful elements such as time pressure and social stigma are involved. Most individuals understand that some practice is necessary but few fully appreciate the extent that is required for consistent and dependable performance in the many communication situations where fluency failure has been both the expectation and often the reality. For the adolescent, and particularly for the adult who as been stuttering for many years, practice must take place for many months and years before the techniques will begin to become functional and an integrated part of the speaker's ability to manage his or her stuttering. Of course, it is one thing to practice and develop confidence in using new responses to stuttering within the clinical environment and quite another to make the transition to the variety of everyday speaking situations in which the support provided by that environment is absent.

The research of Brundage and her associates in exploring the use of virtual reality may hold promise for assisting speakers to make this difficult transition. The control and options provided by this technology have been found useful for assisting individuals with a variety of problems (e.g., anxiety reduction related to fear of flying, enhancement of motor skills, weight loss) in successfully transitioning to gradually more difficult activities beyond the therapeutic environment (Brundage, 2007). The highly realistic, three-dimensional virtual experiences provide a realistic immersion in an environment that has been found to be comparable to live experiences in terms of the physiologic, cognitive, emotional, and behavioral responses (Brundage, 2007; Brundage & Graap, 2004; Brundage, Hancock, Kiselewich, & Stallings, 2006; Duncko, Brundage, Graap, Kling, & Gold, 2006), including the amount of stuttering and communication apprehension (Brundage, Graap, Gibbons, Ferrer, & Brooks, 2006; Brundage, et al., 2006).

The system makes use of a head-mounted display, combined with headphones for auditory input, as well as a tracking system that provides for changing views that correspond to the speaker's head movements. It is possible to develop a variety of virtual situations that occur in the person's everyday experiences at school, work, or social activities. Importantly, these situations can be controlled for extraneous distractions that tend to occur in real-world situations, allowing the speaker to focus on events and stimuli that have particular meaning for them. Experiences can be organized in a hierarchical manner and repeated as often as necessary in order for the individual to achieve desensitization and to explore a variety of responses to the situation. For example, an individual can enter a virtual classroom to find one of several different groups of people in the audience. Beyond the size of the audience, the response of the individuals in the room can be altered according to such factors as the attentiveness of the listeners, their response to the speaker, background noise, and time pressure. As Brundage and colleagues describe (Brundage, 2007; Brundage, & Graap, 2004; Brundage et al., 2006), the virtual environment provides a realistic experience for practice and exploration but without the risks inherent in live performances. Speakers have the opportunity to develop a sense of empowerment in speaking experiences that they would otherwise avoid. It may well be that this technology and evolving software will provide the clinician with many applications for both assessment and treatment activities.

As the speaker progresses from the security of the treatment setting to beyond-treatment environments, successful management will help to prevent plateaus or regression. The self-motivated requirement of continued practice may be the hardest lesson that many speakers have to learn. Each individual has a choice to make about the price they want to pay for enhanced fluency and communicative facility. The good news is that highly successful management of stuttering is possible and that, over time, the work becomes easier.

Clinical Insight

One of our teenage clients who was beginning to realize how much he was going to have to practice his treatment techniques brought this story back from a skiing trip to Colorado. He had been watching people learning to negotiate a hill with a series of moguls and wondered out loud to a nearby instructor how long it would take to master such a difficult section. After considering the question for a moment, the instructor responded by saying, "Well, if you practiced every day for about six hours and you did that for about six months you would be pretty good. But you still wouldn't master it." Only after hearing that description did the young man fully appreciate how much he was going to have to practice so that he would become "pretty good" at using his therapy techniques during more difficult speaking situations.

Clinical Insight

Another story about the degree of practice and overlearning that must take place in order to master difficult and complex activities was related by Daly (1999). He described how every spring he and his friends charter a sailboat and spend a week on the Chesapeake Bay. One year one of the friends wasn't able to come along and another person took his place. The new fellow happened to be a professional oboe player. Each morning he would come up on deck and practice his oboe. His playing was enjoyable for everyone but eventually one of the crew members asked him why he continued to practice even though he was on a vacation. He responded by saying, "If I didn't practice for one day, I would know it. If I didn't practice for two days, the oboe section would know it. And if I didn't practice for three days, the entire orchestra would know it."

Developing Perspective Through Humor

As the speaker is able to achieve success in the management of his stuttering, many associated cognitive changes are reflected by the presence and acknowledgement of humor. As we suggested in Chapter 1, the clinician can lead the way in identifying and appreciating the humorous aspects of a situation by providing "new eyes" for viewing the old problem. As the speaker is able to externalize and achieve some distance from his or her relationship with stuttering, the clinician can be on the lookout for indicators of the client's ability to provide a

Clinical Insight

James, a middle-aged man, had attended therapy for only a short time but was already considerably desensitized to his stuttering. One day during group therapy, he related how, during his college years, he had eventually worked up the courage to call a young woman he had noticed in one of his classes for a date. He rarely used the telephone and never had telephoned a woman's dormitory before. [Note: Although it may be difficult for some of today's readers to appreciate, in those days there was only a single telephone located in the hallway of each floor of the woman's dorm.] The coed James wanted to call was named Harriet, and rather than risk saying an entire sentence such as "May I speak to Harriet?" he decided to simply say "Harriet?" to whoever happened to answer the telephone. He dialed the dormitory and the telephone began ringing. After a few moments, a woman came to the phone and answered it. James froze, and the very best he could do was produce a series of breathy sounds as he kept repeating the initial "H" of Harriet's name. After this went on for several seconds, he heard the coed partially cover the phone and announce to the other women in the hall, "It's him again!"

humorous interpretation of events. Such opportunities occur frequently during group sessions, where a humorous story by one client often leads to a change in perspective by others in the group. With the distance afforded by the passage of time, behavioral mastery, and cognitive changes in perspective resulting from therapeutic success, the client is able to release the damaging effects of the experience and see his or her previous experiences with new eyes. Listener reactions from the past, from mildly inappropriate to obviously patronizing, as painful as they may have been when first experienced, lose some of their bite when distance and objectivity are applied to the wound. The entire group can share the experience and participate in a new interpretation of an old predicament. Along with the examples found in Chapter 1, here are two additional examples of the many stories people have provided over the years.

Clinical **Insight**

Walt had recently graduated from college and had enrolled himself in an intensive treatment program at a local university. As part of a group assignment, clients were to pair up and walk across campus to the streets of the college town and keep a record of listener reactions as they asked for directions from strangers. Walt and his partner decided they would ask for the location of the police station. Still in the early stages of treatment and clearly stuttering, he viewed his task as daunting one. He attempted to find the listener who posed the least possible threat. Entering the first street adjacent to the campus, he spied the best of all possible targets. Coming around the corner and approaching him on the street was an elderly woman. As he approached her, he positioned himself so that even if he stuttered, she would have no alternative but to stop. She was the prototypical grandmother. She wore a cloth coat and a hat with a veil. She was carrying a shopping bag in each hand, along with an umbrella. As Walt began to ask his question, she stopped. She looked up at him and placed both shopping bags on the sidewalk. Walt continued stuttering his way through his required question asking about the location of the police station. As he completed his sentence, she responded. Yes, she did know the location of the police station. She spoke very slowly, a fact that was enhanced by her lipstick-red mouth as well as the veil attached to the front of her hat. "See the . . . big . . . red . . . light?" she asked, as she turned and pointed to the stoplight one block behind her. She continued, even slower now, "When you get to that big . . . red . . . light . . . turn . . . (and she paused even longer here as she took the elbow of his right arm) . . . left." At that same moment, to emphasize her instructions, she spun him around to his left. Somewhat wide-eyed and mortified for the moment, he pondered these events as he made his way back to the group meeting. As he shared his experience with the other group members, everyone, including Walt, appreciated the humorous telling of his story. There was genuine empathy and laughter all around as each member of the group shared similar experiences with well-meaning but overly patronizing listeners.

Considerations for Concluding Formal Treatment

For children, the decision of terminating formal therapy is reasonably straight forward. As described in Chapter 9, once the child is able to maintain easy, fluent speech in a variety of situations at home and in school for several weeks or months, the decision to conclude treatment becomes obvious. The Stage 2 criteria of the Lidcombe Program described in Chapter 9 provide a reasonable approach for phasing-out weekly therapy meetings (e.g., home severity ratings [SR] of less than 2.0 and 1.0%SS during clinic visits for several weeks). Some monitoring in the form of meetings, telephone calls, and emails—perhaps as long as two years following the conclusion of formal treatment—is frequently recommended.

For adults, the issue is usually a little more complex for, as we have described, patterns of coping with stuttering have been well-established and are usually more difficult to change. For those who take part in intensive treatment programs that are organized over a period of weeks, the participants are enrolled for a set period and follow-up sessions and support are typically provided. Many individuals are unable to take part in intensive programs and choose, instead, to attend treatment on a once- or twice-a-week basis. In this situation there is often no preset determination or discussion about when treatment is likely to be concluded. As discussed at the outset of this chapter, it is probably reasonable to conceive of the process as a period of formal or professional assistance followed by a lifelong period of informal or self-therapy. Still, there are no uniform criteria that have been recommended for terminating formal treatment.

Van Riper (1973) suggested that if the speaker becomes bored and unenthused about treatment or even about maintaining fluency, it may be time to terminate formal treatment. Certainly it is better to anticipate the end of treatment and to schedule a final exit meeting or two than to have the client simply cease attending. Apart from the effect on the client, such lack of closure provides the clinician with less opportunity to learn from the therapeutic encounter. Like Adams and Runyan (1981), who suggest that dismissal can take place when the client's speech is indistinguishable from typically fluent speakers, Bloodstein (1987) suggests that successful treatment should result in speech that sounds not only natural but also spontaneous, and that subjects should be free of the need to monitor his or her speech. St. Louis and Westbrook (1987) propose that clients should be free from stuttering before being dismissed from treatment. Whether it is realistic to expect adults who have stuttered for most of their lives to be able to achieve such goals before being dismissed from formal treatment is questionable. While it is possible that a high level of spontaneous and natural-sounding fluency may be a realistic goal for some speakers it is not the case for many adults. Obviously, there should be a clinically significant reduction in stuttering as formal treatment is concluded, but there are still likely to be occasions where some form of stuttering will take place. Patterns of avoidance and stress reactions during particularly difficult communication situations are likely to persist, depending on the extent to which speakers challenge themselves in expanding their speaking experiences and confidence.

Discussing the criteria for termination with the speaker at or near the outset of treatment is one possible solution to this problem. It is probably never too soon for the clinician to begin asking the client to address the issue of terminating or phasing out formal treatment. A request to the speaker to consider some operational definitions about when he or she will be able to be on his or her own is a valid issue from the outset. Often the client will respond with, "You're the expert, you tell me." Of course, the clinician is the expert about fluency disorders in a generic sense, but as we indicate on many occasions throughout this book, the client must become the authority concerning his or her own situation and therapeutic goals. Certainly, we can obtain several measures of the speaker's progress that will be helpful in making the decision to end formal treatment. But, in a high-quality therapeutic alliance, our client will be likely to tell us when he or she is ready.

Continued treatment beyond what is necessary may serve to reinforce the client's dependency. In addition, there is a law of diminishing returns whereby, at a certain point, the cost of treatment, financial or otherwise, is no longer worth the effect. If the client has reached a plateau and little progress is noted for several weeks, such leveling-off may suggest that the client—not to mention the clinician—needs a break. A break from treatment also may be indicated if the client becomes bored or other issues such as financial constraints or the logistics of attending treatment become preeminent. Just as in the case of attending graduate school or beginning a period of arduous athletic training, pushing ahead at full speed is not always the best strategy. Sometimes "less is more," and it may be best to back away for a while. A break may provide the opportunity to reassess priorities and evaluate and regain motivation. It may be that a vacation from treatment is the best investment for future growth. Temporary dismissal from treatment may not be an easy decision, for there is the chance that we will lose contact with the person and progress may cease. Nonetheless, forgoing treatment for a time can be an essential step in the overall process. When termination of treatment is discussed, the clinician can make it clear that group treatment or consultation on a less formal basis is available. If the speaker has not already done so, joining a support group can serve to keep his or her momentum going and foster desensitization and an assertive approach concerning the achievement of fluency.

Conclusion

The consistent findings from in-depth studies of the experiences provided by people who stutter indicate themes of suffering, struggle, helplessness, anxiety, low self-worth and highly restricted lives (Finn, 1996; Corcoran & Stewart, 1998; Crichton-Smith, 2002; Anderson-Felsenfeld, 2003; Plexico, Manning & DiLollo, 2005). The descriptions are dominated by the individuals' overall response to their global life experience and their self-interpretation as communicators and as human beings. From the speaker's perspective, the experience of stuttering is represented by these intrinsic features as much or more than it is by the more obvious surface behaviors. These findings strongly indicate that a successful therapeutic outcome should include validation by the client of changes in the intrinsic features of the problem (see also, Conture, 1996). Recent findings by Langevin et al. (2006) also provide convincing support for a model of treatment effectiveness that incorporates input from clients and significant others as well as clinicians and researchers.

The process of change both within and beyond the therapeutic environment is most often indicated in the form of small victories. Change often begins once the speaker begins to recognize the need for help and begins to take action for obtaining assistance. For most speakers, multiple factors must be considered when tracking successful change for a multidimensional problem such as stuttering. Trivial criteria are likely to yield convincing but inaccurate views of success. The surface features of the problem in the form of less frequent, easier, and more open stuttering clearly indicate success. Alterations in cognitive and affective responses also indicate important, sometimes substantial, changes as speakers develop more insightful, less reflexive and fearful responses to the possibility as well as the reality of their stuttering. The speaker brings to the therapeutic experience a history of abilities and speech-related problems that will interact with the therapeutic alliance and the particular treatment strategy. It is not surprising that success will look and sound somewhat different for each individual given the interplay of these factors. Regardless of the therapeutic program, speakers achieve excellent, modest, or, particularly if they terminate the program prematurely, little success.

Peck, in a discussion of the psychotherapeutic process, indicates that "the majority of patients, even in the hands of the most skilled and loving therapists, will terminate their therapy at some point far short of completely fulfilling their potential" (Peck, 1978, p. 180). Early termination is also sometimes characteristic of intervention for fluency disorders. Not all clients make as much progress as we would like, at least during the time that we share with them. But nearly any person who is ready and motivated enough to approach rather than avoid the problem is likely to make progress. As clients meet with an experienced clinician, they begin to learn something about themselves and their communication problem. They are likely to become desensitized to the problem over time. As they develop a more accurate and broader view of their situation, they are more likely to begin coping in ways that are more agentic and less influenced by the habitual and typically less efficient responses.

As treatment progresses, it becomes increasingly important for indicators of change to accurately reflect the speaker's ability to enter into and successfully communicate in speaking situations beyond the therapy setting. Many individuals quickly adapt to and become fluent within the supportive therapeutic environment. Clues to successful change in daily speaking situations can be indicated by self-report devices and, of course, by clinician observation. Perhaps the most salient clues are provided by the speaker's written or verbal descriptions of their experiences. All of these sources provide information about clients' ability to accomplish improved levels of self-monitoring, practice and self-discipline, approach behavior, open and effortless speech, self-confidence and esteem, and a new and often humorous perspective of themselves and their situation. As a result of these accomplishments the individual is able to elaborate an increasingly agentic lifestyle.

Ideally, the decision to gradually phase out of and terminate the formal support provided by the clinician and the therapy program should be made by the speaker. It can be difficult for the clinician to see some clients leave, for the therapeutic alliance is often a positive experience for everyone involved. Therapy that is unnecessary, beyond the obvious ethical issues, may serve to reinforce the client's dependency. As we discuss in the final chapter, some speakers will need additional contact with the clinician in one form or another. Should additional individual or group treatment become necessary, it is helpful for the speaker to interpret the decision as an opportunity for continued growth and support rather than as dependency.

Topics for Discussion

1. How would you explain what you consider to be the primary principles of therapeutic change to an adult who stutters?

2. Describe the factors that are likely to facilitate or detract from the possibility of therapeutic success.

3. How would you document attitudinal, behavioral, and cognitive indicators of successful therapeutic change for (a) children and (b) adults who stutter?

4. What are examples of the "little victories" that are demonstrated by a speaker whom you are particularly interested in highlighting and rewarding?

5. Using a three-minute sample of spontaneous speech, rate five non-stuttering adult speakers using the 9-point naturalness rating scale described in this chapter. Also rate recorded samples of speakers who are approaching the conclusion of treatment.

6. Explain your criteria for considering the termination of formal treatment for an adolescent or adult who has been coming to you for treatment.

Recommended Readings

Hillis, J. W. (1993). Ongoing assessment in the management of stuttering: A clinical perspective. *American Journal of Speech-Language Pathology, 2*(1), 24–37.

Langevin, M., Hunick, W. J., Kully, D., Peters, H. F. M., Lomheim, H., & Tellers, M. (2006). A cross-cultural, long-term outcome evaluation of the ISTAR Comprehensive Stuttering Program across Dutch and Canadian adults who stutter. *Journal of Fluency Disorders, 31,* 229–256.

Manning, W. H. (1999a). Progress under the surface and over time. In N. B. Ratner & E. C. Healey (Eds.), *Stuttering Research and Practice: Bridging the Gap* (pp. 123–129). Mahwah, NJ: Lawrence Erlbaum.

Starkweather, C. W. (1999). The effectiveness of stuttering therapy: An issue for science? In N. B. Ratner and E. C. Healey (Eds.), *Stuttering Research and Practice: Bridging the Gap* (pp. 231–244). Mahwah, NJ: Lawrence Erlbaum.

CHAPTER 12

Indicators of Successful Change Following Treatment

Speaking to people is not just a way of making a living for me; it's an affirmation of the ability that we all share to face an adversary or challenge without fear. And I enjoy it every bit as much as I enjoyed competing in basketball. . . . As I've traveled across the country telling my story and trying to get people to draw on their own inner strength and to fight to realize their dreams, I've received as many compliments, as much praise, as I ever received in basketball. While it's seldom publicized and not as dramatic as being chosen to play in an NBA All-Star game or having my jersey retired, it's every bit as rewarding as anything I experienced on the basketball court. (p. 198)

Bob Love (2000). The Bob Love Story.
Chicago, IL: Contemporary Books.

Chapter Objectives

The objectives of this final chapter are to consider the critical issue of maintaining the changes that have taken place during the formal therapy experience and to respond to the possibility of relapse, a circumstance that is common to many human conditions. Following a period of successful intervention for a problem (or instruction to achieve a level of skill or fitness) it is common for a person to experience some degree of regression to a pretherapy level. How might we conceptualize such regression and what is the probability of a brief lapse or a more profound and longer-lasting relapse taking place? A further objective of this chapter is to describe ways of predicting a relapse or, conversely, the likelihood of long-term enhancement of the desirable behavioral skills and cognitive problem-solving and coping abilities that have been achieved. Drawing on the suggestions of experienced clinicians, a variety of maintenance activities are suggested and the empowering effect of support groups is emphasized.

Recovery or Successful Management?

Is it realistic to think of adolescents and adults *recovering* as a result of treatment for fluency disorders? Although young children are more likely to recover with little or no memory of having stuttered, it may be more reasonable to think of older speakers as undergoing an evolving process of successful management, as is often the case with other complex human problems. Although investigators of treatment efficacy and relapse indicate that substantial changes take place during treatment for the majority of people, a review of this literature suggests that, with many important exceptions, relatively few people who stutter into adulthood become completely spontaneous and fluent speakers. Having stuttered for decades, the evolution of new ways of speaking and thinking are going to take some practice and adjustment (and as discussed in Chapter 3, time to reorganize cortical and subcortical neural functioning). Even for individuals who attain fluent speech there are likely to be some residual effects in the form of avoidance and anxiety related to communicating. Nearly all autobiographical accounts written by people who have undergone successful treatment contain descriptions of the long-term effects of being a person who stutters (e.g., Chmela, 1998; Daly, 1998; Johnson, 1930; Krall, 1998; Manning, 1991b, 1998; Murray & Edwards, 1980; Quesal, 1998; Ramig, 1998; St. Louis, 1998). Nevertheless, these effects can be countered with vigilance, practice, support, and continued expansion of fluency and communication skills. It is also important to emphasize that many speakers report a variety of positive effects from being someone who has spend several years journeying through life as a person who stutters. These speakers genuinely appreciate the fluency they have earned and enjoy their ability to communicate with others. The lessons learned from successfully coping with adversity are applied to other aspects of their lives. In addition, there are many examples of individuals who, having stuttered during the earlier decades of their lives, are able to become highly accomplished communicators and successful public speakers.

The ability to successfully manage stuttering is similar to other areas of clinical intervention where relapse is a common phenomenon such as drug addiction, alcoholism, weight reduction, smoking cessation, and marital problems (Lefcourt, 1976). For example, one-year success rates for intensive smoking-cessation programs range from 20% to 40%. For nonintensive interventions, success rates range from 10% to 20% (DiClemente, 1993). On a somewhat more optimistic note, a review of the relapse literature by Craig (1998) indicates that relapse for individuals with addictive disorders have decreased from

70% by 12 months post-intervention in the 1960s and 1970s to 12-month rates of 40%–60% in the 1990s. This improvement has been attributed to the incorporation of anti-relapse programs, including follow-up programs, enhancement of self-efficacy, and involvement with self-help support groups.

After formal treatment is concluded the process of change becomes self-directed. This informal or maintenance phase of the process for the adult who stutters may continue for the rest of the speaker's life. During maintenance, the person who stutters must be ready to accept full responsibility for self-management, a role that should be considered as early as possible during formal treatment. Because subsequent self-directed maintenance is by far the longest stage in the therapeutic process—typically with little or no contact with a clinician or researcher—it is a part of the process that is least understood. The emphasis for the speaker is on the consolidating the gains of therapy, coping with relapse, and the continuing evolution of the speaker's ability to live an agentic life style.

Our Limited View of Change

As discussed in Chapter 1, student clinicians rarely have the opportunity to observe speakers for more than one or two semesters. As a result, students are apt to see only a small window of the behavioral and cognitive changes that are taking place for the speaker. Professional clinicians will also see a relatively small window of change if they have little or no contact with the individual following the termination of treatment, a time when significant lifestyle changes are likely to occur. Certainly some people do maintain contact with their clinician, but mostly—as Van Riper (1973) points out—these are clients who need additional help. The majority go off on their own, leaving the clinician with no idea about their progress over the years. Boberg (1981, 1986) was one of the first clinical researchers to recognize this problem and suggested that comprehensive clinical programs should have a system for assisting the client in the maintenance of clinical gains as well as providing refresher programs emphasizing client self-management of cognitive and attitudinal changes.

One of the major considerations as the speaker begins the period of self-management following successful therapeutic change is the possibility of relapse. This is especially true during the first few months or years following the termination of formal intervention. It is during this time when the ability of the speaker to perform self-directed change determines the ultimate effectiveness of the formal therapy experience. To the listener, relapse is likely to be first observed in the surface features of the problem in terms of the quantity and quality of the speaker's fluency. However, for the speaker, relapse begins with the return of the old and ingrained responses of fear and avoidance. Thus, just as the assessment of stuttering is multidimensional, the determination of the speaker's ability to maintain change must be multidimensional as well. Concentration on a single feature such as the frequency of stuttering tends to exclude the important affective and cognitive features of the problem, features that those who stutter perceive as vital (Krauss-Lehrman & Reeves, 1989, 1970; Yaruss et al., 2002; Reeves, 2006; St. Louis, 2006; Yaruss, Quesal, & Murphy, 2002). In any case, maintenance of the many changes that take place during formal treatment is apt to be somewhat more difficult when the client is on his or her own doing battle against a long history of stuttering and the well-learned coping techniques that have been relied on for years.

Transfer and Maintenance

Of the three basic stages of treatment—establishment of fluency, transference of new abilities to extra-treatment speaking situations, and maintenance of the new abilities following formal treatment—maintenance is typically regarded as the most challenging aspect of the treatment process (Boberg, 1981). Maintenance is burdensome for the client, for he or she is working against many forces that are pulling in the direction of pretreatment performance and cognition.

Maintenance is often enigmatic for the clinician because it is often difficult to maintain contact with the client. Even when some form of contact is maintained, there are practical and ethical issues that make it difficult to obtain accurate data concerning post-treatment performance. Maintenance of the changes achieved during informal treatment will be more likely to occur if, during the period of formal treatment, the clinician has provided opportunities that enable the client to focus on the transfer of cognitive, affective, and behavioral changes to a variety of speaking experiences beyond the treatment setting. As Gregory points out, "The essence of effective therapy is transfer" (1995, p. 199). It is unnecessary to wait until the speaker achieves partial or complete fluency in the treatment environment before taking the speech to the street. Most people can benefit from these activities from the outset of treatment. Early on, the speaker can begin the process of becoming desensitized to a wide variety of environmental stimuli that have elicited habitual coping patterns of avoidance and fear. The clinician can help the speaker to successfully predict and identify listener reactions. Experiences in speaking situations beyond the immediate therapy environment can help the speaker to self-monitor and eventually vary the characteristic behavioral patterns of their stuttering. Something as basic as a tape recorder can function as a stimulus for achieving success in extra-treatment speaking situations (Howie, Woods, & Andrews, 1982). Of course, a most powerful stimulus for providing the speaker with cues and support in daily speaking situations is the participation of the clinician. Objects (books, games, work-related items) and individuals (family members, friends, colleagues) that are brought to the treatment setting can serve as powerful discriminative stimuli that help to cue the client for achieving success when he or she ventures beyond the treatment room.

As discussed in earlier chapters, the lack of homogeneity among clients is a major variable that contributes to the variable effects of treatment. This lack of client, as well as environmental, homogeneity may also help to explain the difficulty of successful speaker maintenance following treatment. For example, Boberg (1986) suggested that differences in long-term progress are as likely to be due to personality factors and the ability of the clients as they are to the nature of the treatment program or even the quality of the clinician. Huinck et al. (2006) provided support for this suggestion with an investigation of 25 adults who underwent intensive treatment in the Comprehensive Stuttering Program (CPS; Boberg and Kully, 1985). They classified speakers as severe or mild (based on the Stuttering Severity Instrument, Riley, 1980) and three measures of emotional and cognitive reactions to their stuttering. Although the speakers rated as severe made larger treatment gains than speakers who were classified as mild, they also demonstrated higher levels of regression during follow-up one and two years later. These results support the idea that individuals with mild stuttering are likely to profit most from treatment that helps them put their stuttering into perspective and decreases negative emotions and cognitions, while those with more severe profiles may first need to focus on reducing stuttering.

The Nature of Regression and Relapse

By discussing the nature of relapse with the client and preparing him or her for the possibility of regression, is the clinician creating a self-fulfilling prophecy? If the topic of regression is never mentioned, is relapse less apt to occur? Or does the clinician have an obligation to prepare the client for something that, in some form at least, is likely to happen? The literature consistently indicates that for adult speakers, some degree of relapse is a possibility following successful treatment and that the clinician is responsible for preparing the client to respond to it if it occurs.

Many authors have recognized relapse as a common event following treatment for adults who stutter (Bloodstein & Bernstein Ratner, 2008; Craig, 1998; Kuhr & Rustin, 1985; Martin, 1981; Perkins, 1979; Silverman, 1981; Van Riper, 1973). Prins (1970) found that about 40% of clients taking part in an intensive residential program experienced some regression following treatment. Although Prins noted that clients believed that maximum regression occurred within six months after the termination of formal treatment, other writers have suggested that clients should be followed for at least two to five years following formal treatment (Bloodstein & Bernstein Ratner, 2008; Conture & Guitar, 1992;

Young, 1975). Martin (1981) reviewed the literature and estimated relapse at approximately 30%. Craig and Hancock (1995) found that 71.7% of 152 adults surveyed experienced relapse but that the majority found that they subsequently regained fluency. Craig and Hancock also noted that relapse tended to be cyclical, occurring up to three times in a year.

Cooper (1977) views relapse as part of the human condition. Silverman (1981) suggests that relapse is likely to occur with a 40% to 90% probability. A survey of members of the National Stuttering Association support group by Yaruss et al. (2002) found that 40 of the 67 respondents (59.7%) indicated that they did not maintain their fluency after treatment (regardless of the treatment approach) and that 35 (52.2%) stated that they were not able to achieve the same fluency in daily life as they did in the treatment room. Van Riper states, "Relapses and remissions are the rule, not the exception, for the adult stutterer if long-term follow-up investigations are conducted" (1973, p. 178). St. Louis and Westbrook report that "relapse is a ubiquitous and familiar problem in stuttering therapy" (1987, p. 252). Perkins states that "maintenance of fluency is the perennial weak link in the therapeutic chain" (1979, p. 119) of stuttering treatment. Finally, as Bloodstein (1995) maintains, although we are adept at making people who stutter fluent, we know little about how to keep them that way.

Thus for most clients, some type of follow-up is necessary. The learning curve is long, and as Van Riper was fond of saying, our old habits are always the strongest. Clients should at least have the option of continuing treatment in some form for as long as they feel that it is necessary. This, of course, is not likely to happen if coming back to the clinic is viewed, by the clinician or the client, as an indication of failure. If learning how to successfully manage stuttering is viewed as a long-term process—which in the majority of cases it surely is—then the client returning for follow-up sessions is not a sign of failure. Rather, it is a natural and acceptable part of the process of change. Additional treatment, more than anything else, simply means that those involved are wise enough to recognize that they are likely to benefit from further effort and growth. Fortunately, many clients do not require a return to intensive individual treatment. Often, group treatment sessions or support group meetings once or twice a month will enable many clients to get back on track and continue making progress.

Somewhat less is known about relapse for children or adolescents. Craig et al. (1996) followed 97 children (aged 9–14) for one year post-treatment and found that 3 of 10 children experienced relapse (2%SS). In a subsequent study, Hancock and Craig (1998) followed 77 of these same children in order to identify possible predictors of relapse (2%SS). A regression analysis indicated that only pretreatment %SS and immediate post-treatment trait anxiety were significant predictors (accounting for 14.4% and 8% of the variance, respectively). That is, children who stuttered to a greater degree prior to treatment were more likely to relapse, a finding similar to the more recent study by Huinck et al. (2006)

with adults. Surprisingly, the children who indicated higher immediate post-treatment measures of trait anxiety (within the normal range) were less likely to relapse. The authors concluded that perhaps the normal but heightened anxiety resulted in the children being more willing to work on their fluency skills. A variety of other variables (age and sex of the children, number of years stuttered, family history of stuttering) had little predictive value. Although we are unaware of any investigations of the phenomena, we have encountered many college-age students who, although they report what appeared to be successful treatment in the early elementary grades, experience an increase in stuttering behavior as they approach their early twenties.

Defining Relapse

Defining relapse following formal treatment is nearly as difficult as determining the severity of the stuttering at the outset. As Craig (1998) points out, a medical definition that defines relapse using an all-or-none criterion (the presence or absence of a disease) clearly does not work well for stuttering. An all-or-none criterion may be used for some addictive behaviors (such as setting a threshold of total abstinence for the use of alcohol or cigarettes). However, it is clear that most people who stutter will have residual attitudes and behaviors following treatment, and zero stuttering is not likely to be the case.

However, many investigators who have studied relapse in stuttering have used the presence of overt stuttering as the one—and often the only—measure of relapse. Some investigators have considered the percentage of syllables stuttered (%SS) and have used a relapse criteria of 2% SS (Craig, Franklin, & Andrews, 1984; Craig & Hancock, 1984; Evesham & Fransella, 1985) or 4% SS (Boberg, 1981). Blood (1995) and Ladouceur, Caron, and Caron (1989) used 3% SS to define treatment success. If the focus of change is going to be on the frequency of stuttering, perhaps a better approach is to consider follow-up fluency levels in terms of both pre- and immediate post-treatment fluency levels (adding 3% to follow-up percentages to account for expected regression) as suggested by Langevin et al. (2006) (see Chapter 11).

As we have suggested, the frequency of stuttering is usually not the initial or only indicator of regression. As Van Riper stated, "Stuttering does not mean relapse. Another moment of fear is no catastrophe" (1973, p. 209). Changes in the attitudinal and cognitive aspects of the problem, often in the form of negative self-talk, may take the lead in the progression of relapse. As an example, Craig and Hancock (1995) found that adults with significantly raised levels of trait anxiety were three times more likely to experience relapse. When elements of avoidance and fear begin to multiply and increasingly influence the speaker's decision making, overt stuttering will not be far behind. Recognizing the great variability of stuttering frequency and the variability of fluency across different speaking situations, Craig and Calver (1991) defined relapse as "stuttering to a degree which was not acceptable to yourself for at least a period of one week" (p. 283), a definition that is probably more realistic and functional than many others.

Relapses may take many forms and may range from brief periods that are mildly irritating to long episodes that are extremely handicapping. The clinician may be able to determine that the client has reached the threshold of a relapse based on observable affective, behavioral, and cognitive aspects of the problem. However, the presence and degree of relapse are probably best determined by the speaker. When speakers get to the point where they believe they are no longer confident of managing their speech on their own or their decisions are increasingly based on the possibility of stuttering, relapse has reached a clinical level. At that point, it is both reasonable and desirable to seek additional professional help.

Possible Causes of Relapse

While describing the shadow side of implementing change, Egan (2007) briefly discusses the idea of "entropy," the tendency of things to break down or fall apart. Applied to humans who are attempting therapeutic or self-directed change, this may be thought of as the tendency to give up on a course of action that has been initiated, something we have all experienced. We intend to lose some weight, we get in a little better shape and then we fall back a bit . . . or maybe a lot. As we begin a process of learning and change, the actions we are taking seem reasonable, often exciting as we hope for success in the endeavor. However, with the routine requirements of hard work, enthusiasm fades and a lack of time and other priorities soon interfere. As Egan describes, we are distracted or become discouraged and flounder. Citing Brownell et al. (1986), he makes the important distinction between the clinician preparing clients for the mistakes they may make and "giving them permission" to make mistakes and implying that they are inescapable. Perhaps even more important, he suggests that there is a critical distinction between a "lapse" (a slip or a mistake) and a "relapse" (a complete cessation of a program of change). A minor regression of earlier confidence and performance does not need to result in a relapse. Finally, Egan comments that the idea that accepting that entropy is common and expected is not a defeatist attitude, it is realism. "Attrition, noncompliance, and relapse are the name of the game" (2007; p. 352); and as clinicians, we should recognize this. Despite a lapse or even a relapse, the speaker, with the assistance of the clinician, can choose what is necessary to keep moving in the desired direction.

Silverman (1981) suggested a number of possible reasons for relapse. Clients who are especially likely to relapse are those who, following treatment, believe themselves to be cured. Believing they have experienced a cure, they are less likely to continue the rigorous process of self-management. Other clients may regress as they come to lose confidence in the treatment program, something that is more apt to occur if they have experienced relapse following previous treatment experiences. As Silverman points out, people tend to expect events to replicate themselves.

Another possible reason for relapse may be that the clinician and the client have thresholds for fluency breaks that are too liberal. In this case, small fluency breaks are accepted and left unchanged. Relapse is also more likely to occur if clients are released from treatment too soon, although just how soon is "too soon" is difficult to assess. It may be worthwhile seeing the client through at least one period of relapse while the support of the clinician is still available. For some speakers, the return of stuttering at some level may be acceptable if it has been the norm for decades. In some cases the presence of stuttering can provide an escape from responsibilities, including work. This probably does not occur enough to explain relapse in most people, but, no doubt, it is one force that can nudge the client back into old, reflexive coping patterns. Disruptive life events may sap the motivation and strength for continued self-management. Daly, Simon, and Burnett-Stolnack (1995) suggest that this may be especially true for adolescents where an emotional crisis precipitates the loss of self-esteem and negatively impacts fluency. As Daly, et al. indicate, adolescent clients are likely to see many negative events, be they social-, academic-, or treatment-related, as catastrophic.

Neurophysiological Loading

For many years, researchers who have studied the etiology, spontaneous recovery, and relapse for subjects with fluency disorders have suggested that some of these speakers possess an underlying physiological or neurophysiological condition (Boberg, 1986; Moore & Haynes, 1980; Perkins, Kent, & Curlee, 1990; Zimmerman, 1980, 1981). The findings from recent neuroimaging studies described in Chapter 3 provide examples of anatomical and physiological differences in adults as well as some children who stutter. Although the implications of these findings are not yet clear, they indicate that at least some individuals who stutter may be working with cortical and subcortical systems that do not readily facilitate speech fluency. The possibilities of such differences may be especially likely for clients with "genetic loading" who have a family history of stuttering. Longitudinal studies by Yairi and Ambrose (2005) have supported earlier suggestions by perceptive clinicians concerning the likelihood of genetic factors in the recovery from or the persistence of stuttering (Boberg, 1986; Sheehan & Martyn, 1966). It may also be that some speakers are genetically predisposed to relapse (Cooper, 1972; Neaves, 1970).

The Natural Variability of Fluency

In Chapters 4 and 5 we discuss how the variability of fluency may make it difficult to diagnose stuttering and to predict future levels of fluency. Kamhi (1982) points out that some people who stutter must expend considerably more effort than others to achieve and maintain fluency, due to the natural variability of their speech-production systems. For some speakers, such variability (including relapses) is more common and perhaps more severe. Kamhi suggests that knowing the stimuli that are likely to induce stress, the speaker can learn to predict and successfully manage these occurrences. The higher the level of fluency desired, the more work is usually required. A related theme is the levels of pretreatment severity estimates. Regardless of how such estimates are made—whether simply estimates of stuttering frequency or a combination of frequency measurements with indicators of various cognitive and behavioral responses to stuttering—investigators typically find that pretreatment severity is a good predictor of post-treatment regression (Eichstaedt, Watt, & Girson, 1998; Huinck et al., 2006).

Speaking in a Nonhabitual Manner

As described in Chapter 11, authors have frequently pointed out that the treatment techniques associated with many treatment protocols result in increased fluency by encouraging the person to speak in a nonhabitual and unnatural manner. Boberg (1981) suggests that, in many ways, the requirements of practicing self-management techniques can be a highly punishing experience that results in a loss of spontaneity. Although altered ways of speaking typically result in rapid increases in fluency, it takes concentration and effort to attain what are clearly nonhabitual respiratory, phonatory, and articulatory patterns. A review of the research on the measurement of speech naturalness for stuttering speakers by Schiavetti and Metz (1997) suggested that some speakers who achieved stutter-free speech sounded as unnatural after treatment as they had prior to treatment. For many years, experienced clinicians have suggested that such techniques tend to have only a temporary impact on a speaker's fluency (Bloodstein, 1949, 1950; Boberg, 1981; Van Riper, 1973, 1990). If the only changes that are emphasized during treatment are the client's speech rate and the related improvement in fluency, it may explain the reasonably high occurrence of relapse with this treatment strategy (Silverman, 1981). Moreover, if, following treatment, the client's speech sounds and feels unnatural and lacks spontaneity, the effects of these changes are not likely to last in the long term (Boberg, 1986; Kalinowski, Nobel, Armson, & Stuart, 1994; Schiavetti & Metz, 1997).

Starke (1994) further points out that the use of artificial speech can also result in prosodic distortion. Although the altered ways of producing speech may promote fluency in a technical sense, they may also result in messages being misperceived. Because of the altered prosody, there is a distinct possibility of a distortion in the speaker's communicative intentions and the relationship between the speaker and the listener, an effect Starke terms "message incompatibility conflict" (1994). Although the speaker may no longer be stuttering in his typical manner, the pragmatics of human communication may suffer unless the listener is able to understand that speech modification techniques are being used.

The Commitment to Ongoing Self-Management

Once formal treatment is concluded, the speaker is likely to feel both internal as well as external pressure to maintain an improved level of fluency. This pressure may be particularly true if the speaker has attended an intensive program away from home and family. Upon returning home, there are apt to be subtle (as well as many not-so-subtle) expectations for the speaker to consistently display their new and much-improved fluency. The occurrence of sporadic stuttering may be viewed as an immediate sign of failure by some ("How awful. After all this time, effort, and money and he still stutters!"). Although many individuals can show much-improved fluency, the fear of even a single fluency break can be immense. One good response to the pressure of others to be fluent when they say such things as, "Your speech is wonderful now that you've had therapy. You don't stutter at all any more, do you?" might be to say something like, "Wwwwell, I'm do-do-doing my best!" (Van Riper, 1971).

Throughout this text we have proposed that success in the treatment of stuttering is possible on many levels. Nevertheless, it must also be stated that changing the surface and intrinsic features of stuttering usually takes considerable effort and time. This effort is apparent throughout the sometimes arduous process of formal treatment. However, for the treatment process to be effective and functional in the longer term, continuing effort and vigilance must occur. As Cooper (1977) points out, it takes a good deal of psychic energy to maintain success. To the extent that treatment results in stuttering that no longer presents a major problem to the speaker, the person may choose decide to devote his finite time and energies to other issues and concerns. Just as students will need to adapt and develop the ideas and techniques they learned during their academic program(s), the person who has undergone fluency treatment will need to elaborate their response to the fact that they have been, or to some degree continue to be, a person who stutters.

There are many reasons why speakers make the choice not to use techniques introduced during treatment. Crichton-Smith (2002) noted that some speakers feel that the effort that must be expended to modify their speech competes with their ability to focus on what it is they want to communicate. This is especially likely to be the case in the early stages of behavioral variation and modification as well as maintenance of these techniques following therapy. It is not surprising that the additional disruption to the linguistic process required by these techniques may not be worth the effort. Crichton-Smith also points out that many therapeutic techniques (and clinicians) overly emphasize the production of fluency, thereby inadvertently promoting the concealment of stuttering, possibly setting the stage for relapse (Sheehan, 1982). This may be especially true for programs that emphasize the achievement of fluency without attending to the cognitive and attitudinal aspects of change (Yaruss et al. 2002). Upon asking a total of 67 individuals about their experiences following treatment, Yaruss et al. found that those who had experienced only fluency-shaping approaches were more likely to report that they had experienced a relapse ($p = .037$) or that treatment was unsuccessful ($p = 0.045$) than those who had taken part in stuttering modification, avoidance reduction, or combined approaches.

Integrating the New Speaking Role—Altering Core Constructs

Joseph Sheehan often commented that for therapy to be successful in the long term the person must eventually make the adjustment of viewing him- or herself as something other than an individual who stutters. For this to occur, Sheehan suggested that the speaker must integrate a new and unfamiliar role as a fluent speaker and "wash the stutterer aspect out of the self-concept" (1970, p. 8). This proposal parallels the frequent comments throughout this text about the principle described in Chapter 8 concerning the value of cognitive restructuring. Still, separating from a self-concept shaped by many years of living the experience of stuttering can be a formidable challenge, as described by the late Marty Jezer, author, and a person who stuttered:

> The potential for stuttering, the fact that we might stutter in the next sentence even though the sentence we are speaking is perfectly fluent, is why so many of us who stutter think of ourselves as stutterers even when we are not stuttering. It would seem, then, that part of our problem lies in how we perceive ourselves as speakers more than in how our listeners react to us when we speak. A stutterer who isn't stuttering may not be a stutterer to the people listening to him, especially if they don't know him. But a stutterer who isn't stuttering often still feels that he is a stutterer, because he knows that fluency is fleeting and stuttering may happen the next time he opens his mouth. (Jezer, 1997, p. 18)

It is not surprising that at the heart of many models of therapeutic and self-directed change is the ability of people to evolve and develop new core constructs about themselves and their possibilities (Boberg, Howie, & Woods, 1979; Dalton, 1987, 1994; Emerick, 1988; Evesham & Fransella, 1985; Fransella, 1972; Fransella & Dalton, 1990; Hayhow & Levy, 1989). Kuhr and Rustin (1985) noted, for example, that following treatment, those clients who were most satisfied with their fluency also made lifestyle changes at many levels. Of course, it takes some time to change habitual coping responses to many old and powerful stimuli. As Fransella (1972) suggests, the speaker is better able to predict how events will transpire when in the role of a person who stutters and, in many instances, less able to predict events when speaking fluently. As Dalton (1987) explains, at some level, the speaker makes a "choice" to stutter, not because he prefers to do so in the usual sense, but because it is what is familiar and consistent with how he understands his world. Given the individual's experience and interpretation of events, the choice is not abnormal. As discussed in Chapter 7, individuals who stutter have learned how to cope and survive in response to emotions such as threat, fear, anxiety, guilt, and hostility. Letting go of such coping responses is difficult. As we have also stressed, it is not likely to happen without the understanding and support of others, including an empathetic clinician.

Given these changes in a person's core constructs, it is not unusual for speakers who have undergone successful treatment to express some anxiety, possibly even vague feelings of guilt, concerning their new fluency. Kuhr and Rustin (1985) found evidence of minor depression in several fluent speakers following treatment. Speakers sometimes express surprise that they are not as content as they thought they would be with their fluency. They may indicate that, on occasion, they feel that they are deceiving others or feel that they are not being themselves. Their unaccustomed fluency and all the responsibility for self-management that comes along with it has changed the self they have grown up with. Even though the speaker enjoys being fluent and feels that the fluency is earned, there may be the sensation of waiting for the other shoe to fall and the tendency to wonder, "Yes, I'm fluent now. But what happens if I lose it?"

The "meaningfulness" of these changes to an individual's core constructs is illustrated by the following quote:

> My hands were trembling as I began. . . . I felt very much alone. So great was my fear that I seemed to go into a trance. It was a kind of out-of-body experience: a fluent person seemed to be speaking out of my mouth. I heard his words, but they did not come from me. When I was finished, the teacher complimented me for my fluency and for my courage. I think the class may even have applauded—not in sarcasm but in appreciation for my triumph and also, I imagine, in relief. My feeling of success was fleeting, however, as at my Bar Mitzvah, I had somehow been fluent. But my fluency mystified me. There was no way to remember how I felt being fluent, because my fluency did not seem to come from me. I was beginning to fear fluency. I knew myself when I was stuttering. But I felt estranged from myself when I was fluent. (Jezer, 1997, p. 108).

While the new fluency may be enjoyable to the listener, it will not always feel comfortable to the speaker, at least not immediately. As Williams (1995) explains from the perspective of personal construct theory, even when fluent, speakers are attempting to gain evidence of support for their new construct of themselves and their world. Individuals are now acting in ways that are not congruent with their long-held view of themselves. It will take some time for the speaker, as well as others in their environment, to adjust to the speaker's new way of communicating and interacting with others.

As described in Chapters 7 and 8, in his theory of personal constructs, Kelly (1955) proposes that cognitive anxiety results from a person's awareness that the events they are experiencing are beyond the comfort level of their system of personal constructs. Consequently, the person is unable to meaningfully integrate and predict the course of events. Recall also that Fransella (1972) proposed that individuals who stutter fail to integrate experiences of fluent speech because the *fluent speaker role* tends to lack any meaningful, predictive quality. DiLollo, Manning, and Neimeyer (2003) found support for Fransella's perspective and the importance of altering the meaningfulness of the fluent-speaker role and thus one's core constructs. DiLollo et al. determined the cognitive anxiety of 29 adults who stuttered (21 males, 8 females, average age of 30.0 years) and a matched group of fluent speakers (21 males, 8 females, average age of 29.1 years). Using content analysis procedures and an adaptation of a *Cognitive Anxiety Scale* (Viney & Westbrook, 1976). DiLollo et al. found that the stuttering individuals demonstrated significantly higher levels ($p < 0.05$) of cognitive anxiety (and hence reduced meaningfulness) for their *fluent speaker role* compared to their *stutterer role*. Measures of cognitive anxiety indicated that both the stuttering and fluent-speaker groups had integrated the dominant speaker role as a "core construct" and that those speaking experiences that ran counter to this role were ignored or discounted. For example, much like the earlier passage by Jezer (1997), the speakers who stuttered typically expressed the view that periods of fluent speech were an "accident" or a "fluke." Two examples from DiLollo et al. provide examples of such interpretations from individuals who stutter in their descriptions of fluent speech.

> Okay, so when is this gonna all come falling down on me? Okay, when am I gonna? I always knew that my speech pattern would get worse and would, you know, begin to struggle again eventually. So I was sort of waiting for, you know. I still have the fears. Let's just say that. I have the fear of speaking and all that. Because I knew eventually that my fluent day or my fluent time of speaking was going to be over soon." (p. 179)

> "Well once again, I'm not fluent. However, I think the way I react to people or the way I did when I had my fluent, my lucky fluency, I kinda felt like

I was one of them and I guess, and it was kinda interesting to be able to talk amongst them without having any difficulty." In this example, the speaker specifically stopped and revised his utterance to include the defensive term "lucky fluency." (p. 179)

The results of DiLollo et al. (2003) indicate the importance of addressing the meaningfulness of the "dominant" speaker role during therapy for people who stutter. Accordingly, an important goal of treatment for individuals who stutter is to assist them in "desconstructing" the dominant role of a *stuttering speaker* in order to begin meaningful integration of fluent speaking experiences and the nondominant *fluent speaker role* into their construct systems. Indications of speakers' reconstruction of their core constructs may be noted by a reduction of statements that defend or protect their *stuttering speaker* role. As suggested by the results of DiLollo et al. (2003) and Williams (1995), individuals who stutter may be attempting to validate their stuttering predictions, even when experiencing considerable achievement in producing fluent speech.

A hallmark of individuals who have achieved successful management of their stuttering is a change from concerns about protecting the self and others to more agentic and approach-oriented strategies. Using a grounded theory procedure, Plexico and Manning (2008a, b) drew on the literature on human coping response to stressors in order to investigate patterns of coping for nine adults who stuttered. Because the speakers believed stuttering to be an uncontrollable and shameful attribute, undesirable coping responses included (1) preventing and (2) escaping from stuttering in order to protect the speaker and assuage the listener. In contrast, more desirable coping responses took the form of (1) speaker elaboration of themselves and their capabilities and (2) the implementation-approach behaviors associated with self-directed behavioral and cognitive goals. That is, successful coping responses involved putting aside self-protection and concern for possible listener reactions and increased interest in their own personal goals and agentic behavior. These changes can be enormous and occur on many levels, and it takes some time for everyone, speakers and listeners alike, to adjust to the many implications of these changes.

A good example of an individual's evolving core constructs are the comments of Alan Badmington and his response to questions about his paper on the 2006 International Stuttering Awareness Day (ISAD) Interactive Computer Conference. The title of his paper was "Technology: A friend or foe of someone who stutters." In response to a question from one of the conference participants, Alan, a retired policeman from Wales, UK, and now a highly successful public speaker, described how, in his fifties he began to change his approach to managing his stuttering (see the following box for Alan's response).

Clinical **Insight**

What influenced me to abandon the Edinburgh Masker [a voice-activated device that provided white noise to both ears of the speaker] and cease avoidances? It's no secret that I knew virtually nothing about stuttering until relatively recent times. Although I had stuttered from childhood, I had absolutely no insight into what was happening. No-one told me. Prior to the advent of the Internet, dissemination of information was relatively sparse.

On April 1, 2000, I witnessed a group of PWS speaking, before an audience, about how they were dealing with their respective stuttering problems. The positive manner in which they spoke had a huge impact upon me (so much so, that I even remember the date). One, in particular, had developed into a successful public speaker. At the time, strange as it may seem, I was not aware of the existence of stuttering associations and had long given up on my stuttering. I was resigned to the fact that it would remain a problem for the rest of my days. Everything changed when I heard him speaking. When he addressed the audience, he was so assured, so confident and so in control of the situation. When he made reference to his public speaking activities and successes, I became even more interested. I wanted to be like him—I wanted to become a public speaker. He became my role model. For the very first time in my life, I believed that it was possible to deal with my stuttering difficulties. He was living proof of that "dream." When British athlete, Roger Bannister, ran the mile in less than four minutes back in the 1950's, the beliefs of other athletes changed overnight. Prior to his record-breaking performance, everyone considered it impossible to break the "four minute mile" barrier. He proved it could be done. Within a relatively short period, many other athletes were regularly achieving the same feat. Within a year, I understand that over 100 had, amazingly, achieved that "impossible" goal. The person I heard speaking became MY Roger Bannister and I shall be, forever, grateful to him for showing me what was possible. He was hugely instrumental in changing the direction of my life. On May 4, 2000 (that date is also indelibly imprinted upon my memory), I joined a particular program that encouraged non-avoidance and expansion of comfort zones. It provided me with a new speaking technique[1] and tools to deal with words that attracted an emotional charge, while also introducing me to the stuttering hexagon concept. This, together with a 24-hour support network, gave me the confidence to discard the mechanical crutch that had been an integral part of my life for more than 20 years. I felt that it was time to walk unaided. The rest is history, as they say—I have not looked back since. Somehow, the successes that I have attained after ceasing to use the Masker have tasted a little sweeter. I valued its assistance for

(continues)

---

[1]The technique(s) are part of the McGuire Program described later in this chapter.

two decades—without it, my life would have embraced so many more avoidance strategies. But, it was great to stand on my own two feet after such a lengthy time. When you achieve something that you, hitherto, considered impossible, it causes you to challenge your self-limiting beliefs. If we conquer something that has challenged our advancement, we grow in stature. That's exactly what I have done during the past six years.

Cited 11 October, 2006. Reprinted with permission of Alan Badmington. ©Alan Badmington 2006.

Listener Adjustment to the New Speaker

Because successful stuttering management also impacts the listener, it may be necessary for those in the client's daily environment to shift their perspective in order to establish a new equilibrium in the relationship. There will be changes in roles as the speaker no longer sees him- or herself in the primary role of a person who stutters (Sheehan, 1970). On occasion, others may not want to change. It is on such occasions that their participation in treatment is especially important. Kuhr and Rustin provide an example of just such a response. They described a wife who felt uncomfortable when her husband returned home with fluent speech, following successful in-patient treatment. His wife's reaction was a negative one, accusing the clinician by stating, "You took him away and made him fluent" (1985, p. 234). To the extent that others in the client's life fail to understand and recognize the nature of changes that are occurring, they will be less likely to understand, appreciate, and reinforce these changes. Near the end of and especially following treatment the responsibility for informing others about these important changes will most likely fall to the speaker. This is more likely to occur in a forthright and effective manner if speakers are desensitized about stuttering and have begun to incorporate their past experiences as a person who stutters into their evolving role as an effective communicator.

There are often many examples of successful adjustment by others in the client's life that contribute much to the continued pattern of growth. In the following example, the client is a middle-aged woman who has stuttered severely for most of her life and only recently began to make even the most routine telephone calls.

Clinician: You say you are beginning to make some of your own telephone calls now?

Client: Oh yes, sometimes I would answer calls when I was at home but I would never place calls. If there was a call that I felt I had to make I would ask my husband to do it.

Clinician: Are you finding that making the calls is becoming less anxiety-producing?

Client: Yes, at least some of them. The other thing that I've begun to do is make some of my husband's calls. You know . . . for things related to his business and our personal travel, airlines reservations and things like that.

Clinician: Wow, that's great. How does he like that?

Client: He thinks it great too. He's busy with his new job and he really appreciates it.

Predicting Long-Term Success

Researchers have found it difficult to predict long-term success following treatment, and there are many behavioral, cognitive, and environmental variables to consider. As discussed earlier, speakers who, based on several behavioral and cognitive indicators, are determined to be more severe prior to treatment show higher levels of regression one and two years later (Huinck et al., 2006). Given the many variables that influence long term change and the unique combination of factors for each speaker, the best approach to this issue is likely to be a multidimensional one. Andrews and Craig (1988), for example, provide support for such an approach. Using a combination of three factors, they found that 97% of the subjects who maintained high skill mastery (0% syllables stuttered), normal speech attitudes as indicated by such measures as the Modified Erickson Scale of Communication Attitudes (S-24) (Andrews & Cutler, 1974), and an internal locus of control as indicated by the Locus of Control of Behavior Scale (LCB) (Craig, Franklin, & Andrews, 1984) were able to maintain success. In fact, no speaker who failed to achieve any of these goals was able to maintain their post-treatment fluency level. Langevin et al. (2006) found that at two years post-treatment, the speakers classified as maintainers consistently had better scores on the S-24; the approach scale of the SESAS; and the struggle, avoidance, and expectancy subscales of the PSI than non-maintainers.

Using a correlation approach, Craig (1988) considered the relationship between %SS 10 to 18 months following treatment (an intensive fluency-shaping approach) and numerous pretreatment variables, including subject demographics (age, sex, and social status), stuttering severity (%SS), speech rate as measured in syllables per minute (SPM), health perceptions, self-reported avoidance and reaction to stuttering, neuroticism and extroversion, locus of control, formal practice, and attendance at self-help meetings, there were small to moderate correlations between follow-up %SS and pretreatment severity, %SS ($r = 0.424$) and SPM ($r = 0.515$). That is, those with greater stuttering and slower speech rates were more likely to stutter at follow-up. Finally, there was no single predictor variable that showed a strong correlation across the subjects.

In summarizing suggestions for preventing relapse and achieving long-term success following treatment, Craig suggests that success involves such things as practice of treatment activities and objectives that are achievable; using positive self-reinforcement; practicing self-monitoring skills; scheduling follow-up treatment; and emphasizing self-responsibility.

The Locus of Control of Behavior Scale (LCB) (Craig, Franklin, & Andrews, 1984) has been considered as a predictor of speakers' ability to maintain the success achieved during formal treatment. Using such a measure is intuitively appealing. Early in treatment, clients typically indicate that stuttering is something over which they have no control (Van Riper, 1982). As treatment programs assist the speaker in the self-management of speech behavior and a cognitive reinterpretation of his or her circumstances (Adams, 1983; Kuhr & Rustin, 1985), the person begins to internalize these changes (Boberg, Howie, & Woods, 1979). Craig, Franklin, and Andrews (1984) as well as Craig and Andrews (1985) demonstrated that changes in speakers' LCB scores toward more internal control during treatment are related to the long-term treatment outcome. In a related investigation, Madison, Budd, and Itzkowitz (1986) found that pretreatment locus of control (LOC) measures corresponded to the degree of change in stuttering following treatment for a group of 7- to 16-year-old children. That is, those children who had a more internal LOC prior to intervention tended to achieve more fluent speech during treatment. However, no significant relationship was found between pretreatment LOC scores and fluency levels during evaluations conducted at both two and six months following treatment. On the other hand, Ladouceur, Caron, and Caron (1989) found no relationship between LCB scores and fluency improvement in nine adults. Surprisingly, they found that some clients became more externally oriented during treatment while also acquiring increased fluency. Ladouceur et al. suggested that the changes in fluency and internal control—at least as gauged by the LCB and behavior—may have had to do with the treatment protocol used and whether or not cognitive changes were a focus of therapy.

Another attempt to predict long-term success using the LCB Scale was conducted by DeNil and Kroll (1994). They considered to what extent adult stutterers' scores on the LCB Scale (Craig, Franklin, & Andrews, 1984) are predictive of their ability to maintain speech fluency both immediately following intensive treatment and approximately two years later. Twenty-one subjects participated in a three-week intensive treatment program based on the Precision Fluency Shaping Program (Webster, 1975). Thirteen subjects who were contacted again two years later participated in a follow-up evaluation, which consisted of the administration of several scales, the reading of a brief passage, and a conversation with a research assistant. All participants were seen by an unfamiliar assistant who was unaware of their previous performance. Furthermore, the assessment took place in a new and unfamiliar location.

While the participants showed a significant long-term improvement in fluency, no predictive relationship was found between scores on the LCB scale and level of fluency, as measured in percent words stuttered, during either post-treatment or follow-up. LCB scores were, however, found to be predictive of the subjects' fluency self-evaluation measured post-treatment and at follow-up. The results of the investigation suggests that while the LCB may contribute to the prediction of the long-term treatment outcome, particularly as perceived by the client, other client and process variables also need to be considered. Although it remains to be seen, the individualized narrative analysis provided by the Pawns and Origins Scales (Westbrook & Viney, 1980) discussed in Chapters 4 may provide a more accurate prediction of long-term success.

The Importance of Support Groups

One of the more important influences on the long-term maintenance of treatment gains may be the client's involvement in self-help groups. Whether these groups are referred to as self-help, support, or advocacy groups, they all provide helpful sources of information and motivation for those who stutter as well as their families and friends. For speakers who have isolated themselves as a result of their stuttering, support groups are likely to be particularly valuable (see Crowe, 1997b). For the first time, the person finds that he or she is among others who share a common problem. The speaker finds that he or she is not alone and that this unique characteristic called stuttering that has, for so long, set him or her apart now provides a way to connect and bond with others. Although an empathetic clinician and successful treatment may promote dramatic decreases in isolation for a client, there is probably nothing as effective as a good support group for increasing people's ability to communicate and expand their world.

The meetings of the local support group chapters also furnish important opportunities to practice techniques and stabilize cognitive changes following formal treatment. The encouragement and support of the other members is difficult to underestimate and often results in enhanced motivation and assertiveness. Group membership can also provide an important social function for some of the members, fostering interaction in an accepting, penalty-free environment. It is a place where members can continue the process of coming to terms with the problem.

The development of self-help groups is closely related to the development and growth of consumerism in the 1960s (Hunt, 1987; Ramig, 1993b). Katz and Bender (1976) provide an often-cited definition (Hunt, 1987; Reeves, 2006) that is recognized by the World Health Organization: Such organizations are typically made up of volunteers who come together for mutual assistance and support in overcoming ". . . a common handicap or life-disrupting problem and

Clinical Insight

I believe that it is important for clinicians who are serious about assisting those who stutter to have the experience of attending at least one of the meetings of the support groups that meet in various cities around the country The largest of these groups in the United States are the National Stuttering Association and Friends. You will find that the experience is unique and distinctly different to any professional meetings you have attended. The primary goal is to provide support by being with others—to observe people as they "let go" of hiding and avoiding and to witness magnificent acts of courage. I'll describe two examples.

At a national meeting of Friends: The National Association of Young People Who Stutter, I wandered into an evening "jam session" where three talented members were playing guitars and inviting others to sing along. After an hour or so of singing, a young girl about 10 years old volunteered to sing a song. She slowly walked up to the front of the room and climbed up onto a stool. As she attempted to begin singing she found herself blocking severely, unable to achieve any airflow or voicing. She was determined to sing her song and attempted to begin many times as the audience patiently waited. Recognizing her plight, another young girl, who appeared to be about the same age, came up from the audience and sat next to her on another stool. They whispered to each other for a moment and then, together, they faced the audience. The second girl began singing the song and was immediately joined by first girl and they sang the song together. It was a wonderful moment and the audience gave them a prolonged standing ovation as they finished.

In the same city some 17 years earlier I attended my first national meeting of the National Stuttering Association. One of the traditional and well-attended events is an "open mike" session. A microphone on a stand is placed in the middle of a large room and people are invited to say whatever they would like. In this instance there were approximately 300 people in the room. Of course, courage is required for most any speaker in accepting such a challenge, but particularly for those who stutter. A few people lined up to take a turn speaking before the large audience, most of them for the first time in their lives. A young woman at the end of the line eventually moved forward to take her turn. She attempted to speak but was able to say only the initial portion of the first word. The audience remained completely silent. Again and again she continued to block on the initial syllable. More than a minute passed before she gradually turned around and with tears streaming down her face, began to walk back to her seat. From somewhere in the audience someone quietly said, "Go ahead," once, twice, and then again. Others quickly joined in and soon the entire audience was repeating "Go ahead!" The woman stopped, gradually turned around, and slowly approached the microphone again. After several more attempts she eventually said her name, explained how happy she was to be attending the meeting and thanked everyone for their support. She also received a standing ovation from the entire audience, many of whom by now also proudly displayed their own tears.

bring about desired social and/or personal change" (p. 141). Through newsletters, Internet discussions, and meetings, the groups provide a variety of members' needs, including the facilitation of personal change, fostering of personal responsibility by members, provision of information and advice, discussion of alternative treatments, fund-raising, and political activities relating to the goals of the group. Coming together with other people who have similar problems and goals is an empowering and exciting experience, and empathy and support from fellow travelers is all but assured. Importantly, this form of help can be obtained at relatively little cost. For all these reasons, Egan (1998) observes that self-help groups are one of the most popular sources of help for people with a variety of problems, and this is certainly the case for those who stutter.

In order to appreciate the nature of such groups, a brief history of two of them is provided here based on a description by Hunt (1987). The British Stammering Association (BSA) was founded in 1968. It is often the case in such groups that the initial development results from the efforts of one person (in this case, Robin Harrison) who is willing to dedicate many years of administrative, public relations, and fund-raising activities in order to get the group organized and functional. The age range of the membership in the BSA was generally from 25 to 40 years, with few teenagers. The average age of people in these groups is greater than those in treatment tends to be, where few clients over the age of 50 are typically found. The size of most local groups was 4 to 6 members, ranging from as small as 2 to a rarely exceeded upper limit of 12. The most common goal reported by individual chapters was to transfer and maintain techniques learned in formal treatment. Although group members often practiced treatment techniques during the meetings, much of the discussion centered on adjusting to the cognitive aspects of being a person who stutters, including fears, anxieties, and feelings of inferiority, powerlessness, and frustration. Hunt (1987) reports that this was especially true for groups with "more mature members" who had achieved some success in managing their speech.

Most of the local chapters tended to be short-lived, lasting for only one or two years. In order for a local group to continue for any length of time, strong leadership is essential. In addition, from time to time, the group needs to elicit the support of local speech-language pathologists for referrals as well as advice. Finally, as Hunt suggests, the group must discipline itself so that it will be more than a social group. It must have specific guidelines and objectives that focus on the self-management of communication and stuttering.

The largest self-help/mutual aid group in the United States is The National Stuttering Association (NSA). Originally founded by Michael Sugarman and Bob Goldman in 1977 and known for more than 20 years as the National Stuttering Project (NSP), the purpose of this group is to provide information and support to children, adolescents, and adults who stutter; their families; and professional clinicians. As Reeves (2006) explains, the NSP became the first truly national consumer-based organization in the USA for individuals who stutter. This was accomplished without professionals, but with no intention of alienating clinicians. The guiding principle of this group is reflected in their statement, "If you stutter, you are not alone." Participation in the NSA group has continued to expand and is composed of several thousand members throughout the United States and approximately 100 local chapters. NSA's monthly publication, *Letting Go*, is sent to all members and provides information and support in the form of informative articles, letters, stories, and reflections written by members. In addition, the NSA office produces news releases and public service announcements; coordinates regional workshops; and develops and distributes brochures, books, and videos. An informative website provides a wide variety of information as well as links to related organizations. All these activities, as well as an annual national convention of 500–600 adults, adolescents, and children who stutter and their families, are designed to educate, advocate, and instill a sense of solidarity and confidence in the members. Continuing education credits are also available for speech-language pathologists at many of the national meetings. The specific goals of NSA are to provide an opportunity for members to share with others their fears, frustrations, and triumphs; practice therapeutic techniques in a safe and supportive environment; take part in speaking experiences they would otherwise be likely to avoid; develop positive cognitive and affective strategies for managing their fluency disorder; and assist members in achieving these goals.

Undoubtedly the greatest virtue of support groups is the ability to provide members with a sense of relief from the feelings of isolation and establishment of contact with others who understand their distress and frustration (Hunt, 1987; Reeves, 2006). A survey conducted by Krauss-Lehrman and Reeves (1989) of 600 National Stuttering Project (NSP) members (142 questionnaires returned) indicated that the *least* important focus of the groups was to provide an adjunct to formal treatment. Ramig (1993b) surveyed 62 support group participants, finding that 49 indicated that their fluency had improved "at least somewhat" as a direct result of their involvement in such groups. More importantly, 55 of the 62 respondents indicated that their participation in support groups had an "at least somewhat positive" or a "very positive" impact on their daily life. The results also suggested that members had to attend something approaching 20 meetings for these changes to take place.

Individuals who stutter and are active members of the National Stuttering Association are somewhat unique among the many individuals who stutter. This is likely to be especially true for those who are able to attend the annual meeting of NSA. It may well be that these people have greater levels of motivation, time, and possibly the financial ability to travel to and attend such meetings. Nevertheless, a survey of 71 individuals who participated in the 1999 annual meeting by Yaruss, et al. (2002) indicated that participation had "very positively" affected their self-image and acceptance of themselves. Only 6.1% of the participants indicated no effect and no respondent indicated a negative impact.

There are a variety of interesting and important issues concerning the functioning of support groups and particularly their interaction with the professional community. For example, a description of self-help groups for individuals who stutter by Reeves (2006) describes a history of hostility regarding professional clinicians by some members of self-help groups. Some members felt (and in some instances rightly so) that they had received poor assistance by clinicians demonstrating a lack of knowledge and understanding about the nature of the stuttering experience. Ben-Ari (2002, as cited in Reeves, 2006) found that members of self-help groups under age 30 were less likely to desire collaboration with professionals than more mature members. As Reeves suggests, some of the younger individuals may have resented the fact that professionals were unable to "fix" them. On the other hand, the older members with more education and experience were more likely to value collaboration with professionals.

In turn, some professional clinicians have been leery of self-help groups and the possibility of some members spreading inaccurate and unhelpful information. In some cases, of course, there is the potential for the promotion of uninformed, inappropriate, or counterproductive attitudes, information, and techniques. However, Cooper (1987), Silverman (1996), and Ramig (1993b) have pointed out that some clinicians tend to have a skeptical view of support groups because they fail to understand the many positive aspects of group membership. Many clinicians recognize that support groups play an important, often critical role, in providing individuals with the support and encouragement essential for success both during and following treatment. It should also be pointed out that, as consumers of treatment services, self-help organizations provide a powerful and effective message to both professional and legislative groups for improved training and service delivery. In recent years there has been a positive and synergistic interaction of the major self-help groups in this country (NSA and Friends) and the professional community. Groups such as the International Stuttering Association (a self-help organization) and the International Fluency Association (a professional organization) have done much to bring together the two communities.

As suggested at the outset of this section, a professional clinician who is serious about understanding and assisting individuals who stutter should attend a local or national meeting of one of the major self-help groups. However, it is good to keep in mind some suggestions about the experience. Gregory (1997) points out that some professionals feel uncomfortable at self-help meetings and wisely suggests that clinicians adopt the role of a cautious consultant rather than turning the experience into a form of group therapy. At most, rather than telling members of the group what they should do, the sensitive clinician might better indicate some of the things that have seemed to work well for some of his or her clients. As Reeves (2006) puts it, "The key factor is whether the focus is on the sharing of experiential knowledge and support rather than professional directed therapy"(p. 260). He further suggests that professional clinicians should focus less on "fixing" or "curing" the person who stutters by eradicating all occurrences of stuttering (which he views as an erroneous expectation for both parties) and think more in terms of providing the opportunity for the person to heal.

The McGuire program (David McGuire) is an international program run by individuals who are recovering or have recovered from stuttering. More than a support group, the program provides a rationale and techniques for therapy provided by the members. Because the members are not professional speech-language clinicians, the philosophy and associated techniques have received little study and, thus, lack empirical support. However, the program incorporates many of the therapeutic goals (increased fluency, improved communication, and greater autonomy/agency) described in Chapter 7. That is, the activities and techniques of the program address not only speech and the achievement of fluency but also altering the many cognitive and affective aspects of the stuttering experience. Intended for persons age 16 or older, attendees of the four-day intensive workshops are offered a holistic approach that emphasizes effective communication and a lifestyle of assertiveness. The therapeutic principles discussed in Chapter 8 (moving toward the problem, assuming responsibility for action, restructuring the cognitive understanding of the self and the problem, and recruiting the support of others) are addressed in a variety of ways. There is also an appreciation of the role of humor when experimenting with new techniques in different settings. To combat the problem of relapse and in recognition that continual practice is necessary, the program includes a support system available to all participants. Comprehensive support in the form of a primary coach is provided for the 12 months following the intensive workshop. In addition, support is provided for the life of the individual and is international in scope, achieved via landline telephone, e-mail, and Skype™ communications software. Individuals are encouraged to attend follow-up workshops in order to consolidate skills and enhance their understanding of techniques, as well as to assist others. Graduates of the program carry cards with a checklist of principles emphasizing effort and perseverance and related techniques such as "do not use tricks and cancel violations; do not avoid words, sounds, or situations; respond (with breathing and speaking techniques) immediately and with great intensity to 'turbulence'; formulate before speaking; resist time pressure; establish eye contact; create air flow; time and coordinate breathing and articulation with forward movement and no holding back." Few programs have such an extensive and thorough system of member support and this undoubtedly contributes to the enthusiastic participation and increasing membership in the McGuire Program.

Maintenance Activities

A basic theme in therapeutic or self-directed change is the requirement that the individual (rather than the clinician) gradually take the major responsibility for identifying and modifying his or her own behaviors and attitudes concerning his or her situation (DiClemente, 1993; Egan, 2007). In the case of fluency disorders, the client must become increasingly sophisticated about stuttering in general, and about his or her own stuttering in particular. The speaker must be able to recognize his or her choices and behaviors and design responses for effectively coping and problem-solving. Moreover, in order for ongoing change to occur, the speaker must do the majority of his or her practice outside the context of the treatment setting. Formal training takes place for only a few hours each week, and changes are not likely to occur until the individual is disciplined enough to practice on his or her own. To the degree that a person does well beyond the treatment environment during formal treatment, he or she will be likely to do well in those same situations during the months and years of informal treatment.

The following is a compilation of suggestions presented by St. Louis and Westbrook (1987) and includes activities suggested by Van Riper (1958, 1973); Boberg (1983); Boberg and Kully (1984); Boberg and Sawyer (1977); Ryan (1979, 1980); Daly (1987); Dell (1980); Shames and Florance (1980); Howie, Tanner, and Andress (1981); St. Louis (1982); Williams, (1983); Craig (1998); and the current author.

- Clinicians should not be surprised when a client experiences a relapse.

- The clinician can stress that it is natural and expected for the client's quantity and quality of his or her fluency to swing from greater to lesser amounts and that this does not need to be interpreted as a disastrous event. Speakers can think of a relapse as a temporary "lapse" and an opportunity to recommit to using cognitive and behavioral techniques.

- The clinician can make it clear to the client that continued consultation and support are available following the termination of formal treatment. Returning to treatment is acceptable.

- Treatment intensity can vary and decrease gradually, with individual sessions gradually occurring less often. Individual treatment sessions may be supplemented or replaced by attendance at group meetings.

- Treatment can be transformed from face-to-face meetings to contact via the telephone, the Internet, and video and audio recordings.

- Recordings made during treatment by the speaker can be used to engender practice and encouragement in the person's home environment.

- Prior to dismissal from formal treatment, the clinician and client can consider the reasons for and indications of relapse and design specific coping responses.

- The speaker can join and become an active member of a national support group for children and adults who stutter, possibly assuming a leadership role.

- Following formal treatment, the speaker can assertively seek new and challenging speaking situations where the envelope of comfort can gradually be expanded. If professional or social contacts do not provide such opportunities, the client may join groups such as Toastmasters or Dale Carnegie.

- The speaker may contact local groups and organizations to talk about his or her interests and professional experiences. Libraries are often interested in finding such speakers.

- The speaker may consider contacting local agencies that need volunteers to read newspapers or books on tape to older people who cannot read or to the blind.

- The speaker can expand his or her assertive and risk-taking behaviors for both speech and nonspeech activities, expanding and cultivating other talents and interests.

- The speaker can continue to reassess opportunities for changes in his or her lifestyle, including possible alteration of interpersonal, vocational, and social roles.

- The speaker can continue to improve and expand on a variety of nonspeaking skills that are likely to enhance his or her participation in life and his or her interaction with others.

- The speaker can continue to monitor and evaluate his positive–negative self-talk, using the stopping and positive redirection activities.

- The speaker can practice the use of positive affirmations on a regular basis.

- The speaker can take part in cognitive-behavioral techniques that decrease anxiety and fear of social interactions.

- Individuals can be taught to identify potentially high-risk situations regarding lifestyle, negative moods, or threatening environments and develop methods of coping with these situations.

- The client can volunteer to work in a treatment setting with adults and children who stutter.

- The client can read selections of the Stuttering Foundation of America's Advice to those who stutter (Publication No. 9) and practice the suggestions contained in the chapters.

Clinical Insight

Adult male, age 53: Basically, I want to share that striving for perfection impeded my improvement. I read about William Jennings Bryan (The Golden Tongued orator) and he was my goal. When I readjusted my sights to become "as fluent as my motor system would allow," then I started to make progress. Gradual progress over a three- or four-year period, with occasional relapses and real breakdowns (like when three people very close to me—one my mother—died within a two-week period). My speech suffered tremendously, but even then I knew that I was grieving and when I grew strong again, and focused attention to my speech again, that I would regain my fluency. I never doubted that. My belief system remained positive that I would speak fluently again, as fluently as my timing system or motor coordination abilities would allow. But striving for perfection was abandoned as unrealistic, and really as unnecessary for success and happiness.

Also, when I took my stuttering out from under the microscope and saw that disfluencies were only a part of me—that helped. When I saw that other qualities (like being a good friend, listener, and caring person to others) was also a part of who and what I was—then I put speech (stuttered or fluent) in a proper perspective. I worked on using light pressure on my first sounds, sure, but also on improving tennis or sailing skills, too—and becoming a better administrator and writer, etc. Putting disfluencies in perspective helped—I realized that our Creator may have more challenges in store for me other than just becoming a perfect speaker. So I decided to work not only on fluency but on other "talents" I have too. That thinking seemed to send me in a more positive direction.

Clinical Insight

Adult male, age 52: I completed an intensive program of treatment in my mid-twenties. That was 28 years ago at this writing. I made obvious progress during the 20-week period of formal treatment. I learned how to decrease my avoidance behaviors (a big part of my stuttering) and to change the way I was stuttering. Very slowly, I began to take charge of my speech, especially specific behaviors associated with my stuttering. I also began to make some preliminary changes in the way I thought about my speech, both my stuttering as well as my fluent speech. But these cognitive changes, what I was telling myself about myself and my speech, came along at a much slower pace. Following my completion of treatment, I continued to expand my new ways of speaking, of stuttering, and thinking in more and more speaking situations. I slowly continued to make progress but it certainly wasn't linear. It was many years, at least 15, before the handicap of stuttering decreased to the point where it was really insignificant.

(continues)

Now, nearly three decades following treatment, I find that I do something that could be classified as stuttering only a few times a year. Nonetheless, I continue to think of myself as someone who stutters—it's just that I don't do it very often. Stuttering is part of who I am and that's perfectly OK. On the rare occasions when I stutter, I regard the situation more with curiosity and as a challenge to myself to stutter openly and easily. And most important, the fact that I might stutter has absolutely no influence on my choices.

Conclusion

Throughout this chapter we have described the importance of activities for transferring and maintaining behavioral techniques and cognitive changes acquired during treatment to communication situations beyond the therapy settings. Most speakers who are beginning therapy have much to learn about themselves and their stuttering and some will require more time than others to become desensitized to stuttering and make better choices. Transfer activities can and should begin as early as possible for both children and adults. Performance during daily activities with the stress of time pressure and competition for communication are the true tests for building confidence in the ability to employ preferred coping responses. Many of the suggestions for continued progress apply to children as well as older speakers. For younger speakers, of course, parent involvement and understanding of the treatment process is critical for supporting and reinforcing the desired progress at all levels of change.

Although many important victories occur throughout treatment, progress must continue long after formal intervention has been completed. Unfortunately, as is the case with many complex human problems, relapse is not unusual, particularly for adults. Emphasis on transfer and maintenance activities beyond the treatment environment will help decrease the possibility of relapse. Following formal treatment, continued persistence, vigilance, and effort are required for continuing success. It is important for the speaker to understand that a small lapse does not mean that a deep and lengthy relapse is imminent. Fluctuations in fluency as well as the speaker's confidence to make good decisions are to be expected. But as those people who have successfully managed their stuttering have informed us, it is important to understand success in the larger context. These speakers have been able to not only achieve improved fluency but also to enhance their ability to communicate with others and achieve an agentic and satisfying lifestyle.

It is also important to realize that other individuals in the client's environment will need to adjust not only to the speaker's newly acquired fluency but also to reformed relationships and altered roles. Family members and friends may need to adapt to a speaker who has become considerably more assertive. Membership in one or more support groups both during and following treatment is highly recommended for maintaining both behavioral and attitudinal changes. There is an ever-increasing source of useful information available from the Internet as well as materials provided by support groups. If treatment is successful, the client must gradually assume the responsibility for self-evaluating and systematically altering both the surface and intrinsic features of stuttering. He or she may also begin to enjoy an ever-expanding participation in many areas of life he or she has so energetically avoided in the past.

A few years ago in one of the Internet discussion groups, I read some insightful comments by an adult female who stuttered (Manning, 1999b). She described her ability to successfully manage her stuttering in terms of the freedom to not hide her stuttering, to talk gently, and be comfortable in speaking situations. Her description of how she manifested this freedom speaks to the central importance of assisting individuals to manage the fear of stuttering and live an agentic lifestyle. Her guidelines included:

- no longer chasing the fluency god,
- obtaining treatment as necessary,
- living without constant fear of uncontrolled stuttering,
- using the telephone without fear,
- speaking without scanning for feared words and situations,
- initiating conversations rather than choosing to be silent,
- speaking for herself rather than relying on others,
- choosing to speak even if she believes she may stutter,
- selecting leisure and career options that require talking without worrying about the possibility of stuttering, and
- stuttering gently without avoidance or shame.

These guidelines nicely summarize the primary goals of both therapeutic and self-directed change for individuals who stutter as described in Chapter 6. Certainly, improving fluency is an obvious goal for people who stutter. But the ability to communicate regardless of the possibility or the reality of stuttering is much more important to many people. Even more important is the ability to achieve a clear decrease in the anxiety and fear associated with the stuttering experience and to fully participate in life as he or she becomes a fully independent and autonomous person.

Topics for Discussion

1. Describe how a clinician's limited view of the speaker during and following treatment may prevent a full understanding about the overall process of therapeutic change.

2. What are some possible causes of post-treatment relapse?

3. What are some of the initial indicators of relapse?

4. Describe several ways to prepare a speaker for the possibility of a lapse or relapse following successful treatment.

5. What speaker characteristics may help to predict relapse (or long-term success) following treatment?

6. Using sources beyond this text, obtain the names, contact information, and goals of the major self-help groups for individuals who stutter around the world.

7. Describe the history and evolving nature of the relationship between self-help and professional communities.

Recommended Readings

Boberg, E. (1983). Behavioral transfer and maintenance programs for adolescent and adult stutterers. In J. Fraser Gruss (Ed.), *Stuttering therapy: Transfer and maintenance* (Publication No. 19) (pp. 41–61). Memphis, TN: Stuttering Foundation of America.

Craig, A. (1998). Relapse following treatment for stuttering: A critical review and correlative data. *Journal of Fluency Disorders, 23,* 1–30.

DiLollo, A., Manning, W. H., & Neimeyer, R. A. (2005). Cognitive complexity as a function of speaker role for adult persons who stutter. *Journal of Constructivist Psychology, 18,* 215–236.

Fransella, F. (1972). *Personal change and reconstruction.* New York: Academic Press.

Hood, S. B. (2003). *Advice to those who stutter* (Publication No. 9). Memphis, TN: Stuttering Foundation of America.

Manning, W. H. (1999a). Progress under the surface and over time. In N. B. Ratner & E. C. Healey (Eds.), *Stuttering Research and Practice: Bridging the Gap* (pp. 123–129). Mahwah, NJ: Lawrence Erlbaum.

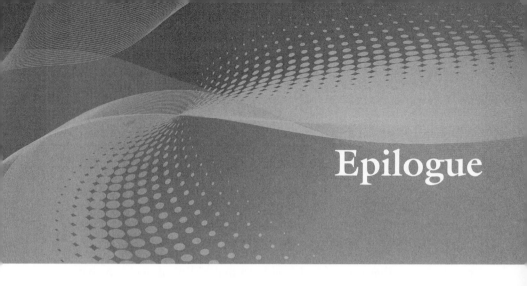

Epilogue

> The trouble with the world is that the stupid are cocksure and the intelligent are full of doubt.
>
> *Bertrand Russell*

I recently heard the comment that when you write a book you are never really done, it's just that you must eventually decide to finish. Of course, the minute you finish the new information that is constantly becoming available begins the aging process of what you have created. But eventually you must decide to stop and let what you have done represent your best effort.

The experience of reading, understanding, and synthesizing the information you discover is continually fascinating and often paradoxical. Writing can be an isolating, sometimes lonely process, as it must be, in order to be alone with your thoughts about what you are reading, synthesizing, and writing. On the other hand, you are connecting with others around the world and across time through the words and ideas in their manuscripts. You find out what you know and you certainly find out what you don't know or clearly understand. Sometimes you are delighted with a section you have written and often, just hours or days later, you are disillusioned as you reread the same section. You are challenged and energized by the creative process of writing for the people who will read the pages you are assembling. But you realize that eventually you will have to let go of what you have crafted.

Throughout the many months of preparing these chapters, particularly on the many occasions when I was unsure of the choices to be made and the direction to take, I returned to the goals described in the Preface. The primary goal that continued to surface above all the others was the development of enthusiasm in those clinicians who desire to assist children, adolescents, and adults who have difficulty communicating fluently. Enthusiasm is often created and enhanced by exploration in the form of continued learning and the development of expertise—not because a professional organization mandates continuing education, but because of the enjoyment of continually expanding our understanding about the possibilities for assisting those who stutter. Just as we encourage those we are trying to help to take action and expand their ability to communicate and to enhance the quality of their lives, the professional clinician must also continually take action by seeking new information and experimenting with alternative strategies and techniques.

With an understanding of the many possibilities and choices of intervention, the experienced and wise clinician is free to focus on the needs of the person who has come to him or her for help. Rather than concentrating on doctrine or techniques, the professional is able to make clinical decisions based on empirically supported research, years of experience, and eventually the moment-by-moment perception of a client's needs and possibilities. As we understand speakers and their stories, we become adept at enabling people to consider and select the options that are best for them. As we have suggested throughout this book, while we may become experts on fluency problems, speakers are the authorities on their own lives.

Clinicians who make the decision to spend a large portion of their lives assisting people with fluency problems need to know that magnificent changes are possible in the speech and the lives of even the most severely involved individual. Timely and effective treatment can help the young child who stutters to live a life free of stuttering. Adults who have stuttered and suffered for decades can achieve the ability to live a life in which speech is spontaneous and enjoyable, and they can learn to communicate as well or better than many normally fluent adults. Perhaps most importantly, they can experience the ability to participate in speaking situations they never dreamed possible and achieve goals they never thought achievable.

Not every speech-language pathologist is equipped to work with people who have fluency problems for, as in each of the specialty areas of our parent field, it takes some unique abilities. For those who choose to come to the assistance of people who stutter and are struggling to communicate with others and to seek fulfillment as human beings, there are many rewarding victories, marvelous colleagues, and great adventures to be enjoyed.

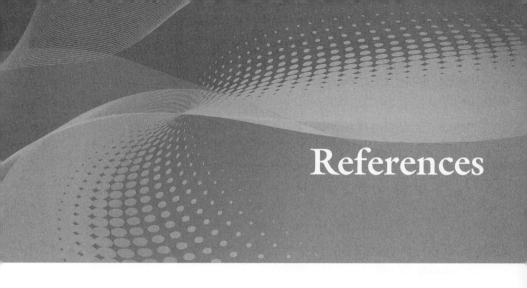

References

Abe, K., Yokoyama, R., & Yorifuji, S., (1993). Repetitive speech disorder resulting from infarcts in the paramedian thalami and mid brain. *Journal of Neurology, Neurosurgery and Psychiatry, 56,* 1024–1026.

Ackoff, R. (1974). *Redesigning the future.* New York: Wiley.

Adams, M. R. (1977a). A clinical strategy for differentiating the normal nonfluent child and the incipient stutterers. *Journal of Fluency Disorders, 2,* 141–148.

Adams, M. R. (1977b). The young stutterer: Diagnosis, treatment and assessment of progress. *Seminars in Speech, Language and Hearing, 1,* 289–299.

Adams, M. R. (1983). Learning from negative outcomes in stuttering therapy: Getting off on the wrong foot. *Journal of Fluency Disorders, 8,* 147–153.

Adams, M. R. (1984). The differential assessment and direct treatment of stuttering, In J. Costello (Ed.), *Speech disorders in children* (pp. 260–295). San Diego, CA: College-Hill Press.

Adams, M. R. (1990). The demands and capacities model I: Theoretical elaborations. *Journal of Fluency Disorders, 15,* 135–141.

Adams, M. R. (1993). The home environment of children who stutter. *Seminars in Speech and Language, 14*(3), 185–191.

Adams, M. R., & Hayden, P. (1976). The ability of stutters and nonstutterers to initiate and terminate phonation during production of an isolated vowel. *Journal of Speech and Hearing Disorders, 19,* 290–296.

Adams, M. R., & Runyan, C. (1981). Stuttering and fluency: Exclusive events or points on a continuum? *Journal of Fluency Disorders, 6,* 197–218.

Agnello, J. G. (1975). Voice onset and voice termination features of stutterers. In L. M. Webster & L. C. Furst (Eds.), *Vocal tract dynamics and disfluency.* New York: Speech and Hearing Institute.

Ahn, H., & Wampold, B. E. (2001). Where oh where are the specific ingredients? A meta-analysis of component studies in counseling and psychotherapy. *Journal of Counseling Psychology, 48,* 251–257.

Ainsworth, S. (Ed.). (1992). *Counseling stutterers* (Publication No. 18, 4th ed.). pp. 171–186. Memphis, TN: Speech Foundation of America.

Albach, J., & Benson, V. (Eds.). (1994). To say what is ours. *The best of 13 years of letting GO*. (3rd Ed.). San Francisco, CA: National Stuttering Project.

Alfonso, P. J., Watson, B. C., & Baer, T. (1987). Measuring stutterers' dynamic vocal tract characteristics by x-ray microbeam pellet tracking. In H. F. M. Peters & W. Hulstijn (Eds.), *Speech motor dynamics in stuttering*. New York: Springer-Verlag.

Allen, G. (1975). Speech rhythm: Its relation to performance universals and articulatory timing. *Journal of Phonetics, 3,* 75–86.

Alm, P. A. (2004). Stuttering and the basal ganglia circuits. *Journal of Communication Disorders, 37,* 325–369.

Alm, P. A. (2005). A new framework for understanding stuttering: The dual premotor model. Presentation to the International Fluency Association, Dublin, Ireland.

Alport, G. W. (1937). *Personality, a psychological interpretation*. New York: Holt.

Alport, G. W. (1961). *Pattern and growth in personality*. New York: Holt, Rinehart & Winston.

Ambrose, N. G. (2004). Theoretical perspectives on the cause of stuttering. *Contemporary Issues in Communication Science and Disorders, 31,* 80–91.

Ambrose, N. G., Cox, N., & Yairi, E. (1997). The genetic basis of persistent and recovered stuttering. *Journal of Speech and Hearing Research, 40,* 567–580.

Ambrose, N. G., & Yairi, E. (1994). The development of awareness of stuttering in preschool children. *Journal of Fluency Disorders, 19,* 229–246.

Ambrose, N. G., & Yairi, E. (1995). The role of repetition units in the differential diagnosis of early childhood incipient stuttering. *American Journal of Speech-Language Pathology, 4*(3), 82–88.

Ambrose, N. G., & Yairi, E., (1999). Normative disfluency data for early childhood stuttering. *Journal of Speech, Language, and Hearing Research, 42,* 895–909.

Ambrose, N. G., Yairi, E., and Cox, N. (1993). Genetic factors in childhood stuttering. *Journal of Speech and Hearing Research, 36,* 701–706.

American Psychiatric Association. (1987). *Diagnostic and statistical manual of mental disorders* (3rd ed.-rev. [DSM-III-R]). Washington, DC: American Psychiatric Association.

American Psychiatric Association. (1994). *Diagnostic and statistical manual of mental disorders* (4th ed.-rev. [DSM-IV]). Washington, DC: American Psychiatric Association.

American Psychiatric Association (2000). *Diagnostic and statistical manual of mental disorders* (4th ed., text revision). Washington, DC: American Psychiatric Association.

American Psychological Association. (1947). Recommended graduate training program in clinical psychology: Report of the committee on training in clinical psychology. *American Psychologist, 2,* 539–558.

American Speech-Language-Hearing Association. (1984). Guidelines for caseload size for speech-language services in the schools. *ASHA, 26,* 53–58.

American Speech-Language-Hearing Association (1995). Guidelines for practice in stuttering treatment. *ASHA, 37*(Suppl. 14): 26–35.

ASHA Omnibus Study (2001). Rockville, MD: American Speech-Language-Hearing Association.

American Speech-Language-Hearing Association (2005). *Evidence-Based Practice in Communication Disorders.* (Position statement). Available at http://www.asha.org/members/deskrefjournals/deskref/default.

Anderson, J. D., & Conture, E.G. (2000). Language abilities of children who stutter: A preliminary study. *Journal of Fluency Disorders, 25,* 283–304.

Anderson, J. D., & Conture, E.G. (2004). Sentence-structure priming in young children who do and do not stutter. *Journal of Speech, Language and Hearing Research, 47,* 552–571.

Amman, J. O. C. (1700/1965). *A dissertation on speech* (reprint). New York: Stechert-Hafner.

Anderson, T. K., & Felsenfeld, S. (2003). A thematic analysis of late recovery from stuttering. *American Journal of Speech-Language Pathology, 12,* 243–253.

Anderson, J., Pellowski, M., Conture, E., & Kelly E. (2003). Temperament characteristics of young children who stutter. *Journal of Speech, Language and Hearing Research, 46,* 1221–1233.

Andrews, G. (1984). Epidemiology of stuttering. In R. F. Curlee & W. H. Perkins (Eds.), *Nature and treatment of stuttering: New directions* (pp. 1–12). San Diego, CA: College Hill Press.

Andrews, G., & Craig, A. (1982). Stuttering: Overt and covert assessment of the speech of treated subjects. *Journal of Speech and Hearing Disorders, 47,* 96–99.

Andrews, G., & Craig, A. R. (1985). The prediction and prevention of relapse in stuttering. The value of self-control techniques and locus of control measures. *Behavior Modification, 9,* 427–442.

Andrews, G., & Craig, A. R. (1988). Prediction of outcome after treatment for stuttering. *British Journal of Psychiatry, 153,* 236–240.

Andrews, G., Craig, A., & Feyer, A. M. (1983). *Therapist's manual for the stuttering treatment programme.* Sydney, Australia: Prince Henry Hospital, Division of Communication Disorders.

Andrews, G., & Cutler, J. (1974). Stuttering therapy: The relation between changes in symptom level and attitudes. *Journal of Speech and Hearing Disorders, 39,* 312–319.

Andrews, G., Guitar, B., & Howie. P. (1980). Meta-analysis of the effects of stuttering treatment. *Journal of Speech and Hearing Disorders, 45,* 287–307.

Andrews, G., & Harris, M. (1964). *The syndrome of stuttering* (Clinics in Developmental Medicine No. 17). London: Spastics Society Medical Education and Information Unit, in association with W. Heinemann Medical Books.

Andrews, G., & Harvey, R. (1981). Regression to the mean in pretreatment measures of stuttering. *Journal of Speech and Hearing Disorders, 46,* 204–207.

Andrews, G., & Neilson, M. (1981). Stuttering: A state of the art seminar. Presentation to the annual meeting of the Speech-Hearing Association, Los Angeles, CA.

Andrews, G., Quinn, P. T., & Sorby, W. A. (1972). Stuttering: An investigation into cerebral dominance of speech. *Journal of Neurology, Neurosurgery, and Psychiatry, 25,* 414–418.

Andrews, G., Yates-Morris, A., Howie, P., & Martin, N. G. (1991). Genetic factors in stuttering confirmed. *Archives of General Psychiatry, 48*(11), 1034–1035.

Apel, K. (1999). Checks and balances: Keeping the science in our profession. *Language, Speech, and Hearing Services in Schools, 30,* 99–108.

Armson, J., & Kiefte, M. (2008). The effect of SpeechEasy on stuttering frequency, speech rate, and speech naturalness. *Journal of Fluency Disorders, 33,* 120–134.

Armson, J., Kiefte, M., Mason, J., De Croos, D. (2006). The effect of SpeechEasy on stuttering frequency in laboratory conditions. *Journal of Fluency Disorders, 31,* 137–152.

Armson, J., & Stewart, A. (1998). Effect of extended exposure to frequency-altered feedback on stuttering during reading and monologue. *Journal of Speech Language, and Hearing Research, 41,* 479–490.

Arndt, J., & Healey, E. C. (2001). Concomitant disorders in school-age children who stutter. *Language Speech Hearing Services in Schools, 32,* 68–78.

Arnold, G. E. (1960). Studies in tachyphemia: I. Present concepts of etiologic factors. Logos, *3,* 25–45.

Arnott, N. (1928). *Elements of physics.* Edinburgh, Scotland: Adams.

ASHA Omnibus Study (2001). Rockville, MD: American Speech-Language-Hearing Association.

Attanasio, J. (1987). The dodo was Lewis Carroll you see: Reflections and speculations. *Journal of Fluency Disorders, 12,* 107–118.

Attanasio, J. (1997). Was Moses a person who stuttered? Perhaps not. *Journal of Fluency Disorders, 22,* 65–68.

Au-Yeung, J., Howell, P., Davis, S., Charles, N., & Sackin, S. (2000). UCL survey on bilingualism and stuttering. Presentation to the 3rd World

Congress on Fluency Disorders, Nyborg, Denmark, 7–11 August 2000. (May also be accessed from http://www.speech.psychol.ucl.ac.uk/survey1/PAPER/ifapaper.html.)

Ayre, A., & Wright, L. (2008). WASSP: An international review of its clinical application. *International Journal of Speech-Language Pathology.* (in press)

Azrin, N. H., Nunn, R. G., & Frantz, S. E. (1979). Comparison of regulated breathing versus abbreviated desensitization on reported stuttering episodes. *Journal of Speech and Hearing Disorders, 44,* 331–339.

Backus, O. (1947). Intensive group therapy in speech rehabilitation. *Journal of Speech Disorders, 12,* 39–60.

Backus, O. (1957). Group structure in speech therapy. In L. E. Travis (Ed.), *Handbook of speech pathology* (pp. 1025–1064). New York: Appleton-Century-Crofts, Inc.

Backus, O., & Beasley, J. (1951). *Speech therapy with children.* Cambridge, MA: Houghton Mifflin.

Bakker, K., & Brutten, G. J. (1989). A comparative investigation of the laryngeal promoter, adjustment and reaction times of stutterers and nonstutterers. *Journal of Speech and Hearing Research, 32,* 239–244.

Bakker, K. (1995). Two supplemental scoring procedures for diagnostic evaluations with the Speech Situation Checklist. *Journal of Fluency Disorders, 20,* 117–126.

Bakker, K., Raphael, L. J. Myers, F. I., & St. Louis, K. O. (2000). Acoustic and perceptual-phonetic analysis of cluttered and noncluttered speech. Presentation to the Annual Convention of the American Speech-Language-Hearing Association, Washington, D.C.

Bamberg, C., Hanley, J., & Hillenbrand, J. (1990). Pitch and amplitude perturbation in adult stutterers and nonstutterers. Presentation to the annual meeting of the American Speech-Language-Hearing Association, Seattle, WA.

Bandura, A. (1977). Toward a unifying theory of behavior change. *Psychological Review, 1,* 191–215.

Bannister, D. (1966). Psychology as an exercise in paradox. *Bulletin of the British Psychological Society, 19,* 21–26.

Barbara, D. A. (Ed.). (1965). *New Directions in Stuttering: Theory and Practice.* Springfield, IL: Charles C. Thomas.

Barbara, D. A. (1982). *The psychodynamics of stuttering.* Springfield, IL: Charles C. Thomas.

Barrager-Dunne, P. (1997). "Catch the little fish": Therapy utilizing narrative, drama, and dramatic play with young children. In C. Smith & D. Nylund (Eds.), *Narrative therapy with children and adolescents* (pp. 71–110). New York, The Guilford Press.

Baumgartner, J. M. (1999). Acquired Psychogenic Stuttering. In R. Curlee (Ed.), *Stuttering and Related Disorders of Fluency* (2nd ed., pp. 269–288). New York: Thieme Medical Publishers, Inc.

Baumgartner, J., & Duffy, J. (1997). Psychogenic stuttering in adults with and without neurologic disease. *Journal of Medical Speech-Language Pathology, 52,* 75–95.

Beck, J. S. (1995). *Cognitive Therapy: Basics and Beyond.* New York: Guilford Press.

Beck, J. S. (2005). *Cognitive Therapy for Challenging Problems.* New York: Guilford Press.

Beech, H., & Fransella, F. (1968). *Research and experiment in stuttering.* Oxford, England: Pergamon Press.

Bell, A. M. (1853). *Observations on defects of speech, the cure of stammering, and the principles of elocution.* London: Hamilton-Adams.

Bennett, E. M., & Chmela, K. A. (1998). The mask of shame: Treatment strategies for adults who stutter. In E. C. Healey & H. F. M. Peters (Eds.), *Proceedings of the 2nd World Congress on Fluency Disorders* (pp. 340–342). Nijmegen, The Netherlands: Nijmegen University Press.

Berenson, B. G., & Carkhuff, R. R. (1967). *Sources of gain in counseling and psychotherapy.* New York: Holt, Rinehart & Winston.

Berenson, B. G., & Mitchell, K. M. (1974). *Confrontation: For better or worse.* Amherst, MA: Human Resource Development Press.

Benecken, J. (1995). On the nature and psychological relevance of a stigma: The "stutterer" or what happens, when "Grace falls". Presentation to the 1st World Congress on Fluency Disorders, Munchen.

Bernstein Ratner, N. (2004). Fluency and stuttering in bilingual children. In B. Goldstein (Ed.), *Bilingual language development and disorders in Spanish-English speakers* (pp. 286–308). Baltimore: Paul H. Brookes Publishing.

Bieri, J. (1955). Cognitive complexity-simplicity and predictive behavior. *Journal of Abnormal and Social Psychology, 51,* 263–268.

Berkowitz, M., Cook, H., & Haughey, J. (1994). Fluency program developed for the public school setting. *Language, Speech and Hearing Services in Schools, 25,* 94–99.

Berlin, C. I., Lowe-Bell, S. S., Cullen, J. K., Jr., Thompson, C. L., & Loovis, C. F. (1973). Dichotic speech perception: An interpretation of right-ear advantage and temporal offset effects. *Journal of the Acoustical Society of America, 53,* 699–709.

Berlin, C. I., & McNeil, M. R. (1976). Dichotic Listening. In N. J. Lass (Ed.), *Contemporary issues in experimental phonetics.* New York: Academic Press.

Berliner, D. C., (1994). Expertise: The wonder of exemplary performances, In J. N. Mangieri, & C. C. Block, (Eds.), *Creating powerful thinking in teachers and students.* Fort Worth, TX: Holt, Rinehart & Winston.

Berry, M. F. (1938). Developmental history of stuttering children. *Journal of Pediatrics, 11,* 209–217.

Bhatnagar, S.C., & Andy, O.J. (1995). *Neuroscience for the Study of Communicative Disorders.* Baltimore, MD: Williams & Wilkins.

Black, J. W. (1951). The effect of delayed sidetone upon vocal rate and intensity. *Journal of Speech and Hearing Disorders, 16,* 56–60.

Blanton, S., & Blanton, M. G. (1936). *For stutterers.* New York: Appleton–Century.

Bloch, E. L., & Goodstein, L. D. (1971). Functional speech disorders and personality: A decade of research. *Journal of Speech and Hearing Disorders, 36,* 295–314.

Blodgett, E. G., & Cooper, E. B. (1988). Talking about it and doing it: Meta linguistic capacity and prosodic control in three to seven year olds. *Journal of Fluency Disorders, 13,* 283–290.

Blomgren, M., Nagarajan, S. S., Lee, J. N., Li, T., & Alvord, L. (2003). Preliminary results of a functional MRI study of brain activation patterns in stuttering and nonstuttering speakers during a lexical access task. *Journal of Fluency Disorders, 28,* 337–357.

Blood, G. (1995). A behavioral-cognitive therapy program for adults who stutter: Computers and counseling. *Journal of Communication Disorders, 28,* 165–180.

Blood, G. (1995). POWER2: Relapse management with adolescents who stutter. *Language, Speech, and Hearing Services in Schools, 26,* 169–179.

Blood, G. W., & Blood, I. M. (1982). A tactic for facilitating social interacting with laryngectomees. *Journal of Speech and Hearing Disorders, 47,* 416–419.

Blood, G. W., Blood, I. M., McCarthy, J., Tellis, G., & Gabel, R. (2001). An analysis of verbal response patterns of Charles Van Riper during stuttering modification therapy. *Journal of Fluency Disorders, 26,* 129–149.

Blood, G., W., & Blood, I. M. (2004). Bullying in adolescents who stutter: Communicative competence and self-esteem, *Contemporary Issues in Communication Science and Disorders, 31,* 69–79.

Blood, G. W., & Hood, S. B. (1978). Elementary school-age stutterers' disfluencies during oral reading and spontaneous speech. *Journal of Fluency Disorders, 3,* 155–165.

Blood, G., & Seider, R. (1981). The concomitant problems of young stutterers. *Journal of Speech and Hearing Disorders, 46,* 31–33.

Bloodstein, O. (1949). Conditions under which stuttering is reduced or absent: A review of literature. *Journal of Speech and Hearing Disorders, 14,* 295–302.

Bloodstein, O. (1950). Hypothetical conditions under which stuttering is reduced or absent. *Journal of Speech and Hearing Disorders, 15,* 142–153.

Bloodstein, O. (1958). Stuttering as anticipatory struggle reaction. In J. Eisenson (Ed.), *Stuttering: A symposium* (pp. 1–69). New York: Harper & Row.

Bloodstein, O. (1960). The development of stuttering I. Changes in nine basic features. *Journal of Speech and Hearing Disorders, 25,* 219–237.

Bloodstein, O. (1961). The development of stuttering III. Theoretical and clinical implications. *Journal of Speech and Hearing Disorders, 26,* 67–82.

Bloodstein, O. (1974). The rules of early stuttering. *Journal of Speech and Hearing Disorders, 39,* 379–394.

Bloodstein, O. (1987). *A handbook on stuttering* (4th ed.). Chicago: National Easter Seal Society.

Bloodstein, O. (1992). Response to Hamre: Part I. *Journal of Fluency Disorders, 17,* 29–32.

Bloodstein, O. (1993). *Stuttering: The search for a cause and cure.* Needham Heights, MA: Allyn & Bacon.

Bloodstein, O. (1995). *A handbook on stuttering* (5th ed.). San Diego: Singular Publishing Group.

Bloodstein, O., & Bernstein Ratner, N. (2008) *A handbook on stuttering.* (6th ed.).Clifton Park, NY: Thomson Delmar Learning.

Bloodstein, O. (1999). Opening comments to the sixth annual leadership conference of the ASHA Special Interest Division, San Diego, CA.

Bloodstein, O., & Shogun, R. (1972). Some clinical notes on forced stuttering. *Journal of Speech and Hearing Disorders, 37,* 177–186.

Bloom, C. & Cooperman, D. K. (1999). *Synergistic stuttering therapy: A holistic approach.* Boston: Butterworth-Heinemann

Bluemel, C. S. (1932). Primary and secondary stammering. *Quarterly Journal of Speech, 18,* 187–200.

Bluemel, C. S. (1957). *The riddle of stuttering.* Danville, IL: Interstate.

Boberg, E. (1981). In E. Boberg (Ed.), *Maintenance of fluency: An Experimental program* (pp. 71–112). New York: Elsevier/North-Holland.

Boberg, E. (1983). Behavioral transfer and maintenance programs for adolescent and adult stutterers. In J. Fraser Gruss (Ed.), *Stuttering therapy: Transfer and maintenance* (Publication No. 19, pp. 41–61). Memphis, TN: Stuttering Foundation of America.

Boberg, E., Howie, P., & Woods, L. (1979). Maintenance of fluency: A review. *Journal of Fluency Disorders, 4,* 93–116.

Boberg, E., & Kully, D. (1984). Techniques for transferring fluency. In W. H. Perkins (Ed.), *Current therapy of communication disorders: Stuttering disorders* (pp. 178–201). New York: Thieme Medical Publishers Inc.

Boberg, E., & Kully, D. (1994). Long-term result of an intensive treatment program for adults and adolescents who stutter. *Journal of Speech and Hearing Research, 37,* 1050–1059.

Boberg, E., & Sawyer, L. (1977). The maintenance of fluency following intensive therapy. *Human Communication, 2,* 21–28.

Boberg, E., Yeudall, L. T., Schopflocher, D., & Bo Lassen, P. (1983). The effect of an intensive behavioral program on the distribution of EEG alpha power in stutterers during the processing of verbal and visuospatial information. *Journal of Fluency Disorders, 8,* 245–263.

Bobrick, B. (1995). *Knotted tongues.* New York: Simon and Schuster.

Bonelli, P., Dixon, M., & Bernstein Ratner, N. (2000). Child and parent speech and language following the Lidcombe Programme of early stuttering intervention. *Clinical Linguistics and Phonetics, 14,* 427–446.

Bonfanti, B. H., & Culatta, R. (1977). An analysis of the fluency patterns of institutionalized retarded adults. *Journal of Fluency Disorders, 2,* 117–128.

Bordeau, L. A., & Jeffrey, C. H. (1973). Stuttering treated by desensitization. *Journal of Behavior Therapy and Experimental Psychiatry, 4,* 209–212.

Borden, G. D., Kim, D. H., & Spiegler, K. (1991). Acoustics of stop consonant-vowel relationships during fluent and stuttered utterances. *Journal of Fluency Disorders, 12*(3), 175–184.

Bothe, A. K. (2003). Evidence-based treatment of stuttering: V. The art of clinical practice and the future of clinical research. *Journal of Fluency Disorders, 28*(3), 247–258.

Bothe A. K. (2004). Evidence-based, outcomes-focused decisions about stuttering treatment: Clinical recommendations in context. In A. K. Bothe (Ed.), *Evidence-based treatment of stuttering: Empirical bases and clinical applications* (pp. 261–270). Mahwah, NJ: Lawrence Erlbaum Associates.

Bothe, A. K., Davidow, J. H., Bramlett, R. E., Franic, D. M. & Ingham, R. J. (2006) Stuttering treatment research 1970–2005: II. Systematic review incorporating trial quality assessment of pharmacological approaches. *American Journal of Speech-Language Pathology, 15*(4), 342–352.

Bothe, A. K., Davidow, J. H., Bramlett, R. E., & Ingham, R. J. (2006A). Stuttering treatment research 1970–2005: I. Systematic review incorporating trial quality assessment of behavioral, cognitive, and related approaches. *American Journal of Speech-Language Pathology, 15*(4), 321–341.

Bothe, A. K., Finn, P., & Bramlett, R. E. (2007). Pseudoscience and the Speech Easy: Reply to Kalinowski, Saltuklaroglu, Stuart, & Buntupalli (2007). *American Journal of Speech-Language Pathology. 16*(1) 77–83.

Bothe, A. K., Franic, D. M., Ingham, R. J., Davidow, J. H. (2007). Pharmacological approaches to stuttering treatment: Reply to Meline and Harn. *American Journal of Speech-Language Pathology, 17,* 98–101.

Bosshardt, H. (1990). Subvocalization and reading rate differences between stuttering and nonstuttering children and adults. *Journal of Speech and Hearing Research, 33,* 776–785.

Bosshardt, H., & Nandyal, I. (1988). Reading rates of stutterers and non-stutterers during silent and oral reading. *Journal of Fluency Disorders, 13,* 407–420.

Botterill, W., & Cook, F. (1987). Personal construct theory and the treatment of adolescent disfluency. In L. Rustin, H. Purser, & D. Rowley (Eds.), *Progress in the treatment of fluency disorders* (pp. 147–165). London: Taylor & Francis.

Bottrill, W., Kelman, E., & Rustin, L. (1991). Parents and their pre-school stuttering children. In L. Rustin (Ed.), *Parents, families and the stuttering child* (pp. 59–71). San Diego, CA: Singular Publishing Group.

Braithwaite, J. (2002). Rules and principles: A theory of legal certainty. *Australian Journal of Legal Philosophy, 27,* 47–82.

Brady, J. (1991). The pharmacology of stuttering: A critical review. *American Journal of Psychiatry, 148,* 1309–1316.

Brady, J. P., & Berson, J. (1975). Stuttering, dichotic listening, and cerebral dominance. *Archives of General Psychiatry, 32,* 1449–1452.

Branch, C., Milner, B., & Rasmussen, T. (1964). Intercarotid sodium amytol for lateralization of cerebral speech dominance. *Journal of Neurosurgery, 21,* 399–405.

Braun, A. R., Varga, M., Stager, S., Schulz, G., Selbie, S., Maisog, J. M., et al. (1997). Altered patterns of cerebral activity during speech and language production in developmental stuttering, An H215O positron emission tomography study. *Brain, 120,* 761–784.

Bray, M. A., Kehle, T. J., Lawless, K. A., & Theodore, L. A. (2003). The relationship of self-efficacy and depression to stuttering. *American Journal of Speech-Language Pathology, 12,* 425–431.

Breitenfeldt, D. H., & Lorenz, D. R. (1989). *Successful stuttering management program.* Cheney: Eastern Washington University.

Brill, A. A. (1923). Speech disturbances in nervous and mental diseases. *Quarterly Journal of Speech, 9,* 129–135.

Brissette, I., Scheier, M. F., & Carver, C. S. (2002). The role of optimism in social network delopment, coping, and psychological adjustment during life transition. *Journal of Personality and Social Psychology, 82,* 102–111.

Brisk, D. J., Healey, E. C., & Hux, K. A. (1997). Clinicians' training and confidence associated with treating school-age children who stutter: A national survey. *Language, Speech, and Hearing Services in Schools, 28,* 164–176.

Broadbent, D.E., & Gregory, M. (1964). Accuracy of recognition for speech presented to the right and left ears. *Quarterly Journal of Experimental Psychology, 16,* 359–360.

Brocklehurst, P. (2005). "Stammerer" or "person who stammers"? A comparison of the impact of two labels on the general public. Unpublished sociolinguistic project. De Montfort University, Leichester, UK.

Brocklehurst, P. H. (2008). A review of evidence for the covert repair hypothesis of stuttering. *Contemporary Issues in Communication Science and Disorders, 35,* 25–43.

Brown, G. S. (2006). Common factors and therapist effects in therapy outcome. Presentation to the annual meeting of the American Speech-Language-Hearing Association, Miami, FL.

Brown, G., & Cullinan, W. L. (1981). Word-retrieval difficulty and disfluent speech in adult anomic speakers. *Journal of Speech and Hearing Research, 24,* 358–365.

Brown, S., Ingham, R. J., Ingham, J. C., Laird, A. R., & Fox, P. T. (2005). Stuttered and fluent speech production: an ALE meta-analysis of functional neuroimaging studies. *Human Brain Mapping, 25,* 105–117.

Brownell, K.D., Marlatt, G. A., Lichtenstein, E. & Wilson, G. T., (1996). Understanding and preventing relapse. *American Psychologist, 41,* 765–782.

Brundage, S. B. (2007). Virtual reality augmentation for functional assessment and treatment of stuttering. *Topics in language disorders, 27,* 254–271

Brundage, S. B., & Graap, K. (2004). Virtual reality: An exciting new tool to enhance stuttering treatment. *Fluency and Fluency Disorders, 14,* 4–8.

Brundage, S., Graap, K., Gibbons, K., Ferrer, M., & Brooks, J. (2006). Frequency of stuttering during challenging and supportive virtual job interviews. *Journal of Fluency Disorders, 31,* 325–339.

Brundage, S., Hancock, A., Kiselewich, K., & Stallings, L., (2006, November). Frequency of stuttering during speeches given to virtual and live audiances. Presentation to the annual meeting of the American Speech-Language-Hearing Association, Miami, FL.

Brutten, G. (1973). Behavior assessment and the strategy of therapy. In Y. Lebrun & R. Hoops, (Eds.), *Neurolinguistic approaches to stuttering* (pp. 8–17). The Hague: Mouton.

Brutten, G. J. (1975). Stuttering: Topography, assessment, and behavior change strategies. In J. Eisenson (Ed.), *Stuttering: A second symposium* (pp. 201–262). New York: Harper and Row.

Brutten, G. J., & Dunham, S. (1989). The Communication Attitude Test: A normative study of grade school children. *Journal of Fluency Disorders, 14,* 371–377.

Brutten, G. J., & Shoemaker, D. J. (1967). *The modification of stuttering.* Englewood Cliffs, NJ: Prentice–Hall.

Brutten, G., & Vanryckeghem, M. (2003a). Behavior Assessment Battery: *A multi-dimensional and evidenced-based approach to diagnostic and therapeutic decision making for adults who stutter.* Belgium: Stichting Integratie Gehandicapten & Acco Publishers.

Brutten, G., & Vanryckeghem, M. (2003b). Behavior Assessment Battery: *A multi-dimensional and evidenced-based approach to diagnostic and therapeutic decision making for children who stutter.* Belgium: Stichting Integratie Gehandicapten & Acco Publishers.

Brutten, G., & Vanryckeghem, M. (2007). *Behavior Assessment Battery for children who stutter.* San Deigo, CA: Plural Publishing, Inc.

Bryngelson, B. (1935). Method of stuttering. *Journal of Abnormal Psychology, 30,* 194–198.

Bryngelson, B. (1938). Prognosis in stuttering. *Journal of Speech Disorders, 3,* 121–123.

Bryngelson, B., Chapman, B., & Hansen, O. (1944). *Know yourself: A guide for those who stutter.* Minneapolis: Burgess Publishing.

Bullen, A. K. (1945). A cross cultural approach to the problem of stuttering. *Child Development, 16,* 1–88.

Burks, H. (1976). *Burks behavioral rating scales.* Los Angeles: Western Psychological Services.

Burton, A. (1972). *Interpersonal psychotherapy.* Englewood Cliffs, NJ: Prentice–Hall.

Cabanas, R. (1954). Some findings in speech and voice therapy among mentally deficient children. *Folia Phoniatrica, 6,* 34–39.

Calkins, S. D., & Fox, N. A. (1994). Individual differences in the biological aspects of temperament. In J. E. Bates, and T. D. Wachs (Eds.), *Temperament: Individual Differences at the Interface of Biology and Behavior (pp. 199–217).* Washington, D.D.: American Psychological Association.

Camarta, S., (1998). Connecting speech and language: clinical applicatins. In R. Paul (Ed.), *Exploring the speech–language connection,* Baltimore: Brookes.

Carkhuff, R. R., & Berenson, B. G. (1967). *Beyond counseling and psychotherapy.* New York: Holt, Rinehart & Winston.

Carlisle, J. A. (1985). *Tangled tongue: Living with a stutter.* Toronto, Canada: University of Toronto Press.

Caruso, A. J. (1988). Childhood stuttering: A review of behavioral, acoustical, and physiological research [abstract]. *ASHA, 30,* 73.

Caruso, A. J., Abbs, J. H., & Gracco, V.L. (1988). Kinematic analysis of multiple movement coordination during speech in stutterers. *Brain, 111,* 439–456.

Caruso, A. J., Gracco, V. L., & Abbs, J. H. (1987). A speech motor control perspective on stuttering: Preliminary observation. In H. F. M. Peters & Hulstijn (Eds.), *Speech motor dynamics in stuttering* (pp. 245–258). Wien: Springer Verlag.

Caruso, A. J., McClowry, M. T., & Max. L. (1997). Age-related effects on speech fluency. *Seminars in Speech and Language, 18*(2), 171–180.

Cattanach, A. (1992). *Play therapy with abused children*. London: Jessica Kingsley.

Cattanach, A. (1994). *Where the sky meets the underworld*. London: Jessica Kingsley.

Cerf, A., & Prins, D. (1974). Stutterers' ear preference for dichotic syllables. Presentation to the annual meeting of the American Speech-Language-Hearing Association, Las Vegas.

Chang, S., Erickson, K. I., Ambrose, N. G., Hasegawa-Johnson, M. A., & Ludlow, C. L. (2008). Brain anatomy differences in childhood stuttering. *NeuroImage, 39,* 1333–1244.

Chapman, A. H., & Chapman-Santana M. (1995) *The use of humor in psychotherapy*. Arq. Neuropsiquiartr, *53*(1), 153–156.

Cheasman, C. (2007). Revealing and healing—a mindfulness approach to stammering. *Speaking Out,* (Spring), 9–10.

Chmela, K. A. (1998). Thoughts on recovery. In E. C. Healey & H. F. M. Peters (Eds.), *Proceedings of the 2nd World Congress on Fluency Disorders* (pp. 376–378). Nijmegen, The Netherlands: Nijmegen University Press.

Chmela, K. A., & Reardon, N. A. (2001). *The school-age child who stutters: Practical ideas for working with feelings and beliefs about stuttering* (Publication No. 5). Stuttering Foundation of America.

Clark, H. (1971). The importance of linguistics for the study of speech hesitations. In D. Horton & J. Jenkins (Eds.), *The perception of language: Proceedings of the symposium*, University of Pittsburgh. Columbus, OH: Charles E. Merrill.

Cockburn, J. (2004). Adaptation of evidence into practice—can change be sustainable? *Medical Journal of Australia, 180,* 66–67.

Colburn, N. (1985). Clustering of disfluency in stuttering children's early utterances. *Journal of Fluency Disorders, 10,* 51–58.

Cole, L. (1986). The social responsibility of the researcher. In F. H. Bess, B. S. Clark, & H. R. Mitchell (Eds.), *Concerns for minority groups in communication disorders* (ASHA Reports No. *16,* ISSN 0569–8553, pp. 93–100). Rockville, MD: American Speech-Language-Hearing Association.

Collins, C. R., & Blood, G. W. (1990). Acknowledgement and severity of stuttering as factors influencing nonstutterers' perceptions of stutterers. *Journal of Speech and Hearing Disorders, 55,* 75–81.

Combs, A., & Snygg, D. (1959). *Individual behavior.* New York: Harper.

Coloroso, B. (2003). *The bully, the bullied, and the bystander.* New York, NY: HarperCollins Publishers. Inc.

Compas, B. E., Malcarne, V. L., & Banez, G. A. (1992). Coping with psychological stress: A developmental perspective. In B. N. Carpenter (Ed.), *Personal Coping: Theory, Research, and Application* (pp. 93–110). Westport, CT: Praeger Publishers.

Conners, C. K. (1997). *Conners' rating scales—revised.* New York: Multi-Health Systems, Inc.

Conture, E. G. (1982). Stuttering in young children. *Journal of Developmental and Behavioral Pediatrics, 3,* 163–169.

Conture, E. G. (1996). Treatment efficacy: stuttering. *Journal of Speech and Hearing Research, 39,* S18–26.

Conture, E. G. (1997). Evaluating childhood stuttering. In R. Curlee & G. Siegel (Eds.), *Nature and treatment of stuttering, new directions* (2nd ed., pp. 239–256). Needham Heights, MA: Allyn & Bacon.

Conture, E. G. (2001). *Stuttering: Its nature, diagnosis and treatment.* Needham Heights, MA: Allyn & Bacon.

Conture, E., & Caruso, A. (1987). Assessment and diagnosis of childhood disfluency. In L. Ruskin, D. Rowley, & H. Purser (Eds.), *Progress in the treatment of fluency disorders* (pp. 57–82). London, England: Taylor & Francis.

Conture, E., & Guitar, B. (1993). Evaluating efficacy of treatment of stuttering: School-age children. *Journal of Fluency Disorders, 18,* 253–287.

Conture, E. & Kelly, E. (1991). Young stutterers' non-speech behaviors during stuttering. *Journal of Speech and Hearing Research, 34,* 1041–1056.

Conture, E., Louko, L., & Edwards, M. L. (1993). Simultaneously treating stuttering and disordered phonology in children: Experimental therapy, preliminary findings. *American Journal of Speech-Language Pathology, 2*(3), 72–81.

Conture, E. G., McCall, G. N., & Brewer, D. (1977). Laryngeal behavior during stuttering. *Journal of Speech and Hearing Research, 20,* 661–668.

Conture, E., Rothenberg, M., & Molitor, R. (1986). Electroglottographic observations of young stutterers' fluency. *Journal of Speech and Hearing Research, 29,* 384–393.

Conture, E., & Schwartz, H. (1984). Children who stutter: diagnosis and remediation. *Communication Disorders, 9,* 1–18.

Cook, M. J., & Smith, L. M. (2006). Outcomes for adult males using the SpeechEasy fluency device for one year. Presentation to the annual meeting of the American Speech-Language-Hearing Association. Miami, FL.

Cooper, E. B. (1966). Client-clinician relationships and concomitant factors in stuttering therapy. *Journal of Speech and Hearing Disorders, 9,* 194–199.

Cooper, E. B. (1968). A therapy process for the adult stutterer. *Journal of Speech and Hearing Disorders, 33,* 246–260.

Cooper, E. B. (1972). Recovery from stuttering in a junior and senior high school population. *Journal of Speech and Hearing Research, 15,* 632–638.

Cooper, E. B. (1973). The development of a stuttering chronicity prediction checklist: A preliminary report. *Journal of Speech and Hearing Disorders, 38,* 215–223.

Cooper, E. B. (1975a). Clinician attitudes toward stutterers: A study of bigotry? Presentation to the annual meeting of the American Speech-Language-Hearing Association, Washington, DC.

Cooper, E. B. (1975b). *Clinician Attitudes Toward Stuttering Inventory* (CATS). Allen, TX: DLM.

Cooper, E. B. (1977). Controversies about stuttering therapy. *Journal of Fluency Disorders, 2,* 75–86.

Cooper, E. B. (1979a). Intervention procedures for the young stutterer. In H. Gregory (Ed.), *Controversies about stuttering* (pp. 63–96). Baltimore, MD: University Park Press.

Cooper, E. B. (1979b). *Understanding stuttering: Information for parents.* Chicago: National Easter Seal Society for Crippled Children and Adults.

Cooper, E. B. (1985). *Cooper personalized fluency control therapy—revised.* Allen, TX: DLM.

Cooper, E. B. (1986a). The mentally retarded stutterer. In K. O. St. Louis (Ed.), *The atypical stutterer* (pp. 123–154). San Diego, CA: Academic Press.

Cooper, E. B. (1986b). Treatment of dysfluency: Future trends. *Journal of Fluency Disorders, 11,* 317–327.

Cooper, E. B. (1987). The chronic perseverative stuttering syndrome: Incurable stuttering. *Journal of Fluency Disorders, 12,* 381–388.

Cooper, E. B. (1990). *Understanding stuttering: Information for parents.* Chicago: National Easter Seal Society.

Cooper, E. B., Cady, B. B., & Robbins, C. J. (1970). The effect of the verbal stimulus words wrong, right and tree on the disfluency rates of stutterers and nonstutterers. *Journal of Speech and Hearing Research, 13,* 239–244.

Cooper, E. B., & Cooper, C. S. (1965). Variations in adult stutterer attitudes towards clinicians during therapy. *Journal of Communication Disorders, 2,* 141–153.

Cooper, E. B., & Cooper, C. S. (1985a). Clinician attitudes toward stuttering: A decade of change (1973–1983). *Journal of Fluency Disorders, 10,* 19–33.

Cooper, E. B., & Cooper, C. S. (1985b). The effective clinician. In E. B. Cooper and C. S. Cooper, *Personalized fluency control therapy—revised* (handbook) (pp. 21–31) Allen, TX: DLM.

Cooper, E. B., & Cooper, C. S. (1985c). *Personalized fluency control therapy—revised (handbook)*. Allen, TX: DLM.

Cooper, E. B., & Cooper, C. S. (1991a). A fluency disorders prevention program for preschoolers and children in the primary grades. *American Journal of Speech-Language Pathology, 1,* 28–31.

Cooper, E. B., & Cooper, C. S. (1991b). *Multicultural considerations in the assessment and treatment of fluency disorders.* Presentation to the Annual Convention of the American Speech-Language-Hearing Association, Atlanta, GA.

Cooper, E. B., & Cooper, C. S. (1992). Clinician attitudes toward stuttering: two decades of change. Presentation to the annual meeting of the American Speech-Language-Hearing Association, San Antonio, TX.

Cooper, E. B., & Cooper, C. S. (1996). Clinician attitudes towards stuttering: Two decades of change. *Journal of Fluency Disorders, 21,* 119–135.

Cooper, S. (2000). *Sticks and stones.* New York: Times Books.

Corcoran, J. A., & Stewart, M. (1998). Stories of stuttering: A qualitative analysis of interview narratives. *Journal of Fluency Disorders, 23,* 247–264.

Cordes, A. K. (1998). Current status of the stuttering treatment literature. In A. K. Cordes & R. J. Ingham (Eds.), *Treatment efficacy for stuttering: A search for empirical bases.* San Diego, CA: Singular Publishing.

Cordes, A. K., & Ingham, R. J. (1994). Time-interval measurement of stuttering: Effects of training with highly agreed or poorly agreed exemplars. *Journal of Speech and Hearing Research, 37,* 1295–1307.

Cordes, A. K., & Ingham, R. J. (1996). Time-interval measurement of stuttering: Establishing and modifying judgment accuracy. *Journal of Speech and Hearing Research, 39,* 298–310.

Cordes, A. K., & Ingham, R. J. (1998). *Treatment efficacy for stuttering: A search for empirical bases.* San Diego, CA: Singular Publishing.

Coriat, I. H. (1943). Psychoanalytic concept of stammering. *Nervous Child, 2,* 167–171.

Coronary Drug Project Research Group. (1980). Influence of adherence to treatment and response of cholesterol on mortality in the coronary drug project. *New England Journal of Medicine, 303,* 1038–1041.

Costello, J. M. (1983). Current behavioral treatment of children. In D. Prins & R. J. Ingham (Eds.), *Treatment of stuttering in early childhood: Methods and issues* (pp. 69–112). San Diego, CA: College-Hill Press.

Cousins, N. (1979). *Anatomy of an illness.* New York: Norton.

Covey, S. (1989). *The seven habits of highly effective people.* New York: Simon & Schuster.

Cox, J. J., Seider, R. A., & Kidd, K. K. (1984). Some environmental factors and hypotheses for stuttering in families with several stutterers. *Journal of Speech and Hearing Research, 27,* 543–548.

Craig, A. (1990). An investigation into the relationship between anxiety and stuttering. *Journal of Speech and Hearing Disorders, 55,* 290–294.

Craig, A. (1998). Relapse following treatment for stuttering: A critical review and correlative data. *Journal of Fluency Disorders, 23,* 1–30.

Craig, A., & Andrews, G. (1985). The prediction and prevention of relapse in stuttering. The value of self-control techniques and locus of control measures. *Behavior Modification, 9,* 427–442.

Craig, A and Calver, P. (1991) Following up on treated stutterers: Studies on perceptions of fluency and job status. *Journal of Speech and Hearing Research, 34,* 279–284.

Craig, A., Franklin, J., & Andrews, G. (1984). A scale to measure locus of control of behavior. *British Journal of Medical Psychology, 57,* 173–180.

Craig, A., & Hancock, K. (1995). Self-reported factors related to relapse following treatment for stuttering. *Australian Journal of Human Communication Disorders, 23,* 48–60.

Craig, A., & Hancock, K. (1996). Anxiety in children and young adolescents who stutter. *Australian Journal of Human Communication Disorders, 24,* 28–38.

Craig, A., Hancock, K., Chang, E., McCready, C., Shepley, A., McCaul, A., Costello, D., Harding, S., Kehran, R., Masel, C., & Reilly, K. (1996). A controlled trial for stuttering in persons aged 9 to 14 years. *Journal of Speech and Hearing Research, 38,* 808–826.

Craig, A., Hancock, K., Tran, Y., Craig, M., & Peters, K. (2002). Epidemiology of stuttering in the community across the entire life span. *Journal of Speech, Hearing and Language Research, 45,* 1097–1105.

Crichton–Smith, I. (2002). Communicating in the real world: accounts from people who stammer. *Journal of Fluency Disorders, 27,* 333–352.

Crockett, W. H. (1965). Cognitive complexity and impression formation. In B. A. Maher (Ed.), *Progress in experimental personality research (Vol. 2).* (pp. 47–90). NY: Academic Press.

Crosby, B. (1997). *The meanest thing to say.* New York: Scholastic, Inc.

Cross, D. E., & Luper, H. L. (1983). Relation between finger reaction time and voice reaction time in stuttering and nonstuttering children and adults. *Journal of Speech and Hearing Research, 26,* 356–361.

Cross, D. E., Shadden, B. B., & Luper, H. L. (1979). Effects of stimulus ear presentation on the voice reaction time of adult stutterers and nonstutterers. *Journal of Fluency Disorders, 4,* 45–58.

Crowe, T. A. (1997a). Counseling: Definition, history, rationale. In T. A. Crowe (Ed.), *Applications of Counseling in Speech-Language Pathology and Audiology* (pp. 3–29). Baltimore: Williams & Wilkins.

Crowe, T. A. (1997b). Emotional aspects of communicative disorders. In T. A. Crowe (Ed.), *Applications of Counseling in Speech-Language Pathology and Audiology* (pp. 30–47). Baltimore: Williams & Wilkins.

Crowe, T. A., & Cooper, E. B. (1977). Clinician attitudes toward and knowledge of stuttering. *Journal of Communication Disorders, 10,* 343–357.

Crowe, T. A., DiLollo, A. P., & Crowe, B. T., *Crowe's Protocols: A Comprehensive Guide to Stuttering Assessment.* San Antonio, TX: The Psychological Corporation.

Crowe, T. A., & Walton, J. H. (1981). Teacher attitudes toward stuttering. *Journal of Fluency Disorders, 6,* 163–174.

Crystal, D. (1987). Towards a "bucket" theory of language disability: Taking account of interaction between linguistic levels. *Clinical Linguistics and Phonetics, 1,* 7–22.

Cuadrado, E. M., & Weber-Fox, C. M. (2003). Atypical syntactic processing in individuals who stutter: Evidence from event-related brain potentials and behavioral measures. *Journal of Speech, Language and Hearing Research, 46,* 960–976.

Culatta, R., & Goldberg. S. A. (1995). *Stuttering therapy: An integrated approach to theory and practice.* Boston: Allyn & Bacon.

Curlee, R. (1984). Counseling with adults who stutter. In W. Perkins (Ed.), *Stuttering disorders.* New York: Thieme Medical Publishers, Inc.

Curlee, R. (1985). Training students to work with stutterers. In E. Boberg (Ed.), *Stuttering: Part one. Seminars in Speech and Language, 6*(2), 131–144. New York: Thieme Medical Publishers, Inc.

Curlee, R. (1993). Evaluating treatment efficacy for adults: Assessment of stuttering disability. *Journal of Fluency Disorders, 18,* 319–331.

Curlee, R. (2000). Demands-Capacities versus Demands-Performance. *Journal of Fluency Disorders, 25*(4), 329–336.

Curlee, R., & Yairi, E. (1997). Early intervention with early childhood stuttering: A critical examination of the data. *American Journal of Speech-Language Pathology, 6,* 8–18.

Curry, F., & Gregory, H. (1969). The performance of stutterers on dichotic listening tasks thought to reflect cerebral dominance. *Journal of Speech and Hearing Research, 12,* 73–81.

Dalton, P. (1987). Some developments in personal construct therapy with adults who stutter. In C. Levy (Ed.), *Stuttering therapies: Practical approaches* (pp. 61–70). London: Croom Helm.

Dalton, P. (1994). A personal construct approach to communication problems. In P. Dalton (Ed.), *Counseling people with communication problems* (pp. 15–27). London: Sage Publications.

Daly, D. A. (1981). Differentiation of stuttering subgroups with Van Riper's developmental tracks: A preliminary study. *Journal of the American Student Speech and Hearing Association, 9,* 89–101.

Daly, D. A. (1986). The clutterer. In K. O. St. Louis (Ed.), *The atypical stutterer* (pp. 155–192). Orlando, FL: Academic Press.

Daly, D. A. (1987). Use of the home VCR to facilitate transfer of fluency. *Journal of Fluency Disorders, 12,* 103–106.

Daly, D. A. (1988). *Freedom of fluency.* Tucson, AZ: LingaSystems.

Daly, D. A. (1992). Helping the clutterer: Therapy considerations. In F. Myers & K. St. Louis (Eds.), *Cluttering: A clinical perspective* (pp. 27–41). San Diego, CA: Singular Publishing Group, Inc.

Daly, D. A. (1993). Cluttering: Another fluency syndrome. In R. Curlee (Ed.), *Stuttering and Related Disorders of Fluency* (pp. 151–175). New York: Thieme Medical Publishers.

Daly, D. A. (1994). Practical techniques that work with children and adolescents who stutter. Presentation to the annual meeting of the American Speech-Language-Hearing Association, New Orleans.

Daly, D. A. (1996). *The Source for Stuttering and Cluttering,* East Moline, IL: LinguiSystems, Inc.

Daly, D. A. (1998). Stuttering: Recovering or recovered. In E. C. Healey & H. F. M. Peters (Eds.), *Proceedings of the 2nd World Congress on Fluency Disorders* (pp. 379–380). Nijmegen, The Netherlands: Nijmegen University Press.

Daly, D. A. (1999). Personal Communication.

Daly, D. A., & Burnett, M. L. (1996) Cluttering: assessment, treatment planning, and case study illustration. *Journal of Fluency Disorders, 21,* 239–248.

Daly, D. A., & Burnett, M. L. (1999). Cluttering: Traditional views and new perspectives. In R. Curlee (Ed.), *Stuttering and Related Disorders of Fluency* (2nd Edition, pp. 222–254). New York: Thieme Medical Publishers, Inc.

Daly, D., Guitar, B., Manning, W., Murphy, B., Nelson, L., Quesal, R., Ramig, P., & St. Louis, K. (1996, Nov.) Successful Treatment of Fluency Disorders: Examples of Long-Term Change. Presentation to the Annual Convention of the American Speech-Language-Hearing Association, Seattle, WA.

Daly, D. A., & Kimbarow, M. L. (1978). Stuttering as operant behavior: Effects of the verbal stimuli wrong, right, and tree on the disfluency rates of school-age stutterers and nonstutterers. *Journal of Speech and Hearing Research, 21,* 589–597.

Daly, D., Riley, J., & Riley, G. (2000). *Speech motor exercises.* Austin, TX: ProEd.

Daly, D., Simon, C., & Burnett-Stolnack, M. (1995). Helping adolescents who stutter focus on fluency. *Language, Speech, and Hearing Services in Schools, 26,* 162–168.

Davidson, R. J. (1994). Affect, cognition, and hemisphereic specialization. In E. Izard, J. Kagan, and R. Zajonc (Eds.), *Emotion, Cognition and Behavior.* New York: Cambridge University Press.

Davidson, R. J. (1995). Cerebral asymmetry, emotion, and affective style. In R. J. Davidson and K. Hugdahl (Eds.), *Brain Asymmetry* (pp. 361–387). Cambridge, MA: MIT Press.

Davis, J. M., & Farina, A. (1970). Appreciation of humor: An experimental and theoretical study. *Journal of Personality and Social Psychology, 15*(2), 175–178.

Deal, J. L. (1982). Sudden onset of stuttering: A case report. *Journal of Speech and Hearing Disorders, 47,* 301–304.

DeBuck, A. (1970). *Egyptian readingbook, exercises and Middle Egyptian texts.* Leiden, Holland: Nederlands Instituut Voor Nabije Oosten.

Dell, C. (1970). *Treating the school age stutterer: A guide for clinicians* (Publication No. 14). Memphis, TN: Speech Foundation of America.

De Nil, L. F. (1999) Stuttering: A neurophysiological perspective. Chapter 7 In N. B. Ratner & E. C. Healey (Eds.), *Stuttering research and practice: Bridging the gap* (pp. 85–102). Mahwah, NJ: Lawrence Erlbaum.

De Nil, L. F. (2004). Recent developments in brain imaging research in stuttering. In B. Maassen, H. Peters, and R. Kent (Eds.), *Speech motor control in normal and disordered speech* (pp. 113–137). Oxford: Oxford University Press.

De Nil, L. F., & Abbs, J. H. (1990). Influence of rate on stutterers' articulatory movements: A microbeam study. *ASHA, 32, 72.*

De Nil, L. F., & Brutten, G. J. (1991). Speech-associated attitudes of stuttering and nonstuttering children. *Journal of Speech and Hearing Research, 34,* 60–66.

De Nil, L. F., & Kroll, R. M. (1995). The relationship between locus of control and long-term stuttering treatment outcome in adult stutterers. *Journal of Fluency Disorders, 20,* 345–364.

De Nil, L. F., Kroll, R. M., Kapur, S., & Houle, S. (2000). A positron emission tomography study of silent and oral single word reading in stuttering and nonstuttering adults. *Journal of Speech, Hearing, and Language Research, 43,* 1038–1053.

De Nil, L. F., Kroll, R. M., Lafaille, S. J., & Houle, S. (2003). A positron emission tomography study of short- and long-term treatment effects on functional brain activation in adults who stutter. *Journal of Fluency Disorders, 28,* 357–381.

De Nil, L. F., Jokel, R., & Rochon, E., (2007). Etiology symptomatology, and treatment of neurogenic stuttering. In E. Conture & R. Curlee, *Stuttering and Related Disorders of Fluency,* (3rd Edition pp. 326–343). New York: Thieme Medical Publishers, Inc.

Denny, M., & Smith, A.. (1992). Gradations in a pattern of neuro-muscular activity associated with stuttering. *Journal of Speech and Hearing Research, 35,* 1216–1229.

DeVore, J., Nandur, M., & Manning, W. (1984). Projective drawings and children who stutter. *Journal of Fluency Disorders, 9,* 217–226.

Dewar, A., Dewar, A. D., & Anthony, J. F. K. (1976). The effect of auditory feedback masking on concomitants of stammering. *British Journal of Disorders of Communication, 11,* 95–102.

DiClemente, C. C. (1993). Changing addictive behaviors: A process perspective. *Current Directions in Psychological Science, 2*(4), 101–106.

Dietrich, S. (1997). Central auditory processing in males who stutter. *Proceedings of the 2nd World Congress on Fluency Disorders* (pp. 73–76). Nijmegen, The Netherlands: Nijmegen University Press.

Dietrich, S., Jensen, K. H., & Williams, D. E. (2001). Effects of the label "stuttering" on student perceptions. *Journal of Fluency Disorders, 26,* 55–66.

DiLollo, A. (2006). Foxes, scorpions, and stuttering research: How a Constructivist perspective might help us avoid getting stung. Presentation to the Fifth world congress on Fluency Disorders. Dublin, Ireland.

DiLollo, A. & Manning, W. H. (2007). Counseling children who stutter and their parents, In E. Conture & R. Curlee, *Stuttering and Related Disorders of Fluency* (3rd Edition, 115–130). New York: Thieme Medical Publishers, Inc.

DiLollo, A., Manning, W. H., & Neimeyer, R. A. (2002). *The reconstruction workbook,* Unpublished manuscript.

DiLollo, A., Manning, W. H., & Neimeyer, R. A. (2003). Cognitive anxiety as a function of speaker role for fluent speakers and persons who stutter. *Journal of Fluency Disorders, 28*(3), 167–186.

DiLollo, A., Manning, W. H., & Neimeyer, R. A. (2005). Cognitive complexity as a function of speaker role for adult persons who stutter. *Journal of Constructivist Psychology, 18,* 215–236.

DiLollo, A., Manning, W, and Plexico, L. (2004). The content analysis of verbal behavior: Applications to stuttering therapy. In A. Packman, A. Meltzer, & H. M. F. Peters (Eds.), Theory, Research and Therapy in Fluency Disorders (*Proceedings of the Fourth World Congress on Fluency Disorders*; errata supplement, pp. 7–12). Nijmegen, The Netherlands: Nijmegen University Press.

DiLollo, A., & Neimeyer, R. (2008). Talking back to stuttering: Constructivist contributions to stuttering treatment. In J. D. Raskin & S. K. Bridges (Eds.), *Studies in Meaning 3: Constructivist Psychotherapy in the Real World* (pp. 165–182). NY: Pace University Press.

DiLollo, A., Neimeyer, R., & Manning, W. (2002). A personal construct psychology view of relapse: indications for a narrative therapy component to stuttering treatment. *Journal of Fluency Disorders, 27*(1), 19–42.

Donaher, J. (2006). Tourette's syndrome and stuttering. *Fluency and Fluency Disorders, 16*(2), 5–6.

Donaher, J. G., Healey, E. C., Sisskin, V., Daly, D., & Graham, C. (2005). *Fluency: The effect of commonly occurring concomitant disorders on stuttering.* Presentation to the Annual Convention of the American Speech-Language-Hearing Association, San Diego, CA.

Doopdy, I., Kalinowski, J., Armson, J. (1993). Stereotypes of stutterers and nonstutterers in three rural communities in Newfoundland. *Journal of Fluency Disorders, 18,* 363–373.

Dorman, M.F., & Porter, R.J. (1975). Hemispheric lateralization for speech perception in stutterers. *Cortex, 11,* 181–185.

Douglass, E., & Quarrington, B. (1952). The differentiation of interiorized and exteriorized secondary stuttering. *Journal of Speech and Hearing Disorders, 17,* 377–385.

Dranya, D. (2008, personal communication)

Dreyfus, H. L., & Dreyfus, S. E. (1986). *Mind over machine.* New York: Free Press.

Drewery, W., Winslade, J., Monk, G. (2000). Resisting the dominating story: Toward a deeper understanding of narrative therapy. In R. Neimeyer & J. D. Raskin (Eds.). *Constructions of Disorder* (pp. 253–263). Washington, D.C.: American Psychological Association.

Duchin, S. W., & Mysak, E. D. (1987). Disfluency and rate characteristics of young, middle-aged, and older males. *Journal of Communication Disorders, 20,* 245–257.

Duncan, B. L. (2002). The legacy of Saul Rosenweig: The profundity of the dodo bird. *Journal of Psychotherapy Integration, 12*(1) 32–57.

Dunlap, K. (1917). The stuttering boy. *Journal of Abnormal Psychology, 12,* 44–48.

Dunlap, K. (1932). *Habits: Their making and unmaking.* New York: Liveright.

Dworzynski, K., Remington, A., Rijsdijk, F., Howell, P., & Plomin, R. (2007). Genetic etiology in cases of recovered persistent stuttering in an unselected, longitudinal sample of young twins. *American Journal of Speech-Language Pathology, 16,* 169–178.

Dykes, R., & Pindzola, R. (1995). Racial/ethnic differences in the prevalence of school-aged stutterers. Presentation to the annual meeting of the American Speech-Language-Hearing Association, Orlando.

Egan, G. (1990). *The skilled helper: A systematic approach to effective helping* (4th ed.). Pacific Grove, CA: Brooks/Cole Publishing Co.

Egan, G. (1998) *The Skilled Helper: A problem-management approach to helping* (6th ed.). Pacific Grove, CA: Brooks/Cole Publishing Co.

Egan, G. (2002). *The skilled helper: A problem-management and opportunity development approach to helping* (7th ed.). Pacific Grove, CA: Brooks/Cole.

Egan, G. (2007). *The skilled helper: A problem-management and opportunity development approach to helping* (8th ed.). Belmont, CA: Thomson Brooks/Cole.

Eichstaedt. A., Watt, N., & Girson, J. (1998). Evaluation of the efficacy of a stutter modification program with particular reference to two new measures of secondary behaviors and control of stuttering. *Journal of Fluency Disorders, 23,* 231–246.

Eisenson, J., & Ogilvie, M. (1963). *Speech correction in the schools* (2nd ed.). New York: Macmillan.

Ellis, A. (1977). The basic clinical theory of rational-emotive therapy. In A. Ellis & R. Grieger (Eds.), *Handbook of rational-emotive therapy* (pp. 218–250). New York: Springer.

Embrechts, M., Ebben, H., Franke, P., & van de Poel, C. (2000). Temperament: A comparison between children who stutter and children who do not stutter. In H. G. Bosshardt, J. S., Yaruss, & H. F. M. Peters (Eds.), *Proceedings of the Third World Congress on Fluency Disorders* (pp. 557–562). Nijmegen, The Netherlands: Nijmegen University.

Emerick, L. (1974). Stuttering therapy: Dimensions of interpersonal sensitivity. In L. L. Emerick & S. B. Hood (Eds.), *The client-clinician relationship: Essays on interpersonal sensitivity in the therapeutic transaction* (pp. 92–102). Springfield, IL: Charles C. Thomas.

Emerick, L. (1988). Counseling adults who stutter: A cognitive approach. *Seminars in Speech and Language, 9*(3), 257–267.

Epley, N., Keysar, B., Bovan, L. V., & Gilovick, T. (2004). Perspective taking as anchoring and adjustment. *Journal of Personality and Social Psychology, 87,* 327–339.

Epston, D., & White, M. (1999). Termination as a right of passage: Questioning strategies for a therapy of inclusion. In R. A. Neimeyer, and R. J. Mahoney (Eds.) *Constructivism in psychotherapy.* Washington, DC: American Psychological Association.

Erickson, R. L. (1969). Assessing communication attitudes among stutterers. *Journal of Speech and Hearing Research, 12,* 711–724.

Ericsson, A. K & Smith, J. (1991). Prospects and limits of the empirical study of expertise: an introduction. In A. K. Ericsson & J. Smith, J. (Eds.), *Toward a general theory of expertise: prospects and limits* (pp. 1–38). Cambridge: Cambridge University Press.

Evesham, M. (1987). Residential courses for stutterers: Combining technique and personal construct psychology. In C. Levy (Ed.), *Stuttering therapies: Practical approaches* (pp. 61–70). London: Croom Helm.

Evesham, M., & Fransella, F. (1985). Stuttering relapse: The effect of a combined speech and psychological reconstruction programme. *British Journal of Disorders of Communication, 20,* 237–248.

Ezrati–Vinacour, R., & Levin, I. (2001). Time estimation by adults who stutter. *Journal of Speech, Language and Hearing Research, 44,* 144–157.

Ezrati–Vinacour, R., Platzky, R., & Yairi, E. (2001). The young child's awareness of stuttering-like disfluency. *Journal of Speech, Language, and Hearing Research, 44,* 368–380.

Fairbanks, G. (1954). Systematic research in experimental phonetics—I. A theory of the speech mechanism as a servomechanism. *Journal of Speech and Hearing Disorders, 19,* 133–139.

Falsenfeld, S. (1997). Epidemiology and genetics of stuttering. In R. Curlee & G. Siegel (Eds.), *Nature and treatment of stuttering, new directions* (2nd ed., pp. 3–23). Needham Heights, MA: Allyn & Bacon.

Fant, G. (1960). *The acoustic theory of speech production.* The Hague, Holland: Mouton.

Farrelly, F., & Brandsma, J. (1974). *Provocative therapy.* Cupertino, CA: Meta Publications.

Faulkner, R. O. (1962). *A concise dictionary of Middle Egyptian.* Oxford, England: University Press.

Felsenfeld, S., Kirk, K. M., Zhu, G., Statham, D. J., Neale, M. C., & Martin, N. G. (2000). A study of the genetic and environmental etiology of stuttrering in a selected twin sample. *Behavior Genetics, 30,* 359–366.

Fenichel, O. (1945). *The psychoanalytic theory of neurosis.* New York: Norton.

Fey, M., & Johnson, B. (1998). Research to practice (and back again) in speech–language intervention. *Topics in Language Disorders, 18*(2), 23–34.

Fibiger, S. (1994). Did Moses and Demosthenes stutter? *Journal of Fluency Disorders Abstracts of the First World Congress on Fluency Disorders, 19,* 173.

Filmore, C. J. (1979). On fluency. In *Individual differences in language ability and language behavior.* New York: Academic Press.

Finitzo, T., Pool, K. D., Freeman, F. J., Devous, M. D., Sr., & Watson, B. C. (1991). Cortical dysfunction in developmental stutterers. In H. F. M. Peters, W. Hulstijn, & C. W. Starkweather (Eds.), *Speech motor control and stuttering* (pp. 251–262). Amsterdam: Elsevier.

Finn, P. (1997). Adults recovered from stuttering without formal treatment: Perceptual assessment of speech normalcy. *Journal of Speech, Language, and Hearing Research, 40,* 821–831.

Finn, P. (2003). Evidence-based treatment of stuttering: II. Clinical significance of behavioral stuttering treatments. *Journal of Fluency Disorders, 28,* 209–218.

Finn, P., Bothe, A. K., & Bramlett, R. E. (2005). Science and pseudoscience in communication disorders: Criteria and applications. *American Journal of Speech-Language Pathology, 14,* 172–186.

Fish, J. M. (1995). Does problem behavior just happen? Does it matter? *Behavior and Social Issues, 5*(1), 3–12.

Fisher, R., & Ury, W. (1981). *Getting to yes: Negotiating agreement without giving in.* Boston: Houghton Mifflin.

Fitch, J. L., & Batson, E. A. (1989). Hemispheric asymmetry of alpha wave suppression in stutterers and nonstutterers. *Journal of Fluency Disorders, 9,* 47–55.

Flanagan, B., Goldiamond, I., & Azrin, N. (1958). Operant stuttering: The control of stuttering behavior through response-contingent consequences. *Journal of Experimental Analysis of Behavior, 1,* 173–177.

Flanagan, B., Goldiamond, I., & Azrin, N. (1958). Instatement of stuttering in normally fluent individuals through operant procedures. *Science, 130,* 979–981.

Flasher, L., & Fogle, P. (2004). *Counseling skills for the speech-language pathologist and audiologist.* Clifton Park, NY: Thompson-Delmar Learning.

Floyd, J., Zebrowski, P., & Flamme, G. A., (2007). Stages of change and stuttering: A preliminary view. *Journal of Fluency Disorders, 32,* 95–120.

Fosnot, S. (1993). Research design for examining treatment efficacy in fluency disorders, *Journal of Fluency Disorders, 18,* 221–251.

Foundas, A. L., Bolich, A. M., Corey, D. M., Hurley, M. & Heilman, K. M. (2001). Anomalous anatomy of speech-language areas in adults with developmental stuttering. *Neurology, 57,* 207–215.

Foundas, A. L., Bolich, A. M., Feldman, J., Corey, D. M., Hurley, M., Lemen, L. C. & Heilman, K. M. (2004). Aberrant auditory processing and atypical planum temporal in developmental stuttering. *Neurology, 63,* 1640–1646.

Foundas, A. L., Corey, D. M., Angeles, V., Bollich, A. M., Crabtree-Hartman, E., & Heilman, K. M., (2003). Atypical cerebral laterality in adults with persistent developmental stuttering. *Neurology, 61,* 1378–1385.

Fox, P. T., Ingham, R. J., Ingham, J. C., Hirsch, T. B., Downs, J. H., Martin, C., Jerabek, P., Glass, T., & Lancaster, J. L. (1996). A PET study of the neural systems of stuttering. *Nature, 382,* 158–162.

Fox, P. T., Lancaster, J. L., & Ingham, R. J. (1993). On stuttering and global ischemia—Letter to the editor. *Archives of Neurology, 50,* 1287–1288.

Franken, M. C., Boves, L., & Peters, H. F. M. (1997). Evaluation of Dutch precision fluency–shaping program. In E. C. Healey & H. F. M. Peters (Eds.) *International Fluency Association, second world congress on fluency disorders: Proceedings* (pp. 303–307). San Francisco, Nijmegen University Press.

Franken, M. C., Boves, L., Peters, H. F. M., & Webster, R. L. (1992) Perceptual evaluation of speech before and after fluency shaping therapy. *Journal of Fluency Disorders, 17,* 223–241.

Franken, M. C., Van der Schalk, C. J., & Boelens, H. (2005). Experimental treatment of early stuttering: A preliminary study, *Journal of Fluency Disorders, 30,* 189–199.

Fransella, F. (1972). *Personal change and reconstruction.* New York: Academic Press.

Fransella, F. (2003). From theory to research to change. In F. Fransella (Ed.), *International Handbook of Personal Construct Psychology* (pp. 211–222). West Sussex, England: John Wiley & Sons.

Fransella, F., & Dalton, P. (1990). *Personal construct counseling in action.* London: Sage.

Freeman, J., Epston, D., & Lobovits, D. (1997). *Playful approaches to serious problems.* New York: W.W. Norton & Company, Inc.

Freeman, F. J., & Ushijima, T. (1975). Laryngeal activity accompanying the movement of stuttering: A preliminary report of EMG investigations. *Journal of Fluency Disorders, 1,* 36–45.

Freeman, F. J., & Ushijima, T. (1978). Laryngeal muscle activity during stuttering. *Journal of Speech and Hearing Research, 21,* 538–5622.

Freud, S. (1905/1961). Jokes and their relation to the unconscious. In James Strachey (Ed.), *The complete psychological works of Sigmund Freud* (vol. 8). London: Hogarth Press.

Freud, S. (1928). Humor. *International Journal of Psychoanalysis, 9,* 1–6.

Freund, H. (1966). *Psychopathology and the problems of stuttering.* Springfield, IL: Charles C. Thomas.

Froeschels, E. (1943). Pathology and therapy of stuttering. *Nervous Child, 22,* 148–161.

Gaines, N., Runyan, C., & Meyers, S. (1991). A comparison of young stutterers' fluent versus stuttered utterances on measures of length and complexity. *Journal of Speech and Hearing Research, 34,* 37–42.

Geschwind, N., & Galaburda, A. M. (1985). Cerebral lateralization: Biological mechanisms, associations, and pathology: I. A hypothesis and a program for research. *Archives of Neurology, 42,* Part I: 429–459.; II: 34–552; III: 634–654.

Gildston, P. (1967). Stutterers' self-acceptance and perceived self-acceptance. *Journal of Abnormal and Social Psychology, 72,* 59–64.

Gillespie, S. K., & Cooper, E. G. (1973). Prevalence of speech problems in junior and senior high schools, *Journal of Speech and Hearing Research, 16,* 739–743.

Gladwell, M. (2005). *Blink: The power of thinking without thinking.* New York: Little, Brown & Company.

Glasner, P. J. (1949). Personality characteristics and emotional problems in stutterers under the age of five. *Journal of Speech and Hearing Disorders, 14,* 135–138.

Glasner, P. J., & Rosenthal, D. (1957). Parental diagnosis of stuttering in young children. *Journal of Speech and Hearing Disorders, 22,* 288–295.

Glauber, I. P. (1958). The psychoanalysis of stuttering. In Jon Eisenson (Ed.), *Stuttering: A symposium* (pp. 71–119). New York: Harper & Brothers.

Glauber, I. P. (1982). *Stuttering: A psychoanalytic understanding.* New York: Human Sciences Press.

Goldberg, B. (1989). Historic treatment of stuttering: From pebbles to psychoanalysis. *ASHA, 31*(6/7), 71.

Goldberg, G. (1985). Supplementary motor and structure and function: Review and hypotheses. *The Behavioral and Brain Sciences, 8,* 567–616.

Goldman-Eisler, F. (1958). The predictability of words in context and the length of pauses in speech. *Language and Speech, 1,* 226–231.

Goldman-Eisler, F. (1961). The continuity of speech utterance: Its determinants and its significance. *Language and Speech, 4,* 220–231.

Goldstein, J. H. (1976). Theoretical notes on humor. *Journal of Communication, 26,* 104–112.

Goleman, D. (1985). Switching therapists may be best. *Indianapolis News,* p. 9.

Goleman, D. (2006). *Social Intelligence.* New York, NY: Bantam Dell.

Goodstein, L. D. (1958). Functional speech disorders and personality: A survey of the research. *Journal of Speech and Hearing Research, 1,* 359–376.

Gordon, K. C., Hutchinson, J. M., & Allen, C. S. (1976). An evaluation of selected discourse characteristics in normal geriatric subjects. *Idaho State University Laboratory Research Reports, 1,* 11–21.

Gordon, P. (1991). Language task effects: A comparison of stuttering and non-stuttering children. *Journal of Fluency Disorders, 16,* 275–287.

Gordon, P., Luper, H., & Peterson, H. J. (1986). The effects of syntactic complexity on the occurrence of disfluencies in 5 year old nonstutterers. *Journal of Fluency Disorders, 11,* 151–164.

Gottwald, S. R. (1999). Family communication pattern and stuttering development: An analysis of the research literature. In N. B. Ratner & E. C. Healey (Eds.), *Stuttering research and practice: Bridging the gap* (pp. 175–192). Mahwah, NJ: Lawrence Erlbaum Associates.

Gottwald, S. R., & Starkweather, C. W. (1995). Fluency intervention for preschoolers and their families in the public schools. *Language, Speech, and Hearing Services in Schools, 26,* 117–126.

Gottwald, S. R., & Starkweather, C. W. (1999). Stuttering prevention and early intervention: A multi-process approach. In M. Onslow and A. Packman (Eds.), *The handbook of early stuttering intervention* (pp. 53–82). San Diego, CA: Singular Publishing Company.

Gould, S. J. (1995). *Dinosaur in a haystack.* New York: Random House.

Graham, E. (1995). The involvement of sense of humor in the development of social relationships. *Communication Reports, 8*(2), 158–169.

Graham, C. (2006, September) The effect of ADHD on the treatment of stuttering, *Fluency and Fluency Disorders, 16*(2), 10–12.

Grant, A. C., Blousse, V., Cook, A. A., & Newman, N. J. (1999). Stroke-associated stuttering. *Archives of Neurology, 56,* 624–627.

Gregory, H. H. (1972). An assessment of the results of stuttering therapy. *Journal of Communication Disorders, 5,* 320–334.

Gregory, H. H. (1979). Controversial issues: Statement and review of the literature. In H. H. Gregory (Ed.), *Controversies about stuttering therapy* (pp. 1–62). Baltimore, MD: University Park Press.

Gregory, H. H. (1983). *The clinician's attitudes in counseling stutterers* (Publication No. 18). Memphis, TN: Stuttering Foundation of America.

Gregory, H. H. (1984). Prevention of stuttering: Management of the early stages. In R. F. Curlee & W. H. Perkins (Eds.), *Nature and treatment of stuttering: New directions*. San Diego: College-Hill Press.

Gregory, H. H. (1986). *Stuttering: Differential evaluation and therapy*. Austin, TX: ProEd.

Gregory, H. H. (1989). Stuttering therapy: A workshop for specialists. Unpublished manuscript, Evanston, IL: Northwestern University and the Stuttering Foundation of America.

Gregory, H. H. (1991). Therapy for elementary school-age children. *Seminars in Speech and Language, 12,* 323–335.

Gregory, H. H. (1995). Analysis and commentary. *Language, Speech, and Hearing Services in Schools, 26*(2), 196–200.

Gregory, H. H. (2004). *Do you stutter: A guide for teens* (4th ed). Memphis, TN: The Stuttering Foundation, Publication No. 0021, 40.

Gregory, H. H., & Hill, D. (1980). Stuttering therapy for children. In W. Perkins (Ed.), *Stuttering disorders*, (pp. 351–363). New York: Thieme Medical Publishers Inc.

Groopman, J. (2003). The biology of hope, In *The Anatomy of Hope, How people prevail in the face of illness*, (pp. 161–190, New York: Random House.

Guenther, F. H. (2008). Neuroimaging of normal speech production. In R. J. Ingham (Ed.), *Neuroimaging in Communication Sciences and disorders*. (pp. 1–51). San Diego: Plural Publishing Inc.

Guitar, B. (1976). Pretreatment factors associated with the outcome of stuttering therapy. *Journal of Speech and Hearing Research, 18,* 590–600.

Guitar, B. (1997). Therapy for children's stuttering and emotions. In R. F. Curlee & G. M. Siegel (Eds.), *Nature and Treatment of Stuttering: New Directions* (2nd ed., pp. 280–291). Boston, MA: Allyn & Bacon.

Guitar, B. (2006). *Stuttering: An integrated approach to its nature and treatment* (3rd ed.). Baltimore, MD: Williams & Wilkins

Guitar, B. E., & Bass, C. (1978). Stuttering therapy: The relation between attitude change and long-term outcome. *Journal of Speech and Hearing Disorders, 43,* 392–499.

Guitar, B., & Grims, S. (1977). Developing a scale to assess communication attitudes in children who stutter. Presentation to the Annual Convention of the American Speech-Language-Hearing Association, Atlanta, GA.

Guitar, B., & Peters, T. J. (1980). *Stuttering: An integration of contemporary therapies* (Publication No. 16). Memphis, TN: Stuttering Foundation of America.

Haefner, R. (1929). *The educational significance of left-handedness*. New York: Teachers College, Columbia University Press.

Hageman, C. F., & Greene, P. N. (1989). Auditory comprehension of stutterers on a competing message task. *Journal of Fluency Disorders, 14,* 109–120.

Haig, R. A. (1986). Therapeutic use of humor. *American Journal of Psychotherapy XL. 4,* 543–553.

Hall, J. W., & Jerger, J. (1978). Central auditory function in stutterers. *Journal of Speech and Hearing Research, 21,* 324–337.

Hall, K. D., & Yairi, E. (1992). Fundamental frequency, jitter, and shimmer in preschoolers who stutter. *Journal of Speech and Hearing Research, 35,* 1002–1008.

Hall, P. K. (1977). The occurrence of disfluencies in language-disordered school-age children. *Journal of Speech and Hearing Disorders, 42,* 364–369.

Hall, K. D., & Yairi, E. (1992). Fundamental frequency, jitter, and shimmer in preschoolers who stutter. *Journal of Speech, Language, and Hearing Research, 35,* 1002–1008.

Hall, K. D., Amir, O., & Yairi, E., (1999). A longitudinal investigation of speaking rate in preschool children who stutter. *Journal of Speech, Language, and Hearing Research, 42,* 1367–1377.

Ham, R. (1986). *Techniques of stuttering therapy.* Englewood Cliffs, NJ: Prentice–Hall.

Ham, R. E. (1989). What are we measuring? *Journal of Fluency Disorders, 14,* 231–243.

Ham, R. E. (1990). *Therapy of stuttering, preschool through adolescence.* Englewood Cliffs, NJ: Prentice-Hall.

Ham, R. E. (1993). Chronic perseverative stuttering syndrome: constructive or casuistic? *American Journal of Speech-Language Pathology, 2*(3), 16–20.

Ham, R. E. (1999). *Clinical management of stuttering in older children and adults.* Gaithersburg, MD: Aspen Publishers. Ind.

Hamre, C. (1992). Stuttering prevention I: Primacy of identification. *Journal of Fluency Disorders, 17,* 3–23.

Hancock, K., & Craig, A. (1998). Predictors of stuttering relapse one year following treatment for children aged 9 to 14 years. *Journal of Fluency Disorders, 23,* 31–48.

Hancock, K, Craig, A., McCready, C., McCaul, A., Costello, D., Campbell, K., & Gilmore, G. (1998). Two- to six-year controlled-trial stuttering outcomes for children and adolescents. *Journal of Speech, Language, and Hearing Research, 41,* 1242–1252.

Hanson, B. R., Gonhoud, K. D., & Rice, P. L. (1981). Speech situation checklist. *Journal of Fluency Disorders, 6,* 351–360.

Harrison, E., Onslow, M., Rousseau, I., (2007). Lidcombe Program 2007: Clinical Tales and Clinical Trials, In E. Conture & R. Curlee (Eds.), *Stuttering and Related Disorders of Fluency* (3rd Edition, pp. 55–75). Philadelphia, PA: Thieme.

Hastorf, A. H., Windfogel, J., & Cassman, T. (1979). Acknowledgement of handicap as a tactic in social interaction. *Journal of Personality and Social Psychology, 37,* 1790–1797.

Hayden, P. A., Scott, D. A., & Addicott, J. (1977). The effects of delayed auditory feedback on the overt behaviors of stutterers. *Journal of Fluency Disorders, 2,* 235–246.

Hayhow, R., & Levy, C. (1989). *Working with stuttering.* Bicester, Oxon, England: Winslow Press.

Healey, E. C. (1982). Speaking fundamental frequency characteristics of stutterers and nonstutterers. *Journal of Communications Disorders, 15*(1), 21–29.

Healey, E. C. (Ed.). (1995, June). *Division 4 Newsletter, 5*(2). Rockville, MD: American Speech-Language-Hearing Association.

Healey, E. C., & Gutkin, B. (1984). Analysis of stutterers' voice onset times and fundamental frequency contours during fluency. *Journal of Speech and Hearing Research, 27,* 219–225.

Healey, E. C., & Reid, R. (2003). ADHA and stuttering: A tutorial. *Journal of Fluency Disorders, 28,* 79–93.

Healey, E. C., & Scott, L. A. (1995). Strategies for treating elementary school-age children who stutter: An integrative approach. *Language, Speech, and Hearing Services in Schools, 26,* 151–161.

Henri, B. P. (1994, January). Graduate student preparation: Tomorrow's challenge. *ASHA, 36,* 43–46.

Heinze, B. A., & Johnson, K. L. (1985). Easy does it–1: *Fluency activities for young children.* East Moline, IL: LinguiSystems.

Heinze, B. A., & Johnson, K. L. (1987). Easy does it–2: *Fluency activities for school-aged stutterers.* East Moline, IL: LinguiSystems.

Helm, N. A., Butler, R. B., & Canter, G. J. (1980). Neurogenic acquired stuttering. *Journal of Fluency Disorders, 5,* 269–279.

Helm, N. A., Yeo, R., Geschwind, M., Freedman, M., & Wenstein, C. (1986). Stuttering: Disappearance and reappearance with acquired brain lesions. *Neurology, 36,* 1109–1112.

Helm-Estabrooks, N. (1986). Diagnosis and management of neurogenic stuttering in adults. In K. O. St. Louis (Ed.), *The Atypical Stutterer* (pp. 193–217). Orlando, FL: Academic Press.

Helm-Estabrooks, N. (1993). Stuttering associated with acquired neurological disorders. In Curlee, R. (Ed.), *Stuttering and Related Disorders of Fluency.* New York: Thieme Medical Publishers.

Helm-Estabrooks, N. (1999). Stuttering associated with acquired neurological disorders. In R. Curlee (Ed.), *Stuttering and related disorders of fluency* (2nd Edition, pp. 255–268). New York: Thieme Medical Publishers, Inc.

Herder, C., Howard, C., Nye, C. & Vanryckeghem, M., (2006). Effectiveness of behavioral stuttering treatment: A systematic review and meta-analysis. *Contemporary Issues in Communication Science and Disorders, 33,* 61–73.

Hillis, J. W. (1993). Ongoing assessment in the management of stuttering: A clinical perspective. *American Journal of Speech-Language Pathology, 2*(1), 24–37.

Hillis, J., & Manning, W. H. (1996, November). Extraclinical generalization of speech fluency: A social cognitive approach. Presentation to the annual meeting of the American Speech-Language-Hearing Association, Seattle.

Hillis, J., & Manning, W. (1998, November) Multidimensional assessment of self-efficacy for speech fluency. Computer laboratory presentation to the annual meeting of the American Speech-Language-Hearing Association, San Antonio, TX.

Hillman, R. E., & Gilbert, H. R. (1977). Voice onset time for voiceless stop consonants in the fluent reading of stutterers and nonstutterers. *Journal of the Acoustical Society of America, 61,* 610–611.

Hinsie, L. E., & Campbell, R., J., (1970). *Psychiatric dictionary* (4th ed.). New York: Oxford University Press.

Hodson, B. W. (1986). The assessment of phonological processes—Revised. Austin, TX: Pro-Ed.

Hollis, &, Campbell, F. (1999). What is meant by intention to treat analysis? Survey of published randomized controlled trials. *British Medical Journal, 319,* 670–674.

Hood, S. B. (1974). Clients, clinicians and therapy. In L. L. Emerick & S. B. Hood (Eds.), *The client-clinician relationship: Essays on interpersonal sensitivity in the therapeutic transaction* (pp. 45–59). Springfield, IL: Charles C. Thomas.

Hood, S. B. (1998). *Advice to those who stutter* (Publication No. 9). Memphis, TN: Stuttering Foundation of America.

Horsley, I. A., & Fitzgibbon, C. T. (1987). Stuttering children: Investigation of a stereotype. *British Journal of Disorders of Communication, 22,* 19–35.

Howell, P. (2004). Assessment of some contemporary theories of stuttering that apply to spontaneous speech. *Contemporary Issues in Communication Sciences and Disorders, 31,* 123–140.

Howell, P., & Au-Yeung, J. (2002). The EXPLAN theory of fluency control applied to the diagnosis of stuttering. In E. Fava (Ed.), *Pathology and therapy of speech disorders* (pp. 75–94). Amsterdam: John Benjamins.

Howell, P., Sackin, S., & Williams, R. (1999). Differential effects of frequency-shifted feedback between child and adult stutterers. *Journal of Fluency Disorders, 24,* 127–136.

Howie, P. M. (1981). Concordance for stuttering in monozygotic and dizygotic twin pairs. *Journal of Speech and Hearing Research, 24,* 317–321.

Howie, P., Woods, C., & Andrews, J. (1982). Relationship between covert and overt speech measures immediately before and immediately after stuttering treatment. *Journal of Speech and Hearing Disorders, 47,* 419–422.

Howie, P. M., Tanner, S., & Andrews, G. (1981). Short and long term outcome in an intensive treatment program for adult stutterers. *Journal of Speech and Hearing Disorders, 46,* 104–109.

Hubbard, C. P., & Yairi, E. (1988). Clustering of disfluencies in the speech of stuttering and nonstuttering preschool children. *Journal of Speech and Hearing Research, 31,* 228–233.

Hubble, M., Duncan, B., & Miller, S. (2004). Directing attention to what works. In M. Hubble, B. Duncan, & S. Miller (Eds.) *The heart and soul of change: What works in therapy.* Washington DC: American Psychological Association.

Hugh-Jones, S., & Smith, P. K. (1999). Self-reports of short- and long-term effects of bullying on children who stammer. *British Journal of Educational Psychology, 69,* 141–158.

Humke, C., & Schaefer, C. E. (1996). Sense of humor and creativity. *Perceptual and Motor Skills, 82*(2), 544–546.

Huinck, W. J., Langevin, M., Kully, D., Graamans, K., Peters, H. F. M., & Huslstijn, W., (2006). The relationship between pre-treatment clinical profile and treatment outcome in an integrated stuttering program. *Journal of Fluency Disorders, 31*(1) 43–63.

Huinck, W. J., & Peters, H. F. M. (2004). *Effect of speech therapy on stuttering: Evaluating three therapy programs.* Presentation to the IALP Congress, Brisbane.

Hunt, B. (1987). Self-help for stutterers—Experience in Britain. In L. Rustin, H. Purser, & K. D. Rowley (Eds.), *Progress in the treatment of fluency disorders* (pp. 198–212). London: Taylor & Francis.

Hunt, H. (1861/1967). *Stammering and stuttering, their nature and treatment.* New York: Hafner Publishing Company.

Ingham, R. J. (1975). A comparison of covert and overt assessment procedures in stuttering therapy outcome evaluation. *Journal of Speech and Hearing Research, 16,* 246–254.

Ingham, R. J. (1982). The effects of self-evaluation and training and maintenance and generalization during stuttering treatment. *Journal of Speech and Hearing Disorders, 47,* 271–280.

Ingham, R. J. (1984). *Stuttering and behavior therapy: Current status and experimental foundations.* San Diego, CA: College-Hill Press.

Ingham, R. J. (1990). Commentary on Perkins (1990) and Moore and Perkins (1990): On the valid role of reliability in identifying "What is stuttering." *Journal of Speech and Hearing Disorders, 55,* 394–397.

Ingham, R. J. (1993). Stuttering treatment efficacy: Paradigm dependent or independent? *Journal of Fluency Disorders, 18,* 133–145.

Ingham, R. J. (2004). Emerging controversies, findings, and directions in neuroimaging and developmental stuttering: On avoiding petard hoisting in Athens, Georgia. In A. C. Bothe (Ed.), *Evidenced-based treatment of stuttering: empirical basis and clinical applications* (pp. 27–64). Mahwah, New Jersey: Lawrence Erlbaum Associates.

Ingham, R. J., Andrews, G., & Winkler, R. (1972). Stuttering: A comparative evaluation of the short term effectiveness of four treatment techniques. *Journal of Communication Disorders, 5,* 91–117.

Ingham, R. J., & Cordes, A. K. (1992). Interclinic differences in stuttering event counts. *Journal of Fluency Disorders, 17,* 171–176.

Ingham, R. J., & Cordes, A. K. (1999). On watching a discipline shoot itself in the foot: Some observations on current trends in stuttering treatment research. In N. B. Ratner & E. C. Healey (Eds.), *Stuttering research and practice: Bridging the gap.* Mahwah, NJ: Lawrence Erlbaum Associates.

Ingham, R. J., & Cordes, A. K., & Gow, M. (1993). Time-interval measurement of stuttering: Modifying interjudge agreement. *Journal of Speech and Hearing Research, 36,* 503–515.

Ingham, R. J., Cykowski, M., Ingham J. C. & Fox, P. T. (2007). In R. J. Ingham (Ed.), *Neuroimaging in Communication Sciences.* pp. 53–85. San Diego: Plural Publishing Inc.

Ingham, R. J., Fox, P. T., & Ingham, J. C. (1994). Brain image investigation of the speech of stutterers and nonstutterers. *ASHA, 36,* 188.

Ingham, R. J., Fox, P. T., Ingham, J. C., Zamarripa, F., Martin, C., Jerabek, P., & Cotton, J. (1996). Functional-lesion investigation of developmental stuttering with Positron Emission Tomography. *Journal of Speech and Hearing Research, 39,* 1208–1227.

Ingham, R. J., Martin, R. R., Haroldson, S. K., Onslow, M., & Leney, M. (1985). Modification of listener-judged naturalness in the speech of stutterers. *Journal of Speech and Hearing Research, 28,* 495–504.

Ingham, R. J., Moglia, R. A., Frank, P., Ingham, J. C. & Cordes, A. K. (1997). Experimental investigation of the effects of frequency-altered auditory feedback on the speech of adults who stutter. *Journal of Speech, Language and Hearing Research, 40,* 361–372.

Ingham, R. J., & Onslow, M. (1985). Measurement and modification of speech naturalness during stuttering therapy. *Journal of Speech and Hearing Disorders, 50,* 261–281.

Ivy, A. E. (1983). *Intentional interviewing and counseling.* Pacific Grove, CA: Brooks/Cole.

Jacobs, M. K., & Goodman, G. (1989). Psychology and self-help groups: Prediction on a partnership. *American Psychologist, 44,* 536–545.

Janke, L., Hanggi, J. & Steinmetz, H. (2004). Morphological brain differences between adult stutterers and non-stutterers. BMC *Neurology, 4,* 23.

Jezer, M. (1997). *Stuttering: A Life Bound Up in Words.* New York, NY: Basic Books.

Johnson, W. (1930). *Because I stutter.* New York: Appleton-Century-Crofts.

Johnson, W. (1946). *People in quandaries.* New York: Harper Brothers.

Johnson, W. (1956). *Speech handicapped school children.* New York: Harper & Row.

Johnson, W. (1958). The six men and the stuttering. In J. Eisenson (Ed.), *Stuttering* (pp. xi–xxiv). New York: Harper & Brothers.

Johnson, W. (1961). Measurement of oral reading and speaking rate and disfluency of adult male and female stutterers and nonstutterers. *Journal of Speech and Hearing Disorders* (Monograph Supplement 7), 1–20.

Johnson, W. (1962). *An open letter to the mother of a "stuttering" child.* Danville, IL: Interstate Printers and Publishers.

Johnson, W., & Associates. (1959). *The Onset of stuttering.* Minneapolis: University of Minnesota Press.

Johnson, W., Brown, S., Curtis, J., Edney, C., & Keaster, J. (1967). *Speech handicapped school children* (3rd ed.). New York: Harper & Row.

Johnson, W., Darley, F. L., & Spriestersbach, D. C. (1963). *Diagnostic methods in speech pathology.* New York: Harper & Row.

Johnson, W., & Leutenegger, R. R. (Eds.). (1955). *Stuttering in children and adults.* Minneapolis: University of Minnesota Press.

Jokel, R., & De Nil, L. F. (2003). A comprehensive study of acquired stuttering in adults. In K. L. Baker & D. T. Rowley, (Eds.). *Proceedings of the Sixth Oxford Dysfluency Conference,* (pp. 59–64). Oxford, UK: Kevin Baker.

Jokel, R., De Nil, L. F., Sharpe, A. K. (2007). A comparison of speech disfluencies in adults with acquired stuttering associated with stroke and traumatic brain injury. *Journal of Medical Speech-Language Pathology, 15*(3), 243–262.

Jokel, R., De Nil, L., Sharpe, K. (2007). Speech disfluencies in adults with neurogenic stuttering associated with stroke and traumatic brain injury. *Journal of Medical Speech-Language Pathology, 15* (3) 243–261.

Jones, M., Onslow, M., Harrison, E., & Packman, A. (2000). Treating stuttering in young children: Predicting treatment time in the Lidcombe Program. *Journal of Speech, Language, and Hearing Research, 43,* 1440–1450.

Jones, R. (1966). Observations on stammering after localized cerebral injury. *Journal of Neurology, Neurosurgery, and Psychiatry, 29,* 192–195.

Jones, J. E., & Niven, P. (1993) *Voices and Silences,* Charles Scribner's Sons: New York.

Jones, M., Onslow, M., Packman, A., Williams, S., Ormond, T., Schwartz, I., et al. (2005). Randomized controlled trial of the Lidcombe Programme of early stuttering intervention., *British Medical Journal, 331,* 659–661.

Kagan, J., Reznick, J. S., and Snidman, N. (1987). The physiology and psychology of behavioral inhibition in children, *Child Development, 58,* 1459–1473.

Kalinowski, J., Armson, J., Roland-Mieszkowski, M., Stuart, A., & Gracco, V. L. (1993). Effects of alterations in auditory feedback and speech rate on stuttering frequency. *Language and Speech, 36,* 1–16.

Kalinowski, J., Guntupalli, V. K., Stuart, A., & Saltuklaroglu, T. (2004). Self-reported efficacy of an ear-level prosthetic device that delivers altered auditory feedback for the management of stuttering. *International Journal of Rehabilitation Research, 27,* 167–170.

Kalinowski, J., Nobel, S., Armson, J., & Stuart, A. (1994). Pretreatment and posttreatment speech naturalness ratings of adults with mild and severe stuttering. *American Journal of Speech-Language Pathology, 3*(2), 61–66.

Kalinowski, J., Saltuklaroglu, T., Stuart, A., & Guntupalli, V. K. (2007). On the importance of scientific rhetoric in stuttering: a reply to Finn, Bothe, and Bramlett (2005). *American Journal of Speech-Language Pathology. 16*(1): 69–76.

Kalinowski, J., Stuart, A., Sark, S., & Armson, J. (1996). Stuttering amelioration at various auditory delays and speech rates. *European Journal of Disorders of Communication, 31,* 259–269.

Kamhi, A. G. (1982). The problem of relapse in stuttering: Some thoughts on what might cause it and how to deal with it. *Journal of Fluency Disorders, 7,* 459–467.

Kamhi, A. G. (1999). To use or not to use: Factors that influence the selection of new treatment approaches. *Language, Speech, and Hearing Services in Schools, 30,* 92–98.

Kamhi, A. G. (2003). Two paradoxes in stuttering treatment. *Journal of Fluency Disorders, 28,* 187–196.

Kanfer, F. H. (1975). Self-management methods. In F. H. Kanfer & A. P. Goldstein (Eds.), *Helping people change* (pp. 416–431). New York: Pergamon Press.

Kanfer, F. H., & Schefft, B. K. (1988). *Guiding therapeutic change.* Champaign, IL: Research Press.

Katz, A. H., & Bender, E. (1976). *The strength in us: Self-help groups in the modern world.* New York: Franklin Watts.

Katz, G., Lincoln, M., & McCabe, P. (2006). Investigating stuttering in people 55 years and older: Do stuttering behaviors persist into older age? Presentation to the University of Sydney Fifth Health Research Conference, (November) Sydney, Australia.

Katz, G., Lincoln, M., & McCabe, P. (2008). The persistence of stuttering behaviours in older people. *Disability and Rehabilitation,* (1), 1–13. Retrieved March *19,* 2009, from http://www.infomaworld.com/a0.1080/0963280802306299.

Kelly, E. M. (1994). Speech rates and turn-taking behaviors of children who stutter and their fathers. *Journal of Speech and Hearing Research, 37,* 1284–1294.

Kelly, E. M. (2000). Modeling stuttering etiology: clarifying levels of description and measurement. *Journal of Fluency Disorders, 25*(4) 359–368.

Kelly, E. M., Martin, J. S., Baker, K. I., Rivera, N. J., Bishop, J. E., Kriziske, C. B., Stettler, D. B., & Stealy, J. M. (1997). Academic and clinical preparation and practices of school speech-language pathologists with people who stutter. *Language, Speech, and Hearing Services in Schools, 28,* 195–212.

Kelly, G. A. (1955a). *The psychology of personal constructs*, Volume 1. New York: Norton.

Kelly, G. A., (1955b). *The psychology of personal constructs*, Volume 2. New York: Norton.

Kent, R. D. (1983). Facts about stuttering: Neurologic perspectives. *Journal of Speech and Hearing Disorders, 48,* 249–255.

Kent, R. D., & Read, C. (1992). *The acoustic analysis of speech.* San Diego, CA: Singular Publishing Group.

Kertesz, A. (1989). Anatomical and physiological correlations and neuroimaging techniques in language disorders. In A. Ardila & F. Ostrosky-Solis (Eds.) *Brain organization of language and cognitive processes.* New York: Plenum Press.

Khedr, E., El-Nasser, W. A., Abdel Haleem, E. K., Bakr, M. S., & Trakhan, M. N. (2000). Evoked potentials and electroencephalography in stuttering. *Folia phoniatrica, 52,* 178–186.

Kidd, K. K. (1977). A genetic perspective on stuttering. *Journal of Fluency Disorders, 2,* 259–269.

Kidd, K. (1984). Stuttering as a genetic disorder. In R. F. Curlee & W. H. Perkins (Eds.), *Nature and treatment of stuttering: New directions* (pp. 149–169). Boston: Allyn & Bacon.

Kidd, K., Heimbuch, R., Records, M. A., Oehlert, G., & Webster, R. (1980). Familial stuttering patterns are not related to one measure of severity. *Journal of Speech and Hearing Research, 23,* 539–545.

Kidd, K. K., Reich, T., & Kessler, S. (1973). *Genetics,* 74 (Part 2), s137.

Kim, D. M., Wampold, B. E., & Bolt, D. M. (2006). Therapist effects and treatment effects in psychotherapy: Analysis of the National Institute of Mental Health Treatment of Depression Collaborative Research Program. *Psychotherapy Research, 16*(2), 161–172.

Kimmel, D. C. (1974). *Adulthood and aging.* New York: John Wiley & Sons.

Kimura, D. (1961). Cerebral dominance and the perception of verbal stimuli. *Canadian Journal of Psychology, 15,* 166–171.

Kimura, D. (1964). Left-right differences in the perception of melodies. *Quarterly Journal of Experimental Psychology, 16,* 355–358.

Kinsborne, M. (1989). A model of adaptive behavior related to cerebral participation in emotional control. In G. Gianotti and Caltagirone (Eds.), *Emotions and the Dual Brain.* New York: Springer-Verlag.

Kirby, G., Delgadillo, J., Hillard, S., & Manning, W. (1992). Visual imagery, relaxation, and cognitive restructuring integrated in fluency therapy. Presentation to the annual meeting of the American Speech-Language-Hearing Association, San Antonio, TX.

Klich, R. J., & May, G. M. (1982). Spectrographic study of vowels in stutterers' fluent speech. *Journal of Speech and Hearing Research, 25*(3), 364–370.

Klin, A., McPartland, Jj., & Volkmar, F. R., (2005). Asperger syndrome. In F. R. Volkmar, R. Paul, A Klin, & D. Cohen (Eds.), *Handbook of autism and pervasive developmental disorders*. Hoboken, NJ: John Wiley and Sons.

Klin, A., Volkmar, F. R., & Sparow, S.S. (2000). *Asperger syndrome*, New York: Guildford Press.

Kline, M., & Starkweather, C. (1979). Receptive and expressive language performance in young stutterers [Abstract]. *ASHA, 21*, 797.

Kloth, S. A., Kraaimaat, F. W., Janssen, P., & Brutten, G. J. (1999). Persistence and remission of incipient stuttering among high-risk children. *Journal of Fluency Disorders, 24*, 23–265.

Kloth, S. A., Janssen, P., Kraaimaat, F. W. & Brutten, G. J. (1998), Persistence and remission of incipient stuttering among high-risk children. *Journal of Fluency Disorders, 24*, 253–265.

Kolk, H., & Postma, A. (1997). Stuttering as a covert repair phenomenon. In R. Curlee & G. Siegel (Eds.), *Nature and treatment of stuttering: New directions* (2nd ed.) (pp. 182–203). Boston: Allyn & Bacon.

Koszybski, A. (1941). *Science and sanity: An introduction to non-Aristotelian systems and general semantics* (2nd Ed.). New York: Int. Non-Aristotelian Library Publishing Co.

Krall, T. (1998). My long term path toward recovery from stuttering. In E. C. Healey & H. F. M. Peters (Eds.), *Proceedings of the 2nd World Congress on Fluency Disorders* (pp. 388–389). Nijmegen, The Netherlands: Nijmegen University Press.

Kramer, M. B., Green, D., & Guitar, B. (1987). A comparison of stutterers and nonstutterers on masking level differences and synthetic sentence identification tasks. *Journal of Communication Disorders, 20*, 379–390.

Krauss-Lehrman, T., & Reeves, L. (1989). Attitudes toward speech-language pathology and support groups: Results of a survey of members of the National Stuttering Project. *Texas Journal of Audiology and Speech Pathology, 15*(1), 22–25.

Kroll, R., Cook, F., De Nil, L., & Ratner, N. (2006). Preparing clinicians to treat stuttering. Presentation to the Fifth world congress on Fluency Disorders. Dublin, Ireland. See also the 2006 International Stuttering Awareness Conference (www.mnsu.edu/comdis/isad9/papers/kroll9.html)

Kroll, R. M., De Nil, L. F., Kapur, S. & Houle, S. (1997). A positron emission tomography investigation of post-treatment brain activation in stutterers. In H. F. M. Peters & W. Hulstijn, (Eds.), *Proceedings of the Third Speech Motor Production and Fluency Disorders* (pp. 307–320). Amsterdam: Elsevier.

Kubie, L. S. (1971). The destructive potential of humor on psychotherapy. *American Journal of Psychiatry, 127*, 861–866.

Kübler Ross, E. (1969). *On death and dying*. New York: Simon and Schuster.

Kuhlman, T. (1984). *Humor and psychotherapy*. Homewood, IL: Dow Jones-Irwin.

Kuhr, A., & Rustin, L. (1985). The maintenance of fluency after intensive in-patient therapy: Long-term follow-up. *Journal of Fluency Disorders, 10,* 229–236.

Kully, D., & Boberg, E. (1988). An investigation of interclinic agreement in the identication of fluent and stuttered syllables. *Journal of Fluency Disorders, 13,* 309–318.

Ladouceur, R., Caron, C., & Caron, G. (1989). Stuttering severity and treatment outcome. *Journal of Behavior Therapy and Experimental Psychiatry, 20,* 49–56.

Lambert, M. J. (1992). Psychotherapy outcome research: Implications for integrative and eclectic therapists. In J. C. Norcross & M. R. Goldfried (Eds.), *Handbook of psychotherapy integration* (pp. 94–129). New York: Basic Books.

Landfield, A. W., & Leitner, L. M. (1980). Personal Construct Psychology. In A. W. Landfield & L. M. Leitner (Eds.), *Personal Construct Psychology*. New York, NY: John Wiley & Sons.

Langevin, M. (2000). *Teasing and bullying: Unacceptable behaviour*. The TAB program. Edmonton, Alberta: Institute for Stuttering Treatment and Research.

Langevin, L., Bortnick, K., Hammer, T., & Wiebe, E. (1998). Teasing/bullying experienced by children who stutter: Toward development of a questionnaire. *Contemporary Issues in Communication Science and Disorders, 25,* 12–24.

Langevin, M., Huinck, W. J., Kully, D., Peters, H. F. M., Lomheim, H., & Tellers, M. (2006). A cross-cultural, long-term outcome evaluation of the ISTAR Comprehensive Stuttering Program across Dutch and Canadian adults who stutter. *Journal of Fluency Disorders, 31,* 229–256.

Langevin, M.,& Kully, D. (2003). Evidence-based practice treatment of stuttering: III. Evidence-based practice in a clinical setting. *Journal of Fluency Disorders, 28*(3), 219–236.

Langevin, M. Kully, D, Ross-Harold, B. (2007). Treatment of School-Age Children who Stutter: A Comprehensive Approach with Strategies for Managing Teasing and Bullying. In E. Conture & R. Curlee (Eds.), *Stuttering and Related Disorders of Fluency* (3rd Edition, pp. 131–150). Philadelphia, PA: Thieme Medical Publishers Inc.

LaSalle, L. R., & Conture, E. G. (1991). Eye contact between young stutterers and their mothers. *Journal of Fluency Disorders, 16*(4), 173–199.

LaSalle, L. R., & Conture, E. G. (1995). Disfluency clusters of children who stutter: Relation of stutterings to self-repairs. *Journal of Speech and Hearing Research, 38*(5), 965–977.

Lass, N., Ruscello, D. M., Pannbaker, M. D., Schmitt, J., & Everly-Myers, D. (1989). Speech-language pathologists' perceptions of child and adult female and male stutterers. *Journal of Fluency Disorders, 14,* 127–134.

Lass, N. J., Ruscello, D. M., Panbacker, M. D., Schmitt, J. F., Kiser, A., Mussa, A., et al. (1994). School administrators' perceptions of people who stutter. *Language, Speech, and Hearing Services in Schools, 25*, 90–93.

Lass, N. J., Ruscello, D. M., Schmitt, J. F., Pannbacker, M. D., Orlando, M. B., Dean, K. A., Ruziska, J. C., & Bradshaw, K. H. (1992). Teachers' perceptions of stutterers. Language, *Speech and Hearing Services in Schools, 23*, 78–81.

LaValley, M .P. (2003). Intent-to-treat analysis of randomized clinical trials. Presentation to the ACR/ARHP Annual scientific meeting, October, 2003, Orlando, FL

Lee, B. S. (1951). Artificial stutter. *Journal of Speech and Hearing Disorders, 16*, 53–55.

Lavid, N., Franklin, D. L., & Maguire, G. A. (1999). Management of child and adolescent with Olanzapine: *Three case reports. Journal of Clinical Psychiatry, 11*, 233–236.

Leahy, M. M. (2004). Therapy talk: Analyzing therapeutic discourse. *Language, Speech and Hearing Services in Schools, 35*, 70–81.

Leahy, M. M., & Warren, A. (2006). Making stuttering manageable: The use of narrative therapy. Presentation to the Fifth world congress on Fluency Disorders. Dublin, Ireland.

Lee, K., Manning, W. & Herder, C. (2009). Determining successful therapeutic changes with Origin and Pawn scaling. Presentation to the annual meeting of the American Speech-Language Association, New Orleans, LA.

Leeper, L. H., Culatta, R. (1995). Speech fluency: Effect of age, gender, and context. *Folia Phoniatrica, 47*, 1–14.

Lefcourt, H. M. (1976). *Locus of control: Current trends in theory and research.* Hillsdale, NJ: Erlbaum.

Lefcourt, H., & Martin, R. (1989). *Humor and life stress: Antidote to adversity.* New York: Springer-Verlag.

Lefcourt, H., Sordoni, C., & Sordoni C. (1974). Locus of control and the expression of humor. *Journal of Personality, 42*, 130–143.

Lemert, E. M. (1953). Some Indians who stutter. *Journal of Speech and Hearing Disorders, 18*, 168–174.

Lemert, E. M. (1962). Stuttering and social structure in two Pacific societies. *Journal of Speech and Hearing Disorders, 27*, 3–10.

Levelt, W. J. M. (1989). *Speaking: From intention to articulation.* Cambridge, MA: Bradford Books.

Levine, J. (1977). Humour as a form of therapy. In A. J. Chapman & H. C. Foot (Eds.), *It's a funny thing, humour* (pp. 127–137). Oxford, England: Pergamon.

Levitt, H.M., Neimeyer, R. A., Williams, D. (2004). Rules vs. principles in psychotherapy: Implications of the quest for universal guidelines in the movement for empirically supported treatments. *Journal of Contemporary Psychotherapy, 35*(1), 117–129.

Levy, C. (1983). Group therapy with adults. In P. Dalton (Ed.), *Approaches to the Treatment of Stuttering* (pp. 150–171). London and Canberra, Australia: Croom Helm.

Lichtheim, M. (1973). *Ancient Egyptian literature, a book of readings: Volume 1. The Old and Middle Kingdoms.* Berkeley: University of California Press.

Liebetrau, R.M., & Daly, D.A. (1981). Auditory processing and perceptual abilities of "organic" and "functional" stutterers. *Journal of Fluency Disorders, 6,* 219–232.

Lilienfeld, S. O., Lynn, S. J., & Lohr, J. M. (2003). Science and pseudoscience in clinical psychology: Initial thoughts, reflections, and considerations. In S. O. Lilienfeld, S. J. Lynn, & J. M. Lohr (Eds.), *Science and Pseudoscience in Clinical Psychology* (pp. 1–16). New York: Guilford Press.

Lincoln, M. A., Onslow, M., & Reed, V. (1997). Social validity of the treatment outcomes of an early intervention program for stuttering. *American Journal of Speech-Language Pathology, 6,* 77–84.

Lincoln, M., Packman, A., and Onslow. M. (2006). Altered auditory feedback and the treatment of stuttering: A review. *Journal of Fluency Disorders, 31,* 71–89.

Lindaman, E. B., & Lippitt, R. O. (1979). *Choosing the future you prefer: Goal setting guide.* Washington, DC: Development Publications.

Loban, W. (1976). *Language development: Kindergarten through grade twelve.* Urbana, IL: National Council of Teachers of English.

Logan, K, J., & Yaruss, J. S. (1999). Helping parents address attitudinal and emotional factors with young children who stutter. *Contemporary Issues in Communication Science and Disorders, 26,* 69–81.

Longhurst, T. M., & Siegel, G. M. (1973). Effects of communication failure on speaker-listener behaviors. *Journal of Speech and Hearing Disorders, 16,* 128–140.

Louko, L., Edwards, M. E., & Conture, E. (1990). Phonological characteristics of young stutterers and their normally fluent peers: Preliminary observations. *Journal of Fluency Disorders, 15,* 191–210.

Love, L. R., & Jefress, L. A. (1971). Identification of brief pauses in the fluent speech of stutterers and nonstutterers. *Journal of Speech and Hearing Research, 14,* 229–240.

Love, R. E. (2000). *The Bob Love Story.* Chicago, IL: Contemporary Books.

Lowe-Bell, S. S., Cullen, J. K., Jr., Berlin, C. I., Thompson, C. L., & Willett, M. E. (1970). Perceptions of simultaneous dichotic and monotic monosyllables. *Journal of Speech and Hearing Research, 13,* 812–822.

Luborsky, L., Rosenthal, R., Diguer, L., et al. (2002). The dodo bird verdict is alive and well—mostly. *Clinical Psychology: Science and Practice, 9*(1), 2-12.

Luborsky, L., Singer, B., & Luborsky, L. (1975). Comparative studies of psychotherapies: Is it true that "everyone has won and all must have prizes"? *Archives of General Psychiatry, 32,* 995–1008.

Ludlow, C. L., Rosenberg, J., Salazar, A., Grafman, J., & Smutok, M. (1987). Site of penetrating brain lesions causing chronic acquired stuttering. *Annals of Neurology, 22,* 60–66.

Luper, H. L., & Mulder, R. L. (1964). *Stuttering therapy for children.* Englewood Cliffs, NJ: Prentice-Hall.

Luterman, D. (1979). *Counseling parents of hearing impaired children.* Boston: Little, Brown, & Co.

Luterman, D. M. (2001). *Counseling persons with communication disorders and their families.* (4th Ed.). Austin, TX: Pro-Ed.

Mackinnon, S. P., Hall, S., & MacIntyre, P. D. (2007). Origins of the stuttering stereotype: Stereotype formation through inference. *Journal of Fluency Disorders, 32,* 297–309.

Madison, L. S., Budd, K. S., & Itzkowitz, J. S. (1986). Changes in stuttering in relation to children's locus of control. *Journal of Genetic Psychology, 147,* 233–240.

Maguire, G., Riley, G., Franklin, D., & Gottschalk, L. (2000). Risperidone for the treatment of stuttering. *Journal of Clinical Psychopharmacology, 20,* 479–482.

Malecot, A., Johnston, R., & Kizziar, P. A. (1972). Syllabic rate and utterance length in French. *Phonetica, 26,* 235–251.

Mahoney, M. J. (2000). Training future psychotherapists. In C. R. Snyder & R. E. Ingham, *Handbook of Psychological Change,* (pp. 272–735). New York: John Wiley & Sons, Inc.

Mahr, G., & Leith, W. (1992). Psychogenic stuttering of adult onset. *Journal of Speech and Hearing Research, 35,* 283–286.

Mallard, A. R., Gardner, L., & Downey, C. (1988). Clinical training in stuttering for school clinicians. *Journal of Fluency Disorders, 13,* 253–259.

Mallard, A. R., & Westrbook J. B. (1988). Variables affecting stuttering therapy in school settings. *Language, Speech, and Hearing Services in Schools, 19,* 362–370.

Manders, E., & Bastijns, P. (1988). Sudden recovery from stuttering after an epileptic attack: A case report. *Journal of Fluency Disorders, 13,* 421–425.

Manning, W. (1977). In pursuit of fluency. *Journal of Fluency Disorders, 2,* 53–56.

Manning, W. (1991a). Sports analogies in the treatment of stuttering: Taking the field with your client. *Public School Caucus, 10*(2), 1, 10–11.

Manning, W. H. (1991b). Making progress during and after treatment. In W. H. Perkins (Ed.) *Seminars in Speech and Language,* (Vol. *12,* pp. 349–354). New York: Thieme Medical Publishers Inc.

Manning, W. H. (1994). The SEA-Scale: Self-efficacy scaling for adolescents who stutter. Presentation to the annual meeting of the American Speech-Language-Hearing Association, New Orleans, LA.

Manning, W. H. (1995) Paddling in the stream of speech. *Letting GO.* Publication of the National Stuttering Project. (September/October 1995).

Manning, W. H., (1996). *Clinical Decision Making in the Assessment and Treatment of Fluency Disorders,* Albany, NY: Delmar

Manning, W. H. (1998). Long term recovery from stuttering. In E. C. Healey & H. F. M. Peters (Eds.), *Proceedings of the 2nd World Congress on Fluency Disorders* (pp. 381–383). Nijmegen, The Netherlands: Nijmegen University Press.

Manning, W. H. (1999a). Progress under the surface and over time. In N. B. Ratner & E. C. Healey (Eds.), *Stuttering Research and Practice: Bridging the Gap* (pp. 123–129). Mahwah, NJ: Lawrence Erlbaum.

Manning, W. (1999b). Management of adult stuttering. In R. Curlee (Ed.), *Stuttering and related disorders of fluency* (2nd Edition, pp. 160–180). New York: Thieme Medical Publishers, Inc.

Manning, W. (2004a). *Clinical decision making with adolescents who stutter.* ASHA Continuing Education Series, Rockville, MD. (2 CDs)

Manning, W. (2004b). "How can you understand? You don't stutter!" *Contemporary Issues in Communication Science and Disorders, 31,* 58–68.

Manning, W. H. (2006). Therapeutic change and the nature of our evidence: improving our ability to help. Chapter 9 (pp. 125–158). In N. Bernstein Ratner & J. Tetnowski, *Current Issues in Stuttering Research and Practice.* Mahwah, NJ.: Lawrence Earlbaum, Inc.

Manning, W. H., & Beachy, T. S. (1995). Humor as a variable in the treatment of fluency disorders. In C. W. Starkweather & H. F. M. Peters (Eds.), *Stuttering: Proceedings of the first world congress on fluency Disorders* (pp. 414–416). International Fluency Association

Manning, W., Burlison, A., & Thaxton, D. (1999). Listener response to stuttering modification techniques. *Journal of Fluency Disorders, 24,* 267–280.

Manning, W., & Cooper, E. B. (1969). Variations in attitudes of the adult stutterer toward his clinician related to progress in therapy. *Journal of Communication Disorders, 2,* 154–162.

Manning, W., Dailey, D., & Wallace, S. (1984). Attitude and personality characteristics of older stutterers. *Journal of Fluency Disorders, 9,* 207–215.

Manning, W. H., & DiLollo, A. (2007) Management of Stuttering for Adolescents and Adults: Traditional Approaches, In E. Conture & R. Curlee, *Stuttering and Related Disorders of Fluency,* (3rd Edition pp. 233–255). New York: Thieme Medical Publishers, Inc.

Manning, W., Emal, & Jamison, W. (1975). Listener judgments of fluency: The effect of part-word CV repetitions and neutral vowel substitutions. *Journal of Fluency Disorders, 1*(3), 18–23.

Manning, W., Hodak, M., & Plexico, L. (2005, October). *Letters from Sarajevo.* Presentation to the International Stuttering Awareness Day Online Conference (ISAD), accessed from http://www.mankato.msus.edu/dept/comdis/isad/isadcon.html

Manning, W., & Monte, K. (1981). Fluency breaks in older speakers: Implications for a model of stuttering throughout the life cycle. *Journal of Fluency Disorders, 6,* 35–48.

Manning, W., Perkins, D., Winn, S., & Cole, D. (1984). Self-efficacy changes during treatment and maintenance for adult stutterers. Presentation to the annual meeting of the American Speech-Language-Hearing Association, San Francisco, CA.

Manning, W., & Shirkey, E. (1981). Fluency and the aging process. In D. S. Beasley & G. A. Davis (Eds.), *Aging: Communication Processes and Disorders* (pp. 175–189). New York: Grune & Stratton.

Manning W., & Shrum, W. (1973). The concept of control in stuttering therapy: A reappraisal. *Division for Children with Communication Disorders Bulletin, 9*(1), 32–34.

Market, K. E., Montague, J. C., Buffalo, M. D., & Drummond, S. S. (1990). Acquired stuttering: Descriptive data and treatment outcome. *Journal of Fluency Disorders, 15,* 21–34.

Martin, R. A., & Lefcourt, H. (1983). Sense of humor as a moderator of the relation between stressors and moods. *Journal of Personality and Social Psychology, 45,* 1313–1324.

Martin, R. A., & Lefcourt, H. (1984). Situational humor response questionnaire: Quantitative measure of sense of humor. *Journal of Personality and Social Psychology, 47,* 145–155.

Martin, R. R. (1981). Introduction and perspective: Review of published research. In E. Boberg (Ed.), *Maintenance of fluency* (pp. 1–30). New York: Elsevier.

Martin, R. R., & Haroldson, S. K. (1982). Contingent self-stimulation for stuttering. *Journal of Speech and Hearing Disorders, 47,* 407–413.

Martin, R. R., & Haroldson, S. K. (1986). Stuttering as involuntary loss of speech control: Barking up a new tree. *Journal of Speech and Hearing Disorders, 51,* 187–190.

Martin, R. R., & Haroldson, S. K. (1992). Stuttering and speech naturalness: Audio and audiovisual judgements. *Journal of Speech and Hearing Research, 35,* 521–528.

Martin, R. R., Haroldson, S., & Kuhl, P. (1972a). Disfluencies in child-child and child-mother speaking situations. *Journal of Speech and Hearing Research, 15,* 753–756.

Martin, R. R., Haroldson, S., & Kuhl, P. (1972b). Disfluencies of young children in two speaking situations. *Journal of Speech and Hearing Research, 15,* 831–836.

Martin, R. R., Haroldson, S. K., & Triden, K. A. (1984). Stuttering and speech naturalness. *Journal of Speech and Hearing Disorders, 49,* 53–58.

Martin, R. R., Kuhl, P., & Haroldson, S., (1972). An experimental treatment with two preschool stuttering children. *Journal of Speech and Hearing Research, 15,* 743–752.

Martin, R. R., & Lindamood, L. P. (1986). Stuttering and spontaneous recovery; Implications for the speech-language pathologist. *Language, Speech, and Hearing Services in Schools, 17,* 207–218.

Martin, R. R., & Siegel, G. M. (1966a). The effects of response contingent shock on stuttering. *Journal of Speech and Hearing Research, 9,* 340–352.

Martin, R. R., & Siegel, G. M. (1966b). The effects of simultaneously punishing stuttering and rewarding fluency. *Journal of Speech and Hearing Research, 9,* 466–475.

Martin, R., St. Louis, K., Haroldson, S., & Hasbrouck, J. (1975). Punishment and negative reinforcement of stuttering using electric shock. *Journal of Speech and Hearing Research, 18,* 478–490.

Maslow, A. (1968). *Towards a Psychology of Being* (2nd ed.). Princeton, NJ: Van Nostrand.

Masterson, J., & Kamhi, A. (1992). Linguistic trade-offs in school-age children with and without language disorders. *Journal of Speech and Hearing Research, 35,* 1064–1075.

Matkin, N., Ringle, R., & Snope, T. (1983). Master report of surveys discrepancies. In N. Rees & T. Snope (Eds.), *Proceedings of the Conference on Undergraduate, Graduate and Continuing Education* (ASHA Reports No. 13). Rockville, MD: American Speech-Language-Hearing Association.

Max, L., Caruso, A. J., & Gracco, V. L. (2003). Kinematic analysis of speech, orofacial nonspeech, and finger movements in stuttering individuals. *Journal of Speech, Language, and Hearing Research, 46,* 215–232.

Mazzucchi, A., Moretti, G., Carpeggianai, P., Parman, M., & Paini, P. (1981). Clinical observations on acquired stuttering. *British Journal of Disorders of Communication 16,*19–30.

Maxwell, D. (1982). Cognitive and behavioral self-control strategies: Applications for the clinical management of adult stutterers. *Journal of Fluency Disorders, 7,* 403–432.

McCabe, A., & Bliss, L. S. (2003). Patterns of narrative discourse: A multicultural lifespan approach. Boston, MA: Allyn and Bacon.

McCarthy, P., Culpepper, N., & Lucks, L. (1986). Variability in counseling experience and training among ESB accredited programs. *ASHA, 28,* 49–53.

McClean, M., Goldsmith, H., & Cerf, A. (1984). Lowerlip EMG and displacement during bilabial disfluencies in adult stutterers. *Journal of Speech and Hearing Research, 27,* 342–349.

McConnaughy, E. A., Prochaska, J. O., & Velicer, W. F. (1983). Stages of change in psychotherapy: Measurement and sample profiles. *Psychotherapy: Theory Research, and Practice, 29*(3) 368–375.

McDearmon, J. R. (1968). Primary stuttering at the onset of stuttering: A reexamination of data. *Journal of Speech and Hearing Research, 11,* 631–637.

McDonald, E. T., & Frick, J. V. (1954). Store clerks' reactions to stuttering. *Journal of Speech and Hearing Disorders, 19,* 306–311.

McFarland, D. H., & Moore, W. H., Jr. (1982). Alpha asymmetries during an electromyographic biofeedback procedure for stuttering. Presentation to the Annual Convention of the American Speech-Language-Hearing Association, Toronto, Canada.

McFarlane, S., & Goldberg, L. (1987). Factors influencing treatment approaches, prognosis and dismissal criteria for stuttering [Abstract]. *ASHA, 29,* 164–165.

McGhee, P. E., & Goldstein, J. H. (1977). *Handbook of humor research: Volume 1,* Basic issues. New York: Springer-Verlag.

McKenzie, W., & Monk, G., (1997). Learning and teaching narrative ideas. In G. Monk, J. Winslade, K. Crocket, & D. Epston (Eds.) *Narrative therapy in practice.* San Francisco, CA: Jossey-Bass Publishers.

McLelland, J. K., & Cooper, E. B. (1978). Fluency-related behaviors and attitudes of 178 young stutterers. *Journal of Fluency Disorders, 3,* 253–263.

Mehrabian, A., & Reed., H., Meyers, S., Ghatak, L., & Woodford, L. (1990). Case descriptions of nonfluency and loci: Initial and follow-up conversations with three preschool children. *Journal of Fluency Disorders, 14,* 383–398.

Merson, R. M. (2003, October). Auditory sidetone and the management of stuttering: From Wollensack to SpeechEasy, Presentation to the 2003 International Stuttering Awareness Day Conference.

Meyers, S., Hall, N. E., & Aram, D. M. (1990). Fluency and language recovery in a child with a left hemisphere lesion. *Journal of Fluency Disorders, 15,* 159–173.

Meyers, S. C., & Freeman, F. J. (1985). Mother and child speech rates as a variable in stuttering and disfluency. *Journal of Speech and Hearing Research, 28,* 436–444.

Miles, S., & Bernstein Ratner, N. (2001). Parental language input to children at stuttering onset. *Journal of Speech, Language, and Hearing Disorders, 44,* 1116–1130.

Millard, S. K., Nicholas, A., & Cook, F. M. (2008). Is parent–child interaction therapy effective in reducing stuttering? *Journal of Speech, Language, and Hearing Research, 51,* 636–650.

Miller, S. D., Duncan, B. L., & Hubble. M. A. (1997). *Escape from Babel: Toward a unifying language for psychotherapy practice.* New York: W. W. Norton & Company.

Miller, S., & Watson, B. C. (1992). The relationship between communication attitude, anxiety and depression in stutterers and nonstutterers. *Journal of Speech and Hearing Research, 35,* 789–798.

Mineka, S. (1985). Animal models of anxiety-based disorders: Their usefulness and limitations. In A. H. Tuma & J. Mase (Eds.), *Anxiety and the anxiety disorders.* Hillsdale, NJ: Lawrence Erlbaum Associates.

Molt, L. (1996). An examination of various aspects of auditory processing in clutterers. *Journal of Fluency Disorders, 21,* 215–225.

Molt, L., (2006a). SpeechEasy AAF device long-term clinical trial: Attitudinal/ perceptual measures. Presentation to the annual meeting of the American Speech-Language-Hearing Association, Miami, FL.

Molt, L., (2006b). SpeechEasy AAF device long-term clinical trial: Speech fluency and naturalness measures. Presentation to the annual meeting of the American Speech-Language-Hearing Association, Miami, FL.

Molt, L., & Brading, T. (1994). Hemispheric patterns of auditory event-related potentials to dichotic CV syllables in stutterers and normal speakers. In C. W. Starkweather & H. F. M. Peters (Eds.) *Proceedings of the 1st World Congress on Fluency Disorders,* Munich, Germany.

Molt, L. F., & Guilford, A. M. (1979). Auditory processing and anxiety in stutterers. *Journal of Fluency Disorders, 4,* 255–267.

Monk, G., (1997). How narrative therapy works. In G. Monk, J. Winslade, K. Crocket, & D. Epston (Eds.) *Narrative therapy in practice.* San Francisco, CA: Jossey-Bass Publishers.

Monk, G., Winslade, J., Crocket, K, & Epston, D. (1997). *Narrative therapy in practice.* San Francisco, CA: Jossey-Bass Publishers.

Moore, S. E., & Perkins, W. (1990). Validity and reliability of judgements of authentic and simulated stuttering. *Journal of Speech and Hearing Disorders, 55,* 383–391.

Moore, W. (1984). Hemispheric alpha asymmetries during an electromyographic biofeedback procedure for stuttering: A single-subject experimental design. *Journal of Fluency Disorders, 9,* 143–162.

Moore, W., & Haynes, W. (1980). Alpha hemispheric asymmetry and stuttering: Some support for a segmentation dysfunction hypothesis. *Journal of Speech and Hearing Research, 23,* 229–247.

Morgenstern, J. J. (1956). Socio-economic factors in stuttering. *Journal of Speech and Hearing Disorders, 21,* 25–33.

Morreall, J. (1982). *Taking laughter seriously.* Albany: State University of New York Press.

Morrison, J. R., (1995). *DSM-IV made easy: The clinician's guide to diagnosis.* New York: Guilford Press.

Mower, D. E. (1998). Analysis of the sudden onset and disappearance of disfluencies in the speech of a 2 ½ year old boy, *Journal of Fluency Disorders, 23,* 103–118.

Mueller, H. G., & Bright, K. E. (1994). Monosyllabic procedures in central testing. In J. Katz (Ed.), *Handbook of clinical audiology,* 4th ed. Baltimore, MD: Williams & Wilkins.

Mullen, R. (2007). The State of the evidence: ASHA develops levels of evidence for communication sciences and disorders, *The ASHA Leader.* (March 6), 8–9, 24–25.

Muma, J. (1967). Syntax of preschool fluent and disfluent speech: a transformational analysis. *Journal of Speech and Hearing Research, 14,* 428–441.

Murphy, A. T., & Fitzsimons, R. M. (1960). Stuttering and personality dynamics. New York: Ronald Press.

Murphy, W. P. (1998) *The school-age child who stutters: Dealing effectively with shame and guilt.* Videotape No. 86. Memphis, TN: Stuttering Foundation of America.

Murphy, B. (1999). A preliminary look at shame, guilt, and stuttering. In N. B. Ratner & E. C. Healey (Eds.), *Stuttering research and practice: Bridging the gap* (pp. 131–143). Mahwah, NJ: Lawrence Erlbaum.

Murphy, W. P., Yaruss, J. S., & Quesal, R. W., (2007). Enhancing Treatment for school-age children who stutter I: Reducing negative reactions through desensitization and cognitive restructuring. *Journal of Fluency Disorders, 32,* 121–138.

Murphy, W. P., Yaruss, J. S., & Quesal, R. W., (2007). Enhancing Treatment for school-age children who stutter II: Reducing bullying through role-playing and self-disclosure, *Journal of Fluency Disorders, 32,* 139–162.

Murray, F. P., & Edwards, S. G. (1980). *A stutterer's story.* Danville, IL: Interstate Printers and Publishers.

Murray, H. L., & Reed, C. G. (1977). Language abilities of preschool stuttering children. *Journal of Fluency Disorders, 2,* 171–176.

Myers, F. L. (1992). Cluttering: A synergistic framework. In F. L. Myers & K. O. St. Louis (Eds.) *Cluttering: A clinical perspective* (pp. 71–84). Kibworth, Great Britain: Far Communications. (Reissued in 1996 by Singular, San Diego, CA.)

Meyers, F. L. (1996). Cluttering: A mater of perspective. *Journal of Fluency Disorders, 21,* 175–186.

Myers, F. L., & St. Louis, K. O. (1992). Cluttering: Issues and controversies. In F. L. Myers & K. O. St. Louis (Eds.), *Cluttering: A clinical perspective* (pp. 11–22). San Diego, CA: Singular Publishing Group, Inc.

Myers, F. L., St. Louis, K. O., Bakker, K., Raphael, L. J., Wiig, E., et al. (2002a). Putting cluttering on the map: Looking ahead. Seminar presented to the Annual Convention of the American Speech-Language-Hearing Association, Atlanta, GA.

Myers, F. L., St. Louis, K. O., Bakker, K., Raphael, L. J., Wiig, E., et al. (2002b). Putting cluttering on the map: Looking back. Seminar presented at the Annual Convention of the American Speech-Language-Hearing Association, Atlanta, GA.

Mysak, E. D. (1960). Servo theory and stuttering. *Journal of Speech and Hearing Disorders, 25,* 188–195.

National Institute of Mental Health. (2003). Attention deficit hyperactivity disorder. Retrieved May, 9 2008 from http://www.nimh.nih.gov/publicat/NIMHadhdpub.pdf.

Neaves, R. (1970). To establish a basis for prognosis in stammering. *British Journal of Disorders of Communication, 5,* 46–58.

Neeley, J. N. (1961). A study of the speech behavior of stutterers and nonstutterers under normal and delayed auditory feedback. *Journal of Speech and Hearing Disorders* (Monograph Supplement No. 7), 63–82.

Neilson, M., & Neilson, P. (1987). Speech motor control and stuttering: A computational model of adaptive sensory-motor processing. *Speech Communications, 6,* 325–333.

Neimeyer, R. A. (2000). *Lessons of Loss: A guide to coping.* Keystone, FL: Psycho-Educational Resources, Inc.

Neimeyer, R A., & Raskin, J. D. (2000) Constructions of disorder: Meaning-making frameworks for psychotherapy, Washington DC: American Psychological Association.

Neumann, K., Preibisch, C., Euler, H. A., von Gudenberg, A. W., Lanfermann, H., Gall, V., et al. (2005). Cortical plasticity associated with stuttering therapy. *Journal of Fluency Disorders, 30,* 23–39.

Newman, P. W., Harris, R. W., & Hilton, L. M. (1989). Vocal jitter and shimmer in stuttering. *Journal of Fluency Disorders, 14,* 87–95.

Nezu, A., Nezu, C., & Blissett, S. (1988). Sense of humor as a moderator of the relations between stressful events and psychological distress: A prospective analysis. *Journal of Personality and Social Psychology, 54,* 520–525.

Nippold, M., & Rudzinski, M. (1995). Parents' speech and children's stuttering: A critique of the literature. *Journal of Speech and Hearing Research, 38,* 978–989.

Oates, D. (1929). Left-handedness in relation to speech defects, intelligence, and achievement. *Forum of Education, 7,* 91–105.

O'Brian, S., Onslow. M., Cream, A., & Packman, A., (2003). The Camperdown Program: Outcomes of a new prolonged-speech treatment model. *Journal of Speech, Language, and Hearing Research, 46,* 933–946.

O'Donnell, J. J., Armson, J., & Kiefte, M. (2008). The effectiveness of SpeechEasy during situations of daily living. *Journal of Fluency Disorders, 33,* 99–119.

Ojemann, R. (1931). Studies in sidedness: III. Relation of handedness to speech. *Journal of Educational Psychology, 22,* 120–126.

Olweus, D. (1993). *Bullying at school: What we know and what we can do.* Oxford: Blackwell.

Onslow, M. (1992). Identification of early stuttering: Issues and suggested strategies. *American Journal of Speech-Language Pathology, 1*(4), 21–27.

Onslow, M. (1999). Review of Stuttering: An Integrated Approach to Its Nature and Treatment, 2nd Edition, Baltimore, MD: Williams & Wilkins. *Journal of Fluency Disorder, 24,* 319–332.

Onslow, M., & Ingham, R. J. (1987). Speech quality measurement and the management of stuttering. *Journal of Speech and Hearing Disorders, 52,* 2–17.

Onslow, M., Packman, A., & Harrison, E (2003). *The Lidcombe Program of early stuttering intervention: A clinician's guide.* Austin, TX: Pro-Ed.

Ornstein, A., & Manning, W. (1985). Self-efficacy scaling by adult stutterers. *Journal of Communication Disorders, 18,* 313–320.

Orton, S.T. (1927). Studies in stuttering. *Archives of Neurology and Psychiatry, 18,* 671–672.

Ost, L., Gotestam, K. G., & Melin, L. (1976). A controlled study of two behavioral methods in the treatment of stuttering. *Behavior Therapy, 7,* 587–592.

Otsuki, H. (1958). Study on stuttering: Statistical observations. *Otorhinolaryngology Clinic, 5,* 1150–1151.

Otto, F., & Yairi, E. (1976). A disfluency analysis of Down's syndrome and normal subjects. *Journal of Fluency Disorders, 1,* 26–32.

Oyler, M. E., & Ramig, P. (1995, November). *Vulnerability in stuttering children.* Presentation to the Annual Convention of the American Speech-Language-Hearing Association, Orlando, FL.

Oyler, M. E., (1996, November). *Temperament: Stuttering and the behaviorally inhibited child.* Presentation to the Annual Convention of the American Speech-Language-Hearing Association, Seattle, WA.

Pachankis, J. E., & Goldfried, M. R., (2007). An integrative, principle-based approach to psychotherapy. In S. G. Hoffman & J Weinberger (Eds.), *The art and science of psychotherapy: An introduction.* New York: Routledge/Taylor & Francis Group.

Paden, E. P. (1970). *A History of the American Speech and Hearing Association 1925–1958.* Washington, DC: American Speech and Hearing Association.

Paden, E. P., Yairi, E., & Ambrose, N. G. (1999). Early childhood stuttering II: Initial status of phonological abilities. *Journal of Speech, Language, and Hearing Research, 42,* 1113–1124.

Panico, J., & Healey, E. C. (2008). The influence of text type, topic familiarity, and stuttering frequency on listener recall, comprehension, and mental effort. *Journal of Speech, Language and Hearing Research.* (In press).

Pangos, J. M., & Bliss, L. S. (1990). Presuppositions for speech therapy lessons. *Journal of Childhood Communication Disorders, 13*(1), 19–28.

Panelli, C., McFarlane, S., & Shipley, K. (1978). Implications of evaluating and interviewing with incipient stutterers. *Journal of Fluency Disorders, 3,* 41–50.

Patterson, C. H. (1985). *The therapeutic relationship: Foundations for an eclectic psychotherapy.* Pacific Grove, CA: Brooks/Cole.

Pauls, D. L. (1990). *A review of the evidence for genetic factors in stuttering ASHA Reports Series.* American Speech-Language-Hearing Association, *18,* 34–38.

Parry, A., & Doan, R. E. (1994). *Story Re-visions: Narrative Therapy in the Postmodern World.* New York: The Guilford Press

Payne, M. (2000). *Narrative Therapy.* London: Sage Publications.

Peck, M. S. (1978). *The road less traveled.* New York: Simon & Schuster.

Peins, M., McGough, W. E., & Lee, B. S. (1972). Evaluation of a tape-recorded method of stuttering therapy: Improvement in a speaking task. *Journal of Speech and Hearing Research, 15,* 364–371.

Perkins, W., Kent, R. D., & Curlee, R. F. (1990). A theory of neuropsycholinguistic function in stuttering. *Journal of Speech and Hearing Research, 34,* 734–752.

Perkins, W. H. (1973). Replacement of stuttering with normal speech: II. Clinical procedures. *Journal of Speech and Hearing Disorders, 38,* 295–303.

Perkins, W. H. (1979). From psychoanalysis to discoordination. In H. Gregory (Ed.), *Controversies about stuttering therapy,* 97–127. Baltimore, MD: University Park Press.

Perkins, W. H. (1983). The problem of definition: Commentary on stuttering. *Journal of Speech and Hearing Disorders, 48,* 246–249.

Perkins, W. H. (1990). What is stuttering? *Journal of Speech and Hearing Disorders, 55,* 370–382.

Perry, A., & Doan, R. E. (1994). Story re-visions: Narrative therapy in the post modern world. New York: The Guilford Press.

Peters, T. J., & Guitar, B. (1991). *Stuttering, an integrated approach to its nature and treatment.* Baltimore, MD: Williams & Wilkins.

Pickett, J. M. (1980). *The sounds of speech communication.* Baltimore, MD: University Park Press.

Pinsky, S. D., & McAdam, D. W. (1980). Electroencephalographic and dichotic indicies of cerebral laterality in stutterers. *Brain & Language, 11,* 374–397.

Pool, K. D., Devous, M. D., Sr., Freeman, F. J., Watson, B. C., & Finitzo, T. (1991). Regional cerebral blood flow in developmental stutterers. *Archives of Neurology, 48,* 509–512.

Postma, A., & Kol, H. (1990). Speech errors, disfluencies, and self-repairs of stutterers in two accuracy conditions. *Journal of Fluency Disorders, 15,* 291–203.

Plexico, L. & Manning, W. (2004, November). *Locus of control for persons who stutter: A content analysis.* Presentation to the Annual Convention of the American Speech-Language-Hearing Association, Philadelphia, PA.

Plexico, L., & Manning. W. (2008a). Coping responses by adults who stutter: Preventing and escaping the problem. Presentation to the annual meeting of the American Speech-Language-Hearing Association, Chicago, IL.

Plexico, L., & Manning. W. (2008b). Coping responses by adults who stutter: Approaching the problem. Presentation to the annual meeting of the American Speech-Language-Hearing Association, Chicago, IL.

Plexico, L., Manning, W., & DiLollo, A. (2005). A phenomenological understanding of successful stuttering management, *Journal of Fluency Disorders, 30*(1) 1–22.

Pollard, R., Ellis, J. B., Finan, D., & Ramig, P. R. (2009) Effects of the SpeechEasy on objective and perceived aspects of stuttering: a six-month, Phase I clinical trial in naturalistic environments. *Journal of Speech, Hearing and Language Research. 52*(2) 1–18.

Pollard, R., Ramig, P. R., Ellis, J. B., & Finan, D., (2007). *Case study of Speech Easy use combined with traditional stuttering treatment.* Presentation to the American-Speech-Language-Hearing Association, Boston, MA.

Plomin, R., & Crabbe, J. (2002). DNA, *Psychological Bulletin, 126,* 806–828.

Postma, A., & Kolk, H. (1992). Error monitoring in people who stutter: Evidence against auditory feedback defect theories. *Journal of Speech and Hearing Research, 35,* 1024–1032.

Postma, A., & Kolk, H. (1993). The covert repair hypothesis: Prearticulatory repair processes in normal and stuttered disfluencies. *Journal of Speech and Hearing Research, 36,* 472–487.

Postma, A., Kolk, H. H. J., & Povel, D. J. (1990). Speech planning and execution in stutterers. *Journal of Fluency Disorders, 15,* 49–59.

Poulos, M. G., & Webster, W. G. (1991). Family history as a basis for subgrouping people who stutter. *Journal of Speech and Hearing Research, 34,* 5–10.

Preibisch, C., Neumann, K., Raab, P., Euler, H. A., von Gudenberg, A. W., Lanfermann, H., & Giraud, A. (2003). Evidence for compensation for stuttering by the right frontal operculum. *NeuroImage, 20,* 1356–1364.

Preus, A. (1972). Stuttering in Down's syndrome. *Scandinavian Journal of Education Research, 15,* 89–104.

Preus, A. (1981). *Attempts at identifying subgroups of stutterers.* Oslo, Norway: University of Norway Press.

Prins, D. (1970). Improvement and regression in stutterers following short-term intensive therapy. *Journal of Speech and Hearing Disorders, 35,* 123–135.

Prins, D. (1997). Modifying stuttering—The stutterer's reactive behavior: perspectives on past, present, and future. In R. Curlee & G. Siegel (Eds.), *Nature and treatment of stuttering, New directions* (2nd ed., pp. 335–355). Needham Heights, MA: Allyn & Bacon.

Prins, D., & Hubbard, C. (1988). Response contingent stimuli and stuttering: Issues and implications. *Journal of Speech and Hearing Research, 31,* 696–709.

Prizant, B., (2001). Forward, In D. M. Luterman, (Ed.), *Counseling persons with communication disorders and their families.* (4th ed., pp. ix-xi). Austin, TX: Pro-Ed.

Prizant, B., & Rydell, P. J. (1984). Analysis of functions of delayed echolalia in autistic children. *Journal of Speech and Hearing Research, 27,* 183–192.

Prochaska, J. O. & DiClemente, C.C. (1992). Stages of change in the modification of problem behaviors. In Herson, M., Eisler, R., & Miller, P. (Eds.), *Progress in behavior modification* (pp. 184–218). Sycamore, IL: Sycamore Publishing Company.

Prochaska, J. O., DiClemente, C. C., & Norcross, J. C. (1992). In search of how people change: Applications to addictive behaviors. *American Psychologist, 47*(9), 1102–1114.

Proctor, A., Duff, M., Patterson, A., & Yairi, E. (2001, November). Stuttering in African American and European American preschoolers. Presentation to the annual meeting of the American Speech-Language-Hearing Association, New Orleans.

Quarrington, B., Seligman, J., & Kosower, E. (1969). Goal setting behavior of parents of beginning stutterers and parents of nonstuttering children. *Journal of Speech and Hearing Research, 12,* 435–42.

Quesal, R.W. (1989). Stuttering research: Have we forgotten the stutterer? *Journal of Fluency Disorders, 14,* 153–164.

Quesal, R. W. (1998). Knowledge, understanding, and acceptance. In E. C. Healey & H. F. M. Peters (Eds.), *Proceedings of the 2nd World Congress on Fluency Disorders* (pp. 384–387). Nijmegen, The Netherlands: Nijmegen University Press.

Quesal, R.W. (2006, Feb.) Assessing and Treating Adolescents Who Stutter in an EBP World. Invited presentation to the 36th Annual Mid-South Conference on Communicative Disorders, Memphis, TN.

Quesal, R. W., & Yaruss, J. S. (2000). Historical perspective on stuttering treatment: Dean Williams, *Contemporary issues in Communication Science and Disorders, 27,* 178–187.

Ramig, P. R. (1993a). High reported spontaneous recovery rates: Fact or fiction? *Language, Speech, and Hearing in Schools, 24,* 156–160.

Ramig, P. R. (1993b). The impact of self-help groups on persons who stutter: A call for research. *Journal of Fluency Disorders, 18,* 351–361.

Ramig, P. R. (1993c). Parent–clinician–child partnership in the therapeutic process of the preschool and elementary-aged child who stutters. *Seminars in Speech and Language, 14,* 226–236.

Ramig, P. R. (1998). My long-term recovery from stuttering. In E. C. Healey & H. F. M. Peters (Eds.), *Proceedings of the 2nd World Congress on Fluency Disorders* (pp. 390–391). Nijmegen, The Netherlands: Nijmegen University Press.

Ramig, P., & Bennett, E. (1995). Working with 7- to 12-year-old children who stutter: Ideas for intervention in the public schools. *Language, Speech, and Hearing Services in Schools, 26,* 138–150.

Ramig, P. R., & Dodge, D. M. (2005). *The child and adolescent stuttering treatment and activity resource guide.* Clifton Park, NY: Thomson Delmar Learning.

Ramig, P. R., Ellis, J. B., & Pollard, R., Chapter 16 in Application of the SpeechEasy to Stuttering Treatment: Introduction, background, and preliminary observations. In B. Guitar & R. McCauley (Eds.), *Treatment of Stuttering: Traditional and Emerging Approaches* Baltimore: Lippincott, Williams & Wilkins. (in press)

Rao, P R. (1991) Neurogenic stuttering as a manifestation of stroke and a mask of dysnomia. *Clinics in Communication Disorders, 1*(1), 31–37.

Raphael, L. J., Bakker, K., Myers, F. L., St. Louis, K. O., Fichtner, V., & Kostel, M., (2005). An update on diadochokinetic rates of cluttered and normal speech. Presentation to the Annual Convention of the American Speech-Language-Hearing Association, San Diego, CA.

Raphael, L. J., Bakker, K., Myers, F. L., St. Louis, K. O., & MacRoy, M. (2004). *Diadochokinetic rates of cluttered and normal speech.* Presentation to the Annual Convention of the American Speech-Language-Hearing Association, Philadelphia, PA.

Raskin, J. & Lewandowski, A. (2000) The construction of disorder as human enterprise. In R. A. Neimeyer & J. D. Raskin (Eds.), *Constructions of Disorder* (pp. 15–40). Washington. DC, American Psychological Association.

Ratner, N. B.(1993). Parents, children, and stuttering. *Seminars in Speech and Language, 14*(3), 238–247.

Ratner, N. B. (1995). Treating the child who stutters with concomitant language or phonological impairment. *Language, Speech, and Hearing Services in Schools, 26,* 180–186.

Ratner, N. B. (1997). Stuttering: A psycholinguistic perspective. In R. Curlee & Siegel (Eds.), *Nature and Treatment of Stuttering: New Directions* (pp. 99–127) (2nd ed.). Boston: Allyn & Bacon.

Ratner, N. B.(2000). Performance or capacity, the model still requires definitions and boundaries it doesn't have. *Journal of Fluency Disorders, 25*(4), 337–346.

Ratner, N. B. (2005). Evidenced-based practice in stuttering: Some questions to consider. *Journal of Fluency Disorders, 30*(1), 163–188.

Ratner, N. B. (1997). Stuttering: A psycholinguistic perspective. In R. Curlee & G. Siegel (Eds.), *Nature and treatment of stuttering: New directions* (2nd ed.). Boston: Allyn & Bacon.

Ratner, N. B., & Guitar, B. (2006). Treatment of very early stuttering and parent-administered therapy: The state of the art. In N. B. Ratner & J. Tetnowski (Eds.), *Current Issues in Stuttering Research and Practice* (pp. 99–124). Mahwah, NJ: Lawrence Erlbaum Associates.

Ratner, N. B., & Healey, E. C. (1999) Bridging the gap between stuttering research and practice: An overview. In N. B. Ratner & E. C. Healey (Eds.), *Stuttering Research and Practice: Bridging the Gap* (pp. 1–12). Mahwah, NJ: Lawrence Erlbaum Associates.

Ratner, N., & Sih, C. (1987). The effects of gradual increases in sentence length and complexity on children's dysfluency. *Journal of Speech and Hearing Disorders, 52,* 278–287.

Reardon, N. A. (2000). Working with teachers. Presentation to the Stuttering Foundation of America Conference, Stuttering therapy: Practical ideas for the school clinician. Charleston, SC, June 10, 2000.

Reardon, N. A. & Yaruss, J. S. (2004). *The Source for Stuttering Ages 7–18*. East Moline, IL: LinguiSystems.

Reeves, P. L. (2006). The role of self-help/mutual aid in addressing the needs of individuals who stutter. Chapter 11 (pp. 255–278). In N. Bernstein Ratner & J. Tetnowski (Eds.), *Current Issues in Stuttering Research and Practice* Mahwah, NJ: Lawrence Erlbaum.

Reich, A., Till, J. A., & Goldsmith, H. (1981). Laryngeal and manual reaction times of stuttering and nonstuttering adults. *Journal of Speech and Hearing Research, 24*(2), 192–196.

Resnick, P. (1993). Defrocking the fraud: The detection of malingering. *The Israel Journal of Psychology and Related Sciences, 30*(2), 93–101.

Reitzes, P. (2006). *50 great activities for children who stutter*. Austin, TX: Pro-Ed.

Reynolds, C. R., & Richmond, B. O. (1994). *Revised Children's Manifest Anxiety Scale*. Los Angeles: Western Psychological Services.

Riaz, N., Steinberg, S., Ahmad, J., Pluzhnikov, A, Riazuddin, S., Cox, N. J., & Drayna, D. (2005). Genomewide significant linkage to stuttering on chromosome 12. *American Journal of Human Genetics, 76,* 76, 647–651.

Ribbler, N. (2006, February). When a student stutters: Identifying the adverse educational impact. *Perspectives on Fluency Disorders, 16*(1), 15–17. Rockville, MD: American Speech-Language-Hearing Association.

Riley, G. (1981). *Stuttering Prediction Instrument for Young Children* (rev. ed.). Austin, TX: Pro-Ed.

Riley, G., & Riley, J. (1979). A component model for diagnosing and treating children who stutter. *Journal of Fluency Disorders, 4,* 279–293.

Riley, G., & Riley, J. (1983). Evaluation as a basis for intervention. In D. Peins & R. Ingham (Eds.), *Treatment of Stuttering in Early Childhood* (pp. 128–152). San Diego, CA: College-Hill.

Riley, G., & Riley, J. (1984). A component model for treating stuttering in children. In M. Prins (Ed.), *Contemporary Approaches in Stuttering Therapy.* Boston: Little, Brown.

Riley, G., & Riley, J. (1985). *Oral motor assessment and treatment: Improving syllable production.* Austin, TX: ProED.

Riley, G., & Riley, J. (2000). A revised component model for diagnosing and treating children who stutter. *Contemporary Issues in Communication Sciences and Disorders, 27,* 188–199.

Riley, G. D. (1972). A stuttering severity instrument for children and adults. *Journal of Speech and Hearing Disorders, 37,* 314–321.

Riley, G. D. (1994). *Stuttering Severity Instrument for Children and Adults—third edition.* (SSI–3). Austin, TX: Pro-Ed.

Riley, J., Riley, G., & Maguire, G., (2004). Subjective Screening of Stuttering severity, locus of control and avoidance: research edition. *Journal of Fluency Disorders, 29,* 51–62.

Robb, M., & Blomgren, M. (1997). Analysis of F2 transitions in the speech of stutterers and nonstutterers. *Journal of Fluency Disorders, 22,* 1–16.

Robb, M., Blomgren, M., & Chen, Y. (1998). Formant frequency fluctuation in stuttering and nonstuttering adults. *Journal of Fluency Disorders, 23,* 73–84.

Robins, G. (2008). www.cs.virginia.edu/~robins/quotes.html

Robinson, V. M. (1991). Humor and the health professions. Throrfare, NJ: Slack.

Rogers, C. R. (1951). *Client-centered Therapy.* Boston: Houghton Mifflin.

Rogers, C. R. (1961). *On Becoming a Person.* Boston: Houghton Mifflin.

Rogers, C. R. (Ed.). (1967). *The therapeutic relationship and its impact.* Madison: University of Wisconsin Press.

Rogers, C. R. (1980). *A way of Being.* Boston: Houghton Mifflin.

Rogers, C. R. (1986). Rogers, Kohut, and Erickson: A personal perspective on some similarities and differences. *Person-Centered Review, 1,* 125–140.

Rosenbek, J., Messert, B., Collins, M., & Wertz, T. (1978). Stuttering following brain damage. *Brain and Language, 6,* 82–86.

Rosenheim, E. (1974). Humor in psychotherapy: An interactive experience. *American Journal of Psychotherapy, 28,* 584–591.

Rosenzweig, S. (1936). Some implicit common factors in diverse methods of psychotherapy. *American Journal of Orthopsychiatry, 6,* 412–415.

Roth, C. R., Aronson, A. E., & Davis, L. J., Jr. (1989). Clinical studies in psychogenic stuttering of adult onset. *Journal of Speech and Hearing Disorders, 54,* 634–646.

Rousey, C. G., Arjunan, K. N., & Rousey, C. L. (1986). Successful treatment of stuttering following closed head injury. *Journal of Fluency Disorders, 11,* 257–261.

Rubin, H. (1986). Postscript: Cognitive therapy. In G. H. Shames & H. Rubin (Eds.), *Stuttering Then and Now* (pp. 474–486). Columbus, OH: Merrill.

Rubin, H., & Culatta, R. (1971). A point of view about fluency. *ASHA, 13,* 93–116.

Rudolf, S. R., Manning, W. H., & Sewell, W. R. (1983). The use of self-efficacy scaling in training student clinicians: Implications for working with stutterers. *Journal of Fluency Disorders, 8,* 55–75.

Runyan, C. M., & Adams, M.R. (1978). Perceptual study of the speech of "successfully therapeutized stutterers." *Journal of Fluency Disorders, 3,* 25–29.

Runyan, C. M., Bell, J. N., & Prosek, R.A. (1990). Speech naturalness ratings of treated stutterers. *Journal of Speech and Hearing Disorders, 55,* 434–438.

Runyan, C. M., Hames, P. E., & Proseck, R. A. (1982). A perceptual comparison between paired stimulus and single stimulus methods of presentation of the fluent utterances of stutterers. *Journal of Fluency Disorders, 7,* 71–77.

Runyan, C. M., Runyan, S. E., & Hibbard, S. (2006). *The Speech Easy [sic] device: A three year study.* Presentation to the annual meeting of the American Speech-Language-Hearing Association. Miami, FL.

Ruscello, D. M., Lass, N. J., Schmitt, J. F., & Panbacker, M. D. (1994). Special educators' perceptions of stutterers. *Journal of Fluency Disorders, 19,* 12 –132.

Rusk, T. (1989). So you want to change: Helping people help themselves. Presentation given at the Twelfth Annual Conference for Trainers, Consultants, and other HRD Professionals, sponsored by University Associates (San Diego), San Francisco, CA.

Rustin, L. (1987). The treatment of childhood dysfluency through active parental involvement. In L. Rustin, H. Purser, & H. Rowley (Eds.), *Progress in the Treatment of Fluency Disorders* (pp. 166–180). London: Taylor & Francis.

Rustin, L., Botterill, W., & Kelman, E. (1996). *Assessment and therapy for young dysfluent children: Family interaction.* London: Whurr Publishers.

Rustin, L., & Cook, F. (1995). Parental involvement in the treatment of stuttering. *Language, Speech, and Hearing Services in Schools, 26,* 127–137.

Ryan, B. (1979). Stuttering therapy in a framework of operant conditioning and programmed learning. In H. Gregory (Ed.), *Controversies about stuttering therapy* (pp. 129–174). Baltimore, MD: University Park Press.

Ryan, B. (1980). *Programmed Therapy for Stuttering Children and Adults* (1st ed.). Springfield, IL: Charles C. Thomas.

Ryan, B. (2001). *Programmed Therapy for Stuttering Children and Adults* (2nd ed.). Springfield, IL: Charles C. Thomas.

Ryan, B. & Van Kirk Ryan. (1995). Programmed stuttering treatment for children: Comparison of two establishment programs through transfer, maintenance, and follow-up. *Journal of Speech & Hearing Research, 38*(1) 61–75.

Sacco, P. R., Metz, D. E., & Schiavetti, N. (1992). Speech naturalness of non-stutterers and treated stutterers: Acoustical correlates. Presentation to the annual meeting of the American Speech-Language-Hearing Association, San Antonio, TX.

Sackett, D. L., Strauss, S. E., Richardson, W. S., Rosenberg, W., & Hayes, R. B. (2000) *Evidenced-based medicine*. Edinburgh: Churchill-Livingston.

Sagan, C. (1996). *The Demon-haunted World: Science as a Candle in the Dark*. New York: Random House.

Salmelin, R., Schnitzler, A., Schmitz, F., & Freund, H. J. (2000). Single word reading in developmental stutters and fluent speakers. *Brain, 123,* 1184–1202.

Saltuklaroglu, T., & Kully, D. (1998). Further validation of the self-efficacy scale for adult stutterers. University of Alberta (unpublished manuscript).

Satcher, D. (1986). Research needs for minority populations. In F. H. Bess, B. S. Clark, & H. R. Mitchel (Eds.), *Concerns for Minority Groups in Communication Disorders* (pp. 89–92). (ASHA Reports, No. *16,* ISSN 0569–8553). Rockville, MD: American Speech-Language-Hearing Association.

Schaeffer, M. L., & Shearer, W. M. (1968). A survey of mentally retarded stutterers. *Mental Retardation, 6,* 44–45.

Schiavetti, N., & Metz, D. E. (1997). Stuttering and the measurement of speech naturalness. In R. Curlee & G. Siegel (Eds.), *Nature and Treatment of Stuttering, New Directions* (2nd ed., pp. 298–412). Needham Heights, MA: Allyn & Bacon.

Schiff, J. L. (1975). *Cathexis Reader: Transactional Analysis Treatment of Psychosis*. New York: Harper & Row.

Schimel, J. (1978). The function of wit and humor in psychoanalysis. *Journal of the American Academy of Psychoanalysis, 6*(3), 369–379.

Schwartz, H. D. (1999). *A primer of Stuttering Therapy*. Needham Heights, MA: Allyn and Bacon.

Schwartz, H., & Conture, E. (1988). Subgroupings of young stutterers: Preliminary behavioral observations. *Journal of Speech and Hearing Research, 31,* 62–71.

Schwartz, H. D., Zebrowski, P. M., & Conture, E. G. (1990). Behaviors at the outset of stuttering. *Journal of Fluency Disorders, 15,* 77–86.

Scott, K. S., & Sisskin, V. (2007). Part II: Speech disfluency in Autism Spectrum Disorders: Clinical problem solving for pervasive developmental disorder, not otherwise specified and Asperger Syndrome. Presentation to the International Stuttering Awareness Day Online Conference (ISAD). http://www.mankato.msus.edu/dept/comdis/isad/isadcon.html

Scott Trautman, L., & Keller, K. (2000). Bilingual intervention for stuttering: a case in point. Presentation to the Annual Convention of the American Speech-Language-Hearing Association, Washington, D.C.

Scripture, E. W. (1931). *Stuttering, Lisping, and Correction of the Speech of the Deaf.* New York: Macmillan.

Seery, C. H., (2005). Differential diagnosis of stuttering for forensic purposes. *American Journal of Speech-Language Pathology, 14,* 284–297.

Shames, G. H., & Sherrick, C. E., Jr. (1965). A discussion of nonfluency and stuttering as operant behavior. *Journal of Speech and Hearing Disorders, 28,* 3–18.

Shapiro, D. A. (1999). *Stuttering intervention: A collaborative journey to fluency freedom.* Austin, TX: Pro-Ed.

Sheehan, J. (1958). Projective studies of stuttering. *Journal of Speech and Hearing Disorders, 23,* 18–25.

Sheehan, J. (1970). *Stuttering: Research and Therapy.* New York: Harper & Row.

Sheehan, J. (1975). Conflict theory and avoidance-reduction therapy. In J. Eisenson (Ed.), *Stuttering, a Second Symposium* (pp. 97–198). New York: Harper & Row.

Sheehan, J. G. (1980). Problems in the evaluation of progress and outcome. In W. H. Perkins (Ed.), *Seminars in Speech, Language and Hearing* (pp. 389–401). New York: Thieme–Stratton.

Sheehan, J. G. (1982). *Stuttering therapy: Transfer and maintenance.* (Publication No. 16). Memphis: Stuttering Foundation of America

Sheehan, J. G., & Costley, M. S. (1977). A reexamination of the role of heredity in stuttering. *Journal of Speech and Hearing Disorders, 42,* 47–59.

Sheehan, J. G., & Martyn, M. (1966). Spontaneous recovery from stuttering. *Journal of Speech and Hearing Research, 9,* 121–135.

Sheehan, J. G., & Martyn, M. (1970). Stuttering and its disappearance. *Journal of Speech and Hearing Research, 13, 279–289.*

Sheehy, G. (1974). *Passages: Predictable Crises of Adult Life.* New York: Bantam Books.

Shenker, R. C., Conte, A., Gingras, A., Courcey, A., & Polomeno, L. (1998). The impact of bilingualism on developing fluency in a preschool child. In: E. C. Healey, & H. F. M. Peters (Eds.), *Second World Congress on Fluency Disorders Proceedings,* San Francisco, August 12–22 (pp. 200–204). Nijmegen: Nijmegen Univ. Press.

Shields, D. (1989). *Dead languages.* New York: Knopf.

Shine, R. E. (1988). *Systematic Fluency Training for Young Children* (3rd ed.). Austin, TX: ProEd.

Shugart, Y. Y., Mundorff, J., Kilshaw, J., Doheny, K., Doan, B., Wanyee, J., et al. (2004). Results of a genome-wide linkage scan for stuttering. *Am J Med Genet A, 124*(2), 133–135.

Siegel, G. (1970). Punishment, stuttering and disfluency. *Journal of Speech and Hearing Disorders, 13,* 677–714.

Siegel, G. (1993). Research: A natural bridge. *ASHA, 35,* 36–37.

Siegel, G. (2000). "Demands and capacities" or "demands and performance." *Journal of Fluency Disorders, 25*(4), 321–328.

Siegen, G. M., & Martin, R. R. (1966). Punishment of disfluencies in normal speakers. *Journal of Speech and Hearing Research, 9,* 208–218.

Silverman, E. (1973). Clustering: A characteristic of preschoolers' speech disfluency. *Journal of Speech and Hearing Research, 16,* 578–583.

Silverman, E. (1974). Disfluency behavior of elementary-school stutterers and nonstutterers. *Language, Speech, and Hearing Services in Schools, 5,* 32–37.

Silverman, E., & Zimmer, C. (1982). Demographic characteristics and treatment experiences of women and men who stutter. *Journal of Fluency Disorders, 7,* 273–285.

Silverman, F. H. (1975). How "typical" is a stutterer's stuttering in a clinical environment? *Perceptual and Motor Skills, 40,* 458.

Silverman, F. H. (1976). Long-term impact of a miniature metronome on stuttering: An interim report. *Perceptual and Motor Skills, 43,* 398.

Silverman, F. H. (1981). Relapse following stuttering therapy. In N. J. Lass (Ed.), *Speech and Language, Advances in Basic Research and Practice* (Vol. 5, pp. 56–78). New York: Academic Press.

Silverman, F. H. (1988a). Impact of a T-shirt message on stutterer stereotypes. *Journal of Fluency Disorders, 13,* 279–281.

Silverman, F. H. (1988b). The monster study. *Journal of Fluency Disorders, 13,* 225–231.

Silverman, F. H. (1996). *Stuttering and Other Fluency Disorders.* Englewood Cliffs, NJ: Prentice Hall.

Silverman, F. H. (2004). *Stuttering and Other Fluency Disorders,* Long Grove, IL: Waveland Press

Silverman, S. W., & Bernstein Ratner, N. (2002) Measuring lexical diversity in children who stutter: application of *vocd. Journal of Fluency Disorders, 27,* 289–305.

Simon, H. A. & Chase, W. G., (1973). Skill in chess. *American Scientist, 61,* 394–403.

Simmons–Mackie, N. & Schultz, M. (2003). The role of humor in therapy for aphasia. *Aphasiology, 17,* 751–766.

Skinner, B. F., (1953). *Science and human behavior.* New York: McMillian.

Slater, S. C. (1992, August). 1992 Omnibus Survey: Portrait of the professions. *ASHA, 34,* 61–65.

Sisskin, V. (2005). The effect of commonly occurring concomitant disorders on stuttering: Asperger Syndrome, Presentation to the annual meeting of the American Speech-Language-Hearing Association, San Diego, CA.

Sisskin, V. (2006). Speech disfluency in Asperger's Syndrome: Two cases of interest. *Perspectives in Fluency and Fluency Disorders, 16*(2), 12–14.

Sisskin, V., & Scott, K. S., (2007). Part I: Speech disfluency in Autism Spectrum Disorders: Clinical Problem Solving for Autistic Disorders. Presentation to the International Stuttering Awareness Day Online Conference (ISAD). http://www.mankato.msus.edu/dept/comdis/isad/isadcon.html

Smith, A. (1989). Neural drive to muscles in stuttering. *Journal of Speech and Hearing Research, 32,* 252–264.

Smith, A. (1990). Toward a comprehensive theory of stuttering: A commentary. *Journal of Speech and Hearing Disorders, 55,* 398–401.

Smith, A. (1999). Stuttering: A unified approach to a multifactorial, dynamic disorder. In N. B. Ratner and E. C. Healey (Eds.), *Stuttering Research and Practice: Bridging the Gap* (pp. 27–44). Mahwah, NJ: Lawrence Erlbaum.

Smith, A., Denny, M, Shaffer, L, Kelly, E. and Hirano, M. (1996). Activity of intrinsic laryngeal muscles in fluent and disfluent speech. *Journal of Speech and Hearing Research, 39,* 329–348.

Smith, A., Denny, M., & Wood, J. (1991). Instability in speech muscle systems in stuttering. In H. F. M. Peters, W. Hulstijn, & W. Starkweather (Eds.), *Speech Motor Control and Stuttering* (pp. 231–242). New York: Elsevier.

Smith A., & Kelly, E. (1997) Stuttering: A dynamic, multifactoral model. In R. F. Curlee & G. M. Siegel (Eds.), *The Nature and Treatment of Stuttering: New Directions* (2nd Ed., pp. 204–217). Needham Heighs, MA: Allyn & Bacon.

Smith, A., & Kleinow, J. (2000). Kinematic correlates of speaking rate change in stuttering and normally fluent adults. *Journal of Speech, Language, and Hearing Research, 43,* 521–536.

Smith, M. L., & Glass, G. V. (1977). Meta-analysis of psychotherapy outcome studies. *American Psychologist, 32,* 752–760.

Simmons-Mackie, N., & Damico, J. S. (1999). Social role negotiation in aphasia therapy: Competence, incompetence, and conflict. In D. Kovarsky, J. F., Duchan & M. Maxell (Eds.), *Constructing (in) competence: Disabling evaluations in clinical and social interaction* (pp. 313–342). Mahwah, NJ: Erlbaum.

Snidecor, J. C. (1947). Why the Indian does not stutter. *Quarterly Journal of Speech, 33,* 493–495.

Sommer, M., Koch, M. A.., Paulus, W., Weiller, C., & Buchel, C. (2002). Mechanisms of disease. Disconnecting of speech-relevant brain areas in persistent developmental stuttering. *Lancet, 360,* 380–383.

Sommers, R. K., Brady, W., & Moore, W. H., Jr. (1975). Dichotic ear preferences of stuttering children and adults. *Perceptual and Motor Skills, 41,* 931–938.

Sommers, R. K., & Caruso, A. J. (1995). *American Journal of Speech-Language Pathology, 4*(3), 22–28.

Special Section (Evidence-based treatment of stuttering: a series of 5 manuscripts), *Journal of Fluency Disorders, 30,* 197–258.

SpeechEasy Professional Information Packet (2006). Available from Janus Development Group, Inc. 112 Staton Road, Greenville, NC 27843. Phone: 866–551–9042.

Spielberger, C. D., Edwards, C. D., Luschene, R. E., Montuori, J., & Platzek, D. (1972). *STAIC preliminary manual.* New York: Consulting Psychologists Press, Inc.

Springer, S.P., & Deutsch, G. (1989). *Left Brain, Right Brain.* New York: W. H. Freeman and Company.

St. Louis, K. O. (1982). Transfer and maintenance of fluency in stuttering clients. Short course presented to the annual meeting of the American Speech-Language-Hearing Association, Toronto, Ontario.

St. Louis, K. O. (1986). *The Atypical Stutterer: Principles and Practices of Rehabilitation.* Orlando, FL: Academic Press.

St. Louis, K. O. (1992). On defining cluttering. In F. L. Myers & K. O. St. Louis (Eds.), *Cluttering: A Clinical Perspective* (pp. 37–53). San Diego: Singular Publishing Group (reissued in 1996, San Diego: Singular Publishing Group).

St. Louis, K. O., (1998). A typical stutterer's story. In E. C. Healey & H. F. M. Peters (Eds.), *Proceedings of the 2nd World Congress on Fluency Disorders* (pp. 392–393). Nijmegen, The Netherlands: Nijmegen University Press.

St. Louis, K. O. (1999). Person–first labeling and stuttering. *Journal of Fluency Disorders, 24,* 1–24.

St. Louis, K. O. (2001). *Living with Stuttering: Stories, Resources, and Hope.* Morgantown, WV: Populore Publishing Company,

St. Louis, K. O., (2006). Measurement Issues in Fluency Disorders. Chapter 4 (pp. 61 –86). In N. Bernstein Ratner & J. Tetnowski, *Current Issues in Stuttering Research and Practice.* Mahwah, NJ.: Lawrence Earlbaum, Inc.

St. Louis, K. O., & Atkins, C. P. (2006). *Self-Awareness of Speech Index* (SASI). Morgantown, WV: Authors.

St. Louis, K. O., & Durrenberger, C. H. (1992). Clinician preferences for managing various communication disorders. Presentation to the Annual Convention of the American Speech-Language-Hearing Association, San Antonio, TX.

St. Louis, K. O., & Hinzman, A. R. (1986). Studies of cluttering: Perceptions of cluttering by speech-language pathologists and educators, *Journal of Fluency Disorders, 11,* 131–149.

St. Louis, K. O., & Lass, N. J. (1981). A survey of communicative disorders students' attitudes toward stuttering. *Journal of Fluency Disorders, 6,* 49–80.

St. Louis, K. O., Murray, C. D., & Ashworth, M. (1991). Coexisting communication disorders in a random sample of school-aged stutterers. *Journal of Fluency Disorders, 16,* 13–23.

St. Louis, K. O., & Myers, F. (1995). Clinical management of cluttering. *Language, Speech, and Hearing Services in Schools, 26,* 187–195.

St. Louis, K. O., & Myers, F. (1997). Management of cluttering and related fluency disorders. In R. F. Curlee & G. M. Siegel (Eds.). *Nature and treatment of stuttering: New directions* (2nd ed.) (pp. 313–332). New York: Allyn & Bacon.

St. Louis, K. O., Myers, F. L., Bakker, K., & Raphael, L. J. (2007). Understanding and treating cluttering, In E. Conture & R. Curlee, *Stuttering and Related Disorders of Fluency.* (3rd Edition, pp. 297–325). New York: Thieme Medical Publishers, Inc.

St. Louis, K. O., Myers, F. L., Faragasso, K., Townsend, P. S., & Gallaher, A. J., (2004). Perceptual aspects of cluttered speech, *Journal of Fluency Disorders, 29,* 213–235.

St. Louis, K. O., & Rustin, L. (1992). Professional awareness of cluttering. In F. M. Myers & K. O. St. Louis (Eds.), *Cluttering: A Clinical Perspective* (pp. 23–35). San Diego, CA: Singular Publishing Group, Inc.

St. Louis, K. O., & Westbrook, J. B. (1987). The effectiveness of treatment for stuttering. In L. Rustin, H. Purser, & D. Rowley (Eds.), *Progress in the Treatment of Fluency Disorders* (pp. 235–257). London: Taylor & Francis.

Stager, S. V., Jeffries, J. J., & Braun, A. R. (2003). Common features of fluency-evoking conditions studied in stuttering subject sand controls: An H(2)12O PET study. *Journal of Fluency Disorders, 28,* 319–335.

Starke, A. (1995). Why do stutterers reject artificial speech? The message incompatibility conflict. *Proceedings of the 1994 Meeting of the International Fluency Association* (V. II, pp. 445–452). University Press Nijmegen, Netherlands.

Starkweather, C. W. (1987). *Fluency and stuttering.* Englewood Cliffs, NJ: Prentice–Hall.

Starkweather, C. W. (1992). Response and reaction to Hamre, "Stuttering Prevention I." *Journal of Fluency Disorders, 17,* 43–55.

Starkweather, C. W. (July 8, 1995). Personal communication.

Starkweather, C.W. (1997). Therapy for younger children. In R. F. Curlee and G. M. Siegel (Eds.), *Nature and treatment of stuttering* (2nd ed., pp. 257–279). Boston: Allyn and Bacon.

Starkweather, C.W. (1999).The effectiveness of stuttering therapy: An issue for science? In N. B. Ratner and E. C. Healey (Eds.), *Stuttering research and practice: Bridging the gap* (pp. 231–244). Mahwah, NJ: Lawrence Erlbaum.

Starkweather, C. W., & Givens-Ackerman, J. (1997). *Stuttering.* Austin, TX: Pro-Ed.

Starkweather, C. W. & Givens-Ackerman, J. (2000). Personal communication.

Starkweather, C. W., & Gottwald, S. R. (1990). The demands and capacities model II: Clinical implications. *Journal of Fluency Disorders, 15,* 143–157.

Starkweather, C. W., & Gottwald, S. R. (2000). The demands and capacities model: Response to Siegel. *Journal of Fluency Disorders, 25*(4), 369–376.

Starkweather, C. W., Gottwald, S. R., & Halfond, M. H. (1990). *Stuttering prevention: A clinical method.* Englewood Cliffs, NJ: Prentice-Hall.

Starkweather, C. W., Hirschmann, P., & Tannenbaum, R. (1976). Latency of vocalization: Stutterers v. nonstutterers. *Journal of Speech and Hearing Research, 19,* 481–492.

Starkweather, C. W., St. Louis, K. O., Blood, G., Peters, T., & Westbrook, J. (1994). American Speech-Language-Hearing Association (1995, March). *Guidelines for Practice in Stuttering Treatment. ASHA, 37* (Suppl. 14, p. 26).

Stern, E. (1948). A preliminary study of bilingualism and stuttering in four Johannesburg schools. *Journal of Logopaedics, 1,* 15, 15–25.

Stetson, R. H. (1951). *Motor phonetics* (2nd ed.). Amsterdam: North-Holland.

Stewart, T., & Rowley, D. (1996). Acquired stammering in Great Britain. *European Journal of Disorders of Communication, 31,* 109.

Stocker, B. (1980). *The Stocker Probe technique for diagnosis and treatment of stuttering in young children.* Tulsa, OK: Modern Education Corporation.

Stocker, B., & Gerstman, L. (1983). A comparison of the probe technique and conventional therapy for young stutterers. *Journal of Fluency Disorders, 8,* 331–339.

Stocker, B., & Usprich, C. (1976). Stuttering in young children and level of demand. *Journal of Fluency Disorders, 1,* 116–131.

Stuart, A., Kalinowski, J., & Rastatter, M. P. (1997). Effect of monaural and binauaral altered auditory feedback on stuttering frequency. *Journal of the Acoustical Society of America, 101,* 3806–3809.

Stuart, A., Kalinowski, J., & Rastatter, M. Saltuklarglu, T., & Dayalu, V., (2004). Investigations of the impact of altered auditory feedback in-the-ear devices on the speech of people who stutter: Initial fitting and 4-month follow-up. *International Journal of Language and Communication Disorders, 39,* 93–119.

Studdert-Kennedy, M., & Shankweiler, D. (1970). Hemispheric specialization for speech perception. *Journal of the Acoustical Society of America, 48,* 579–594.

Subramanian, A., Yairi, E., & Amir, O. (2003). Second formant transitions in fluent speech of persistent and recovered preschool children who stutter. *Journal of Communication Disorders, 36,* 59–75.

Sugarman, M. (1980). It's O.K. to stutter: A personal account. *Journal of Fluency Disorders, 5,* 149–157.

Suresh, R., Ambrose, N., Roe, C., et al. (2006). New complexities in the genetics of stuttering: Significant sex-specific linkage signals. *The American Journal of Human Genetics, 78,* 554–563.

Sussman, H.M. (1971). The laterality effect in lingual-auditory tracking. *Journal of the Acoustical Society of America, 49,* 1874–1880.

Sussman, H. M., & MacNeilage, P. F. (1975). Hemispheric specialization for speech production and perception in stutterers. *Neuropsychologia, 13,* 19–26.

Sussman, H. M., MacNeilage, P. F., & Lumbley, J. (1974). Sensorimotor dominance and the right-ear advantage in mandibular-auditory tracking. *Journal of the Acoustical Society of America, 56,* 214–216.

Sussman, H. M., MacNeilage, P. F., & Lumbley, J. (1975). Pursuit auditory tracking of dichotically presented tonal amplitudes. *Journal of Speech and Hearing Research, 18,* 74–81.

Tasko, S. M., McClean, M. D., & Runyan, C. M. (2007). Speech motor correlates of treatment-related changes in stuttering severity and speech naturalness. *Journal of Communication Disorders, 40,* 42–65.

Thompson, J. (1983). Assessment of fluency in school-age children (resource guide). Danville, IL: Interstate Printers and Publishers.

Thompson, J. (1984). Update: School-age stutterers. *Journal of Fluency Disorders, 9,* 199–206

Tellis, G. M., Bressler, L., & Emerick, K., (2008). An exploration of clinicians views about assessment and treatment of stuttering. *Perspectives on Fluency and Fluency Disorders, 18,* 16–23.

Throneberg, R. N., & Yairi, E. (1994). Temporal dynamics of repetitions during the early stages of childhood stuttering: An acoustic study. *Journal of Speech and Hearing Research, 37,* 1067–1075.

Throneberg, R. N., Yairi, E., & Paden, E. (1994). Relation between phonologic difficulty and the occurrence of disfluencies in the early stage of stuttering. *Journal of Speech and Hearing Research, 37,* 504–509.

Tiffany, W. R. (1980). The effects of syllable structure on diadochokinetic and reading rates. *Journal of Speech and Hearing Research, 23,* 894–908.

Tiger, R. J., Irvine, T. L., & Reiss, R. P. (1980). Cluttering as a complex of learning disabilities. *Language, Speech, and Hearing Services in the Schools, 11,* 3–14.

Toscher, M. M., & Rupp, R. R. (1978). A study of the central auditory processes in stutterers using the Synthetic Sentence Identification (SSI) test battery. *Journal of Speech and Hearing Research, 21,* 779–792.

Travis, L. E. (1931). *Speech Pathology.* New York: Appleton-Century-Crofts.

Travis, L. E. (1957). The unspeakable feelings of people with special reference to stuttering. In L. E. Travis (Ed.), *Handbook of speech pathology* (pp. 916–946). New York: Appleton-Century-Crofts.

Travis, L. E. (1971). The unspeakable feelings of people with special reference to stuttering. In L. E. Travis (Ed.), *Handbook of speech pathology and audiology* (pp. 1001–1003). New York: Appleton-Century-Crofts.

Travis, L. E. (July 10, 1978). Personal communication.

Travis, L. E., & Knott, J. R. (1936). Brain potentials for normal speakers and stutterers. *Journal of Psychology, 2,* 137–150.

Travis, L. E., Johnson, W., & Shover, J. (1937). The relation of bilingualism to stuttering. *Journal of Speech Disorders, 2,* 185–189.

Travis, L. E., & Knott, J. R. (1937). Bilaterally recorded brain potentials from normal speakers and stutterers. *Journal of Speech Disorders, 2,* 239–241.

Travis, L.E., & Malamud, W. (1937). Brain potentials from normal subjects, stutterers, and schizophrenic patients. *American Journal of Psychiatry, 93,* 929–936.

Tetnowski, J. (1998). Linguistic effects on disfluenchy. In R. Paul (Ed.) *Exploring the speech–language connection,* Baltimore: Brookes.

Trichton, M., & Tetnowski, J. (2006). Perspectives of self-help groups for people who stutter from group leaders. Presentation to the annual meeting of the American Speech-Language-Hearing Association, Miami, FL.

Truax, C. B., & Carkhuff, R. R. (1966). *Toward effective counseling and psychotherapy.* Chicago: Aldine Press.

Tuckman, B. (1965). Developmental sequence in small groups. *Psychological Bulletin, 63,* 384–399.

Tudor, M. (1939). An experimental study of the effect of evaluative labeling on speech fluency. Master's thesis, University of Iowa.

Turnbaugh, K. R., Guitar, B. E., & Hoffman, P. R. (1979). Speech clinicians' attribution of personality traits as a function of stuttering severity. *Journal of Speech and Hearing Research, 22,* 37–45.

Turnbull, J. (2000). The transtheoretical model of change: Examples from stuttering. *Counseling Psychology Quarterly, 3*(1), 13–21.

Tversky, A., & Kahneman, D. (1974). Judgment under uncertainty: Heuristics and Biases. *Science, 185,* 1124–1131.

Valiant, G. E. (1977). *Adaptation to Life.* Boston: Little, Brown & Co.

Van Borsel, J. (1997). Neurogenic stuttering: A review. *Journal of Clinical Speech and Language Studies, 7,* 17–33.

Van Borsel, J., Achten, E., Santens, P., Lahorte, P., & Voet, T. (2003). fMRI of developmental stuttering: A pilot study. *Brain and Language, 85,* 369–377.

Van Borsel, J., Bontinck, C., Coryn, M., Paemeleire, F., & Vandemaele, P. (2007). Acoustic features of palilalia. *Brain and Language, 101,* 90–96.

Van Borsel, J., Maes, E., & Foulon, S. (2001). Stuttering and bilingualism A review. *Journal of Fluency Disorders, 26,* 179–205.

Van Borsel, J., Reunes, G., & Van den Bergh, N. (2003). Delayed auditory feedback in the treatment of stuttering. Clients as consumers. *International Journal of Language and Communication Disorders, 38,* 119–129.

Van Borsel, J., Van Lierde, K., Van Cauwenberge, P., Guldemont, I., & Van Orsho-ven, M., (1998). Severe acquired stuttering following injury of the left supple-mentary motor region: A case report. *Journal of Fluency Disorders, 23,* 49–58.

Van Borsel, J., & Vanryckeghem, M., (2000). Dysfluency and phonic tics in Tourette syndrome: A case report. *Journal of Communication Disorders, 33,* 227–240.

Van Lieshout, P. H. H. M., Hulstijn, W., & Peters, H. F. M. (1996). From planning to articulation in speech production: What differentiates a person who stutters from a person who does not stutter? *Journal of Speech and Hearing Research, 39,* 546–564.

Van Riper, C. (1937). The preparatory set in stuttering. *Journal of Speech Disor-ders, 2,* 149–154.

Van Riper, C. (1939). *Speech correction: Principles and methods* (11th ed.). Engle-wood Cliffs, NJ: Prentice-Hall.

Van Riper, C. (1971). *The nature of stuttering.* Englewood Cliffs, NJ: Prentice-Hall.

Van Riper, C. (1973). *The treatment of stuttering* (2nd ed.). Englewood Cliffs, NJ: Prentice-Hall.

Van Riper, C. (1974). A handful of nuts. *Western Michigan Journal of Speech Therapy, 11*(2), 1–3.

Van Riper, C. (1975). The stutterer's clinician. In Jon Eisenson (Ed.), *Stuttering, a second symposium* (pp. 453–492). New York: Harper & Row.

Van Riper, C. (1977). Adult Stuttering Therapy. A series of eight video tapes produced at Western Michigan University, Kalamazoo, MI. Distributed by The Stuttering Foundation of America.

Van Riper, C. (July *1,* 1978). Personal communication.

Van Riper, C. (1979). *A career in speech pathology.* Englewood Cliffs, NJ: Prentice-Hall.

Van Riper, C. (1982). *The nature of stuttering* (2nd ed.). Englewood Cliffs, NJ: Prentice-Hall.

Van Riper, C. (1984). Henry Freund: 1896–1982. *Journal of Fluency Disorders, 9,* 93–102.

Van Riper, C. (1990). Final thoughts about stuttering, *Journal of Fluency Disor-ders, 15,* 317–318.

Van Riper, C. (1992b). Some ancient history. *Journal of Fluency Disorders, 17,* 25–28.

Vanryckeghem, M. (2007). Behavior Assessment Battery: Evidence-based approach to the assessment and treatment of Children Who Stutter. *Pro-ceedings of 5th World Congress on Fluency Disorders (International Fluency Association): Research, treatment and self-help in fluency disorders: New hori-zons,* 209–214.

Vanryckeghem, M., & Brutten, G. J. (1992). The Communication Attitude Test: A test-retest reliability investigation. *Journal of Fluency Disorders, 17,* 117–190.

Vanryckeghem, M., & Brutten, G. J. (1996). The relationship between communication attitude and fluency failure of stuttering and nonstuttering children. *Journal of Fluency Disorders, 21,* 109–118.

Vanryckeghem, M., & Brutten, G. J. (1997). The speech-associated attitudes of children who do and do not stutter and differential effect of age. *American Journal of Speech-Language Pathology, 6*(4), 67–73.

Vanryckeghem, M., & Brutten, G. J. (2006). *KiddyCAT, Communication Attitude Test for Preschool and Kindergarten Children who Stutter,* San Diego, CA: Plural Publishing Inc.

Vanryckeghem, M., Brutten, G. J., & Herandez, L. M. (2005). A comparative investigation of the speech–associated attitude of preschool and kindergarten children who do and do not stutter. *Journal of Fluency Disorders, 30,* 307–318.

Vanryckeghem, M., Brutten, G. J., Uddin, N. & Van Borsel, J. (2004). A Behavior Checklist comparative investigation of the speech-associated coping responses of adults who do and do not stutter. *Journal of Fluency Disorders, 29,* 237–250.

Vanryckeghem, M., & Herder, C. (2004). Normative investigation of speech-associated coping behaviors of children who do and do not stutter. *ASHA Leader, 9,* 101.

Viney, L. L., & Westbrook, M. T. (1976). Cognitive anxiety: A method of content analysis for verbal samples. *Journal of Personality Assessment, 40,* 140–150.

Viney, L. L., & Westbrook, M. T. (1980). Scales measuring people's perception of themselves as origins and pawns, *Journal of Personality Assessment, 44,* 167–174.

Viswanath, N., Lee, H. S., & Chakraborty, R., (2004). Evidence for a major gene influence on persistent developmental stuttering. *Human Biology, 76,* 401–412.

Viswanath, N. S., Rosenfield, D. B., & Nudelman, H. B. (1992). Stutterers and cerebral blood flow: Letter to the editor. *Archives of Neurology, 49,* 346–347.

Wada, J., & Rasmussen, T. (1960). Intracarotid injection of sodium amytal for the lateralization of cerebral speech dominance. *Journal of Neurosurgery, 17,* 266–282.

Wakaba, Y. (1998). Research on temperament of stuttering children with early onset. In E. C. Healey & H. Peters (Eds.), *Proceedings of the Second World Congress on Fluency Disorders* (pp. 84–87). Nijmegen, The Netherlands: Nijmegen University

Waldrop, J., & Exter, T. (1990). What the 1990 census will show. *American Demographics, 12,* 20–30.

Walker, C., & Black, J. (1950). *The intrinsic intensity of oral phrases (Joint Project Report No. 2).* Pensacola, FL: United States Naval School of Aviation Medicine, Naval Air Station.

Wall, M. J. (1980). A comparison of syntax in young stutterers and nonstutterers. *Journal of Fluency Disorders, 5,* 345–352.

Wall, M. J., & Myers, F. L. (1995). *Clinical management of childhood stuttering* (2nd ed.). Austin, TX: Pro-Ed.

Walle, G. (1975). *The prevention of stuttering, Part 1* (film). Memphis, TN: Stuttering Foundation of America.

Wampold, B. E. (2001). *The Great Psychotherapy Debate: Models, Methods, and Findings.* Lawrence Erlbaum Associates: Mahwah, NJ.

Wampold, B. E., & Brown, G. S. (2005). Estimating variability in outcomes due to the therapist: A naturalistic study of outcomes in managed care. *Journal of Consulting and Clinical Psychology. 73*(5), 914–923.

Wampold, B.E., Mondin, G.W., Moody M., Stich, F., Benson, K. & Ahn, H. (1997). A meta-analysis of outcome studies comparing bona fide psychotherapies: Empirically, "all must have prizes." *Psychological Bulletin, 122,* 203–215.

Watkins, K. E., Smith, S. M., Davis, S., & Howell, P. (2008). Structural and functional abnormalities of the motor system in developmental stuttering. *Brain, 131*(1), 50–59.

Watkins, R. V., Yairi, E., & Ambrose, N. G. (1999). Early childhood stuttering III: Initial status of expressive language abilities. *Journal of Speech, Language, and Hearing Research, 42,* 1025–1135.

Watson, B. C., & Freeman, F. J. (1997). Brain imaging contributions. In R. F. Curlee & G. M. Siegel (Eds.), *Nature and Treatment of Stuttering: New Directions.* Needham Heights, MA: Allyn & Bacon.

Watson, B. C., Freeman, F. J., Devous, M. D., Chapman, S. B., Finitzo, T., & Pool, K. D. (1994). Linguistic performance and regional cerebral blood flow in persons who stutter. *Journal of Speech and Hearing Research, 37,* 1221–1228.

Watson, B. C., Pool, K. D., Devous, M. D., Freeman, F. J., & Finitzo, T. (1992). Brain blood flow related to acoustic laryngeal reaction time in adult developmental stutterers. *Journal of Speech and Hearing Research, 35,* 555–561.

Watson, J. B. (1988). A comparison of stutterers' and nonstutterers' affective, cognitive, and behavioral self-reports. *Journal of Speech and Hearing Research, 31,* 377–385.

Weber-Fox, C. (2001). Neural systems for sentence processing in stuttering. *Journal of Speech, Language and Hearing Research, 44,* 814–825.

Weber-Fox, C., Spencer, R. M. C., Spruill III, J. E., & Smith, A. (2004). Phonological processing in adults who stutter: Electrophysiological and behavioral evidence. *Journal of Speech, Language and Hearing Research, 47,* 1244–1258.

Webster, E. (1966). Parent counseling by speech pathologists and audiologists. *Journal of Speech and Hearing Disorders, 31,* 331–345.

Webster, E. (1968). Procedures for group counseling in speech, pathology and audiology. *Journal of Speech and Hearing Disorders, 31,* 331–345.

Webster, E. (1977). *Counseling with parents of handicapped children.* New York: Grune & Stratton.

Webster, R. L. (1974). A behavioral analysis of stuttering: Treatment and theory. In *Treatment methods in psychopathology.* New York: Wiley.

Webster, R. L. (1975). *Clinicians' program guide: The precision fluency shaping program.* Roanoke, VA: Communication Development Corp.

Webster, R. L. (1979). Empirical considerations regarding stuttering therapy. In H. H. Gregory (Ed.), *Controversies about stuttering therapy* (pp. 209–239). Baltimore, MD: University Park Press.

Webster, R. L. (1986). Postscript: Stuttering therapy from a technological point of view. In G. H. Shames & H. Rubin (Ed.), *Stuttering then and now* (pp. 407–414). Columbus, OH: Merrill.

Weisel, A., & Specktor, G. (1998). Attitudes toward own communication and toward stutterers. *Journal of Fluency Disorders, 23,* 157–172.

Weiss, A. L. (1993). The pragmatic context of children's disfluency. *Seminars in Speech and Language, 14*(3) 215–224.

Weiss, A. L., & Zebrowski, P. M. (1992). Disfluencies in the conversation of young children who stutter: Some answers about questions. *Journal of Speech and Hearing Research, 35,* 1230–1238.

Weiss, D. A. (1964). *Cluttering.* Englewood Cliffs, NJ: Prentice-Hall.

Weiss, D. A. (1967). Similarities and differences between stuttering and cluttering. *Folia Phoniatrica, 19,* 98–104.

West, R., & Ansberry, M. (1968). *The rehabilitation of speech* (4th ed.). New York: Harper & Row.

Westbrook, M. T., & Viney, L. L. (1980). Scales measuring people's perception of themselves as origins and pawns, *Journal of Personality Assessment, 44,* 167–174.

Westen, D., & Morrison, K. (2001). A multidimensional meta-analysis of treatments for depression, panic, and generalized anxiety disorder: An empirical examination of the status of empirically supported therapies. *Journal of Counseling and Clinical Psychology, 69,* 875–899.

Wexler, K. (1982). Developmental disfluency in 2-, 4-, and 6-year-old boys in neutral and stress situations. *Journal of Speech and Hearing Research, 25,* 229–234.

White, E. B. (1954/1960) Some remarks on humor. The second tree from the corner. In J. J. Enck, E. T. Forter, & A. Whitley (Eds.), *The comic in theory and practice* (pp. 102–108). New York: Appleton-Century-Crofts.

White M. (1995). *Externalizing Conversations Exercise.* Adelaide: Dulwich Centre Publications.

White, P. A., & Collins, S. R. C. (1984). Stereotype formation by inference: A possible explanation for the "stutterer" stereotype. *Journal of Speech and Hearing Research, 27*, 567–570.

White, M. & Epston, D. (1990). *Narrative means to therapeutic ends.* New York: Norton.

Williams, D. (1979). A perspective on approaches to stuttering therapy. In H. Gregory (Ed.), *Controversies about stuttering therapy* (pp. 241–268). Baltimore, MD: University Park Press.

Williams, D. (1983). Working with children in the school environment. In J. Fraser Gruss (Ed.), *Stuttering therapy: Transfer and maintenance* (Publication No. 19). Memphis, TN: Stuttering Foundation of America.

Williams, D. (1985). Talking with children who stutter. In J. Fraser (Ed.), *Counseling stutterers* (pp. 35–45). Memphis, TN: Stuttering Foundation of America.

Williams, D. E. (1957) A point of view about 'stuttering'. *Journal of Speech and Hearing Disorders, 22*(3), 390–397.

Williams, D. E. (1971). Stuttering therapy for children. In L. E. Travis (Ed.), *Handbook of speech pathology* (pp. 1073–1093). New York: Appleton-Century-Crofts.

Williams, D. E. (1995). A clinical failure: Susan (pp. 130–131). In *Stuttering: Successes and failures in therapy.* Memphis: Stuttering Foundation.

Williams, D. E. (2004). *The Genius of Dean Williams.* (Publication 425). Memphis: Stuttering Foundation.

Williams, D. E., & Silverman, F. H., (1968). Note concerning articulation of school-age stutterers. *Perceptual and Motor Skills, 27,* 713–714.

Williams, D. E., Silverman, F. H., & Kools, J. A. (1968). Disfluency behavior of elementary school stutterers and nonstutterers: The adaptation effect. *Journal of Speech and Hearing Research, 11,* 622–630.

Williams, D. E., Wener, D. L. (1996). Cluttering and stuttering exhibited in a young professional: Post hoc case study (clinical impressions). *Journal of Fluency Disorders, 21,* 1–9.

Williams, J. D., & Martin, R. B. (1974). Immediate versus delayed consequences of stuttering responses. *Journal of Speech and Hearing Research, 17,* 569–575.

Williams, R. (1995). Personal construct theory in use with people who stutter. In M. Fawcus (Ed.), *Stuttering: From theory to practice.* London: Whurr Publishers.

Wingate, M. (1959). Calling attention to stuttering. *Journal of Speech and Hearing Research, 2,* 326–335.

Wingate, M. (1964a). A standard definition of stuttering. *Journal of Speech and Hearing Disorders, 29,* 484–489.

Wingate, M. E. (1964b). Recovery from stuttering. *Journal of Speech and Hearing Disorders, 29,* 312–321.

Wingate, M. (1968). Research trends in stuttering. *Voice,* (Journal of the California Speech and Hearing Association), *17,* 2–6.

Wingate, M. E. (1969). Sound and pattern in "artificial" fluency. *Journal of Speech and Hearing Research, 12,* 677–686.

Wingate, M. E. (1971). The fear of stuttering. *Journal of the American Speech-Language-Hearing Association, 13,* 3–5.

Winslade, J., & Monk, G. (1999). *Narrative counseling in schools: Powerful and brief.* Thousand Oaks, CA: Corwin Press, Inc.

Winslow, M. & Guitar, B. (1994). The effects of structured turn-taking on disfluencies: A case study. *Language, Speech, and Hearing Services in Schools, 25,* 251–257.

Wittke-Thompson, J, K., Ambrose, N., Yairi, E., Roe, C., Cook, E. H., Ober, C., & Cox, N. J. (2007). Genetic studies of stuttering in a founder population. *Journal of Fluency Disorders, 32,* 33–50.

Wolf, A. E. (1991). *Get Out of My Life, But First Could You Drive Me and Cheryl to the Mall? A parent's guide to the new teenager.* New York: The Noonday Press.

Wood, F., Stump, D., McKeehan, A., Sheldon, S., & Proctor, J. (1980). Patterns of regional cerebral blood flow during attempted reading aloud by stutterers both on and off Haloperidol medication: Evidence for inadequate left frontal activation during stuttering. *Brain and Language, 9,* 141–144.

Woods, C. L., & Williams, D. E. (1976). Traits attributed to stuttering and normally fluent males. *Journal of Speech and Hearing Research, 19,* 267–278.

Woolf, G. (1967). The assessment of stuttering as struggle, avoidance and expectancy. *British Journal of Disorders of Communication, 2,* 158–171.

World Almanac and Book of Facts. (1995). Mahwah, NJ: Funk and Wagnalls Corp.

World Health Organization. (1977). *Manual of the international statistical classification of diseases, injuries, and causes of death* (Vol. 1). Geneva: World Health Organization.

World Health Organization. (1980). *International classification of impairments, disabilities, and handicaps: A Manual of classification of classification relating to the consequences of disease.* Geneva, Switzerland: World Health Organization.

Wright, L., & Ayre, A. *The Wright and Ayre Stuttering Self-Rating Profile (WASSP),* Oxon, UK: Winslow Press Ltd.

Wu, J. C., Maguire, G., Riley, G., Fallon, J., LaCasse, L., Chin, S., Klein, E., Tang, C., Cadwell, S., & Lottenberg, S. (1995). A positron emission tomography deoxyglucose study of developmental stuttering. *NeuroReport, 6,* 501–505.

Wyatt, G. L. (1969). *Language learning and communication disorders in children.* New York: Free Press.

Yairi, E. (1981). Disfluencies of normally speaking two-year-old children. *Journal of Speech and Hearing Research, 24,* 490–495.

Yairi, E. (1982). Longitudinal studies of disfluencies in two-year-old children. *Journal of Speech and Hearing Research, 25,* 155–160.

Yairi, E. (1983). The onset of stuttering in two- and three-year-old children. *Journal of Speech and Hearing Disorders, 48,* 171–177.

Yairi, E. (1993). Epidemiologic and other considerations in treatment efficacy research with preschool-age children who stutter. *Journal of Fluency Disorders, 18*(2–3), 197–219.

Yairi, E. (1997a). Disfluency characteristics of early childhood stuttering. In R. F. Curlee & G. M. Siegel (Eds.), *Nature and treatment of stuttering: New directions* (2nd ed., pp. 49–78). Boston: Allyn & Bacon.

Yairi, E. (1997b). Home environment and parent–child interaction in childhood stuttering. Curlee & G. Siegel (Eds.), *Nature and treatment of stuttering, New directions* (2nd ed., pp. 24–48). Needham Heights, MA: Allyn & Bacon.

Yairi, E. (2004). The formative years of stuttering: A changing portrait. *Contemporary Issues in Communication Science and Disorders, 31,* 92–104.

Yairi, E., & Ambrose, N. G. (1992a). A longitudinal study of stuttering in children: A preliminary report. *Journal of Speech and Hearing Research, 35,* 755–760.

Yairi, E., & Ambrose, N. G. (1992b). Onset of stuttering in preschool children: Selected factors. *Journal of Speech and Hearing Research, 35,* 782–788.

Yairi, E., & Ambrose, N. G. (1999). Early childhood stuttering I: Persistency and recovery rates. *Journal of Speech, Language, and Hearing Research, 42,* 1097–1112.

Yairi, E., & Ambrose, N. G. (1999b). Spontaneous recovery and clinical trials research in early childhood stuttering: A response to Onslow and Packman (1999). *Journal of Speech, Language, and Hearing Research, 42,* 402–410.

Yairi, E., & Ambrose, N. G. (2005). *Early Childhood Stuttering, For Clinicians by Clinicians,* Austin, TX: Pro-Ed.

Yairi, E., Ambrose, N. G., & Niermann, R. (1993). The early months of stuttering: A developmental study. *Journal of Speech and Hearing Research, 36,* 521–528.

Yairi, E., Ambrose, N. G., Paden, E. P., & Throneberg, R. N. (1996). Predictive factors of persistence and recovery: Pathways of childhood stuttering. *Journal of Communication Disorders, 29,* 51–77.

Yairi, E., & Carrico, D. (1992). Pediatricians' attitudes and practices concerning early childhood stuttering. *American Journal of Speech-Language Pathology, 1,* 54–62.

Yairi, E., & Clifton, N. F. (1972). Disfluent speech behavior of preschool children, high school seniors and geriatric persons. *Journal of Speech and Hearing Research, 15,* 714–719.

Yairi, E., & Hall, K. D. (1993). Temporal relations within repetitions of preschool children near the onset of stuttering: A preliminary report. *Journal of Communication Disorders, 26,* 231–244.

Yairi, E., & Lewis, B. (1984). Disfluencies at the onset of stuttering. *Journal of Speech and Hearing Research, 27,* 155–159.

Yairi, E., & Williams, D. (1971). Reports of parental attitudes by stuttering and nonstuttering children. *Journal of Speech and Hearing Research, 14,* 596–604.

Yaruss, J. S. (1997a). Clinical measurement of stuttering behaviors. *Contemporary Issues in Communication Science and Disorders, 24,* 33–44.

Yaruss, J. S. (1997b). Improving assessment of children's oral motor development in clinical settings. In W. Hulstijn, H. F. M. Peters, & P. H. H. M. Van Lieshout (Eds.), *Speech production:Motor control, brain research, and fluency disorders* (pp. 565–571). Amsterdam: Elsevier Science.

Yaruss, J. S. (1998). Describing the consequences of disorders: Stuttering and the international classification of impairments, disabilities, and handicaps. *Journal of Speech, Language, and Hearing Research, 41,* 249–257.

Yaruss, J. S. (2000). The role of performance in the demands and capacities model. *Journal of Fluency Disorders, 25*(4), 347–358.

Yaruss, J. S., Coleman, C., & Hammer, D. (2006). Treating preschool children who stutter: Description and preliminary evaluation of a family-focused treatment approach. *Language, Speech and Hearing Services in Schools, 37,* 118–136.

Yaruss, J. S., & Conture, E. G. (1995). Motor and child speaking rates and utterance lengths in adjacent fluent utterances. *Journal of Fluency Disorders, 20,* 257–278.

Yaruss, J. S., Murphy, B., Quesal, R. W., & Reardon, N. A. (2004). *Bullying and Teasing: Helping children who stutter.* National Stuttering Association, New York.

Yaruss, S. & Quesal, R. (2002). Academic and clinical education in fluency disorders: an update. *Journal of Fluency Disorders, 27,* 43–63

Yaruss, S. & Quesal, R. (2006). Overall assessment of the speaker's experience of stuttering (OASES). *Journal of Fluency Disorders, 31,* 90–115.

Yaruss, J. S., & Quesal, R. W., (2004). Stuttering and the International Classification of Functioning, Disability, and Health (ICF): An Update. *Journal of Communication Disorders, 37,* 35–52.

Yaruss, J. S., Quesal, R., W., & Murphy, W. (2002). National Stuttering Association members' opinions about stuttering treatment. *Journal of Fluency Disorders, 27,* 227–241.

Yaruss, J. S., Quesal, R. & Reeves. L. (2007). Self-help and mutual aid groups as an adjunct to stuttering therapy. In E. Conture & R. Curlee, *Stuttering and related disorders of fluency* (3rd Edition, pp. 256–276). New York: Theime Medical Publishers.

Yaruss, J. S., Quesal, R. W., Reeves, L, Molt, L. F., Kluetz, B., Caruso, A. J., McClure, J. A., & Lewis, F. (2002). Speech treatment and support group experiences of people who participate in the National Stuttering Association. *Journal of Fluency Disorders, 27,* 115–134.

Yates, A. J. (1963). Delayed auditory feedback. *Psychological Bulletin, 60,* 213–232.

Yeakle, M. K., & Cooper, E. B. (1986). Teacher perceptions of stuttering. *Journal of Fluency Disorders, 11,* 345–359.

Young, M. A. (1975). Onset, prevalence, and recovery from stuttering. *Journal of Speech and Hearing Disorders, 40,* 49–58.

Young, M. A. (1981). A reanalysis of "Stuttering therapy: The relation between attitude change and long-term outcome." *Journal of Speech and Hearing Disorders, 46,* 221–222.

Zebrowski, P. M. (1997). Assisting young children who stutter and their families: Defining the role of the speech-language pathologist. *American Journal of Speech-Language Pathology, 6*(2), 19–28.

Zebrowski, P. M. (2002). Building clinical relationships with teenagers who stutter. *Contemporary Issues in Communication Science and Disorders, 29,* 91–100.

Zebrowski, P. M. (2007) Treatment factors that influence therapy outcomes for children who stutter. In E. Conture & R. Curlee, *Stuttering and Related Disorders of Fluency.* (3rd Edition, pp. 23–38). New York: Thieme Medical Publishers, Inc.

Zebrowski, P. M., Conture, E. G., & Cudahy, E. A. (1985). Acoustic analysis of young stutterers' fluency: Preliminary observations. *Journal of Fluency Disorders, 10,* 173–192.

Zebrowski, P., Moon, J. & Robin, D. (1997). Visuomotor tracking abilities of stuttering and nonstuttering children. In H. Peters, W. Hulstijn & P. van Lieshout (Eds.), *Speech Production: Motor Control, Brain Research, and Fluency Disorders.* Proceedings of the 3rd International Conference on Speech Motor Production and Fluency Disorders, Nijmegen, The Netherlands. (pp. 579–584). Amsterdam: Elsevier Science Publishers.

Zenner, A., Ritterman, S., Bowden, S., & Gronhovd, D. (1978). Measurement and comparison of anxiety levels of parents of stuttering, articulatory defective and normal-speaking children. *Journal of Fluency Disorders, 3,* 273–284.

Zimmerman, G. (1980). Stuttering: A disorder of movement. *Journal of Speech and Hearing Research, 23,* 122–136.

Zimmerman, G. (1981). Stuttering: In need of a unifying conceptual framework. *Journal of Speech and Hearing Research, 24,* 25–31.

Zinker, J. (1977). *Creative process in Gestalt therapy.* New York: Random House.

Zinsser, W. (1988). *Learning to write.* New York: Harper and Row.

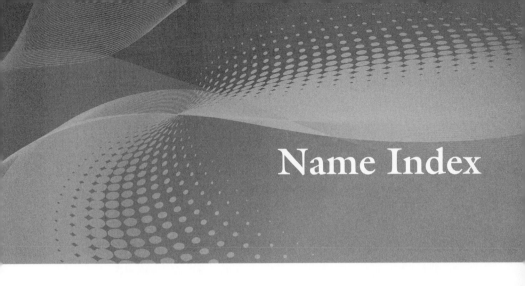

Name Index

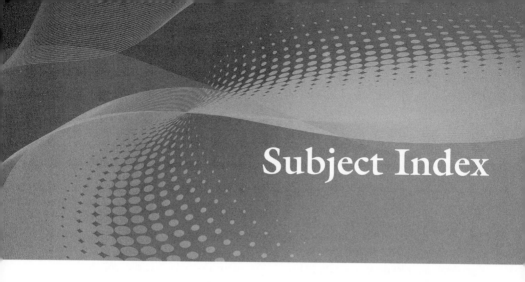

Subject Index

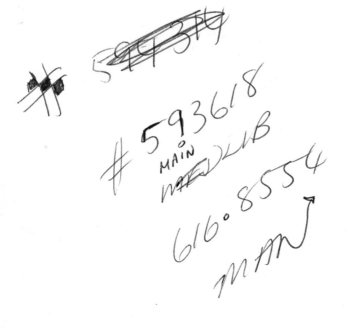

593618
MAIN MEDLIB
616.8554
MAN